£45.00
09

CLINICAL EMERGENCY MEDICINE CASEBOOK

Unlike the comparatively calm and orderly world of many specialties and subspecialties in medicine, emergency medicine is not divided into specific areas of practice. Emergency patients come in all shapes and sizes, at any time of day or night, with a wide range and acuity of maladies. Emergency physicians must become experts in diverse areas of medicine. They are required to make prompt, informed and often lifesaving decisions about patient care. A cornerstone of emergency medicine training is the constant study of clinical scenarios and simulated cases. This book offers a unique yet underutilized strategy for learning: a case-based approach from real patients and actual events. Each case provides the opportunity for learning essential clinical concepts. Focused exclusively on the needs of emergency physicians in training, students and nurses, the book covers more than 100 common and unusual emergency medicine case scenarios. The procedures and learning have been class-tested by the Stanford/Kaiser EM Residency Program and are supplemented with high-quality clinical photographs and images.

Joel T. Levis, M.D., Ph.D., FACEP, FAAEM, is Clinical Instructor of Emergency Medicine (Surgery) at Stanford University School of Medicine and Senior Emergency Physician for The Permanente Medical Group, Kaiser Santa Clara, California. Dr. Levis is Medical Director, Foothill College Paramedic Program, Los Altos Hills, California.

Gus M. Garmel, M.D., FACEP, FAAEM, is Clinical Associate Professor of Emergency Medicine (Surgery) at Stanford University School of Medicine and Senior Emergency Physician for The Permanente Medical Group, Kaiser Santa Clara, California. Dr. Garmel is coeditor of *An Introduction to Clinical Emergency Medicine: Guide for Practitioners in the Emergency Department*, published in 2005 by Cambridge University Press, and author of *Career Planning Guide for Emergency Medicine*, 2nd ed., published in 2007 by EMRA.

CLINICAL EMERGENCY MEDICINE CASEBOOK

JOEL T. LEVIS, M.D., Ph.D., FACEP, FAAEM

Clinical Instructor, Department of Surgery, Division of Emergency
   Medicine, Stanford University
Senior Emergency Physician, The Permanente Medical Group, Kaiser Santa Clara, CA
Medical Director, Foothill College Paramedic Program, Los Altos Hills, CA

GUS M. GARMEL, M.D., FACEP, FAAEM

Co-Program Director, Stanford/Kaiser EM Residency
Clinical Associate Professor, Department of Surgery, Division of
   Emergency Medicine, Stanford University
Medical Student Clerkship Director, Emergency Medicine (Surg 313D),
   Stanford University School of Medicine
Director, Emergency Medicine Clerkship for Rotating Interns, Kaiser Santa Clara, CA
Senior Emergency Physician, The Permanente Medical Group, Kaiser Santa Clara, CA
Senior Editor, *The Permanente Journal*, Portland, OR

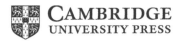

CAMBRIDGE
UNIVERSITY PRESS

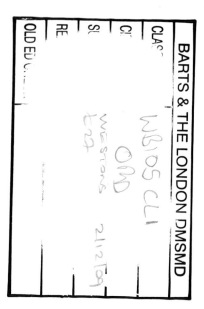
CAMBRIDGE UNIVERSITY PRESS
Cambridge, New York, Melbourne, Madrid, Cape Town, Singapore, São Paulo, Delhi

Cambridge University Press
32 Avenue of the Americas, New York, NY 10013-2473, USA

www.cambridge.org
Information on this title: www.cambridge.org/9780521719643

First published 2009

Printed in the United States of America

A catalog record for this publication is available from the British Library

Library of Congress Cataloging in Publication data

Levis, Joel T., 1964–
Clinical emergency medicine casebook / Joel T. Levis, Gus M. Garmel.
    p. ; cm.
Includes bibliographical references and index.
ISBN   978-0-521-71964-3 (pbk.)
1. Emergency medicine – Case studies.   I. Garmel, Gus. M.   II. Title.
[DNLM: 1. Emergency Treatment – methods – Case Reports.   2. Emergency
Treatment – methods – Problems and Exercises.   3. Emergencies – Case Reports.
4. Emergencies – Problems and Exercises.   5. Emergency Medicine – methods –
Case Reports.   6. Emergency Medicine – methods – Problems and Exercises.
WB 18.2 L666c 2009]
RC86.7.L49   2009
616.02′5–dc22   2008047232

ISBN   978-0-521-71964-3 paperback

Dedication

Joel T. Levis, M.D., Ph.D.

To my mother, Eileen Levis: For your constant support, encouragement and sacrifices throughout the years.

To my colleagues at Kaiser Santa Clara and Stanford University, and the residents of the Stanford/Kaiser Emergency Medicine Residency Program: You are all such wonderful clinicians and talented people, and you continue to inspire me.

To Gus: A superb mentor, phenomenal educator, tremendous clinician and true friend; without your efforts, this textbook would not have happened.

And to my wife Estelle: For your encouragement and love that gives me strength to pursue my dreams. Without you, the rewards of life would have little meaning.

Gus M. Garmel, M.D.

To my residents, students and colleagues in emergency medicine, nursing and other specialties: Because of you, outstanding patient care happens.

To The Permanente Medical Group, Kaiser Santa Clara, and Stanford University: The organization and institutions that support my academic pursuits and encourage me to excel in all aspects of my professional life.

To Joel, a former resident and chief resident: Your enthusiasm for our specialty is refreshing, and your work ethic unparalleled. I am honored to be your colleague, mentor and friend, and to have collaborated with you on this and prior scholarly projects.

To my parents, siblings and friends: Thanks for encouraging me to follow my dreams.

And to Laura, my true passion in life.

Contents

IV. GASTROENTEROLOGY

V. GENITOURINARY AND GYNECOLOGY

VI. NEUROLOGY/NEUROSURGERY

VII. TRAUMA

VIII. ORTHOPEDICS

XIII. MISCELLANEOUS

Preface

Emergency medicine is a tremendously challenging medical specialty. Fortunately, this field is profoundly rewarding. It gives health care professionals the unique opportunity to help individuals at their time of greatest need. Sometimes, simply offering reassurance, kindness or compassion is all that we can do; the importance of which should never be underestimated.

In emergency medicine, health care professionals assist individuals whose pain, anxiety and stress levels are high. Often, our quick decisions and actions are life-saving. Emergency medicine personnel continuously use their extraordinary skills, knowledge and experience to "make things happen" and "get the job done," in an attempt to positively impact patients and their families, significant others, friends and persons important to them.

In reality, physicians, nurses, mid-level providers, paramedics, residents and medical students generally have time to look up information from various sources. Yet emergency personnel have the responsibility to provide services not available to individuals at that moment anywhere other than an emergency department. Therefore, our purpose is even more vital.

Practitioners with the most experience often provide the best care, which suggests that lifelong learning and learning from errors is crucial to medical practice (perhaps why it is called "practice"). Educators of and mentors for residents, medical students, nurses, mid-level providers, paramedics and support staff recognize that the amount of knowledge one must possess is overwhelming. Often, knowing how and where to obtain information at a moment's notice is critical to successful patient care outcomes. With *Clinical Emergency Medicine Casebook*, we attempt to offer what we consider to be an essential yet underutilized strategy for learning: a case-based approach from real patients and actual events. There is agreement in medicine that patients teach us a great deal; this textbook will provide the opportunity for significant learning to occur at one's leisure. Using carefully selected cases with key teaching points, each learning opportunity (case) illustrates important clinical concepts that can expand even the most sophisticated learner's knowledge base.

Our goal is not to offer a definitive encyclopedia of emergency medicine (if such a book were possible). Rather, we have produced a unique textbook that gives readers the chance to intelligently work through cases, rehearsing the approach they might take for a similar patient in their clinical setting, and what actions they might initiate to render outstanding patient care. Each case is arranged by organ system or special category and is included because of its educational value and interest to clinicians. These cases are not exclusive to emergency medicine practice, even though each occurred at a single high-volume, high-acuity emergency department. The variety of cases offered should assist health care professionals in diverse fields who wish to improve their diagnostic and clinical skills. It is our hope that you, our colleagues, will benefit from our efforts. Without question, future patients will benefit from your efforts.

   With great admiration and respect for our specialty and those active in its practice, we hope you enjoy *Clinical Emergency Medicine Casebook*.

Gus M. Garmel, M.D.
Joel T. Levis, M.D., Ph.D.

Acknowledgments

Joel T. Levis and Gus M. Garmel wish to express gratitude to their emergency medicine colleagues at Kaiser Santa Clara, California, for expertly caring for the patients presented in this unique case-based textbook. We appreciate the assistance of several of our specialty colleagues from our medical center, whose input helped make this textbook a far superior resource for a much broader audience. Our medical staff colleagues who cared for these patients in the hospital and after discharge are to be praised for their efforts. Sonia Y. Johnson, M.D., an emergency medicine colleague and gifted artist, offered beautiful illustrations that detail key points in several cases. Drs. Levis and Garmel are especially grateful to Amal Mattu, M.D., FACEP, FAAEM, Program Director for the Emergency Medicine Residency, Co-Program Director for the Emergency Medicine/Internal Medicine Combined Residency and Associate Professor of Emergency Medicine, University of Maryland School of Medicine. An incredibly talented author and educator himself, his enthusiasm for this project demonstrates his commitment to our specialty and his respect for us as leaders in medical education. Thank you, Amal, for your friendship, and for sharing your passion by contributing the foreword to our textbook. Finally, we appreciate the complete confidence that Marc Strauss and the staff at Cambridge University Press had in us and in our emergency medicine case-based resource.

Foreword

Sir William Osler once said, "He who studies medicine without books sails an uncharted sea, but he who studies medicine without patients does not go to sea at all." Osler championed the importance of providing clinical correlations to the learning provided by books. In recent years, medical schools have come to recognize the importance of clinical correlations. The majority of medical schools in the United States have increased patient interactions for even first- and second-year medical students. Education has become much more problem-based, using simulated cases and case presentations. However, the authors and editors of textbooks have been much slower to adapt to this change. The majority of medical textbooks, including those in the specialty of emergency medicine, remain disease-oriented rather than patient-oriented. In other words, readers are expected to improve their practice of medicine by reading about diseases rather than by reading about patients. As a result, most textbooks occupy prominent positions on dusty bookshelves, rarely used, let alone read cover-to-cover. Fortunately, those of us who are teachers and students of emergency medicine are in luck. Two outstanding educators have stepped forward to provide a text that will not be relegated to those dusty bookshelves but will instead be relished and appreciated for its ability to help us navigate those uncharted seas that Osler spoke of many years ago.

Drs. Gus Garmel and Joel Levis have been teaching emergency medicine for many years. Both have proven track records of success in medical education. Dr. Garmel has received several prestigious national teaching awards and scholarships and has published several important textbooks, many book chapters and numerous articles. Dr. Levis has also been recognized among his peers for his scholarly activities, including teaching, authorship and research. These dedicated educators have already produced several successful academic collaborations. Congratulations to them for having the insight to produce a novel textbook that allows readers to study emergency medicine with the patient in mind.

Clinical Emergency Medicine Casebook presents the reader with real-life case presentations that cover the entire spectrum of the specialty of emergency medicine. These cases are presented in a succinct manner, with just enough information and relevant visual clues that the patient seems to magically appear from within the pages. The reader is then prompted for a diagnosis and, with a flip of the page, the clinically oriented teaching begins. The authors provide a diagnosis, followed by a concise discussion of the condition, including management plans and a set of concluding "Key Teaching Points" that reinforce the essentials of the case. Their detailed and thoughtful discussions frequently address myths, pitfalls and risk management pearls useful for readers at every level, from student through experienced practitioner. Following the discussion and teaching points is a brief set of references and suggestions for further reading. The cases are organized in sections important to clinical practice. Within each section, the randomness of case presentations simulates the randomness of actual emergency medicine practice, forcing readers to remain focused and "stay on their toes."

The quality of the cases selected is a particular strength of the text. Drs. Levis and Garmel have chosen cases that practicing emergency physicians are likely to see in a busy emergency department. Some cases are relatively common; for these, the authors provide critical teaching points that are often not well known. They have also included cases that are less commonly encountered in routine practice yet are equally important because of their likelihood for morbidity or mortality. For these cases, the authors focus on methods to minimize risk and improve patient outcomes. Esoteric cases have been specifically excluded in favor of maximizing practical teaching.

Another obvious strength of the book is the quality of the visuals throughout the text. The electrocardiograms, radiographs, photos and illustrations are crisp and unambiguous in their demonstration of important findings, a rare quality in most medical texts. The text is therefore incredibly useful for gaining visual diagnosis skills. Overall, students, residents, mid-level providers and experienced emergency physicians will find this book useful for improving their clinical practice and practical knowledge base.

Kudos to Drs. Levis and Garmel, who have written a special textbook. *Clinical Emergency Medicine Casebook* represents a valuable addition to the emergency medicine literature. Students and clinicians will find this unique book practical, easy to read and downright enjoyable. My sincere hope is that this text will serve as a model to other authors regarding the importance of bringing the patient to the reader.

Amal Mattu, M.D., FAAEM, FACEP
Director, Emergency Medicine Residency
Co-Director, Emergency Medicine/Internal Medicine Combined
    Residency
Associate Professor, Department of Emergency Medicine
University of Maryland School of Medicine
Coauthor, ECGs for the Emergency Physician, Volumes 1 and 2
Coeditor, Electrocardiography in Emergency Medicine
Coeditor, Emergency Medicine: Avoiding the Pitfalls and
    Improving the Outcomes
Consulting Editor, Emergency Medicine Clinics of North America

PART I

HEENT (HEAD, EYES, EARS, NOSE AND THROAT)

Sore throat in a 29-year-old male

HISTORY OF PRESENT ILLNESS

A 29-year-old male with a medical history significant for type I diabetes presented to the ED complaining of a sore throat, inability to swallow solids and fevers to 103°F (39.4°C) for two days. He noted a hoarse voice and was able to tolerate only small sips of liquids. He denied significant neck swelling or stiffness, and was able to tolerate his secretions. He had immigrated to the United States from Mexico as a teenager, and his immunization status was unknown.

PHYSICAL EXAM

GENERAL APPEARANCE: The patient was a well-developed, nontoxic, moderately obese male who appeared slightly dehydrated, sitting upright and in no acute distress.

VITAL SIGNS

Temperature	103°F (39.4°C)
Pulse	100 beats/minute
Blood pressure	145/85 mmHg
Respirations	22 breaths/minute
Oxygen saturation	100% on room air

HEENT: Oropharynx was pink and moist, no erythema, exudates, tonsillar or uvular swelling noted.

NECK: Supple, anterior cervical lymphadenopathy noted, tenderness to palpation over cricoid cartilage noted.

LUNGS: Clear to auscultation bilaterally.

CARDIOVASCULAR: Regular rate and rhythm without rubs, murmurs or gallops.

ABDOMEN: Soft, nontender, nondistended.

EXTREMITIES: No clubbing, cyanosis or edema.

A peripheral intravenous line was placed and blood was drawn and sent for laboratory testing. Laboratory tests were significant for a leukocyte count of 24 K/μL (normal 3.5–12.5 K/μL) with 92% neutrophils (normal 50–70%). A soft-tissue lateral neck radiograph was obtained (Figure 1.1).

What is your diagnosis?

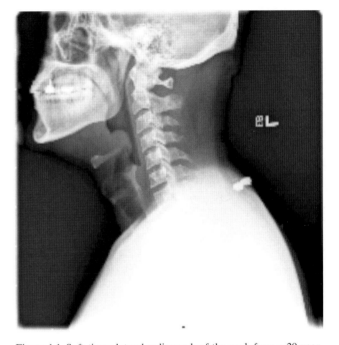

Figure 1.1 Soft-tissue lateral radiograph of the neck from a 29-year-old male with sore throat and inability to swallow solids.

ANSWER

The diagnosis is epiglottitis. The soft-tissue lateral neck radiograph demonstrates swelling of the epiglottis ("thumbprint" sign, Figure 1.2). The Ear, Nose and Throat (ENT) specialist was urgently consulted, and bedside nasopharyngoscopy demonstrated a swollen, red epiglottis with 90% obstruction of the upper airway. The patient received ceftriaxone 1 gm and decadron 10 mg intravenously, normal saline 1 liter IV bolus, and was admitted to the ICU for close monitoring and observation. The patient was discharged on hospital day #4 after his symptoms had improved. Repeat nasopharyngoscopy demonstrated significant improvement of the epiglottic swelling. He was continued on cefpodoxime proxetil (Vantin™) orally for ten days following discharge.

Epiglottitis in adults

Acute epiglottitis is a potentially life-threatening condition that results from inflammation of the supraglottic structures.[1,2] Commonly considered a pediatric disease, the current incidence of epiglottitis in adults is 1 to 2 cases per 100,000, which is presently 2.5 times the incidence in children.[1] Epiglottitis occurs most frequently in men in the fifth decade; the disease is more common in countries that do not immunize against *Haemophilus influenzae* type B. Currently, the most common cause of epiglottitis is infection, although sources such as crack cocaine use have also been implicated.[1] Common pathogens include *H. influenzae* (Hib), β-hemolytic streptococci and viruses.

The clinical presentation of adult epiglottitis may differ significantly from that of the classic drooling child seated in a tripod position. The most common symptoms in adults are sore throat, odynophagia and muffled voice.[3] Sore throat is the chief complaint in 75–94% of cases, whereas odynophagia may be present in as many as 94% of cases.[4] The presence of stridor significantly increases the need for emergent airway intervention.[5] Unlike children with epiglottitis, where emergency airway management is essential, most cases of adult epiglottitis do not require acute airway intervention due to the greater diameter of the adult airway.

The leukocyte count is greater than 10,000 in 80% of cases of adult epiglottitis. Soft-tissue lateral neck radiography, which may show an enlarged, misshapen epiglottis ("thumbprint" sign), has a sensitivity of 88% in establishing the diagnosis.[3] Patients who appear ill or are in extremis should not leave the ED for radiographs, and airway management in patients in extremis should be the first and foremost responsibility. Direct laryngoscopy is the most accurate investigation to establish a diagnosis of epiglottitis.[3] Management focuses on two important aspects: close monitoring of the airway with intubation (if necessary) and treatment with intravenous antibiotics.[6] Antibiotics should be directed against Hib in every patient, regardless of immunization status. Cefotaxime, ceftriaxone or ampicillin/sulbactam are appropriate choices. Steroids are commonly used in the management of

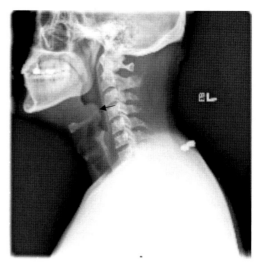

Figure 1.2 Soft-tissue lateral radiograph of the neck from a 29-year-old male with epiglottitis, demonstrating "thumbprint" sign (arrow).

acute epiglottitis, although no randomized trials to date support this practice.[6]

KEY TEACHING POINTS

1. Acute epiglottitis is a potentially life-threatening condition resulting from inflammation of the supraglottic structures, with a current incidence of 1 to 2 cases per 100,000 adults in the United States.
2. Sore throat is the chief complaint in 75–94% of cases of adult epiglottitis, whereas odynophagia may be present in as many as 94% of cases.
3. Soft-tissue lateral neck radiography, which may show an enlarged, misshapen epiglottis ("thumbprint" sign), has a sensitivity of 88% in establishing the diagnosis.
4. The definitive diagnosis is made through direct laryngoscopic visualization of an enlarged, inflamed epiglottis.
5. Treatment of epiglottitis includes intravenous antibiotics and close airway monitoring in an ICU setting. Most clinicians treat acute cases with intravenous steroids.

REFERENCES

[1] Belleza WG, Kalman S. Otolaryngologic emergencies in the outpatient setting. *Med Clin N Am* 2006;90:329–53.
[2] Berger G, Landau T, Berger S, et al. The rising incidence of adult acute epiglottitis and epiglottic abscess. *Am J Otolaryngol* 2003;24:374–83.
[3] Tan C-K, Chan K-S, Cheng K-C. Adult epiglottitis (Clinical Vistas Briefs). *CMAJ* 2007;176:602.
[4] Bitner MD, Capes JP, Houry DE. Images in emergency medicine: adult epiglottitis. *Ann Emerg Med* 2007; 49:560,563.
[5] Katori H, Tsukuda M. Acute epiglottitis: analysis of factors associated with airway intevention. *J Laryngol Otol* 2005;119:967–72.
[6] Alcaide ML, Bisno AL. Phayrngitis and epiglottitis. *Infect Dis Clin N Am* 2007;21:449–69.

Left eye pain and discharge in a 44-year-old male

HISTORY OF PRESENT ILLNESS

A 44-year-old male with no significant medical history presented to the ED with several days of worsening left eye pain, discharge and decreased vision, as well as swelling and redness to the eyelid and surrounding tissue. He did not wear contact lenses or eyeglasses. The patient currently could not see from his left eye. He denied fevers, headaches or recent trauma to the eye, although he did report a foreign body sensation to the eye several days prior to the onset of these symptoms. He denied experiencing similar symptoms in the past.

PHYSICAL EXAMINATION

GENERAL APPEARANCE: The patient appeared to be in no acute discomfort.

VITAL SIGNS

Temperature	98.1°F (36.7°C)
Pulse	75 beats/minute
Blood pressure	135/85 mmHg
Respirations	22 breaths/minute
Oxygen saturation	100% on room air

EYES: The visual acuity of the right eye was 20/40; the right pupil was round and reactive to light. No vision or light perception was elicited from the left eye. The left upper and lower eyelids were swollen and erythematous. A thick yellow-green discharge exuded from the left orbit; the pupil could not be examined secondary to the thickness and adherence of the exudates. The left eye was proptotic (Figure 2.1).

What is your diagnosis?

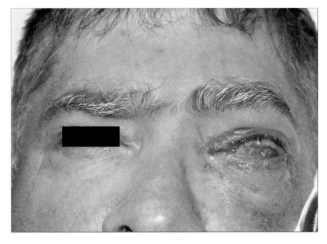

Figure 2.1 A 44-year-old male with several days of swelling, redness and exudate of his left eye.

ANSWER

The diagnosis is endophthalmitis and orbital cellulitis of the left eye. A CT scan of the orbits revealed a markedly proptotic left ocular globe, as well as a markedly distended left anterior chamber with mild posterior displacement of the hyperdense lens (Figure 2.2). The CT also demonstrated enhancing infiltrate of the preseptal and periorbital soft tissues associated with the left orbit, consistent with orbital cellulitis. It was surmised that the patient had recently incurred a penetrating injury to the globe, which resulted in endophthalmitis with extension to orbital cellulitis.

The patient was started on intravenous antibiotics (ceftriaxone 1 gm q12 h and vancomycin 1 gm q12 h), as well as antibiotic eye drops (cefazolin and tobramycin, one drop each q1 h) and aggressive lubrication of the eye. He was admitted to the medical service with close ophthalmology involvement. By hospital day #10, no improvement in the patient's symptoms occurred despite aggressive antibiotic therapy, and the decision was made to surgically enucleate the left eye.

Periorbital cellulitis, orbital cellulitis and endophthalmitis

Periorbital cellulitis (also called preseptal cellulitis) is an infection that occurs anterior to the orbital septum. The orbital septum is a layer of fibrous tissue arising from the periosteum of the skull and continues into the eyelids. Because this layer provides an effective barrier against the spread of infection from the preseptal tissues into the orbit, periorbital cellulitis does not progress to orbital cellulitis.[1] Periorbital tissue may become infected either by trauma or due to primary bacteremia, which is especially common in young children at high risk for pneumococcal bacteremia.[1]

Orbital cellulitis is post-septal, with involvement of the orbit itself. It is most commonly the result of a complication of ethmoid sinusitis, which accounts for more than 90% of all cases.[2] Orbital cellulitis can also be caused by the direct extension of infection from the globe, eyelids, ocular adnexae and other periocular tissues, in addition to the sinuses. Orbital cellulitis is more common in children but can also occur in adults.[3] Along with eyelid edema and erythema seen in periorbital cellulitis, patients with orbital cellulitis have proptosis, chemosis (edema of the bulbar conjunctiva), impairment of and pain with extraocular movements, and decreased extraocular movements.[1-4] The presence of fever, systemic signs, and toxicity is variable in patients with orbital cellulitis.[4] Bacterial causes of orbital cellulitis are most commonly *Streptococcus* species, *Staph aureus* and *Haemophilus influenzae* Type B.[2] *Pseudomonas, Klebsiella, Eikenella* and *Enterococcus* are less common culprits. Polymicrobial infections with aerobic and anaerobic bacteria are more common in patients 16 years or older.[2]

Endophthalmitis is a serious intraocular inflammatory disorder resulting from infection of the vitreous cavity.[5] Exogenous endophthalmitis occurs when infecting organisms gain entry into the eye by direct inoculation, such as from

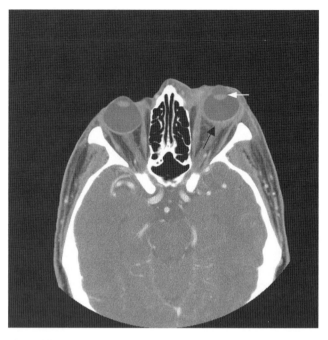

Figure 2.2 CT of the orbits of a 44-year-old male demonstrating a markedly proptotic left ocular globe (dark arrow), as well as a markedly distended left anterior chamber with mild posterior displacement of the hyperdense lens (white arrow).

intraocular surgery, penetrating trauma, or contiguous spread from adjacent tissues. Endogenous endophthalmitis occurs when infectious agents are hematogenously disseminated into the eye from a distant focus of infection.[6] Progressive vitritis is a hallmark of any form of endophthalmitis. Histologically, there is massive infiltration of the vitreous cavity with inflammatory cells, primarily neutrophils.[5] In most instances, vitreous infiltration is accompanied by progressive intraocular inflammation associated with loss of vision, pain, and hypopyon. Further progression may lead to panophthalmitis, corneal infiltration and perforation, orbital cellulitis, and phthisis bulbi (atrophy and degeneration of a blind eye).[5] Decreased vision and permanent loss of vision are common complications of endophthalmitis. Patients may require enucleation to eliminate a blind and painful eye. The most important laboratory studies are Gram stain and culture of the aqueous and vitreous humor.[6]

Diagnostic testing for orbital cellulitis starts with contrast-enhanced CT imaging of the orbits.[3] Findings on CT indicating orbital cellulitis include any of the following: proptosis, inflammation of the ocular muscles, subperiosteal abscess or frank orbital abscess.[1] Ipsilateral (or bilateral) sinusitis should also be evident (except in cases where orbital cellulitis is caused by extension of endophthalmitis). Sinus disease is important in the pathogenesis of orbital cellulitis but not of periorbital cellulitis.[1] Purulent material from the nose should be collected with cotton or calcium alginate swabs and submitted for Gram stain and culture on aerobic and anaerobic media; any material obtained from the sinuses or directly from an orbital abscess should be assessed in the same manner.[2]

Uncomplicated post-traumatic periorbital cellulitis can generally be treated with oral antimicrobials directed against Gram-positive bacteria (e.g., cephalexin, dicloxacillin or clindamycin).[1] The patient with orbital cellulitis should be promptly hospitalized for treatment, with ophthalmology and infectious disease consultations. Historically, the presence of subperiosteal or intraorbital abscess was an indication for surgical drainage in addition to antibiotic therapy; however, medical management alone is successful in many cases.[2] Intravenous broad-spectrum antibiotics (e.g., second- and third-generation cephalosporins or ampicillin/sulbactam) should be started immediately until antibiotics can be tailored to pathogens identified on culture.[2,3] Typically, intravenous antibiotic therapy should be continued for 1 to 2 weeks, followed by oral antibiotics for an additional 2 to 3 weeks.[1–3]

Treatment of traumatic endophthalmitis includes admission to the hospital with ophthalmologic consultation, intravenous antibiotics (including vancomycin and an aminoglycoside or third-generation cephalosporin) and topical fortified antibiotics.[6] Intravitreal antibiotics should be administered by an ophthalmologist, with consideration for pars plana vitrectomy.[5,6] Tetanus immunization is necessary if immunization is not current.

KEY TEACHING POINTS

1. Clinical signs and symptoms of orbital cellulitis include eyelid edema and erythema, proptosis, chemosis, pain with extraocular movements and ophthalmoplegia.

2. The diagnostic test of choice for orbital cellulitis is a contrast-enhanced CT scan of the orbits, demonstrating proptosis, inflammation of the ocular muscles, and subperiosteal or orbital abscess.

3. Treatment of orbital cellulitis includes administration of broad-spectrum intravenous antibiotics with close ophthalmology involvement.

4. Endophthalmitis, a serious intraocular inflammatory disorder resulting from infection of the vitreous cavity, may progress to orbital cellulitis.

5. Treatment of traumatic endophthalmitis includes hospital admission and administration of intravenous, topical and intravitreal antibiotics.

REFERENCES

[1] Givner LB. Periorbital versus orbital cellulitis. *Pediatr Infect Dis J* 2002;21:1157–8.

[2] Harrington JN. Cellulitis, orbital. eMedicine Web site. Available at http://www.emedicine.com/oph/topic205.htm. Accessed June 21, 2008.

[3] Pasternak A, Irish B. Ophthalmologic infections in primary care. *Clin Fam Pract* 2004;6:19–33.

[4] Wald ER. Periorbital and orbital infections. *Infect Dis Clin N Am* 2007;21:393–408.

[5] Lemley CA, Han DP. Endophthalmitis: a review of current evaluation and management. *Retina* 2007;27:662–80.

[6] Peters JR, Egan DJ. Endophthalmitis. eMedicine Web site. Available at http://www.emedicine.com/emerg/topic880.htm. Accessed June 21, 2008.

3

Sudden, monocular vision loss in a 62-year-old female

HISTORY OF PRESENT ILLNESS

A 62-year-old female with no significant medical history presented to the ED complaining of seeing "floaters" and flashing lights in her right eye associated with loss of vision in the right inferolateral visual field (affecting only her right eye) for the past three days. She did not wear eyeglasses or contact lenses, and denied pain, redness or discharge from the eye. She denied trauma to the eye or headaches.

PHYSICAL EXAMINATION

GENERAL APPEARANCE: The patient appeared well developed and in no acute discomfort.

VITAL SIGNS

Temperature	98.6°F (37°C)
Pulse	80 beats/minute
Blood pressure	135/85 mmHg
Respirations	20 breaths/minute
Oxygen saturation	100% on room air
Visual acuity	OD 20/100
	OS 20/20
	OU 20/40

EYES: PERRL, EOMI and no afferent pupillary defect. Lids, lashes and lacrimal glands normal, no conjunctival or scleral injections, no ocular discharge. The cornea was clear, without edema, fluorescein uptake or cloudiness. No cell or flare on slit lamp examination. Right inferolateral visual field deficit affecting the right eye only. Retinal examination of both undilated eyes was normal. Intraocular pressures were 12 mmHg OD and 16 mmHg OS, respectively.

A linear, 10-MHz ultrasound probe was gently placed over the closed right eye using a small amount of water-soluble gel (Figure 3.1).

What is your diagnosis?

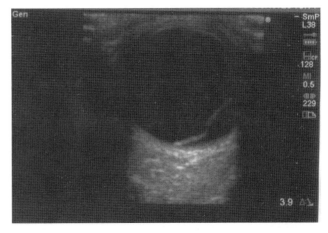

Figure 3.1 Ultrasound image of the right eye from a 62-year-old female with 3 days of floaters and an inferolateral visual field deficit of the right eye.

ANSWER

The diagnosis is retinal detachment. The ultrasound image demonstrates an inferolateral detachment of the retina (arrow, Figure 3.2). The ophthalmologist was urgently consulted, and confirmed the presence of retinal detachment upon dilated retinal examination of the right eye. The patient underwent microsurgical repair of the retinal detachment, regaining normal vision of her right eye.

Retinal detachment

Retinal detachment (RD) involves separation of the retina from the underlying retinal epithelium (Figure 3.3). It affects approximately 2 in 10,000 people per year.[1] Risk factors for the development of RD include increasing age, previous cataract surgery, focal retinal atrophy, myopia, trauma, diabetic retinopathy, family history of RD, uveitis, and prematurity.[1] Patients complain of new floaters, squiggly lines or cobwebs that appear abruptly, associated with visual field loss.[2] Over time, the patient may report a shadow in the peripheral visual field, which, if ignored, may spread to involve the entire visual field in a matter of days.[3] Vision loss may be filmy, cloudy, irregular or curtain-like.

Examination of the eyes should begin with an assessment of the visual acuity. The external eye examination should include inspection for any signs of trauma and confrontational visual field testing; the latter can assist in isolating the location of the RD.[3] Pupillary reaction should be checked, and a slit lamp biomicroscopy performed. Intraocular pressures should be measured in both eyes, as hypotony of more than 4–5 mmHg less than the unaffected eye is common in RD.[3] Finally, a funduscopic examination with ophthalmoscopy is required. This examination may not reveal the RD, particularly in an undilated eye, as the detachment may be at the periphery of the retina where the retina is the thinnest.[2]

Patients with new onset visual loss can be rapidly assessed for RD using bedside ultrasound, readily performed by

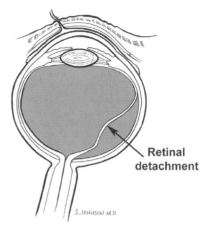

Figure 3.3 Retinal detachment.

emergency physicians.[4–8] The diagnosis of retinal detachment can be made using almost any ultrasonographic probe, although a linear probe such as the 7.5- to 10-MHz probe is preferred. The patient is asked to look straight ahead with closed, but not clenched, eyelids. The probe is placed perpendicular to the orbit, using conduction gel and minimal pressure to obtain the image.[5] Care should be taken to avoid placing excessive pressure on the globe while performing the scan, particularly if there is concern for globe rupture (in the setting of trauma).

RD requires urgent consultation with an ophthalmologist. Surgical repair of retinal detachments, typically performed by a retinal specialist, has a high success rate.[1] More invasive therapies, such as scleral buckling and posterior vitrectomy, have success rates of nearly 90%, whereas less invasive therapies, such as pneumatic retinopexy, may be performed in an office setting in select cases. If the repair is technically successful, visual acuity is often restored to predetachment levels.[1]

KEY TEACHING POINTS

1. Retinal detachment (RD) involves separation of the retina from the underlying retinal epithelium, and affects approximately 2 in 10,000 people per year.
2. RD is an ophthalmologic emergency, requiring urgent ophthalmology consultation.
3. Patients with RD complain of new floaters, squiggly lines or cobwebs that appear abruptly, associated with visual field loss.
4. Key components of the ocular examination include visual acuity testing, gross and slit lamp inspection of both eyes, visual field confrontation and extraocular movement assessment, pupillary response to light and accommodation, testing of intraocular pressures, and fundoscopic examination (best performed on a dilated eye).
5. Bedside ultrasound is a useful and readily available tool for making the diagnosis of RD in the emergency department.

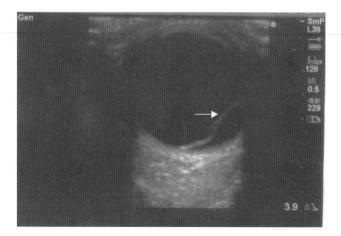

Figure 3.2 Ultrasound image of right eye from a 62-year-old female demonstrating inferolateral retinal detachment (arrow).

REFERENCES

[1] Vortmann M, Schneider JI. Acute monocular visual loss. *Emerg Med Clin N Am* 2008;26:73–96.

[2] Magauran B. Conditions requiring emergency ophthalmologic consultation. *Emerg Med Clin N Am* 2008;26:233–8.

[3] Larkin GL. Retinal detachment. eMedicine Web site. Available at http://www.emedicine.com/EMERG/topic504.htm. Accessed July 10, 2008.

[4] Blaivas M, Theodoro DL, Sierzenski PR. A study of bedside ocular ultrasonography in the emergency department. *Acad Emerg Med* 2002;9:462b–3b.

[5] Lewin RM, Williams SR, Ahuja Y. Ultrasonographic diagnosis of retinal detachment in the emergency department. *Ann Emerg Med* 2005;45:97–8.

[6] Kahn An, Kahn Am, Corinaldi C. Retinal detachment diagnosed by bedside ultrasound in the emergency department. *West J Emerg Med* 2005;6:47–51.

[7] Babineau MR, Sanchez LD. Ophthalmologic procedures in the emergency department. *Emerg Med Clin N Am* 2008;26:17–34.

[8] Shinar Z. Images in emergency medicine: Retinal detachment. *West J Emerg Med* 2008;9:54.

4

Syncope and monocular vision loss in a 76-year-old female

HISTORY OF PRESENT ILLNESS

A 76-year-old female with a medical history significant for hypertension, hypothyroidism, hyperlipidemia and chronic renal insufficiency presented to the ED after fainting while shopping. She reported feeling lightheaded and dizzy while walking in a grocery store, at which time she experienced a brief loss of consciousness. She fell to the floor, bystanders called emergency services but she quickly regained consciousness. She denied head trauma or neck pain after the fall. She also denied chest pain but had been experiencing some shortness of breath with exertion over the past several weeks, as well as low back pain and bilateral thigh pain worse in the morning. She also noted gradually worsening vision in her right eye over the past week, increasing redness to that eye, and a mild, right-sided headache; her vision prior to this had been normal. Upon presentation to the ED, she could perceive light and vague shapes with the right eye. Her medications included metoprolol, hydrochlorothiazide, Cozaar, levothyroxine, lovastatin and ibuprofen 400 mg orally twice daily for low back pain. She denied tobacco use, drank alcohol occasionally, lived alone and drove a car for transportation.

PHYSICAL EXAMINATION

GENERAL APPEARANCE: The patient appeared well hydrated and well nourished, and in no acute discomfort.

VITAL SIGNS

Temperature	98°F (36.6°C)
Pulse	54 beats/minute
Blood pressure	138/53 mmHg
Respirations	22 breaths/minute
Oxygen saturation	98% on room air
Visual acuity	OS 20/50
	OD light perception and hand motion only (unable to count fingers)

HEENT: Atraumatic, normocephalic, PERRL, EOMI, no afferent pupillary defect. Sclera of the right eye red and injected, no discharge. Tenderness to palpation over right forehead. No facial lesions or asymmetry noted.

NECK: Supple, no jugular venous distension.

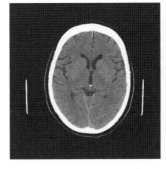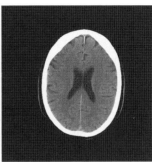

Figure 4.1 Noncontrast CT of the brain from a 76-year-old female with syncope and monocular vision loss.

CARDIOVASCULAR: Bradycardic rate, regular rhythm without rubs, murmurs or gallops.

LUNGS: Clear to auscultation bilaterally.

ABDOMEN: Soft, nontender, nondistended.

RECTAL: Normal tone, brown stool, hemoccult negative.

EXTREMITIES: No clubbing, cyanosis or edema.

NEUROLOGIC: Visual acuity deficit of right eye (cranial nerve II) as described; remaining neurologic examination nonfocal.

A peripheral intravenous line was placed and blood was drawn and sent for laboratory testing. A 12-lead ECG demonstrated sinus bradycardia, rate 56, without the presence of ST-T wave changes. A noncontrast CT of the brain was obtained (Figure 4.1). Laboratory tests were significant for a leukocyte count of 12.6 K/μL (normal 3.5–12.5 K/μL) with 81% neutrophils (normal 50–70%), hematocrit of 27% (normal 34–46%), creatinine of 1.7 mg/dL (normal < 1.1 mg/dL), erythrocyte sedimentation rate (ESR) of 120 mm/hr (normal 0–20 mm/hr) and C-reactive protein (CRP) of 18.2 mg/dL (normal < 0.9 mg/dL). The electrolytes, glucose and troponin I were within normal limits, and a urinalysis did not show signs of infection.

What is your diagnosis?

ANSWER

The diagnosis is temporal arteritis and normochromic, normocytic anemia. The CT scan of her brain was normal. Her syncope was attributed to her anemia. The patient was admitted to the medicine service and transfused with two units of packed red blood cells. Her post-transfusion hematocrit improved to 33%. Ophthalmology was urgently consulted and the patient was started on oral prednisone 50 mg per day, with the first dose given in the ED. She was discharged on hospital day #2 without visual improvement of the right eye. She underwent an outpatient temporal artery biopsy two days later, which confirmed the diagnosis of temporal arteritis. The patient's oral prednisone dose was increased to 80 mg daily at that time. By six weeks, her CRP had normalized and the ESR had decreased to 56 mm/hr; minimal improvement in her right eye's vision was noted, whereas no visual changes had occurred in the left eye. A gradual taper of prednisone was done over three months. Over this period, her vision slowly improved but not completely back to her baseline.

Temporal arteritis

Temporal arteritis, also called giant-cell arteritis (GCA), is a granulomatous arteritis of the aorta and its major branches with a predilection to affect the extracranial branches of the carotid artery.[1] Although it can be seen in a variety of populations, there is an epidemiologic predilection for people of Northern European decent and those living at higher latitudes.[2] Women are twice as likely to be affected as men. Cases are rare before 50 years of age; the incidence increases with age, peaking in the eighth decade.[2] The incidence of temporal arteritis is 15 to 25 per 100,000 in adults over 50 years of age in the United States, and peaks at 1100 per 100,000 persons at 85 years of age.[2]

In giant-cell arteritis, transmural inflammation of the arteries induces luminal occlusion through intimal hyperplasia.[3] Clinical symptoms reflect end-organ ischemia. Branches of the external and internal carotid arteries are particularly susceptible. Their involvement leads to the classic manifestations of blindness, headache, scalp tenderness and jaw claudication.[3] Systemic symptoms (fatigue, malaise, anorexia, fever) are present in about half of patients.[4] A headache is probably the most frequent symptom, occurring in two-thirds of patients.[2,4] The pain is frequently severe and tends to be located over the temporal or occipital areas; however, it may be less well-defined. Scalp tenderness is usually confined to the temporal and, less commonly, occipital arteries, but may be diffuse. On physical examination, the frontal or parietal branches of the superficial temporal arteries may be thickened, nodular, tender or occasionally erythematous.[4] Pulses may be decreased or absent. Nearly half of patients suffer jaw claudication. In rare cases, vascular narrowing may lead to infarction of the scalp or tongue.[4]

Unilateral or bilateral blindness (resulting from arteritis of the intraorbital posterior ciliary and central retinal arteries) is the most common dreaded complication if temporal arteritis is left untreated or inadequately treated. This complication may be seen in up to half of patients.[5] Affected patients typically report partially-obscured vision ("a shade covering one eye"), which may progress to total blindness.[4] If untreated, the other eye is likely to become affected within 1 to 2 weeks. Once established, visual impairment is usually permanent. Blurring, diplopia or amaurosis fugax occurs in 65% of patients before the development of permanent visual loss.[2] The progression to permanent visual loss occurs an average of 8.5 days after these early findings.[2]

The ESR is a well-known marker for inflammatory conditions, including GCA. Most patients with GCA have an ESR greater than 50 mm/hr.[2] Although GCA studies have not established a well-defined normal ESR, past studies have suggested a normal value of ($age/2$) for men and ($age + 10$)/2 for women.[2,6] A 2002 meta-analysis found that only 4% of patients with biopsy-proven GCA had normal ESRs.[6] As a nonspecific marker of inflammation, an ESR greater than 50 has a reported specificity of 48%.[2] The CRP level has been found to be a more sensitive indicator of disease than the ESR both at diagnosis and during relapse.[4] One small study found that a CRP greater than 6 mg/dL occurred in 49 of 55 cases of GCA.[7] There is conflicting literature on the accuracy of CRP or ESR to diagnose and follow GCA, with some authors favoring CRP and others favoring ESR.[2] Following both may be helpful.

The presence of normocytic, normochromic anemia is another helpful finding. Although pooled data have shown only 44% sensitivity for positive biopsy, anemia can be helpful when evaluating disease activity.[8] Studies have shown a negative correlation between the presence of anemia and the likelihood to progress to ischemic complications, such as permanent vision loss.[2]

Temporal artery biopsy confirms GCA in 50–80% of cases, demonstrating a panmural mononuclear cell infiltration that can be granulomatous with histiocytes and giant cells.[1] To increase yield, the length of the biopsy specimen should be at least 3–5 cm and sampled at multiple levels.[1] Biopsy does not need to be performed urgently in the ED; it can be performed as an outpatient.[9] In patients suspected of having GCA, treatment with steroids should be instituted immediately to preserve vision while a prompt temporal artery biopsy is arranged.[1] Although steroid therapy may affect biopsy results, inflammatory changes usually persist for 2 to 4 weeks after initiation of treatment.[9]

Steroids prevent visual complications in GCA, and bring about rapid improvement in clinical symptoms.[1] The optimal initial dosage remains controversial, but most investigators support that prednisone be initiated at a dose of 40–60 mg/day.[1] Symptomatic improvement usually occurs within the first 1 to 2 weeks following the initiation of prednisone, accompanied by a reduction in ESR over the first month. The duration of maintenance therapy with prednisone (following a taper) may last for one year or more, depending upon the patient's response.[9] Although thromboembolic occlusion is not a likely mechanism in the development of GCA, therapeutic benefit in its treatment has been reported with the use of low-dose aspirin.[3] Prevention of platelet aggregation is potentially effective, even in patients with partial luminal occlusion.

KEY TEACHING POINTS

1. Symptoms of temporal arteritis (also known as giant-cell arteritis) may be nonspecific, including headache, scalp tenderness, jaw claudication and gradual vision loss.

2. If left untreated, temporal arteritis can result in unilateral or bilateral blindness.

3. The erythrocyte sedimentation rate (ESR) and C-reactive protein (CRP) are the most useful laboratory tests in diagnosing and following the clinical course of temporal arteritis.

4. Temporal artery biopsy is the gold standard for the diagnosis of temporal arteritis.

5. Prednisone is the mainstay of treatment for temporal arteritis, and should be started once the diagnosis of temporal arteritis is considered, before a temporal artery biopsy is performed or the results are known.

REFERENCES

[1] Langford CA. Vasculitis in the geriatric population. *Clin Geriatr Med* 2005;21:631–47.

[2] Donnelly JA, Torregiani S. Polymyalgia rheumatica and giant cell arteritis. *Clin Fam Pract* 2005;7:225–47.

[3] Weyand CM, Goronzy JJ. Mechanisms of disease: medium- and large-vessel vasculitis. *N Engl J Med* 2003;349:160–9.

[4] Salvarani C, Cantini F, Boiardi L, et al. Medical progress: polymyalgia rheumatica and giant-cell arteritis. *N Engl J Med* 2002;347:261–71.

[5] Younger DS. Headaches and vasculitis. *Neurol Clin N Am* 2004;22:207–28.

[6] Smetana GW, Shmerling RH. Does this patient have temporal arteritis? *JAMA* 2002;287:92–101.

[7] Kyle V, Cawston TE, Hazleman BL. Erythrocyte sedimentation rate and C reactive protein in the assessment of polymyalgia rheumatica: giant cell arteritis on presentation and during follow up. *Ann Rheum Dis* 1989;48:667–71.

[8] Evans JM, O'Fallon WM, Hunder GG. Increased incidence of aortic aneurysm and dissection in giant cell (temporal) arteritis: a population-based study. *Ann Intern Med* 1995;122:505–7.

[9] Egland AG, Jackson LW. Temporal arteritis. eMedicine Website. Available at http://www.emedicine.com/EMERG/topic568.htm. Accessed June 24, 2008.

5

Eye pain and blurred vision in an 89-year-old female

HISTORY OF PRESENT ILLNESS

An 89-year-old female with an ophthalmologic history significant for open angle glaucoma in both eyes, who had failed medical management and had undergone trabeculectomy with mitomycin C treatment to the left eye six months earlier, presented to the ED with several days of progressively worsening vision, redness, pain, photophobia and discharge from her left eye. She denied trauma or new eye drops and did not wear contact lenses.

PHYSICAL EXAMINATION

GENERAL APPEARANCE: The patient was an elderly female in no acute discomfort.

VITAL SIGNS

Temperature	98.6°F (37°C)
Pulse	88 beats/minute
Blood pressure	150/90 mmHg
Respirations	18 breaths/minute
Oxygen saturation	99% on room air

EYES: Visual acuity: 20/40 OD; finger counting at 5 feet OS.

PERRL, EOMI. Intraocular pressures measured 10 mmHg OD and 18 mmHg OS, respectively.

Gross inspection of the left eye: redness and swelling to lids, conjunctival injection, mucoid discharge, layering of milky material to inferior portion of cornea (Figure 5.1).

What is your diagnosis?

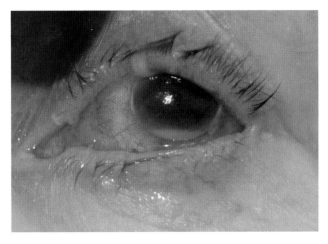

Figure 5.1 Left eye of an 89-year-old female with progressively worsening vision, redness, pain and photophobia.

ANSWER

The diagnosis is endophthalmitis with hypopyon. Figure 5.1 demonstrates several of the findings of this condition: a red eye with circumlimbal flush, a hypopyon (inflammatory cells and exudates [pus] layered in the anterior chamber of the eye), and purulent discharge on the lid margin and eyelashes. The patient received gatifloxacin 0.3% eye drops to the left eye, and her eye was subsequently dilated with tropicamide 1% and phenylephrine 2.5% drops. The patient was taken to the OR emergently by the ophthalmologist, where a vitrectomy with intravitreal injection of antibiotics was performed. The patient was discharged that same day to continue gatifloxacin and prednisolone eye drops every hour while awake, with a follow-up appointment with the ophthalmologist the following day.

Endophthalmitis

Endophthalmitis is an infection involving the deep structures of the eye, namely the anterior, posterior and vitreous chambers.[1] Noninfectious (sterile) endophthalmitis may result from various causes, such as retained native lens material after an operation or from toxic agents.[2] The two classifications of endophthalmitis are endogenous and exogenous. Endogenous endophthalmitis results from the hematogenous spread of organisms from a distant source of infection (e.g., endocarditis).[2] Exogenous endophthalmitis results from direct inoculation of the eye as a complication of ocular surgery, foreign bodies, or blunt or penetrating trauma.[1,2]

Acute postoperative endophthalmitis refers to infectious endophthalmitis that occurs shortly after ocular surgery. Most patients present within 1 to 2 weeks of surgery, often within a few days. Initial symptoms are often rapidly progressive, including pain, redness, ocular discharge and blurring.[3] Common signs include decreased visual acuity, lid swelling, conjunctival and corneal edema, anterior chamber cells and fibrin, hypopyon, vitreous inflammation, retinitis, and blunting of the red reflex.[3] Common pathogens of endophthalmitis are *Staphylococcus*, *Streptococcus* and *Bacillus*[1]. Endophthalmitis caused by *H. influenza* has been documented, occurring from 6 days up to 18 months after invasive eye surgery.[4]

Treatment with empiric antibiotics must be prompt because endophthalmitis can result in a poor visual outcome if not treated aggressively.[4] Emergent consultation with an ophthalmologist is necessary once this diagnosis is entertained. Endophthalmitis is an ophthalmologic emergency, as the patient is in danger of losing his or her vision.[2] Emergency treatment should begin with a dose of broad-spectrum intravenous antibiotics. Intravitreal antimicrobial therapy remains the mainstay of treatment.[3] The majority of patients require intravitreal injections, vitreous tap, subconjunctival steroids or vitrectomy to prevent loss of the eye.[4]

KEY TEACHING POINTS

1. Endophthalmitis is an ophthalmologic emergency requiring a high index of suspicion and prompt consultation with an ophthalmologist.
2. Initial symptoms of endophthalmitis include pain, redness, ocular discharge and blurring of vision.
3. Common signs include decreased visual acuity, lid swelling, conjunctival and corneal edema, anterior chamber cells and fibrin, hypopyon, vitreous inflammation, retinitis, and blunting of the red reflex.
4. Intravitreal antimicrobial therapy remains the mainstay of treatment for infectious endophthalmitis; the majority of patients require intravitreal injections, vitreous tap, subconjunctival steroids or vitrectomy to prevent loss of the eye.

REFERENCES

[1] Burnette DD. Ophthalmology. In: Marx JA, Hockberger RS, Walls RM, et al. (eds). *Rosen's Emergency Medicine: Concepts and Clinical Practice*, 6th ed. Mosby, 2006:1052.
[2] Egan DJ, Radin PJ, Peak DA. Endophthalmitis. eMedicine Website. Available at http://www.emedicine.com/emerg/topic880.htm. Accessed June 27, 2008.
[3] Lemley CA, Han DP. Endophthalmitis: a review of current evaluation and management. *Retina* 2007;27:662–80.
[4] Naradzay J, Barish RA. Approach to ophthalmologic emergencies. *Med Clin N Am* 2006;90:305–28.

PART II

CARDIOVASCULAR

6

Palpitations and chest heaviness in a 26-year-old female

HISTORY OF PRESENT ILLNESS

A 26-year-old female with no significant medical history presented to the ED complaining of two hours of palpitations, mild chest pressure and general body weakness. She denied shortness of breath, nausea, sweating or leg swelling. She denied drugs, alcohol or tobacco use, as well as pregnancy.

PHYSICAL EXAMINATION

GENERAL APPEARANCE: The patient was well nourished and well hydrated, appeared tired but easily arousable.

VITAL SIGNS

Temperature	97.2°F (36.2°C)
Pulse	142 beats/minute
Blood pressure	123/70 mmHg
Respirations	20 breaths/minute
Oxygen saturation	100% on room air

HEENT: Unremarkable.

NECK: Supple, no jugular venous distension.

CARDIOVASCULAR: Tachycardic rate, regular rhythm, no rubs, murmurs or gallops.

LUNGS: Clear to auscultation bilaterally.

ABDOMEN: Soft, nontender, nondistended.

EXTREMITIES: No clubbing, cyanosis or edema; radial pulses were rapid and weak.

NEUROLOGIC: Nonfocal.

The patient was placed on the cardiac monitor, a peripheral intravenous line was placed and a 12-lead ECG was obtained (Figure 6.1).

What is your diagnosis?

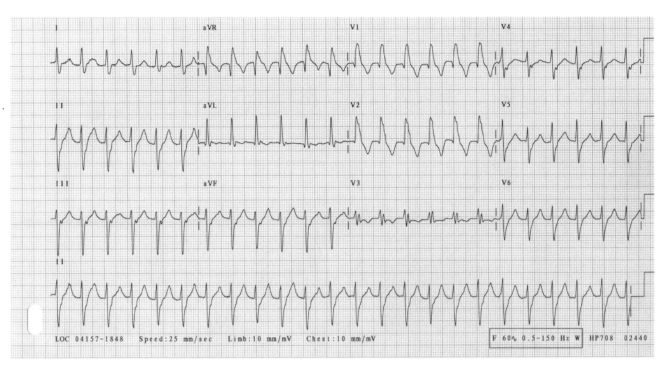

Figure 6.1 12-lead ECG from a 26-year-old female with palpitations and chest pressure.

ANSWER

The diagnosis is idiopathic fascicular ventricular tachycardia (IFVT). The ECG in Figure 6.1 shows a tachycardia without obvious P waves, widened QRS complexes with a regular rhythm and rate of 142, and a right bundle branch block pattern with a left anterior fascicular block. The patient was initially given adenosine IV without any affect on the rate or rhythm. The patient was then given IV diltiazem, which caused a slowing of the ventricular rate. A repeat ECG (Figure 6.2) was obtained, which demonstrated P waves independent of QRS complexes. This finding is consistent with AV dissociation and ventricular tachycardia arising in the His-Purkinje system. Shortly thereafter, her rhythm spontaneously converted to normal sinus rhythm (Figure 6.3). A bedside echocardiogram performed in the ED after cardioversion demonstrated normal left ventricular function with an ejection fraction of 55%. The patient was admitted to the telemetry unit for continued monitoring overnight, and was started on flecainide and metoprolol orally. She was discharged from the hospital the following day in normal sinus rhythm with normal vital signs, with close follow up in the cardiology clinic.

Idiopathic fascicular ventricular tachycardia

Idiopathic monomorphic ventricular tachycardia (VT) can be subdivided into three distinct subgroups: fascicular, adenosine-sensitive, and automatic (propranolol-sensitive) VT.[1] Idiopathic fascicular ventricular tachycardia (IFVT) is characterized by a relatively narrow QRS complex and a right bundle branch block pattern.[2] The QRS axis depends on which fascicle is involved in re-entry. Left axis deviation is noted with left posterior fascicular tachycardia; right axis deviation is present with left anterior fascicular tachycardia. IFVT shows a typical rSR′ morphology in lead V1.[3] This type of idiopathic ventricular tachycardia is also known as intrafascicular tachycardia, verapamil-sensitive VT, or Belhassen tachycardia.[3]

Fascicular tachycardia is typically seen in individuals without structural heart disease, usually occurring in patients 15–40 years old. It occurs more frequently in men than women.[1–3] Patients tend to present with paroxysmal sustained tachycardia; initiation of tachycardia may occur with exercise. Termination usually requires administration of an intravenous antiarrhythmic medication.[3] Sometimes the tachycardia can be incessant, resulting in tachycardia-induced cardiomyopathy. Symptoms may range from none to palpitations, shortness of breath, fatigue or dizziness; syncope or sudden death is extremely rare in these patients.[3]

Intravenous verapamil is effective in terminating the IFVT;[1–3] in 1981, Belhassen et al. were among the first to report termination or suppression of IFVT by the calcium-channel blocker, verapamil.[4] However, the efficacy of oral verapamil in preventing tachycardia relapse is variable.[2] Calcium-channel blockers should be used with extreme caution, especially if a wide-complex tachycardia is present or the diagnosis of IFVT is in question. In these cases, an adenosine trial should occur first. Although fascicular tachycardias do not generally respond to adenosine, termination of VT originating from the left anterior fascicle by intravenous adenosine has been documented.[1] Radiofrequency catheter ablation procedures have demonstrated a 90% success rate for the treatment of fascicular tachycardia with minimal complications.[3]

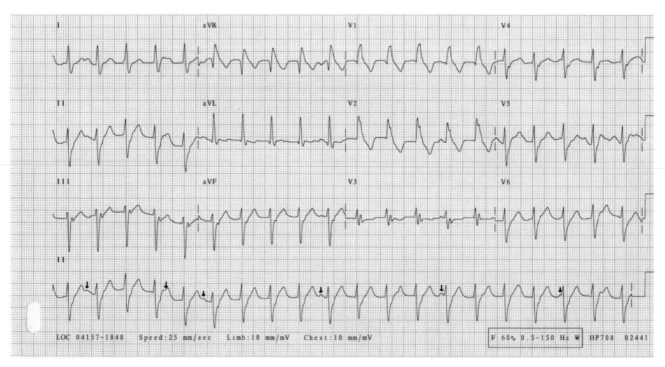

Figure 6.2 12-lead ECG from a 26-year-old female with palpitations after treatment with IV diltiazem (arrows on lead II identify P waves).

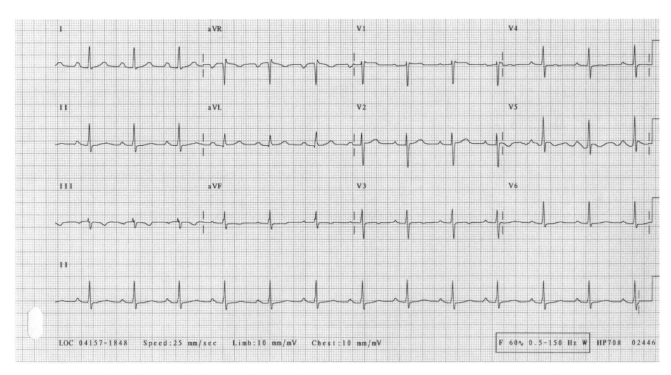

Figure 6.3 12-lead ECG from a 26-year-old female with palpitations demonstrating normal sinus rhythm.

KEY TEACHING POINTS

1. Idiopathic fascicular ventricular tachycardia (IFVT) is an important cardiac dysrhythmia with specific electrocardiographic features (a relative narrow QRS complex and a right bundle branch block pattern) and therapeutic options (verapamil, diltiazem or adenosine).
2. IFVT usually occurs in young patients from 15–40 years of age without structural heart disease.
3. Symptoms of IFVT range from none to palpitations, shortness of breath, fatigue or dizziness. Syncope or sudden death is extremely rare in these patients.
4. Intravenous verapamil is effective in terminating IFVT, whereas catheter ablation procedures demonstrate a 90% success rate for the long-term suppression of these dysrhythmias.
5. Caution should be taken in using calcium-channel blockers as first-line treatment for any wide-complex tachycardia, including ventricular tachycardia. Despite being the treatment for IFVT, adenosine is a safer first-line agent.

REFERENCES

[1] Kassotis J, Slesinger T, Festic E, et al. Adenosine-sensitive wide-complex tachycardia: an uncommon variant of idiopathic fascicular ventricular tachycardia – a case report. *Angiology* 2003;54:369–72.
[2] Johnson F, Venugopal K, Khadar SA, et al. Idiopathic fascicular ventricular tachycardia. *Indian Pacing Electrophysiol J* 2004;4:98–103.
[3] Chiu C, Sequeira IB. Diagnosis and treatment of idiopathic ventricular tachycardia. *AACN Clinical Issues* 2004;15:449–61.
[4] Belhassen B, Rotmensch H, Laniado S. Response of recurrent sustained ventricular tachycardia to verapamil. *Br Heart J* 1981;46:679–82.

7

Chest pain in a 26-year-old male

HISTORY OF PRESENT ILLNESS

A 26-year-old male with no significant medical history presented to the ED complaining of several hours of substernal chest pain after using cocaine daily for the preceding six days. His last cocaine use was 24 hours prior to presentation. He described the chest pain as central, pressure-like, constant and nonradiating. He also reported associated palpitations, shortness of breath and diaphoresis, as well as several days of insomnia and anorexia. He had been drinking tequila for the past 24 hours in an effort to "calm himself down."

PHYSICAL EXAMINATION

GENERAL APPEARANCE: The patient appeared well developed and well nourished, anxious and diaphoretic, and in no acute discomfort.

VITAL SIGNS

Temperature	99.1°F (37.3°C)
Pulse	132 beats/minute
Blood pressure	150/92 mmHg
Respirations	24 breaths/minute
Oxygen saturation	98% on room air

HEENT: PERRL, EOMI, dry mucous membranes.

NECK: Supple, no jugular venous distension.

CARDIOVASCULAR: Tachycardic rate, regular rhythm without rubs, murmurs or gallops.

LUNGS: Clear to auscultation bilaterally.

ABDOMEN: Soft, nontender, nondistended.

EXTREMITIES: No clubbing, cyanosis or edema, brisk radial and dorsalis pedis pulses.

SKIN: Warm and moist, no rashes.

NEUROLOGIC: Nonfocal.

The patient was placed on the cardiac monitor, a peripheral intravenous line was placed and blood was drawn and sent for laboratory testing. A 12-lead ECG was obtained (Figure 7.1).

What is your diagnosis?

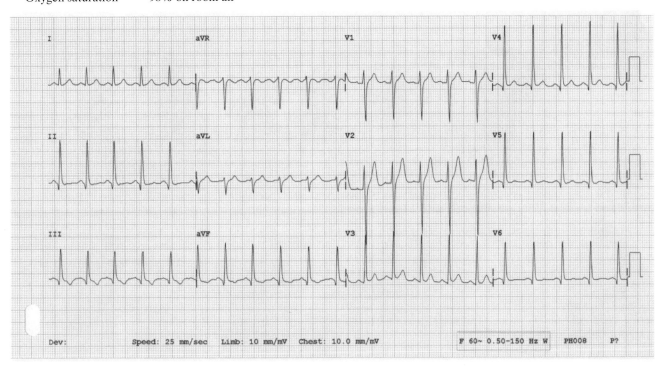

Figure 7.1 12-lead ECG from a 26-year-old male with several hours of chest pain.

ANSWER

The diagnosis is cocaine-associated chest pain. The ECG (Figure 7.1) demonstrates sinus tachycardia, rate 142, with nonspecific ST-T wave changes. The patient received a total of 3 liters normal saline IV infusion, three 1-mg doses of lorazepam IV, aspirin 162 mg orally, and was observed for eight hours in the ED. His chest pain resolved with intravenous fluids and lorazepam. Laboratory tests revealed an initial troponin I less than 0.02 ng/mL (normal 0.00–0.09 ng/mL), CK 120 U/L (normal 38–174 U/L), creatinine of 1.36 mg/dL (normal 0.8–1.5 mg/dL) and hematocrit of 52% (normal 39–51%), with the remainder of laboratory tests within normal limits. A repeat troponin I obtained four hours following the first was also normal (< 0.02 ng/mL). On discharge, the patient was symptom-free with a pulse of 90 beats/minute and a blood pressure of 126/80 mmHg. The patient was instructed to avoid cocaine and was scheduled for an outpatient ECG treadmill, which subsequently did not demonstrate any evidence of exercise-induced ischemia.

Cocaine-associated chest pain

In two separate studies of patients presenting to the ED with cocaine-associated chest pain, the incidence of acute myocardial infarction (AMI) in these patients was found to be 6%.[1,2] Several mechanisms have been proposed for the manner in which cocaine causes cardiac ischemia and infarction in individuals who use cocaine. These mechanisms include coronary vasoconstriction, increased platelet aggregation, thrombus formation leading to MI, myocardial toxicity and increased cardiac demand for oxygen resulting from adrenergic stimulation.[3] In addition, chronic cocaine users may be prone to premature atherosclerosis of their coronary arteries.

The initial stabilization and nonpharmacological treatment of patients with cocaine-associated chest pain is similar to that of patients with typical angina or MI resulting from atherosclerotic coronary artery disease (CAD): bed rest, oxygen, cardiac monitor and IV. Patients whose chest pain may be caused by ischemia should receive aspirin if there are no contraindications (e.g., known allergy or suspected subarachnoid hemorrhage).[4] Benzodiazepines (diazepam or lorazepam) should be administered, particularly in the agitated patient and in those with hyperdynamic vital signs (common with recent cocaine use).[3] Benzodiazepines have been demonstrated to reduce the heart rate and systemic arterial pressure in cocaine-intoxicated patients. Beta-blockers are contraindicated in the setting of cocaine-associated myocardial ischemia.[3–5] Cocaine decreases left coronary artery diameter and coronary sinus blood flow while increasing coronary vascular resistance, effects that are exacerbated by beta-adrenergic blockade. These effects presumably occur through unopposed alpha-adrenergic stimulation.

Nitroglycerin has been shown to alleviate cocaine-induced vasoconstriction in patients with CAD.[6] Furthermore, the early use of lorazepam in combination with nitroglycerin seems to be more efficacious than nitroglycerin alone in relieving chest pain associated with cocaine use.[7] Patients who continue to have chest pain despite the administration of oxygen, benzodiazepines, aspirin and nitroglycerin may be treated with low-dose IV phentolamine (1 mg).[4] Phentolamine has been shown to reverse cocaine-induced coronary artery vasoconstriction in humans.

A prospective study has attempted to validate the use of 9- to 12-hour observation periods in low- to moderate-risk patients who experience cocaine-associated chest pain.[8] Patients with normal troponin I levels, no evidence of new ischemic changes on ECG and no cardiovascular complications (AMI, dysrhythmias or recurrent symptoms) were discharged from the observation unit. During the 30-day follow-up period, none of the 302 patients in the cohort died from a cardiovascular event, and only 4 patients with detailed follow-up had a MI (1.6%); all four nonfatal MIs occurred in patients who continued to use cocaine. These results suggest that an observation period of 9–12 hours for low- to moderate-risk patients presenting with cocaine-associated chest pain appears to be safe, and that continued use of cocaine may result in a small percentage of nonfatal MIs in low- to moderate-risk individuals.

KEY TEACHING POINTS

1. The rate of AMI in patients presenting to an ED with cocaine-associated chest pain is approximately 6%, although the overall prevalence is likely to be lower as not all individuals seek medical attention or admit to using cocaine.
2. Benzodiazepines should be given, particularly to an agitated patient or one with hyperdynamic vital signs.
3. The early use of lorazepam in combination with nitroglycerin seems to be more efficacious than nitroglycerin alone in relieving chest pain associated with cocaine use.
4. Beta-blockers are contraindicated in the setting of cocaine-associated chest pain or myocardial ischemia.
5. An observation period of 9–12 hours for low- to moderate-risk patients presenting with cocaine-associated chest pain appears to be safe; continued use of cocaine may result in a small percentage of nonfatal MIs in low- to moderate-risk individuals.

REFERENCES

[1] Hollander JE, Hoffman RS, Gennis P, et al. Prospective multicenter evaluation of cocaine-associated chest pain. *Acad Emerg Med* 1994;1:330–9.
[2] Weber JE, Chudnofsky CR, Boczar M, et al. Cocaine-associated chest pain: how common is myocardial infarction? *Acad Emerg Med* 2000;7:873–7.

[3] Levis JT, Garmel GM. Cocaine-associated chest pain. *Emerg Med Clin N Am* 2005;23:1083–103.

[4] Hahn IH, Hoffman RS. Diagnosis and treatment of acute myocardial infarction: cocaine use and acute myocardial infarction. *Emerg Med Clin N Am* 2001;19:1–18.

[5] McCord J, Jneid H, Hollander JE, et al. Management of cocaine-associated chest pain and myocardial infarction. A scientific statement from the American Heart Association Acute Cardiac Care Committee of the Council on Clinical Cardiology. *Circulation* 2008;117:1897–907.

[6] Brogan WC, Lange RA, Kim AS, et al. Alleviation of cocaine-induced coronary vasoconstriction by nitroglycerin. *J Am Coll Cardiol* 1991;18:581–6.

[7] Honderick T, Williams D, Seaberg D, et al. A prospective, randomized, controlled trial of benzodiazepines and nitroglycerin or nitroglycerin alone in the treatment of cocaine-associated acute coronary syndromes. *Am J Emerg Med* 2003;21:39–42.

[8] Weber JE, Shofer FS, Larkin L, et al. Validation of a brief observation period for patients with cocaine-associated chest pain. *N Engl J Med* 2003;348:510–7.

8

Palpitations in a 36-year-old male

HISTORY OF PRESENT ILLNESS

A 36-year-old male with no significant medical history presented to the ED complaining of 30 minutes of palpitations, described as a rapid, irregular heart beat. The patient reported mild shortness of breath and fatigue but denied chest pain, nausea or sweating. He described several similar episodes in the past, which had always resolved spontaneously within two hours. Earlier that day, the patient had exercised strenuously and did not drink much water afterward. He denied tobacco, intravenous drugs, cocaine or methamphetamine use, and drank alcohol only occasionally.

PHYSICAL EXAMINATION

GENERAL APPEARANCE: The patient appeared well nourished, well developed and in no acute distress.

VITAL SIGNS

Temperature	97°F (36.1°C)
Pulse	125 beats/minute
Blood pressure	147/80 mmHg
Respirations	18 breaths/minute
Oxygen saturation	100% on room air

HEENT: Unremarkable.

NECK: Supple, no jugular venous distension.

CARDIOVASCULAR: Tachycardic rate with an irregularly irregular rhythm; no rubs, murmurs or gallops.

LUNGS: Clear to auscultation bilaterally.

ABDOMEN: Soft, nontender, nondistended.

EXTREMITIES: No clubbing, cyanosis or edema.

NEUROLOGIC: Nonfocal.

The patient was placed on the cardiac monitor and a 12-lead ECG was obtained (Figure 8.1). A peripheral intravenous line was placed, blood was drawn and sent for laboratory testing, and intravenous fluids (normal saline 2-liter bolus) were administered. Laboratory tests, including a complete blood count, electrolyte panel, creatinine, glucose and troponin I, were within normal limits. A portable chest radiograph was normal.

What is your diagnosis?

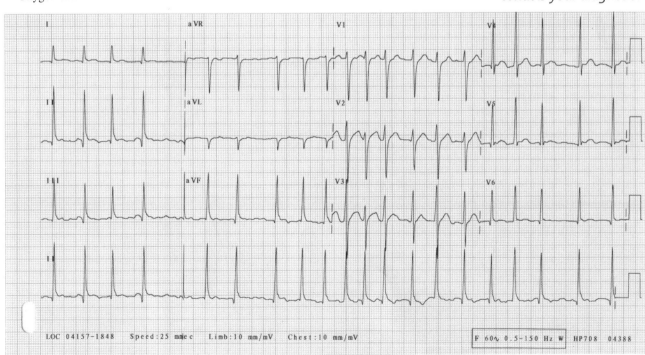

Figure 8.1 12-lead ECG from a 36-year-old male with palpitations.

ANSWER

The diagnosis is rapid atrial fibrillation. The ECG (Figure 8.1) demonstrates atrial fibrillation with a rapid ventricular response of approximately 131 beats/minute. Two 10-mg IV doses of diltiazem were given for rate control. After three hours, the patient stated his symptoms had resolved, and a repeat ECG was obtained (Figure 8.2).

The repeat ECG demonstrated normal sinus rhythm, rate of 81 beats/minute, without acute ST-T wave changes. The patient was discharged from the ED, started on atenolol with close follow up in the cardiology clinic.

Atrial fibrillation

Electrocardiographically, atrial fibrillation is characterized by the presence of rapid, irregular fibrillatory waves that vary in size, shape and timing.[1] This set of findings is usually associated with an irregular ventricular response, although regularization may occur in patients with complete heart block, an accelerated junctional or idiopathic rhythm, or a ventricular-paced rhythm. Atrial fibrillation is the most common dysrhythmia that requires treatment, with an estimated prevalence in the United States of 2.3 million patients in 2001.[2] This prevalence increases with age – atrial fibrillation occurs in 3.8% of people 60 years of age and older and in 9.0% of those over 80 years.[2]

The most devastating consequence of atrial fibrillation is stroke, due to thromboembolism typically emanating from the left atrial appendage. The rate of stroke varies but may range from 5.0–9.6% per year among patients at high risk taking aspirin (but not warfarin).[2] Patients with paroxysmal atrial fibrillation (i.e., self-terminating) and persistent atrial fibrillation (i.e., lasting more than seven days or requiring cardioversion) appear to have a risk of stroke that is similar to that of patients with permanent atrial fibrillation.[3] Atrial fibrillation is associated with an increase in the relative risk of death ranging from 1.3 to 2.6, independent of other risk factors.[1,4]

In most cases, atrial fibrillation is associated with cardiovascular disease (i.e., hypertension, coronary artery disease, cardiomyopathy, and valvular disease). In some cases, atrial fibrillation results from another supraventricular tachycardia (e.g., Wolff-Parkinson-White syndrome). Other predisposing conditions include excessive alcohol intake, hyperthyroidism, and pulmonary disorders, including pulmonary embolism.[2] "Lone" atrial fibrillation (i.e., occurring in the absence of a cardiac or other explanation) is common, particularly in patients with paroxysmal atrial fibrillation – up to 45% of such patients have no underlying cardiac disease.[2]

Patients with atrial fibrillation may have palpitations, dyspnea, fatigue, lightheadedness or syncope. These symptoms are usually related to the elevated heart rate, and in most patients can be mitigated with the use of pharmacologic therapy.[1,2] The patient's history and physical examination should focus on the potential causes of atrial fibrillation. The "minimum evaluation" recommended at diagnosis should include a 12-lead ECG, chest radiograph, transthoracic echocardiography, and serologic tests of thyroid function.[2,5]

Patients presenting in rapid atrial fibrillation with significant hemodynamic instability or with signs and symptoms of ongoing cardiac ischemia should be emergently cardioverted using synchronized, electrical cardioversion (after

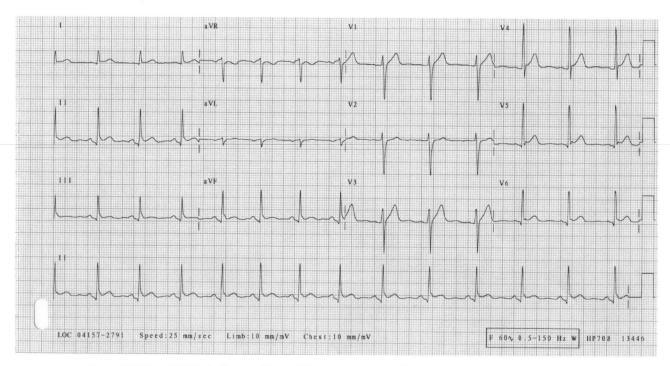

Figure 8.2 12-lead ECG of a 36-year-old male following two doses of diltiazem and resolution of palpitations.

careful assessment of the airway, breathing and circulation). In patients who are hemodynamically stable and without ischemia, rate control is the first priority. A number of pharmacologic agents are available to control the heart rate and rhythm. First-line therapy for rate control includes intravenous β-adrenergic blockers (e.g., metoprolol IV) or calcium-channel blockers (e.g., diltiazem IV). Digoxin is useful in combination with other agents, or when β-adrenergic blocking agents and calcium-channel blockers are not well tolerated.[6] Current guidelines recommend a target ventricular rate during atrial fibrillation of 60–80 beats/minute at rest and 90–115 beats per minute during exercise.[2,5]

A number of agents may maintain sinus rhythm (e.g., β-adrenergic blockers, amiodarone, procainamide, flecainide, sotalol).[2] The use of β-adrenergic blocking agents may be effective in adrenergically-mediated and paroxysmal atrial fibrillation. With the exception of β-adrenergic blocking agents, most antiarrhythmic drugs carry a risk of serious adverse effects. Antiarrhythmic therapy should be chosen on the basis of the patient's underlying cardiac condition.[2]

Spontaneous conversion to sinus rhythm within 24 hours after the onset of atrial fibrillation is common, occurring in up to two-thirds of patients.[1] Once the duration of atrial fibrillation exceeds 24 hours, the likelihood of conversion decreases. Synchronized, direct-current cardioversion or early drug therapy to restore sinus rhythm should be considered in patients in whom the dysrhythmia has lasted less than 48 hours or who take long-term warfarin therapy. In many patients, the precise time of onset of atrial fibrillation cannot be determined accurately. In these circumstances, it is recommended to administer anticoagulation therapy to the patient before attempting cardioversion. There are two alternative approaches: outpatient systemic anticoagulation with warfarin to achieve an international normalized ratio of 2.0–3.0 for at least three weeks, followed by cardioversion or cardioversion guided by transesophageal echocardiography. Regardless of which of these approaches is taken, anticoagulation therapy is mandatory for a minimum of three to four weeks after cardioversion.[1]

KEY TEACHING POINTS

1. Electrocardiographically, atrial fibrillation is characterized by the presence of rapid, irregular fibrillatory waves that vary in size, shape and timing.
2. The most devastating consequence of atrial fibrillation is stroke due to thromboembolism; the rate of stroke may range from 5.0–9.6% per year among patients at high risk not taking warfarin.
3. Patients presenting in rapid atrial fibrillation with significant hemodynamic instability or with signs and symptoms of acute cardiac ischemia should be emergently cardioverted using synchronized, electrical cardioversion.
4. Rate control with pharmacologic agents (e.g., beta- or calcium-channel blockers) is the primary goal in hemodynamically stable patients presenting in rapid atrial fibrillation.
5. Spontaneous conversion to sinus rhythm within 24 hours after the onset of atrial fibrillation is common, occurring in up to two-thirds of patients.

REFERENCES

[1] Falk RH. Medical progress: atrial fibrillation. *N Engl J Med* 2001;344:1067–78.
[2] Page RL. Clinical practice: newly diagnosed atrial fibrillation. *N Engl J Med* 2004;351:2408–16.
[3] Hart RG, Pearce LA, Rothbart RM, et al. Stroke with intermittent atrial fibrillation: incidence and predictors during aspirin therapy. *J Am Coll Cardiol* 2000;35:183–7.
[4] Benjamin EJ, Wolf PA, D'Agostino RB, et al. Impact of atrial fibrillation on the risk of death: the Framingham Heart Study. *Circulation* 1998;98:946–52.
[5] Fuster V, Ryden LE, Asinger RW, et al. ACC/AHA/ESC guidelines for the management of patients with atrial fibrillation: executive summary. *J Am Coll Cardiol* 2001;38:1231–66.
[6] Farshi R, Kistner D, Sarma JS, et al. Ventricular rate control in chronic atrial fibrillation during daily activity and programmed exercise: a cross-over open-label study of five drug regimens. *J Am Coll Cardiol* 1999;33:304–10.

9

Chest pressure for two days in a 37-year-old male

HISTORY OF PRESENT ILLNESS

A 37-year-old male with a medical history significant for Becker's muscular dystrophy, cardiomyopathy and congestive heart failure presented to the ED with two days of chest pressure. He reported the pressure as constant, rated at a level of 3 (on a scale of 0 to 10), and described the pressure as slightly worsening on deep inspiration. He described increased shortness of breath with exertion and a cough productive of clear sputum but denied fevers, chills, nausea, lightheadedness or sweating.

PHYSICAL EXAMINATION

GENERAL APPEARANCE: The patient was a pale, obese male who appeared in no acute discomfort.

VITAL SIGNS

Temperature	97.5°F (36.4°C)
Pulse	118 beats/minute
Blood pressure	102/72 mmHg
Respirations	18 breaths/minute
Oxygen saturation	96% on room air

HEENT: Unremarkable.

NECK: Supple, mild jugular venous distension noted.

CARDIOVASCULAR: Distant heart sounds, audible S1 and S2, unable to assess for rubs, murmurs or gallops.

LUNGS: Rales at the lung bases bilaterally, no rhonchi or wheezes.

ABDOMEN: Soft, nontender, nondistended.

EXTREMITIES: Trace lower extremity edema bilaterally to mid-anterior shin.

NEUROLOGIC: Nonfocal.

The patient was placed on the cardiac monitor, a peripheral intravenous line was placed and blood was drawn and sent for laboratory testing. A 12-lead ECG (Figure 9.1) and a portable chest radiograph were obtained (Figure 9.2, panel A). Laboratory tests were significant for a leukocyte count of 18 K/µL (normal 3.5–12.5 K/µL) with 90% neutrophils (normal 50–70%), hematocrit of 31% (normal 39–51%), creatinine of 1.5 mg/dL (normal < 1.3 mg/dL) and a positive D-dimer. The troponin I was within normal limits. A bedside echocardiogram was obtained (Figure 9.3).

What is your diagnosis?

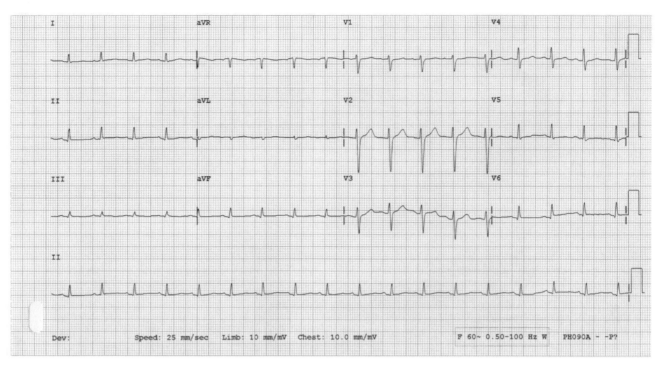

Figure 9.1 12-lead ECG from 37-year-old male with chest pressure for two days.

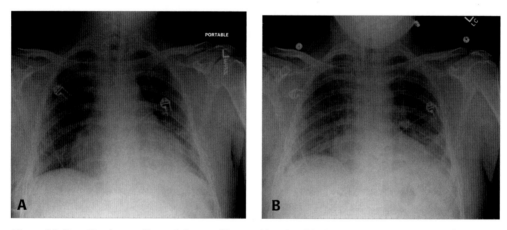

Figure 9.2 Portable chest radiograph from a 37-year-old male with chest pressure for two days (panel A); comparison with a portable chest radiograph obtained from the same patient five days earlier (panel B).

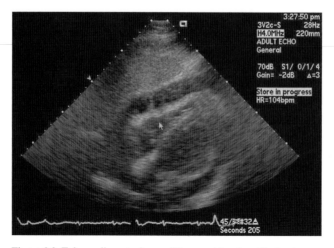

Figure 9.3 Echocardiogram from a 37-year-old male with chest pressure for two days (arrow, right ventricle).

ANSWER

The diagnosis is pericardial effusion with cardiac tamponade. The ECG demonstrates low voltage and poor R wave progression (Figure 9.1), whereas the chest radiograph shows marked cardiomegaly compared with a portable chest radiograph five days previously during a chest pain evaluation (Figure 9.2, panels A and B). The bedside echocardiogram demonstrates a moderate circumferential pericardial effusion with signs of tamponade (evidence of right atrial collapse, Figure 9.3). The patient was taken to the OR and underwent a pericardial window procedure using video-assisted thoracoscopic surgery (VATS) performed by the cardiothoracic surgeon to relieve the tamponade and drain the pericardial effusion. Seven hundred milliliters of straw-colored fluid was removed during VATS; bacterial and fungal cultures of the pericardial fluid returned negative. The etiology of the pericardial fluid and resulting tamponade was determined to be viral.

Cardiac tamponade

Cardiac tamponade is the result of compression of the myocardium by the contents of the pericardium. This compression is generally caused by fluid but in rare cases may be caused by gas, pus, blood, or a combination of materials.[1] Cardiac tamponade is a continuum reflecting the amount of fluid (or other material), its rate of accumulation, and the condition of the heart. The three stages necessary for cardiac tamponade to develop include fluid filling the recesses of the parietal pericardium, fluid accumulating faster than the rate of the parietal pericardium's ability to stretch, and fluid accumulating faster than the body's ability to increase blood volume to support right ventricle filling pressures.[1] The final result of these processes is increased pericardial pressure, which causes decreased cardiac compliance and decreased blood flow into the heart, which leads to decreased cardiac output. The most important factor in the development of tamponade is the rate of fluid accumulation.[1] The main pathophysiologic derangement of cardiac tamponade is reduced cardiac output.

In the United States, malignant disease is the most common cause of pericardial effusion with tamponade.[2] Other causes of pericardial effusions that may result in tamponade include infection, connective tissue disease, heart failure, valvular heart disease, myocardial infarction, uremia, cardiac surgery, trauma and idiopathic.[3] Although malignancy is the most common etiology of pericardial effusion in developed countries (including the United States), tuberculosis should be considered in endemic areas. Acute pericardial tamponade occurs in approximately 2% of penetrating chest trauma; this condition is rarely seen in blunt trauma.[2]

Cardiac tamponade symptoms are usually nonspecific. The patient may complain of chest pain, cough or dyspnea.[1] The classic triad of cardiac tamponade described by Beck is hypotension, distended neck veins, and muffled heart sounds. These signs may be absent if tamponade develops quickly or if the patient is hypovolemic.[1] Initially, the heart responds to tamponade by increasing the heart rate to maintain cardiac output. This compensatory mechanism is maintained until late in the course; decompensation may occur quickly.

In cardiac tamponade, the ECG classically shows decreasing voltage or electrical alternans, although the latter is rare.[1] Electrical alternans on the ECG is pathognomonic of cardiac tamponade. It is characterized by alternating levels of ECG voltage of the P waves, QRS complexes and T waves, the result of the heart swinging in a large effusion. The chest radiograph may demonstrate an enlarged cardiac silhouette after as little as 200 mL of fluid accumulation.[2] This enlarged cardiac silhouette occurs in patients with slow fluid accumulation, compared to a normal cardiac silhouette seen in patients with rapid fluid accumulation and tamponade. Thus, the chronicity of the effusion may be suggested by the presence or absence of an enlarged cardiac silhouette.[2]

Echocardiography is the diagnostic procedure of choice to identify pericardial effusions and cardiac tamponade.[3] In the normal pericardium, there is approximately 30–50 mL of fluid between the visceral and parietal pericardium.[4] This amount of fluid is usually not visible on ultrasound. The pericardium should appear echogenic. If an effusion is present, an anechoic (dark) space will be evident between the pericardium and the beating heart. With a large or rapidly developing pericardial effusion, this anechoic space surrounding the heart may be associated with diastolic collapse of the right atrium or right ventricle.[4] Right atrial collapse is virtually 100% sensitive for cardiac tamponade but is less specific.[3] Duration of right atrial collapse exceeding one-third of the cardiac cycle increases specificity without sacrificing sensitivity. Left atrial collapse is seen in about 25% of patients and is specific for cardiac tamponade.[3] Left ventricular collapse is less common due to the muscularity of the left ventricle's wall.

Initial treatment of cardiac tamponade includes intravenous fluids to augment volume to the right ventricle, which increases the filling pressure in an effort to overcome the pressure of pericardial constriction.[1] Pericardiocentesis, preferably ultrasound-guided, is the treatment of choice. Enough fluid should be withdrawn to result in hemodynamic stability. If tamponade recurs, pericardiocentesis may be repeated or a drainage catheter can be left in the pericardial space.[1] A pericardiotomy may ultimately be necessary. Cardiac tamponade often has a high mortality rate, depending on the severity and nature of the underlying disease, the time course of onset, and the rapidity of diagnosis and successful intervention.[1]

KEY TEACHING POINTS

1. Cardiac tamponade results from increased pericardial pressure due to a rapidly accumulating pericardial effusion, which causes decreased cardiac compliance and decreased blood flow into the heart, in turn leading to decreased cardiac output.

2. In the United States, malignancy is the most common cause of pericardial effusion with tamponade; other causes

include infection, connective tissue disease, heart failure, valvular heart disease, myocardial infarction, uremia, cardiac surgery, trauma and idiopathic.

3. The classic triad of cardiac tamponade (hypotension, distended neck veins, and muffled heart sounds) is seen in less than 40% of patients with cardiac tamponade.

4. In cardiac tamponade, the ECG may show evidence of low voltage or electrical alternans, whereas the chest radiograph may demonstrate an enlarged cardiac silhouette.

5. Echocardiography is the study of choice for diagnosing cardiac tamponade; the treatment of cardiac tamponade is volume augmentation and pericardiocentesis.

REFERENCES

[1] Jouriles NJ. Pericardial and myocardial disease. In: Marx JA, Hockberger RS, Walls RM, et al. (eds). *Rosen's Emergency Medicine: Concepts and Clinical Practice*, 6th ed. Mosby, 2006;1285–6.

[2] Valley VT, Fly CA. Pericarditis and cardiac tamponade. eMedicine Website. Available at http://www.emedicine.com/emerg/topic412.htm. Accessed June 26, 2008.

[3] Hold BD. Pericardial disease and pericardial tamponade. *Crit Care Med* 2007;25:S355–64.

[4] Tang A, Euerle B. Emergency department ultrasound and echocardiography. *Emerg Med Clin N Am* 2005;23:1179–94.

10

Low back pain and leg weakness in a 40-year-old male

HISTORY OF PRESENT ILLNESS

A 40-year-old male with a history of hypertension and medication noncompliance presented to the ED complaining of the sudden onset of low back pain associated with weakness and numbness of his left leg. The pain occurred suddenly as the patient was bending over to pick up his son. He described his back pain as a "tearing" with radiation down his left leg, and rated the pain at a level of 10 (on a scale of 0 to 10). The patient denied abdominal or chest pain, shortness of breath, fevers, or bowel or bladder incontinence. He reported some nausea without vomiting. He denied any history of previous back trauma or back problems. He had a history of hypertension for which he was prescribed medication but stopped it some time ago. He denied tobacco or intravenous drug use, and drank alcohol occasionally.

PHYSICAL EXAMINATION

GENERAL APPEARANCE: The patient was a well-developed male in significant discomfort.

VITAL SIGNS

Temperature	97.7°F (36.5°C)
Pulse	59 beats/minute
Blood pressure	268/119 mmHg
Respirations	22 breaths/minute
Oxygen saturation	100% on room air

HEENT: Unremarkable.

NECK: Supple, no jugular venous distension.

CARDIOVASCULAR: Regular rate and rhythm without rubs, murmurs or gallops.

LUNGS: Clear to auscultation bilaterally.

ABDOMEN: Soft, nontender, nondistended, no pulsatile masses.

BACK: No thoracic or lumbar spine tenderness or erythema; no costovertebral angle tenderness.

EXTREMITIES: Left leg was pale and cool; left femoral, dorsalis pedis and posterior tibialis pulses were absent.

NEUROLOGIC: Notable for left lower extremity paralysis (left leg strength 0/5 proximal and distal) with decreased sensation over the entire left leg.

A peripheral intravenous line was placed, blood was drawn and sent for laboratory testing. Laboratory tests were significant for a leukocyte count of 18.1 K/μL (normal 3.5–12.5 K/μL), creatinine of 1.4 mg/dL (normal < 1.3 mg/dL), potassium of 2.8 mEq/L (normal 3.5–5.3 mEq/L), bicarbonate of 19 mEq/L (normal 22–30 mEq/L) and lactic acid of 4.2 mmol/L (normal 0.7–2.1 mmol/L). A CT angiogram (CTA) of the chest, abdomen and pelvis was obtained (Figures 10.1 and 10.2).

What is your diagnosis?

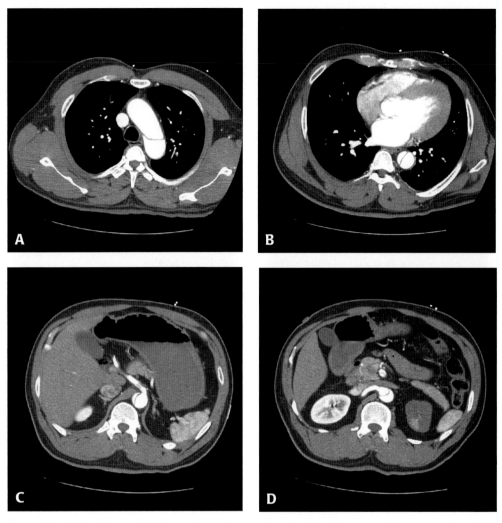

Figure 10.1 CTA of chest and abdomen from a 40-year-old male with sudden onset of low back pain and left leg paralysis (panels A–D represent superior to inferior transverse images).

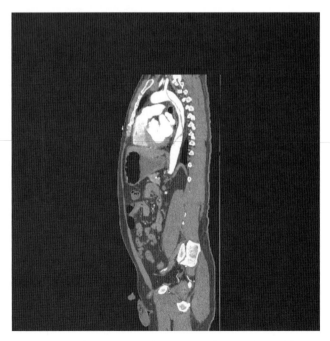

Figure 10.2 Sagittal reconstruction image of CTA of chest, abdomen and pelvis from a 40-year-old male with sudden onset low back pain and left leg paralysis.

ANSWER

The diagnosis is type B aortic dissection. The CTA demonstrates a type B aortic dissection, beginning distal to the take-off of the left subclavian artery, extending throughout the thoracic aorta and into the left common iliac, left external iliac and left femoral artery (Figures 10.1 and 10.2). An intimal flap is also seen in the celiac axis, superior mesenteric artery and left renal artery (Figure 10.1, panels C and D). Decreased perfusion of the left kidney is apparent compared to the right kidney.

An esmolol and nitroprusside drip were started for blood pressure control, and the patient was given Dilaudid™ and Zofran™ for pain and nausea control. The vascular surgery service was consulted emergently. The patient was taken to the OR where endovascular stents of the distal aorta and left iliac artery were successfully placed, resulting in return of palpable distal pulses in the left lower extremity (Figure 10.3).

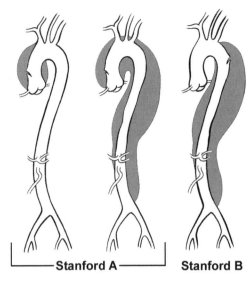

Figure 10.4 Stanford classification for aortic dissections.

Aortic dissection

Aortic dissection is a longitudinal cleavage of the aortic media created by a dissecting column of blood.[1,2] Acute aortic dissection has been estimated to affect 14–20 million individuals globally per year, with an incidence of 2.9 per 100,000 population per year.[3] Dissections predominantly affect males (male/female ratio 5:1). Two-thirds involve the ascending aorta (proximal), with a peak incidence for proximal dissections being 50–60 years of age and 60–70 years of age for distal dissections.[3] Hypertension, the most common risk factor associated with aortic dissection, is seen in most patients. Aortic dissection is uncommon before age 40 except in association with congenital heart disease, Ehlers-Danlos or Marfan syndrome, giant cell arteritis and pregnancy. More than 2000 cases of aortic dissection occur each year in the United States; it is the most common acute illness of the aorta.[4] Common misdiagnoses include myocardial infarction, atypical chest pain, congestive heart failure and gastrointestinal bleeding.[4]

Anatomic classification is important for diagnosis and therapy. The Stanford classification is based on the involvement of the ascending aorta (Figure 10.4). Type A dissections involve the ascending aorta; type B dissections do not. Dissections that involve the ascending aorta are much more lethal than those limited to the distal aorta, and call for a different therapeutic approach. In the International Registry of Acute Aortic Dissection (IRAD), 62% of dissections are type A and 38% are type B.[1] Patients with distal dissections tend to be older, heavy smokers with chronic lung disease, and more often have generalized atherosclerosis and hypertension compared with patients who have proximal aortic dissections.[1]

The classic presenting symptom of aortic dissection is abrupt onset of chest pain. With distal dissections, the pain is located in the back and is characterized as "tearing" in half of cases. Two-thirds of these cases additionally present with "sharp" pain, and approximately one-fifth present with "migratory" pain. In almost half of cases, the pain primarily involves or includes the abdominal area.[3] Syncope is much more commonly associated with dissections involving the ascending aorta or retrograde arch. Paralysis is reported to occur in 2–8% of patients with distal dissection, and hypertension is much more common than hypotension (more than 70% versus more than 5%, respectively).[3] Approximately 14% of patients who have dissections involving the distal aorta present with femoral pulse deficits.[3]

Routine chest radiograph will be abnormal in 80–90% of patients but the abnormalities are nonspecific and rarely diagnostic.[1] Mediastinal widening occurs in greater than 75% of cases, and may occur in the ascending aorta, aortic arch or the descending portion of the thoracic aorta; it may be difficult to differentiate from aortic tortuosity that is associated with chronic hypertension. The "calcium sign" (defined as a separation of the intimal calcium deposit from the outermost portion of the aorta by more than 5 mm) is an uncommon radiographic manifestation of aortic dissection. Up to 12% of patients with aortic dissection have a normal chest radiograph;

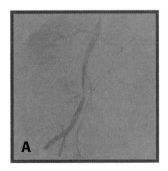
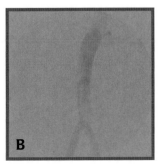

Figure 10.3 Intraoperative aortic angiogram from a 40-year-old male with type B aortic dissection (panel A) demonstrating endovascular placement of distal aortic stent (panel B).

therefore, a plain chest radiograph is inadequate to rule out aortic dissection.[1]

Imaging modalities to confirm aortic dissection include aortography, CT scanning, MRI and echocardiography.[1–5] CT scanning is useful in hemodynamically-stable patients but has potential limitations in patients with contrast allergy. MRI is as accurate as CT but is limited to hemodynamically-stable patients. Transesophageal echocardiography (TEE) is preferable to transthoracic echocardiography (TTE) and is as accurate as CT or MRI for detection of aortic dissection. Advantages of TEE include its portability and that it does not require contrast.

Opioids should be administered for pain control and to decrease sympathetic tone in patients with acute aortic dissection. The two goals of medical management are to reduce blood pressure and to decrease the rate of arterial pulse increase (dP/dt) to diminish shearing forces. Sodium nitroprusside should be titrated to maintain the systolic blood pressure at 100–120 mmHg or at the lowest level to maintain vital organ perfusion. Because nitroprusside increases the heart rate and may also increase dP/dt, a beta-blocker must be started before or in conjunction with sodium nitroprusside. Esmolol is an ultrashort-acting beta-blocker that is easily titrated. Esmolol is typically administered as a continuous infusion of 50–300 µg/kg/min, with a 500 µg/kg loading dose given over 1 minute before the infusion is begun or the rate is increased.[6] Labetalol has both alpha-blocking and beta-blocking activity and can be used as monotherapy. A suggested dose is an initial 20 mg IV bolus every 5 to 10 minutes, incrementally increased to 80 mg until a target heart rate has been reached or a total of 300 mg is given.[1,2]

Type A acute aortic dissections require prompt surgical treatment. Definitive treatment of type B acute aortic dissections is less clear. At most institutions, medical therapy with aggressive antihypertensive agents and beta-blockers is used in the ICU setting.[7] Operative intervention for acute type B dissections is reserved for life-threatening complications, such as progression of the dissection, rapid expansion, end-organ ischemia caused by side-branch compromise, ongoing pain, uncontrolled hypertension or rupture.[7] Open surgical interventions involve a combination of graft replacement, closure of the open entry site or fenestration to create a re-entry tear.[7] Endovascular stent grafting in patients with type B dissections has demonstrated promising short- and mid-term results. Proposed advantages of this less-invasive approach include shorter operative times, decreased need for general anesthesia, lack of aortic cross-clamping, avoidance of cardiopulmonary bypass, avoidance of major thoracic or thoracoabdominal incisions, less pain, quicker recovery, and shorter hospital and ICU stays.[7] Endovascular stenting may also play a role in patients with uncomplicated type B dissections. A retrospective analysis of 80 patients with type B aortic dissection treated endovascularly compared with 80 patients treated medically yielded a two-year survival rate of 94.9% using the endovascular approach versus 67.5% in the medically-treated group.[8]

KEY TEACHING POINTS

1. Acute aortic dissection is a true emergency requiring prompt diagnosis and vascular surgery consultation.
2. Hypertension is the most common risk factor for aortic dissection.
3. Stanford type A dissections involve the ascending aorta, whereas Stanford type B dissections do not.
4. Symptoms and signs of aortic dissection can include tearing chest pain radiating to the back, back pain, limb pain, weakness or numbness, syncope, pulse deficits, and hypertension that is difficult to control or refractory to medical management.
5. CTA is most useful in making the diagnosis of aortic dissection in stable patients. Other diagnostic modalities include MRI, transesophageal echocardiography and conventional aortography.
6. Immediate treatment of patients with aortic dissection involves opioid analgesia and strict blood pressure control with esmolol and sodium nitroprusside (or Labetalol™ as a single agent).
7. Definitive treatment of type A dissection is surgical. Type B dissection may be medically managed in uncomplicated cases, whereas complicated cases (progression of the dissection, rapid expansion, end-organ ischemia, ongoing pain, uncontrolled hypertension or rupture) require an open surgical approach or endovascular repair.

REFERENCES

[1] Ankel F. Aortic Dissection. In: Marx JA, Hockberger RS, Walls RM, et al. (eds). *Rosen's Emergency Medicine: Concepts and Clinical Practice*, 6th ed. Philadelphia: Mosby, 2006;1324–9.

[2] Osinuga O, Kesari S, Hmidi A, et al. Aortic dissection. eMedicine Website. Available at http://www.emedicine.com/MED/topic2784.htm. Accessed June 25, 2008.

[3] Karmey-Jones R, Simeone A, Meissner M, et al. Descending thoracic aortic dissections. *Surg Clin N Am* 2007;87:1047–86.

[4] Rogers RL, McCormack R. Aortic disasters. *Emerg Med Clin N Am* 2004;22:887–908.

[5] Nienaber CA. The diagnosis of thoracic aortic dissection by noninvasive imaging procedures. *N Engl J Med* 1993;328:1–9.

[6] Frakes MA. Esmolol: a unique drug with ED applications. *J Emerg Nurs* 2001;27:47–51.

[7] Lee JT, White RA. Current status of thoracic aortic endograft repair. *Surg Clin N Am* 2004;84:1295–318.

[8] Nienaber CA, Zannetti S, Barbieri B, et al. Investigation of stent grafts in patients with type B Aortic Dissection: design of the INSTEAD trial – a prospective, multicenter, European randomized trial. *Am Heart J* 2005;149:592–9.

11

Acute chest pain in a 42-year-old male

HISTORY OF PRESENT ILLNESS

A 42-year-old male with a medical history significant for hypertension and hyperlipidemia presented to the ED complaining of substernal chest pain that started four hours prior to presentation. The pain was located in the left upper chest and was described as dull and constant. He rated his pain at a level of 4 (on a scale of 0 to 10), with radiation to his back. The pain was aggravated by movement and worsened on deep inspiration. He denied any nausea, vomiting, sweating or shortness of breath, as well as recent cough or fevers. He also denied recent long trips or leg swelling. The patient had undergone an exercise treadmill test six months earlier, which revealed no evidence of exercise-induced ischemia.

PHYSICAL EXAMINATION

GENERAL APPEARANCE: The patient appeared well developed, well hydrated, and in no acute distress.

VITAL SIGNS

Temperature	97.6°F (36.4°C)
Pulse	56 beats/minute
Blood pressure	142/74 mmHg
Respirations	22 breaths/minute
Oxygen saturation	97% on room air

HEENT: Unremarkable.

NECK: Supple, no jugular venous distension.

CARDIOVASCULAR: Regular rate and rhythm without rubs, murmurs or gallops.

LUNGS: Clear to auscultation bilaterally.

ABDOMEN: Soft, nontender, nondistended.

EXTREMITIES: No clubbing, cyanosis or edema.

NEUROLOGIC: Nonfocal.

A 12-lead ECG was obtained (Figure 11.1), and the patient was placed on the cardiac monitor. A peripheral intravenous line was placed, and blood was drawn and sent for laboratory testing. The patient received aspirin 162 mg orally and morphine sulfate IV for his pain. A portable chest radiograph was obtained (Figure 11.2). Laboratory results were significant for a positive D-dimer; the remainder of the laboratory tests (complete blood count, electrolytes, creatinine, glucose and troponin I) were normal. A CT angiogram of the chest did not demonstrate evidence of pulmonary embolism. A second troponin I obtained eight hours after the onset of symptoms was normal (<0.02 ng/mL).

The patient was discharged from the ED with the diagnosis of chest pain, not otherwise specified. The patient's pain had not completely resolved and progressively worsened after discharged. The patient returned to the ED later that same evening, a repeat ECG was obtained (Figure 11.3), and a repeat troponin I obtained 13 hours after the onset of the pain was normal.

What is your diagnosis?

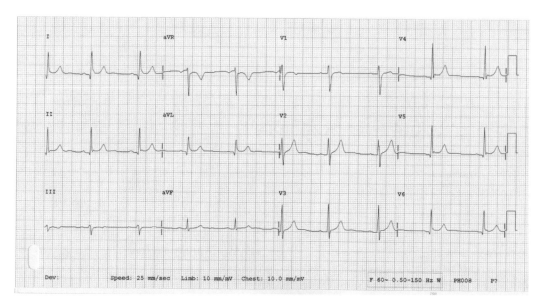

Figure 11.1 12-lead ECG from a 41-year-old male with left-sided chest pain for four hours.

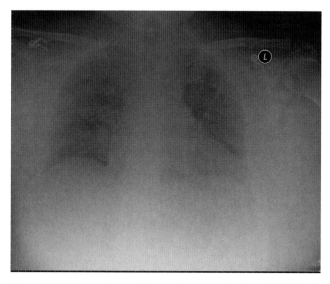

Figure 11.2 Chest radiograph from a 41-year-old male with left-sided chest pain for four hours.

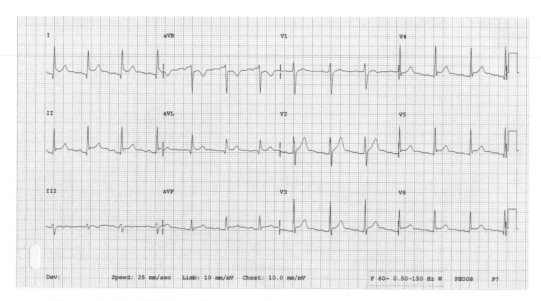

Figure 11.3 12-lead ECG from a 41-year-old male 13 hours after the onset of left-sided chest pain.

The diagnosis is acute pericarditis. The initial ECG obtained demonstrates minimal ST-segment elevation in leads I, II, V_4-V_6, with PR-segment elevation in lead aVR, findings consistent with early pericarditis. The chest radiograph was evaluated as low lung volumes without infiltrate or effusion. The repeat ECG obtained 13 hours after the onset of symptoms demonstrates diffuse ST-segment elevation, concave-upward in appearance, PR depression in leads I, II, V3-V6, with PR-segment elevation in lead aVR, indicative of acute pericarditis. The patient received morphine sulfate IV in the ED and was started on indomethacin 25 mg orally every eight hours at discharge. On a follow-up visit with his primary care physician four days later, the patient reported marked improvement in his symptoms.

Acute pericarditis

Acute pericarditis, a diffuse inflammation of the pericardial sac and superficial myocardium, has a number of underlying causes. These include infection (primarily viral), immunologic disorders, uremia, trauma, malignancy, cardiac ischemia and acute myocardial infarction.[1] In clinical practice using a traditional diagnostic approach, idiopathic and viral acute pericarditis is found in 80–90% of cases in immunocompetent patients from developed countries.[2] The incidence of pericarditis in postmortem studies ranges from 1–6%, whereas it is diagnosed antemortem in only 0.1% of hospitalized patients and in 5% of patients seen in EDs with chest pain without myocardial infarction.[3] The possible sequelae of pericarditis include cardiac tamponade, recurrent pericarditis and pericardial constriction.[3]

More than half of patients with pericarditis will present complaining of chest pain that may radiate to the back, neck or shoulders.[4] If pain radiates to one or both trapezius muscle ridges, it may be due to pericarditis because the phrenic nerve (which innervates these muscles) traverses the pericardium.[3] In contrast to acute coronary syndromes, pericardial pain typically worsens with inspiration and is improved while sitting up and leaning forward. Approximately 25–40% of patients with pericarditis will complain of dyspnea, and 17% of fever.[4]

The most common physical finding in patients with pericarditis is a pericardial friction rub, which occurs in approximately 50–85% of cases.[3-5] A pericardial friction rub is best heard at the lower sternal border or apex when the patient is sitting forward on his or her hands and knees. Other findings on physical exam may include fever (may reach 104°F/40°C), cardiac dysrhythmias (e.g., premature atrial and ventricular contractions), tachypnea and dyspnea.[5] Individuals with associated cardiac tamponade may show jugular venous distension, tachycardia, hypotension or pulsus paradoxus.

The 12-lead ECG in patients with acute pericarditis classically shows widespread upward concave ST-segment elevation and PR-segment depression.[3] In addition, lead aVR on the ECG can demonstrate ST-segment depression and PR-segment elevation.[1] The ECG abnormalities evolve

through four classic stages.[6] Stage I is characterized by ST-segment elevation, prominent T waves and PR-segment depression. Stage II is characterized by a normalization of the initial abnormalities, namely resolution of the ST-segment elevation. Stage III involves T wave inversion, usually in the same distribution where ST-segment elevation was encountered. Finally, Stage IV is a normalization of all changes with a return to the baseline ECG. Persistent ST-segment elevation and pathologic Q waves are not encountered in patients with pericarditis – these ECG findings should suggest another etiology.[6]

Although the white cell count, erythrocyte sedimentation rate (ESR) and serum C-reactive protein (CRP) concentrations usually are elevated in patients with acute pericarditis, these tests provide little insight into the cause of the disease.[3] Troponin levels are elevated in 35–50% of patients with pericarditis, a finding thought to be caused by epicardial inflammation rather than myocyte necrosis.[3,7] The magnitude of the elevation in the serum troponin concentration appears to correlate with the magnitude of the ST-segment elevation, and the concentration usually returns to normal within one to two weeks after diagnosis. An elevated troponin does not predict an adverse outcome, although a prolonged elevation (lasting longer than two weeks) suggests myocarditis, which has a worse prognosis.[3,7]

The diagnostic test of choice for large effusions, cardiac tamponade and constrictive pericarditis is two-dimensional Doppler echocardiography.[8] This imaging modality can demonstrate moderate or large effusions. In cardiac tamponade, Doppler examination may show the characteristic swinging motion of the heart that gives rise to electrical alternans on the ECG. Doppler studies are helpful in differentiating pericarditis from restrictive cardiomyopathy.[8] Transthoracic echocardiography is generally not required in patients with unequivocal evidence of pericarditis and no poor prognostic indicators.[3]

Most patients with idiopathic pericarditis can be managed conservatively, with a nonsteroidal anti-inflammatory drug (NSAID) such as indomethacin, ibuprofen or aspirin. These agents are believed to be equally effective.[8] Colchicine (administered at a dose of 0.6 mg twice daily) appears to be effective alone or in combination with ibuprofen in treating acute pericarditis, although it has not been tested in randomized trials; it is preferred in patients who have recurrent pericarditis.[3] Patients who do not respond to an NSAID may need a short course of prednisone (5–10 mg per day for one to two weeks).[8] Rarely, patients do not respond to this therapy or show evidence of recurrent pericarditis; these patients require a prolonged corticosteroid course (i.e., several months).

Most patients with acute pericarditis have a brief and benign course, and can be managed as an outpatient with NSAIDs. Indicators of a poor prognosis in patients with pericarditis include temperature above 100.4°F (38°C), a subacute onset, an immunosuppressed state, pericarditis associated with trauma, a history of oral anticoagulation therapy, myopericarditis, a large pericardial effusion or cardiac tamponade.[3] Patients with one or more of these criteria are at increased risk for serious complications and should be admitted to the hospital.

KEY TEACHING POINTS

1. Pain from pericarditis typically worsens on inspiration and improves while sitting up and leaning forward.
2. The most common physical finding in patients with pericarditis is a pericardial friction rub, which occurs in approximately 50–85% of cases.
3. The 12-lead ECG in acute pericarditis classically shows widespread upward concave ST-segment elevation, PR-segment depression and PR-segment elevation in lead aVR.
4. Plasma troponin levels are elevated in 35–50% of patients with pericarditis, a finding thought to be caused by epicardial inflammation rather than myocyte necrosis.
5. The treatment of choice for idiopathic pericarditis is NSAIDs.

REFERENCES

[1] Williamson K, Mattu A, Plautz CU, et al. Electrocardiographic applications of lead aVR. *Am J Emerg Med* 2006;24:864–74.
[2] Imazio M, Cecchi E, Demichelis B, et al. Indicators of poor prognosis of acute pericarditis. *Circulation* 2007;115:2739–44.
[3] Lange RA, Hillis LD. Acute pericarditis. *N Engl J Med* 2004;351:2195–202.
[4] Ringstrom E, Freedman J. Approach to undifferentiated chest pain in the emergency department. *Mt Sinai J Med* 2006;73:499–505.
[5] Valley VT, Fly CA. Pericarditis and cardiac tamponade. eMedicine Website. Available at http://www.emedicine.com/emerg/topic412.htm. Accessed July 10, 2008.
[6] Brady WJ. ST segment and T wave abnormalities not caused by acute coronary syndromes. *Emerg Med Clin N Am* 2006;24:91–111.
[7] Bonnefoy E, Gordon P, Kirkorian G, et al. Serum cardiac troponin I and ST-segment elevation in patients with acute pericarditis. *Eur Heart J* 2000;21:832–6.
[8] Goyle KK, Walling AD. Diagnosing pericarditis. *Am Fam Physician* 2006;66:1695–702.

12

Rapid heart rate in a 47-year-old male

HISTORY OF PRESENT ILLNESS

A 47-year-old male with a medical history significant for diabetes, hypertension and chronic obstructive pulmonary disease (COPD) presented to the ED complaining of two hours of palpitations and rapid heart rate associated with mild, substernal chest pain and shortness of breath. The patient denied lightheadedness or dizziness and had not experienced similar episodes in the past. He reported that his symptoms had started suddenly while at work.

PHYSICAL EXAMINATION

GENERAL APPEARANCE: The patient was a moderately obese male, slightly diaphoretic but in no acute distress.

VITAL SIGNS

Temperature	98.0°F (36.6°C)
Pulse	198 beats/minute
Blood pressure	150/90 mmHg
Respirations	22 breaths/minute
Oxygen saturation	100% on room air

HEENT: Unremarkable.

NECK: Supple, no jugular venous distension.

CARDIOVASCULAR: Tachycardic rate, regular rhythm, unable to assess for rubs, murmurs or gallops.

LUNGS: Clear to auscultation bilaterally.

ABDOMEN: Soft, nontender, nondistended.

EXTREMITIES: No clubbing, cyanosis or edema; brisk capillary refill.

NEUROLOGIC: Nonfocal.

The patient was placed on the cardiac monitor, and a 12-lead ECG was obtained (Figure 12.1). A peripheral intravenous line was placed, and blood was drawn and sent for laboratory testing.

What is your diagnosis?

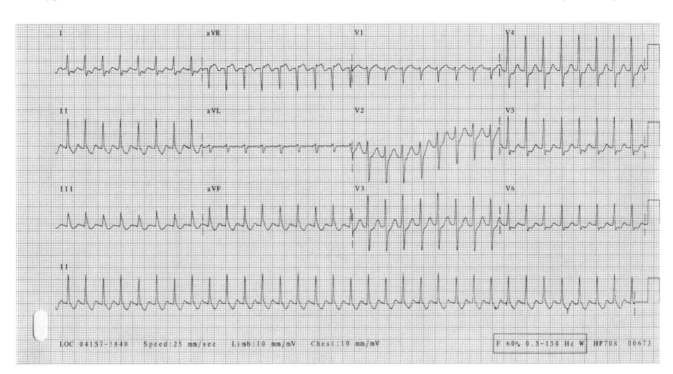

Figure 12.1 12-lead ECG from a 47-year-old male with rapid heart rate.

ANSWER

The diagnosis is supraventricular tachycardia (SVT). The patient was given 6 mg adenosine IV rapidly while the 12-lead ECG was continuously recording (Figure 12.2). The patient converted to normal sinus rhythm, and a repeat ECG was obtained (Figure 12.3). Laboratory tests revealed a normal complete blood count, electrolytes, BUN, creatinine, glucose, and troponin I. A second troponin I drawn eight hours after the onset of symptoms was also within normal limits. The patient remained in normal sinus rhythm and was discharged from the ED without complications after several hours of observation.

Supraventricular tachycardia

The term supraventricular tachycardia (SVT) refers to paroxysmal tachydysrhythmias that require atrial or atrioventricular nodal tissue (or both) for their initiation and maintenance.[1] The incidence of SVT is about 35 cases per 100,000 persons per year; the prevalence is about 2.25 per 1000.[1] SVT is often recurrent, occasionally persistent, and a frequent cause of visits to EDs and primary care physician offices. SVTs are not usually associated with structural heart disease, although there are exceptions (e.g., the presence of accessory pathways associated with hypertrophic cardiomyopathy or Ebstein's anomaly, atrial tachycardias in patients with congenital or acquired heart disease). Re-entry dysrhythmias are usually induced by premature atrial or ventricular ectopic beats. Precipitating factors such as hyperthyroidism, excessive intake of caffeine, alcohol or recreational drugs increase the risk of recurrence.[1]

Common symptoms of SVT include palpitations, anxiety, lightheadedness, chest pain, pounding in the neck and chest, and dyspnea; syncope is uncommon. SVTs have a sudden onset and termination, in contrast to sinus tachycardias, which accelerate and decelerate gradually. Physical examination during episodes may reveal the "frog sign" – prominent jugular venous A waves due to atrial contraction against the closed tricuspid valve.[2] The usual presentation of SVT on ECG is a narrow complex tachycardia (QRS interval less than 120 msec) with a rate of 140–280 beats/minute.[3] In less than 10% of cases, wide complex tachycardia is the manifestation of SVT.[1] After restoration of sinus rhythm, the 12-lead ECG should be examined for the presence of delta waves, which indicate an accessory pathway (bypass tract). If delta waves are present, referral to a cardiologist should occur.

When a patient presents in SVT and is hemodynamically stable, attempting a therapeutic/diagnostic maneuver with vagal stimulation is reasonable.[4] The maneuvers include

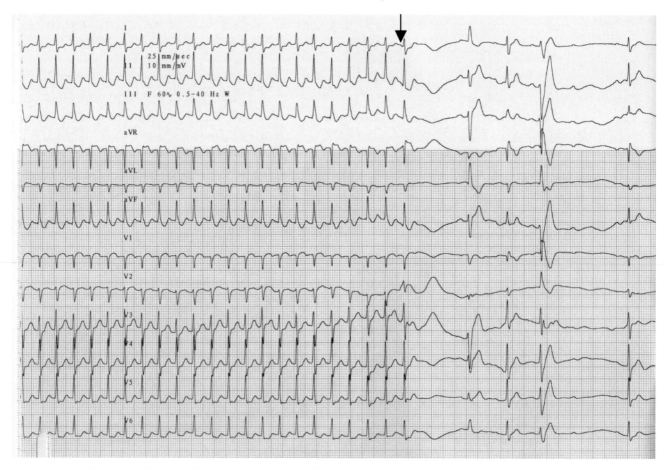

Figure 12.2 12-lead ECG showing conversion of SVT to normal sinus rhythm after administration of 6 mg adenosine IV rapid bolus (arrow indicates adenosine administration).

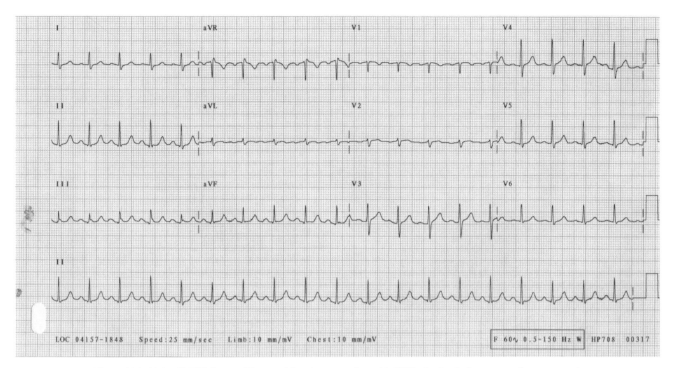

Figure 12.3 12-lead ECG from a 47-year-old male presenting with SVT, obtained after conversion to normal sinus rhythm.

carotid massage (in patients without carotid bruits or known carotid artery disease), Valsalva maneuver, and application of ice bag to the face (stimulates the diving reflex). These maneuvers increase vagal tone, thus slowing conduction through the atrioventricular (AV) node.[1,4,5] A continuous 12-lead ECG recording of the episode should be obtained during vagal maneuvers because the way in which the dysrhythmias resolve may provide clues to their mechanism. In rare cases, episodes of SVT are so poorly tolerated (e.g., result in hemodynamic instability) that they require immediate electrical cardioversion.

If the dysrhythmia is not terminated by vagal maneuvers, adenosine (6 or 12 mg IV) will usually cause AV-nodal block, either terminating the dysrhythmia or allowing visualization of the underlying mechanism.[5] Data from randomized trials shows that SVT is terminated in 60–80% of patients treated with 6 mg adenosine, and in 90–95% of those treated with 12 mg.[6] In patients with atrial tachycardia, adenosine causes a transient AV-nodal block or interrupts the tachycardia. ECG monitoring is required during the administration of adenosine, and resuscitation equipment should be available in the event that the rare complications of bronchospasm or ventricular fibrillation occur.[7] Adenosine is contraindicated in heart transplant recipients and should be used cautiously in patients with severe obstructive lung disease.[1]

If SVT is refractory to adenosine or rapidly recurs, the tachycardia can usually be terminated by the administration of an intravenous calcium-channel blocker (e.g., diltiazem, verapamil) or a beta-blocker (e.g., metoprolol).[1] As a next step, procainamide, ibutilide, propafenone or flecainide can be given intravenously if the blood pressure is stable.[8] Sequential

trials with different antidysrhythmic agents should occur only after careful consideration of their possible negative hypotensive, bradycardic and proarrhythmic effects. At any point, electrical cardioversion is an alternative; this technique is generally considered in hemodynamically stable patients if AV-nodal blocking agents fail.

In ambulatory patients with frequent episodes of SVT (two or more per month), ECG recordings or event recorders may be useful to document dysrhythmias in the outpatient setting. In patients presenting with SVT, an outpatient echocardiogram should be considered to rule out structural heart disease, even though this is uncommon. Because electrolyte abnormalities and hyperthyroidism may contribute to SVT, it is reasonable to check potassium and serum thyrotropin levels; however, these tests generally have a low yield. SVT presents infrequently as a wide complex tachycardia, in which there is an associated bundle-branch block or conduction over an accessory pathway. Wide QRS complex, regular tachycardias should routinely be treated as ventricular tachycardia, unless the diagnosis of SVT with aberrant conduction or SVT with preexcitation is certain.[1] Adenosine and other AV-nodal blocking agents are generally ineffective and potentially deleterious in patients with ventricular tachycardia.

KEY TEACHING POINTS

1. SVT frequently occurs in young, healthy individuals and is usually not associated with structural heart disease.
2. Common symptoms of SVT include palpitations, anxiety, lightheadedness, chest pain, pounding in the neck and chest, and dyspnea; syncope is uncommon.

3. Hemodynamically unstable patients in SVT require immediate electrical cardioversion.
4. Treatment for hemodynamically stable patients in SVT should begin with vagal maneuvers, followed by intravenous adenosine, which has both diagnostic and therapeutic value.
5. SVT infrequently presents as a wide complex tachycardia. Wide QRS complex, regular tachycardias should routinely be treated as ventricular tachycardia unless the diagnosis of SVT with aberrancy or SVT with preexcitation is certain.

REFERENCES

[1] Delacretaz E. Clinical practice: supraventricular tachycardia. *N Engl J Med* 2006;354:1039–51.
[2] Gursoy S, Steurer G, Brugada J, et al. The hemodynamic mechanism of pounding in the neck in atrioventricular nodal reentrant tachycardia. *N Engl J Med* 1992;327:772–4.
[3] Stahmer SA, Cowan R. Tachydysrhythmias. *Emerg Med Clin N Am* 2006;24:11–40.
[4] Haro LH, Hess EP, Decker WW. Arrhythmias in the office. *Med Clin N Am* 2006;90:417–38.
[5] Hood RE, Shorofsky SR. Management of arrhythmias in the emergency department. *Cardiol Clin* 2006;24:125–33.
[6] DiMarco JP, Miles W, Akhtar M, et al. Adenosine for paroxysmal supraventricular tachycardia: dose ranging and comparison with verapamil: assessment in placebo-controlled, multicenter trials. *Ann Intern Med* 1990;113:996.
[7] Xanthos T, Ekmektzoglou KA, Vlachos IS, et al. A prognostic index for the successful use of adenosine in patients with paroxysmal supraventricular tachycardia in emergency settings: a retrospective study. *Am J Emerg Med* 2008;26:304–9.
[8] Glater KA, Dorostkar PC, Yang Y, et al. Electrophysiologic effects of ibutilide in patients with accessory pathways. *Circulation* 2001;104:1933–9.

13

Chest pain and syncope in a 48-year-old male

HISTORY OF PRESENT ILLNESS

A 48-year-old male with a medical history significant for tobacco use was brought to the ED by paramedics after a syncopal episode. The patient reported substernal chest pressure followed by the onset of lightheadedness, at which time he experienced a transient loss of consciousness. Upon arousal by his coworkers, he was still experiencing chest pressure and lightheadedness. The patient was found to have a heart rate of 50 beats/minute with a blood pressure of 80/40 mmHg and was transported to the ED code III. A peripheral intravenous line was established en route, and aspirin 162 mg orally, atropine 1 mg and 500 mL normal saline IV were administered by the paramedics without significant improvement in his blood pressure or heart rate.

PHYSICAL EXAMINATION

GENERAL APPEARANCE: The patient appeared well developed and well hydrated, spoke in full sentences, and was in moderate distress.

VITAL SIGNS

Temperature	98.6°F (37°C)
Pulse	50 beats/minute
Blood pressure	80/40 mmHg
Respirations	22 breaths/minute
Oxygen saturation	99% on room air

HEENT: Unremarkable.

NECK: Supple, no jugular venous distension.

CARDIOVASCULAR: Bradycardic rate, regular rhythm, without rubs, murmurs of gallops. Weak radial and dorsalis pedis pulses.

LUNGS: Clear to auscultation bilaterally.

ABDOMEN: Soft, nontender, nondistended.

EXTREMITIES: No clubbing, cyanosis or edema.

NEUROLOGIC: Nonfocal

The patient was placed on the cardiac monitor, supplemental oxygen was administered (2 liters by nasal cannula) and a 12-lead ECG was obtained (Figure 13.1).

What is your diagnosis?

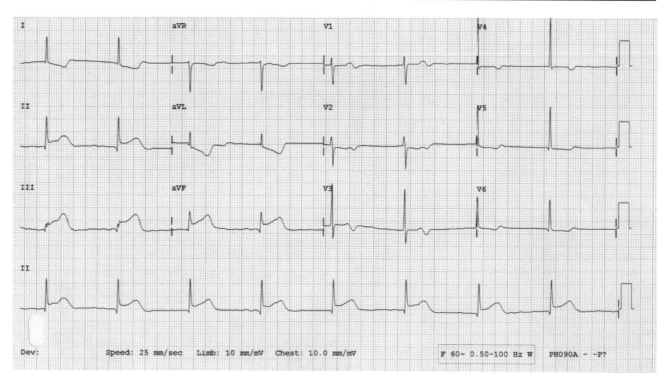

Figure 13.1 12-lead ECG from a 48-year-old male with chest pain and hypotension following a syncopal episode.

ANSWER

The diagnosis is inferior wall myocardial infarction (MI) with complete (third-degree) heart block. The 12-lead ECG (Figure 13.1) demonstrates significant ST-segment elevation in leads II, III and aVF, with reciprocal ST-segment depression in leads I and aVL, consistent with an inferior wall myocardial infarction, as well as a junctional escape rhythm (ventricular rate 50 beats/minute). Transcutaneous pacing was initiated with improvement of the heart rate to 60 beats/minute and blood pressure to 110/70 mmHg. An interventional cardiologist was immediately notified, the patient received eptifibatide and heparin IV and was urgently transported to the cardiac catheterization laboratory. Coronary angiogram revealed a 100% occlusion of the proximal right coronary artery (RCA) and moderate to severe disease of the ostial and proximal left anterior descending (LAD) artery. Successful percutaneous coronary intervention (PCI) with aspiration thrombectomy and stent placement of the proximal RCA occlusion occurred, along with temporary pacemaker insertion. A repeat ECG obtained two hours following admission demonstrated a normal sinus rhythm with resolution of acute ischemic changes (Figure 13.2). The patient was discharged on hospital day #5 in good condition, with close follow up in the cardiology clinic.

Inferior wall myocardial infarction and complete heart block

In inferior wall ST-segment elevation myocardial infarction (STEMI), the leads showing the greatest magnitude of ST-segment elevation, in descending order, are leads III, aVF and II. A total of 80–90% of patients who have ST-segment elevation in these inferior leads have an occlusion of the RCA; however, an occlusion of the left circumflex coronary artery (LCx) can produce a similar ECG pattern. In addition to ST-segment elevation in the inferior leads (II, III and aVF), reciprocal ST-segment depression in lead aVL is seen in almost all patients who have an acute inferior STEMI.[1]

Acute inferior wall STEMI is often complicated by high-degree atrioventricular (AV) block, the incidence reported to be 6–13%.[2] Patients with complete heart block (CHB) are significantly more likely to die during hospitalization than patients without CHB (likely related to infarct size rather than the presence of heart block).[3,4] The heart block may be a gradual delay of conduction or the abrupt onset of third-degree heart block.[4] Most patients will develop heart block within 24 hours of admission. The duration of CHB varies dramatically from a few minutes to more than 10 days; permanent pacemaker implantation is seldom required. Additionally, the duration of hospitalization is significantly longer for patients with CHB than those without CHB.[3]

Treatment of patients with inferior wall STEMI and CHB involves immediate stabilization of the airway, breathing and circulation (ABCs). Intravenous atropine (0.5–1.0 mg) may be administered in hemodynamically unstable patients to improve the heart rate and blood pressure. If unsuccessful, temporary transcutaneous pacing should be initiated. Treatment of STEMI includes oral aspirin, heparin, a glycoprotein IIb/IIIa inhibitor (such as eptifibatide, abciximab or tirofiban) and emergent cardiac catheterization. If a cardiac catheterization laboratory is not immediately available,

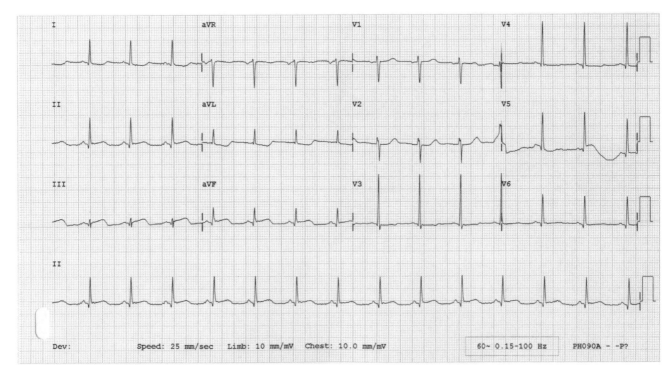

Figure 13.2 12-lead ECG from a 48-year-old male with chest pain and hypotension post-PCI.

fibrinolytic agents (thrombolytics) are recommended. Beta-blockers (e.g., metoprolol) and nitrates should not be administered to patients who are already bradycardic and hypotensive.

The exact cause of heart block in inferior wall MI is unclear but is likely due to ischemia without necrosis of the AV node.[3] CHB in inferior MI usually involves the supra-Hisian AV junction due to hypoperfusion of the AV-nodal artery (virtually all inferior MIs have occlusion proximal to the AV-nodal artery).[1,3] An alternative hypothesis involves increased vagal tone, called the Bezold-Jarisch reflex.[3] This mechanism does not explain the correlation of increased infarct size with heart block or the cases of sudden CHB without sinus slowing. Others have suggested that high levels of potassium and adenosine near the conducting tissue after cardiac cell infarction might cause transient blocks.[1,3]

KEY TEACHING POINTS

1. In acute inferior wall MI, the leads showing the greatest magnitude of ST-segment elevation, in descending order, are leads III, aVF and II. Patients with ST-segment elevation in these inferior leads have an occlusion of the RCA (80–90% of the time) or the LCx artery (10–20%).

2. Acute inferior wall myocardial infarction (MI) is complicated by high-degree atrioventricular (AV) block in 6–13% of cases.

3. Treatment of patients with inferior wall MI and CHB involves stabilization of the ABCs, attempts to override the block (IV atropine and transcutaneous pacing), and treatment of the underlying cause (STEMI).

4. Medications that lower the heart rate or blood pressure (e.g., metoprolol, nitroglycerin) should be used with extreme caution (or not at all) in patients with inferior wall MI and CHB.

5. The exact cause of heart block in inferior wall MI is unclear but is likely due to ischemia without necrosis of the AV node.

REFERENCES

[1] Altar S, Barbagelata A, Birnbaum Y. Electrocardiographic diagnosis of ST-elevation myocardial infarction. *Cardiol Clin* 2006;24:343–65.

[2] Ramamurthy S, Anandaraja S, Matthew N. Percutaneous coronary intervention for persistent complete heart block complicating inferior myocardial infarction. *J Invasive Cardiol* 2007;19:E372–4.

[3] Chiu C-A, Youssef AA, Wu C-J, et al. Impact of PercuSurge GuardWire device on prevention and reduction of recovery time from complete heart block in patients with acute inferior myocardial infarction undergoing primary percutaneous coronary intervention. *Int Heart J* 2007;48:35–44.

[4] Rotondo N, Pollack ML, Chan TC. Electrocardiographic manifestations: acute inferior wall myocardial infarction. *J Emerg Med* 2004;26:433–40.

15

Palpitations and shortness of breath in a 69-year-old male

HISTORY OF PRESENT ILLNESS

A 69-year-old male with a medical history significant for a previous myocardial infarction, two-vessel coronary artery bypass graft, diabetes, congestive heart failure and ischemic cardiomyopathy (ejection fraction 40%) presented to the ED by ambulance complaining of palpitations and shortness of breath. The patient experienced a brief syncopal episode when getting up from bed immediately before his wife called emergency services. In the ED, the patient appeared awake, alert and in no acute distress. His medications included aspirin, felodipine, furosemide, insulin and Flomax®. In the ED, the patient denied chest pain or shortness of breath but reported palpitations and feeling lightheaded.

PHYSICAL EXAMINATION

GENERAL APPEARANCE: The patient was an elderly-appearing male lying supine on the gurney, awake, alert and in no acute discomfort.

VITAL SIGNS

Temperature	98.1°F (36.7°C)
Pulse	180 beats/minute
Blood pressure	110/70 mmHg
Respirations	22 breaths/minute
Oxygen saturation	98% on room air

HEENT: Unremarkable.

NECK: Supple, no jugular venous distension.

CARDIOVASCULAR: Tachycardic, regular heart sounds, unable to appreciate rubs, murmurs or gallops. Palpable and rapid radial and dorsalis pedis pulses.

LUNGS: Clear to auscultation bilaterally.

ABDOMEN: Soft, nontender, nondistended.

RECTAL: Brown stool, hemoccult negative.

EXTREMITIES: No clubbing, cyanosis or edema.

NEUROLOGIC: Nonfocal.

A 12-lead ECG was obtained (Figure 15.1) and the patient was placed on the cardiac monitor. A peripheral intravenous line was placed, and blood was drawn and sent for laboratory testing.

What is your diagnosis?

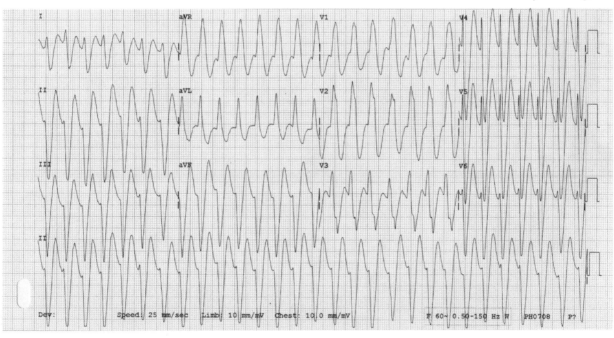

Figure 15.1 12-lead ECG from a 69-year-old male with palpitations and shortness of breath.

ANSWER

The ECG demonstrated a wide complex tachycardia (QRS >150 msec, rate 174), consistent with ventricular tachycardia. The patient was given amiodarone 150 mg intravenously over 10 minutes, followed by the initiation of an amiodarone IV drip at 1 mg/min. The patient converted to sinus rhythm shortly after initiation of the amiodarone drip, with a repeat ECG demonstrating first-degree AV block and ST-segment depression in leads II, aVF, V_5 and V_6 (Figure 15.2). An initial troponin I obtained on presentation was 0.05 ng/mL (normal 0.00–0.09 ng/mL). Because of the ST-segment depression note on the repeat ECG, a heparin infusion was initiated. A repeat troponin I obtained eight hours after presentation peaked at 5.2 ng/mL. The patient underwent placement of an internal cardioverter-defibrillator (ICD) the following day.

Wide complex tachycardia

Tachycardias (rate greater than 100 beats/minute) can be divided into two categories based on the width of the QRS complexes: narrow complex (QRS duration ≤120 msec) or wide complex (QRS duration >120 msec) tachycardias.[1,2] If the dysrhythmia has a narrow QRS complex, it is by definition a supraventricular tachycardia (SVT). These dysrhythmias are often well tolerated by patients in good health. These patients can be treated using vagal maneuvers, intravenous adenosine or calcium-channel blockers, and discharged from the ED to complete their evaluation as an outpatient if the SVT converts to sinus rhythm with a controlled rate.[1] If the tachycardia has a wide QRS complex, it is either ventricular

tachycardia (VT) or, less commonly, an SVT with aberrant conduction. Other rare causes of wide complex tachycardia (WCT) include medications (e.g., tricyclic antidepressants, digitalis, lithium, cocaine, diphenhydramine), hyperkalemia, post-cardiac arrest and WCTs with pre-excitation syndromes (i.e., Wolff-Parkinson-White syndrome).[2]

In several large series concerned with the differential diagnosis of wide QRS tachycardias, the overwhelming majority of cases are VT (up to 80%); the next largest group is SVT with aberrancy, with other diagnoses contributing a small fraction of cases.[3] From a practical standpoint, it is clear that the major differential diagnosis of WCT is between VT and SVT with aberrancy. A frequently used diagnostic algorithm by Brugada to identify VT on ECG incorporates many previously published morphologic criteria in a step-wise algorithm. It has been demonstrated to have good sensitivity and specificity in the absence of pre-existing intraventricular conduction abnormalities (Table 15.1).[4,5]

With regard to distinguishing VT from SVT with aberrancy, most clinical situations of WCT will be VT in etiology (more than 70% of the time). A corollary to this is if there is doubt as to the etiology of the WCT, the safest approach is to treat the rhythm as VT.[3] Most patients who present with VT have underlying heart disease. Individuals with previous myocardial infarction (MI) or known coronary artery disease (CAD) are approximately four times more likely to present with ventricular rather than supraventricular etiologies of their WCT.[6]

Patients in VT without a pulse require immediate defibrillation. If the patient has a pulse and is hemodynamically unstable, synchronized cardioversion should be performed as

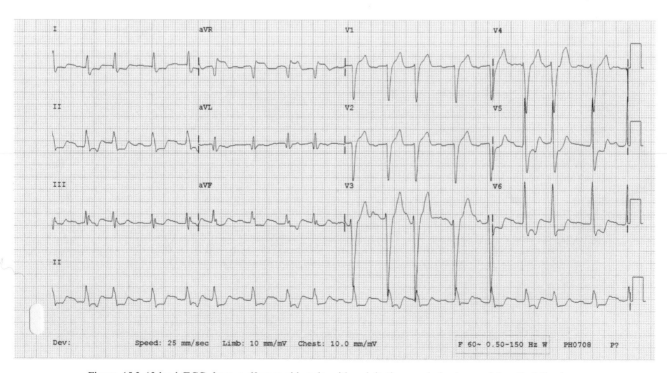

Figure 15.2 12-lead ECG from a 69-year-old male with palpitations and shortness of breath following treatment with IV amiodarone.

TABLE 15.1 Diagnosis of wide QRS complex tachycardia

Step 1: Is there absence of an RS complex in all precordial leads V_1 to V_6?
If yes, then the rhythm is VT.
Step 2: Is the interval from the onset of the R wave to the nadir of the S wave greater than 100 msec (0.10 sec) in any precordial leads?
If yes, then the rhythm is VT.
Step 3: Is there AV dissociation?
If yes, then the rhythm is VT.
Step 4: Are morphology criteria for VT present (Table 15.2)?
If yes, then the rhythm is VT.

From Stahmer SA, Cowan R, Emerg Med Clin North Amer 2006;24:11–40.

quickly as possible (consider sedation). The patient should be supported using advanced cardiac life support (ACLS) guidelines. In a stable patient with sustained, monomorphic VT, pharmacologic therapy may augment cardioversion. In the acute phase of treatment, the intravenous drug of choice is amiodarone, particularly in patients with an impaired cardiac ejection fraction.[1,7] Amiodarone should be administered as a 150 mg IV bolus over 10 minutes, followed by an infusion at 1 mg/min for six hours, decreasing to 0.5 mg/min subsequently. Other medications that can be used include procainamide, which may be especially useful when atrial fibrillation with pre-excitation is suspected. Once stabilized, all patients who have VT should be admitted to the hospital for further evaluation and treatment.

In elderly patients with VT, definitive therapy often mandates placement of an implantable cardioverter-defibrillator (ICD). With a two-year mortality rate of 30% after MI, ICDs are common in elderly patients. The MADIT and AVID trials demonstrated that ICDs are superior to pharmacologic therapy alone.[7–9]

KEY TEACHING POINTS

1. In greater than 70% of cases of wide complex QRS tachycardia, the diagnosis will be ventricular tachycardia (VT); therefore, when in doubt, treat as VT.
2. Amiodarone is the drug of choice for patients presenting with stable VT, particularly in those with impaired ejection fractions.
3. Pulseless VT mandates defibrillation; unstable patients presenting with VT with a pulse require immediate electrical cardioversion.
4. All patients presenting with VT should be admitted for further evaluation and treatment.
5. Definitive therapy of VT or VF in selected patients (e.g., elderly, post-myocardial infarction, post-resuscitation from near fatal ventricular dysrhythmias) involves placement of an implantable cardioverter-defibrillator (ICD).

REFERENCES

[1] Hood RE, Shorofsky SR. Management of arrhythmias in the emergency department. *Cardiol Clin* 2006;24:125–33.
[2] Hollowell H, Mattu A, Perron AD, et al. Wide-complex tachycardia: beyond the traditional differential diagnosis of ventricular tachycardia vs supraventricular tachycardia with aberrant conduction. *Am J Emerg Med* 2005;23:876–89.
[3] Miller JM, Das MK, Yadav AV, et al. Value of the 12-lead ECG in wide QRS tachycardia. *Cardiol Clin* 2006;24:439–51.
[4] Brugada P, Brugada J, Mont L, et al. A new approach to the differential diagnosis of a regular tachycardia with a wide QRS complex. *Circulation* 1991;83:1649–59.
[5] Stahmer SA, Cowan R. Tachydysrhythmias. *Emerg Med Clin N Am* 2006;24:11–40.
[6] Garmel GM. Wide complex tachycardias: understanding this complex condition. Part I – epidemiology and electrophysiology. *West J Emerg Med* 2008;9:28–39.
[7] Gupta R, Kaufman S. Cardiovascular emergencies in the elderly. *Emerg Med Clin N Am* 2006;24:339–70.
[8] Moss AJ, Hall WJ, Cannom DS, et al. Improved survival with an implanted defibrillator in patients with coronary disease at high risk for ventricular arrhythmia. *N Engl J Med* 1996;335:2933–40.
[9] AVID Investigators. A comparison of antiarrhythmic-drug therapy with implantable defibrillators in patients resuscitated from near fatal ventricular arrhythmias. *N Engl J Med* 1997;337:1576–83.

TABLE 15.2 Morphology criteria for ventricular tachycardia

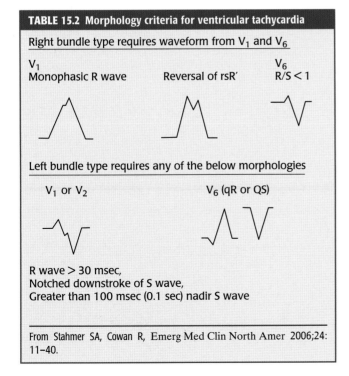

Right bundle type requires waveform from V_1 and V_6

V_1
Monophasic R wave   Reversal of rsR′ V_6
R/S < 1

Left bundle type requires any of the below morphologies

V_1 or V_2 V_6 (qR or QS)

R wave > 30 msec,
Notched downstroke of S wave,
Greater than 100 msec (0.1 sec) nadir S wave

From Stahmer SA, Cowan R, Emerg Med Clin North Amer 2006;24: 11–40.

16

Chest pain following emotional stress in a 70-year-old female

HISTORY OF PRESENT ILLNESS

A 70-year-old female with a medical history significant for hypertension, hypercholesterolemia and paroxysmal atrial fibrillation presented to the ED complaining of chest pain for several hours after being emotionally distressed over her husband's recent illness and hospitalization. She described her pain as pressure-like, located centrally without radiation, and rated it at a level of 8 (on a scale of 0 to 10). The pressure was associated with diaphoresis but was not associated with shortness of breath or nausea. Her medications included Cozaar®, diltiazem, hydrochlorothiazide, warfarin and simvastatin. She did not drink or smoke, and lived with her husband.

PHYSICAL EXAMINATION

GENERAL APPEARANCE: The patient appeared well nourished, well hydrated, was tearful and in moderate discomfort.

VITAL SIGNS

Temperature	98°F (36.6°C)
Pulse	80 beats/minute
Blood pressure	160/90 mmHg
Respirations	20 breaths/minute
Oxygen saturation	100% on room air

HEENT: Unremarkable

NECK: Supple, no jugular venous distension.

CARDIOVASCULAR: Regular rate and rhythm without rubs, murmurs or gallops.

LUNGS: Clear to auscultation bilaterally.

ABDOMEN: Soft, nontender, nondistended.

RECTAL: Normal tone, brown stool, hemoccult negative.

EXTREMITIES: No clubbing, cyanosis or edema.

NEUROLOGIC: Nonfocal.

The patient was placed on the cardiac monitor, a 12-lead ECG was obtained (Figure 16.1) and compared to an ECG from six months earlier (Figure 16.2). A peripheral intravenous line was placed, blood was drawn and sent for laboratory testing, and the patient was given aspirin, intravenous heparin and eptifibatide (Integrilin®). The initial troponin I returned elevated at 4.2 ng/mL (normal 0.00–0.09 ng/mL). The patient was taken emergently for coronary angiography, which demonstrated normal coronary arteries as well as mild inferior and anterior wall hypokinesis and apical left ventricular ballooning.

What is your diagnosis?

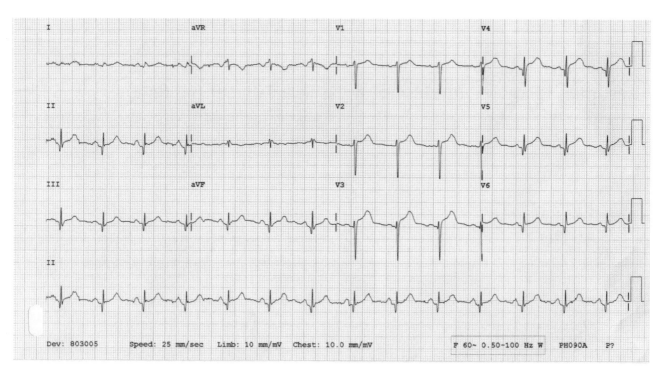

Figure 16.1 12-lead ECG from a 70-year-old female with chest pressure for several hours.

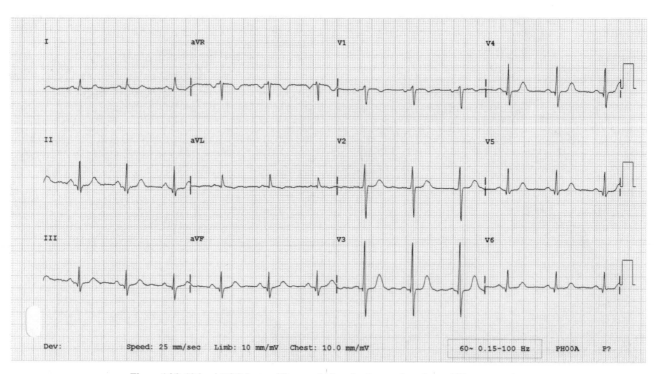

Figure 16.2 12-lead ECG from a 70-year-old female six months prior to ED presentation.

ANSWER

The diagnosis is Takotsubo cardiomyopathy ("broken heart syndrome") due to emotional stress and adrenergically mediated myocardial injury. The ECG (Figure 16.1) demonstrates ST-segment elevation in the anterolateral leads (V_1–V_6), which were new compared to a prior ECG from this patient (Figure 16.2). The patient was discharged on hospital day #2 and instructed to continue her previous medications, and begin aspirin and clopidogrel for one month. An echocardiogram performed one week after discharge demonstrated globally decreased left ventricular function, as well as wall motion abnormalities of the inferior, apical and lateral walls.

Takotsubo cardiomyopathy

Takotsubo cardiomyopathy is a transient cardiomyopathy characterized by marked apical hypokinesis and ballooning in the absence of significant coronary artery disease.[1] *Takotsubo*, from *tako* (octopus) and *tsubo* (jar), is a Japanese term for a round-bottomed, narrow-necked jar used to trap octopus in Japan.[1] Similar to this octopus jar, the heart's appearance on a left ventriculogram in Takotsubo cardiomyopathy appears wide at the apex during end systole, with narrowing where there is basilar hyperkinesis.[1] Typically, patients with Takotsubo cardiomyopathy present with symptoms consistent with acute myocardial infarction, including chest pain, ST-segment changes and positive cardiac enzymes following a exposure to emotional stress.[2] Receiving news of a sudden death, participating in an argument, attending a funeral, observing an armed robbery and even a surprise party have been documented as precipitating events occurring shortly before the onset of cardiac symptoms.[2]

A striking preponderance of female patients with this syndrome (often postmenopausal) compared with male patients (6:1) has been identified.[3] The clinical background associated with transient apical ballooning is remarkably similar in most cases. The patient is typically a female in her seventh decade, evaluated for the sudden onset of cardiac symptoms such as dyspnea or chest pain.[4] In most instances, these symptoms occur close in time to an identified "trigger." This precipitating event is commonly, but not exclusively, an emotional one but may also be an acute medical illness, such as a severe asthmatic attack.[4] The majority of patients exhibit chest pain and ECG changes that suggest myocardial ischemia; however, most do not develop Q waves.[4] ECG presentations can be quite variable: ST-segment elevations similar to those in ST-segment elevation myocardial infarction (STEMI) are common but not the rule.[3] Often, deep T-wave inversions follow where the ST-segment elevations occurred in the acute setting rather then the classic pattern of Q wave development. The most common leads demonstrating ST-segment elevation are leads V_1–V_3 and, occasionally, leads I and aVL.[3] Myocardial enzyme release is less than expected given the ECG findings and wall motion abnormalities demonstrated.

On coronary angiography, patients do not show evidence of obstructive coronary artery disease. In addition, repeat echocardiography demonstrates complete resolution of left ventricular (LV) dysfunction, usually within two to four weeks, with a normal ejection fraction and no residual wall motion abnormalities.[2] Takotsubo cardiomyopathy is strongly suggested by the following four key clinical criteria:

- a setting of acute emotional stress;
- symptoms and findings suggestive of acute coronary syndrome (ACS) with normal coronary arteries on angiography;
- echocardiographic demonstration of LV dysfunction with preserved function at the base and akinesia of all other segments; and
- restoration of normal LV function within several weeks of symptom onset.[2]

The precise mechanism that causes this type of LV dysfunction is unknown. The most commonly discussed mechanism for this condition is stress-induced catecholamine release.[5] Studies have shown plasma catecholamine levels in patients with Takotsubo cardiomyopathy to be 2–3 times greater than those in patients with classic myocardial infarction, and 7–34 times greater than published normal values.[2,6] Elesber et al. demonstrated that impaired myocardial perfusion due to abnormal microvascular blood flow is frequently present in patients with apical ballooning syndrome (ABS), and correlates with the extent of myocardial injury, indicating that microvascular dysfunction plays a pivotal role in the pathogenesis of myocardial stunning in this syndrome.[7] Fortunately, the prognosis is favorable for patients with Takotsubo cardiomyopathy who survive the initial heart failure episode using general symptomatic and supportive measures; LV systolic function typically returns to normal within a few weeks.[2]

KEY TEACHING POINTS

1. Takotsubo cardiomyopathy is a transient cardiomyopathy characterized by marked apical hypokinesis and ballooning in the absence of significant coronary artery disease. However, it is a diagnosis of exclusion.
2. Patients with Takotsubo cardiomyopathy present with symptoms of acute myocardial infarction (AMI), including chest pain, ST-segment changes and positive cardiac enzymes following exposure to acute emotional stress.
3. On coronary angiography, patients with Takotsubo cardiomyopathy do not show evidence of obstructive coronary artery disease.
4. Elevation of plasma catecholamine levels and abnormal microvascular blood flow most likely play important roles in the development of Takotsubo cardiomyopathy.
5. The prognosis is favorable for patients with Takotsubo cardiomyopathy, with LV systolic function typically returning to normal within a few weeks.

REFERENCES

[1] Kolkebeck TE. Takotsubo cardiomyopathy: an unusual syndrome mimicking an ST-elevation myocardial infarction. *Am J Emerg Med* 2007;25:92–5.

[2] Mitchell SA, Crone RA. Takotsubo cardiomyopathy: a case report. *J Am Soc Echocardiogr* 2006;19:1190.e9–10.

[3] Geninatti M, Thames M. All stressed out and no pump to go. *Am J Emerg Med* 2007;25:202–7.

[4] Aurigemma GP, Tighe DA. Echocardiography and reversible left ventricular dysfunction. *Am J Med* 2006;119:18–21.

[5] Merchant EE, Johnson SW, Nguyen P, et al. Takotsubo cardiomyopathy: a case series and review of the literature. *West J Emerg Med* 2008;9:104–11.

[6] Wittstein IS, Theimann DR, Lima JAC, et al. Neurohormonal features of myocardial stunning due to sudden emotional stress. *N Engl J Med* 2005;352:539–48.

[7] Elesber A, Lerman A, Bybee KA, et al. Myocardial perfusion in apical ballooning syndrome correlate of myocardial injury. *Am Heart J* 2006;152:469.e9–13.

17

General body weakness and slow heart rate in a 72-year-old male

HISTORY OF PRESENT ILLNESS

A 72-year-old male with a medical history significant for coronary artery disease, hypertension, hyperlipidemia and diabetes presented to the ED complaining of two months of gradually worsening fatigue and general body weakness. The patient saw his primary care provider (PCP) one week earlier and had his metoprolol dose reduced from 50 mg orally daily to 25 mg orally daily secondary to fatigue and poor medication tolerance. One week prior to presentation, he discontinued his metoprolol without resolution of his symptoms. On the day of presentation to the ED, he noted a slow heart rate when checking his radial pulse. He denied chest pain or shortness of breath, abdominal pain, nausea and vomiting but felt lightheaded when standing.

PHYSICAL EXAMINATION

GENERAL APPEARANCE: The patient appeared well nourished, well hydrated and in no acute distress.

VITAL SIGNS

Temperature	97.8°F (36.5°C)
Pulse	37 beats/minute
Blood pressure	150/90 mmHg
Respirations	20 breaths/minute
Oxygen saturation	98% on room air

HEENT: Unremarkable.

NECK: No jugular venous distension.

CARDIOVASCULAR: Bradycardic, regular rate without rubs, murmurs or gallops.

LUNGS: Clear to auscultation bilaterally.

ABDOMEN: Soft, nontender, nondistended.

EXTREMITIES: No clubbing, cyanosis or edema.

NEUROLOGIC: Nonfocal.

The patient was placed on the cardiac monitor, a 12-lead ECG was obtained (Figure 17.1), a peripheral intravenous line was placed, and blood was drawn and sent for laboratory testing.

What is your diagnosis?

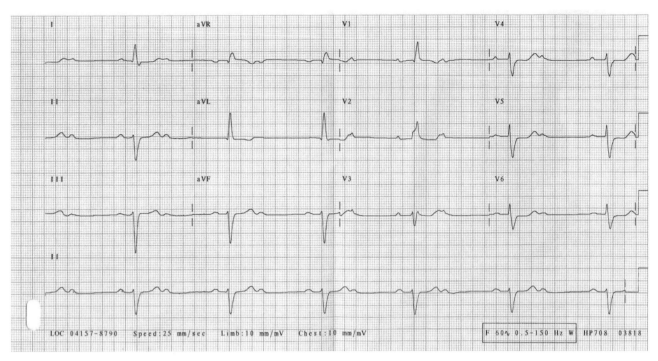

Figure 17.1 12-lead ECG from a 72-year-old male with fatigue and general body weakness.

ANSWER

The diagnosis is 2:1 atrioventricular block (one conducted atrial complex for every nonconducted beat). Based upon this ECG alone, it is impossible to determine whether the patient has Mobitz Type I or Type II conduction. Laboratory tests were normal (complete blood count, electrolytes, BUN, creatinine, glucose, troponin I). The patient was admitted to telemetry for monitoring. He continued to maintain a heart rate in the 30s with a normal blood pressure and without symptoms. A cardiology consult was obtained, and the patient was diagnosed with a high-grade second-degree atrioventricular (AV) block. The patient underwent a permanent pacemaker placement with resolution of the block and was discharged feeling much improved on hospital day #4.

Atrioventricular (AV) blocks

In first-degree AV block, the PR interval is prolonged, with a duration greater than 0.20 sec, and is constant without progressive change.[1] The P wave has normal morphology and precedes every QRS complex. The QRS complex usually has a normal morphology and axis. Every atrial complex is conducted to the ventricles. First-degree AV block can be a normal finding, especially in healthy young adults or athletes.[2] It may occur pathologically because of conduction disease in the AV node or the His-Purkinje system, acute myocardial infarction (particularly inferior MI), myocarditis, electrolyte disturbances and the use of AV nodal-blocking agents.[2]

Second-degree AV block refers to a disorder of the cardiac conduction system in which some atrial impulses are not conducted to the ventricles.[3] Electrocardiographically, some P waves are not followed by a QRS complex. Second-degree AV block is composed of two types: Mobitz I (Wenckebach) block and Mobitz II. Mobitz I second-degree AV block is characterized by a progressive prolongation of the PR interval, which results in a progressive shortening of the R–R interval. Ultimately, the atrial impulse fails to conduct, a QRS complex is not generated and there is no ventricular contraction. The PR interval is the shortest in the first beat in the cycle, whereas the R–R intervals between conducted beats are constant.[3] Mobitz I block is caused by conduction delay in the AV node (72% of patients) or the His-Purkinje system (the remaining 28%).[3]

Mobitz II second-degree AV block is characterized by an unexpected nonconducted atrial impulse.[3] Thus, the PR and R–R intervals between conducted beats are constant. In Mobitz II block, the conduction delay occurs infranodally. The QRS complex is likely to be wide, except in patients where the delay is localized to the bundle of His. The usual pattern of dropped beats in Mobitz II block ranges from two conducted atrial complexes for every nonconducted beat (3:1), up

to combinations of 4:1 or 3:2 patterns.[2] Mobitz Type II carries a worse prognosis than Mobitz Type I, and may require permanent pacemaker placement if the patient is symptomatic.

When the ratio of AV conduction is 2:1, it is impossible to determine whether the patient has Mobitz Type I or Type II conduction. In this case, some authors recommend describing the 2:1 conduction pattern without categorizing it as Type I or Type II.[2] Nonetheless, the physician should initially "assume the worst" in situations of 2:1 conduction; that is, the block is Mobitz II unless proven otherwise.[1]

Third-degree AV block (complete heart block) occurs when no atrial impulses reach the ventricles.[4] The atria and ventricles thus function independently (i.e., there is AV dissociation), and the atrial rate is faster than the ventricular rate because the latter is an escape rhythm. The atrial impulses (P waves) "march" out on the ECG, as do the ventricular depolarizations (QRS complexes), yet they are unrelated. Ventricular escape rhythms are usually associated with a worse prognosis and are more commonly caused by acquired (noncongenital) conditions. It is possible that no escape rhythm is generated, resulting in asystole.[4]

KEY TEACHING POINTS

1. First-degree AV block can be a normal finding, especially in healthy young adults or athletes.
2. For second-degree AV blocks, Mobitz Type II carries a worse prognosis than Mobitz Type I, and may require permanent pacemaker placement if the patient is symptomatic.
3. When the ratio of AV conduction is 2:1, it is impossible to determine whether the patient has Mobitz Type I or Type II conduction; assume that the block is Mobitz II unless proven otherwise.
4. Third-degree AV block (complete heart block) occurs when no impulses from the atria reach the ventricles, resulting in AV dissociation. This requires permanent pacemaker placement.

REFERENCES

[1] Brady WJ, Harrington RA. Atrioventricular block. In: Chan TC, Brady WJ, Harrigan RA, et al. (eds). *ECG in Emergency Medicine and Acute Care*. Philadelphia: Elsevier, 2005;85–9.

[2] Patel PM, Wu W-C. The electrocardiogram in the primary care office. *Prim Care Clin Office Pract* 2005;32:901–30.

[3] Levine MD. Heart block, second degree. eMedicine Website. Available at http://www.emedicine.com/emerg/topic234.htm. Accessed June 30, 2008.

[4] Ufberg JW, Clark JS. Bradydysrhythmias and atrioventricular conduction blocks. *Emerg Med Clin N Am* 2006;24:1–9.

18

Headache, neck pain and chest pain in a 73-year-old male

HISTORY OF PRESENT ILLNESS

A 73-year-old male with a medical history significant for hypertension, coronary artery disease and prior myocardial infarction presented to the ED complaining of a headache, neck pain and chest pain for one hour. The patient was leaning over his bathroom sink when he experienced the sudden onset of a severe, bitemporal headache that quickly radiated down his posterior neck and into his back, left chest and sternum. The patient described the pain as a heaviness and rated it at a level of 8 (on a scale from 0 to 10). He reported associated sweating and shortness of breath, but denied nausea or vomiting, dizziness, focal weakness, numbness, visual changes or slurred speech. He had taken three sublingual nitroglycerin tablets prior to arrival without improvement in his symptoms, as well as 81 mg of aspirin. His medications included aspirin, clonidine, lisinopril, lovastatin and bisoprolol/hydrochlorothiazide. He denied tobacco, alcohol or recreational drug use. He was a practicing Jehovah's Witness.

PHYSICAL EXAMINATION

GENERAL APPEARANCE: The patient appeared awake and alert, and in mild discomfort.

VITAL SIGNS

Temperature	97.4°F (36.3°C)
Pulse	75 beats/minute
Blood pressure	189/73 mmHg
Respirations	20 breaths/minute
Oxygen saturation	98% on room air

HEENT: PERRL, EOMI.

CARDIOVASCULAR: Regular rate and rhythm with II/VI diastolic murmur at the left upper sternal border, no rubs or gallops.

LUNGS: Bilateral rales at the bases without wheezes or rhonchi.

ABDOMEN: Soft, nontender, nondistended.

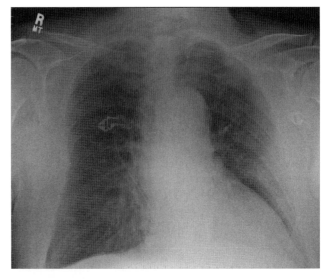

Figure 18.1 Portable chest radiograph of a 73-year-old male with headache, neck pain and chest pain.

EXTREMITIES: 2+ pitting edema of bilateral lower extremities. Strong and equal peripheral pulses in upper and lower extremities.

NEUROLOGIC: Nonfocal.

A peripheral intravenous line was placed, and blood was drawn and sent for laboratory testing. An ECG was obtained that demonstrated a normal sinus rhythm with a ventricular rate of 82, multiple premature ventricular contractions, as well as ST-segment depression in leads I, II and V_4 through V_6, all new compared to a previous ECG obtained one year earlier. Laboratory tests (complete blood count, chemistry panel and troponin I) were all within normal limits. The patient was given sublingual nitroglycerin for his chest pain, and a portable chest radiograph was obtained (Figure 18.1).

What is your diagnosis?

ANSWER

The diagnosis is aortic dissection, Stanford type A. The chest radiograph demonstrated a widened mediastinum. A chest CT with intravenous contrast was obtained, which demonstrated a type A aortic dissection arising just above the level of the aortic valve and involving the ascending, transverse and descending thoracic aorta, extending into the abdominal aorta, terminating just above the iliac bifurcation (Figure 18.2). The vascular surgeon was urgently consulted. An esmolol and nitroprusside IV drip were begun for blood pressure control, and the patient was taken urgently to the OR for definitive surgical treatment of the dissection.

Aortic dissection

An aortic dissection refers to the separation of the layers of the aortic wall (the intima, media and adventitia) with entry of blood into the aortic media, creating a false lumen.[1] The dissection usually originates from a tear in the aortic intima. It can then propagate proximally or distally, leading to many clinical features of dissection. Aortic dissections are classified by the portion of the aorta involved. In the Stanford system, type A dissections involve the ascending aorta, either alone or with the descending aorta; type B dissections are confined to the descending aorta (Figure 18.3).[1] Dissections are also classified as acute (if present less than two weeks) or chronic (if present longer than two weeks). The majority of thoracic aortic dissections presenting to the ED are acute, presenting with chest or back pain.

More than 2000 cases of thoracic aortic dissection (TAD) occur annually in the United States.[2] It is the most common acute illness of the aorta. Most cases occur in patients 50–70 years old, with males predominating. Ascending aortic dissection left untreated carries a 75% mortality rate within the first two weeks alone; if the diagnosis remains unrecognized, the mortality reaches 90% at one year.[2,3] Estimated mortality rates are 1–2% per hour for the first 24–48 hours.[2]

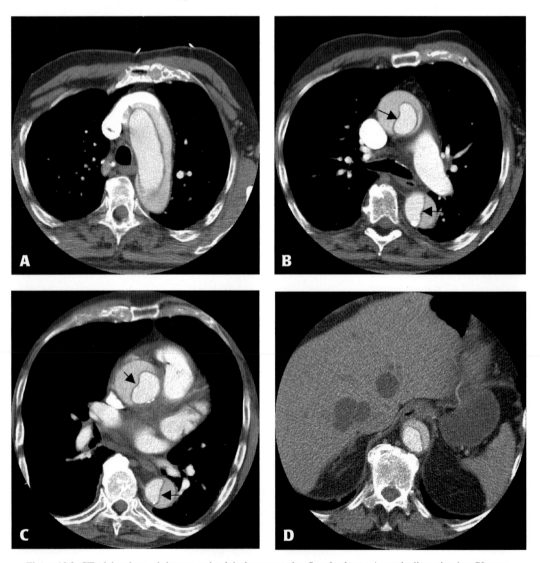

Figure 18.2 CT of the chest, abdomen and pelvis demonstrating Stanford type A aortic dissection in a 73-year-old male, with dissection from the aortic arch (panel A), extending into the ascending and descending aorta (panels B and C, arrows) and into the abdominal aorta (panel D).

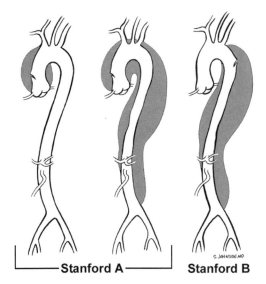

Figure 18.3 Stanford classification for aortic dissections.

Risk factors for thoracic aortic dissection include hypertension, advanced age, male gender, pregnancy, bicuspid aortic valve, coarctation of the aorta, connective tissue diseases such as Marfan's syndrome and cocaine use.[2] Ninety-five percent of patients with TAD report pain; most often, the pain is abrupt in onset, located in the anterior chest, posterior chest or back.[1–3] The pain may be described as ripping or tearing; however, these terms are only used by 50% of patients.[3] TAD is associated with syncope in as many as 13% of patients; this may be the sole presenting symptom in 3% of patients.

On physical examination, approximately 50% of patients with TAD are hypertensive (SBP $\geq$150 mmHg), whereas 16% are hypotensive or in shock.[3] The diastolic murmur of aortic insufficiency is present in less than one-third of patients, whereas focal neurologic deficits suggestive of cerebrovascular accident are found in 5–17% of patients.[3,4] Measurement of the blood pressure in both arms and the thigh demonstrates a systolic pressure differential of more than 20 mmHg in 20–40% of patients.[1] Myocardial infarction is a relatively rare complication of proximal aortic dissection, estimated to occur in approximately 1–7% of all cases. ECGs obtained in such cases may show ST-segment elevation or depression consistent with infarction or ischemia.[2,4]

The chest radiograph is abnormal in 85–90% of patients.[1] Mediastinal widening (more than 8 cm) is the most common finding, occurring in 63% of type A dissections and 56% of type B dissections.[1] Other common CXR findings include separation of calcium (more than 5 mm) from the edge of the aortic wall, a blurred aortic knob, a left pleuroapical cap, a left pleural effusion, deviation of the paraspinous line, shift and elevation of the right mainstem bronchus, and deviation of the trachea or esophagus to the right.

Bushnell and Brown published an extensive review of the literature examining the usefulness and accuracy of medical history, physical examination and chest radiograph for detecting acute TAD.[5] They concluded that pain of abrupt onset, pulse deficits and neurologic deficits increase the likelihood of TAD, whereas a normal chest radiograph and the absence of acute-onset pain appear to decrease its likelihood. However, because the presentation of TAD is highly variable, the diagnosis cannot be ruled out based on medical history, physical examination or plain radiography findings; further diagnostic testing is required to confirm or rule out the diagnosis.[5]

The strategy employed to confirm the diagnosis of TAD depends on the resources available, the patient's clinical condition and one's pretest suspicion. Unstable patients with a high pretest probability must not leave the ED (except to go to the operating room). In such patients, transesophageal echocardiography (TEE) can be performed at the bedside by a cardiologist. TEE is quick, portable, does not require exposure to contrast, and can be performed in the ED.[1] It is highly accurate in experienced hands, with a sensitivity as high as 98% and a specificity reported between 63–96%.[1] The main disadvantage is its lack of universal availability.

Chest CT is fast, universally available, noninvasive, less operator dependent and highly accurate, with a sensitivity of 94% and a specificity of 87–100%.[1] Multidetector row CT scanners have a sensitivity of 99% for detecting TAD.[3] Additionally, CT provides information about other potential diagnoses. Disadvantages of CT include the need for contrast dye and the need to leave the ED. Aortography was the gold standard for diagnosis of TAD but has been supplanted by CT scanning and TEE. Aortography has a sensitivity of 87% and a reported specificity of 75–94%.[1] Disadvantages to aortography are that it is invasive, time-consuming and exposes patients to a high volume of contrast dye. Finally, MRI is an extremely accurate diagnostic modality for the diagnosis of TAD – its use will likely increase in the future.

The initial management of patients with TAD is aggressive heart rate and blood pressure control. In hypertensive patients, therapy begins with a short-acting, rapid-onset beta-blocker, such as esmolol or metoprolol, with the goal of lowering the heart rate to a target of 60 beats/minute.[1] Following the initiation of beta-blocker therapy, a potent IV vasodilator such as nitroprusside is added and titrated to a goal SBP of 100–120 mmHg. Monotherapy with IV labetalol is an excellent alternative. Pain should be controlled with narcotics. Hypotensive patients must be aggressively resuscitated with normal saline; however, inotropic agents should be avoided as they increase shear stress. Despite the presence of cardiac ischemia in patients with TAD, anticoagulation and fibrinolytic therapy must be withheld as the consequences of such therapy can be devastating.[1]

Further management of TAD is determined by the type of dissection and complications. Proximal dissections are a surgical emergency. Seventy-two percent of patients with type A dissection are treated operatively, with an operative mortality at experienced centers varying from 7–36%.[1] Type B dissections are usually managed nonoperatively. Indications for surgery include propagation of the dissection, increasing size of the hematoma, compromise of major branches of the aorta, impending rupture or bleeding into the pleural cavity. Endovascular therapy with stent placement in some centers is becoming increasingly popular for both type A and B dissections in the appropriate setting. Given the high morbidity and mortality and need for close monitoring, all patients with aortic dissections must be managed in the ICU.

KEY TEACHING POINTS

1. Ascending aortic dissection left untreated has a 75% mortality rate within the first two weeks alone; if the diagnosis remains unrecognized, the mortality reaches 90% at one year.
2. Risk factors for TAD include hypertension, advanced age, male gender, pregnancy, bicuspid aortic valve, coarctation of the aorta, connective tissue diseases and cocaine use.
3. Because the presentation of TAD is highly variable, the diagnosis cannot be ruled out based on medical history, physical examination or plain radiography; further diagnostic testing is required with chest CT or TEE to confirm or rule out the diagnosis.

4. The initial management patients with TAD is aggressive heart rate and blood pressure control, whereas further management of TAD is determined by the type of dissection and complications (surgery for type A dissections, medical management for type B dissections).
5. Endovascular stent placement has become an option for the treatment of aortic dissections in the appropriate setting.

REFERENCES

[1] Gupta R, Kaufman S. Cardiovascular emergencies in the elderly. *Emerg Med Clin N Am* 2006;24:339–70.
[2] Rogers RL, McCormack R. Aortic disasters. *Emerg Med Clin N Am* 2004;22:887–908.
[3] Kelly BS. Evaluation of the elderly patient with acute chest pain. *Clin Geriatr Med* 2007;23:327–49.
[4] Haro LH, Krajicek M, Lobl JK. Challenges, controversies, and advances in aortic catastrophes. *Emerg Med Clin N Am* 2005;23:1159–77.
[5] Bushnell J, Brown J. Rational clinical examination abstract: clinical assessment for acute thoracic aortic dissection. *Ann Emerg Med* 2005;46:90–2.

19

Near syncope, tachycardia and chest pain in a 74-year-old female

HISTORY OF PRESENT ILLNESS

A 74-year-old female with a history of hyperlipidemia, hypertension, and dyspnea of unclear etiology complained to her husband of mild chest pressure and lightheadedness while brushing her teeth. Her husband checked her blood pressure and found it to be 74/50 mmHg with a heart rate of 110 beats/minute per automatic blood pressure cuff, so he called emergency services. The patient had undergone a stress thallium test six months prior to presentation, which showed evidence of moderate to severe stress-induced myocardial ischemia in the septum and inferior wall. A coronary artery catheterization shortly afterward demonstrated a 45% ejection fraction with an area of focal basal inferior hypokinesis but no obstructive coronary disease. Her prior ECG showed a first-degree heart block with right bundle branch block and left posterior fascicular blocks. Approximately one week prior to presentation, the patient complained of being lightheaded, which prompted reduction of her metoprolol in half to 12.5 mg once daily.

Upon arrival to the patient's residence, the paramedics found the patient awake and in a wide complex tachycardia at 200 beats/minute with a monomorphic, uniform and regular QRS morphology (Figure 19.1, panel A). The patient was given intravenous lidocaine, which resulted in the rhythm noted in Figure 19.1, panel B. The patient's blood pressure improved slightly to a systolic pressure of 100 mmHg. She was transported code III to the ED, where she continued to complain of mild lightheadedness but denied chest pain or shortness of breath.

PHYSICAL EXAMINATION

GENERAL APPEARANCE: The patient was awake and alert, and in no acute distress.

VITAL SIGNS
Temperature	98.6°F (37°C)
Pulse	53 beats/minute
Blood pressure	100/60 mmHg
Respirations	22 breaths/minute
Oxygen saturation	99% on room air

HEENT: Unremarkable

NECK: Supple, no jugular venous distension.

CARDIOVASCULAR: Bradycardic rate, regular rhythm without rubs, murmurs or gallops.

LUNGS: Clear to auscultation bilaterally.

ABDOMEN: Soft, nontender, nondistended.

EXTREMITIES: No clubbing, cyanosis or edema; weak peripheral pulses.

NEUROLOGIC: Nonfocal.

The patient was placed on the cardiac monitor, a peripheral intravenous line was placed, and blood was drawn and sent for laboratory testing. A 12-lead ECG revealed continuation of the rhythm noted in Figure 19.1, panel B, without obvious ST-T wave changes. Laboratory tests (including a complete blood count, electrolytes, creatinine, glucose and troponin I) were within normal limits.

What is your diagnosis?

73

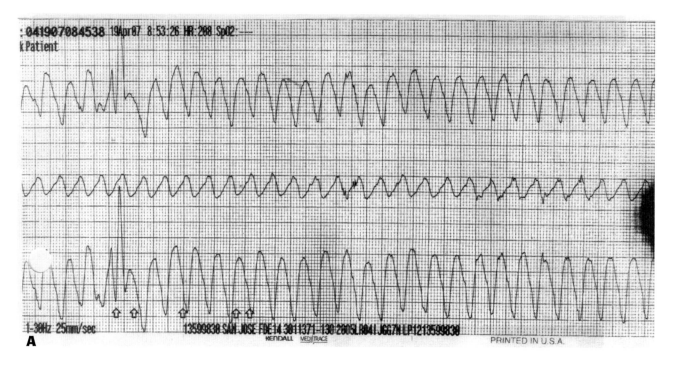

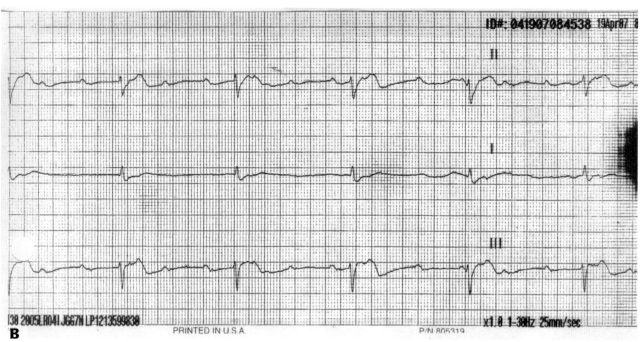

Figure 19.1 Rhythm strip of a 74-year-old female before (panel A) and after (panel B) administration of pre-hospital IV lidocaine.

ANSWER

The diagnosis is complete atrioventricular (AV) block (third-degree heart block) following conversion from ventricular tachycardia with lidocaine. Upon presentation to the ED, she remained in third-degree heart block with what appeared to be a junctional escape rhythm at 53 beats/minute. A temporary jugular venous pacing wire was placed in the ED. Despite adjustments to the pacemaker's sensitivity, the pacer spikes were falling on the T waves, at which time the pacemaker was temporarily turned off while the pacemaker wire was repositioned. Approximately three minutes later, the patient lost consciousness and became pulseless. The resultant rhythm shown in Figure 19.2 (panel D) is polymorphic ventricular tachycardia consistent with *torsades de pointes*. The patient was immediately defibrillated at 200 Joules (biphasic), which restored her rhythm to second-degree heart block. The patient regained consciousness and her pacemaker was immediately turned back on with the rate set at 90 to override her intrinsic rhythm. The patient was admitted to the ICU and ultimately underwent permanent internal cardioverter-defibrillator (ICD) placement.

Trifascicular block, complete heart block and lidocaine

Intraventricular conduction abnormalities (IVCA) comprise a group of abnormalities seen on the ECG that may confuse clinicians and can conceal potentially lethal disease entities, such as acute myocardial infarction (AMI).[1] There are multiple types of IVCAs, each with its unique clinical significance. It is useful to categorize conduction abnormalities (blocks) by the number of fascicles involved. Electrical conduction from the bundle of His is relayed to the right bundle and the anterior and posterior divisions of the left bundle.[2] Unifascicular blocks, such as right bundle branch block (RBBB), left anterior fascicular block (LAFB) and left posterior fascicular block (LPFB), are the result of a conduction disturbance in one fascicle. Bifascicular blocks, such as left bundle branch block (LBBB), the combination of RBBB and LAFB, or RBBB and LPFB, occur when two of the three fascicles are involved. Trifascicular block denotes a block in all three fascicles.[1]

Trifascicular block can present as a bifascicular block plus a third-degree AV block. If the block in one of the fascicles is incomplete, the ECG generally demonstrates a bifascicular block and a first- or second-degree AV block. If conduction in the dysfunctional fascicle also fails, complete heart block ensues. Patients who have multifascicular block have advanced conduction system disease that may progress to complete heart block and sudden cardiac death. The cumulative three-year rate of sudden death in patients who have bifascicular block has been estimated to be 35% in patients who have LBBB, 11% in patients who have RBBB and LAFB, and 7% in patients who have RBBB and LPFB.[1]

Lidocaine blocks sodium channels, predominantly in the open (or possibly inactivated) state. It has rapid onset and offset, and does not affect normal sinus node automaticity in usual doses. In Purkinje fibers in vitro, lidocaine depresses normal as well as abnormal forms of automaticity, as well as early and late after-depolarizations.[3] It can convert areas of unidirectional block into bidirectional block during ischemia and prevent development of VF by preventing fragmentation of organized large wave fronts into heterogeneous wavelets. In vivo, lidocaine has minimal effect on automaticity or conduction except in unusual circumstances. Patients with pre-existing sinus node dysfunction, abnormal His-Purkinje conduction, or junctional or ventricular escape rhythms can develop depressed automaticity or conduction following IV lidocaine.[3] Occasional sinus node depression and His-Purkinje block have been reported with its use.

In this patient, a previous ECG demonstrated an incomplete trifascicular block (bifascicular block with first-degree AV block), placing her at increased risk to progress to third-degree (complete) AV block. In addition, as the patient had known disease of the His-Purkinje system, the use of lidocaine to suppress ventricular tachycardia resulted in additional suppression of conduction through this diseased system, resulting in complete heart block. Finally, it is possible that the patient was experiencing AV nodal blockade during the week prior to presentation when she described feeling lightheaded to her doctor, at which time the dose of her beta-blocker was reduced.

KEY TEACHING POINTS

1. Patients who have multifascicular block have advanced conduction system disease that may progress to complete heart block and sudden cardiac death.
2. All patients with third-degree heart block require admission to either a telemetry floor (if hemodynamically stable and transcutaneous pacing achieves capture) or an intensive care unit. The decision on telemetry versus intensive care should be made in conjunction with the cardiologist, based on hospital resources.
3. Patients with complete AV block and concomitant acute MI, active myocardial ischemia, congestive heart failure, wide complex escape rhythm or symptoms of hypoperfusion may require early placement of a permanent pacemaker, particularly if difficulty obtaining capture from an external or transvenous pacemaker is encountered.[4]
4. Patients with pre-existing sinus node dysfunction, abnormal His-Purkinje conduction, or junctional or ventricular escape rhythms can develop depressed automaticity or conduction following IV lidocaine administration.

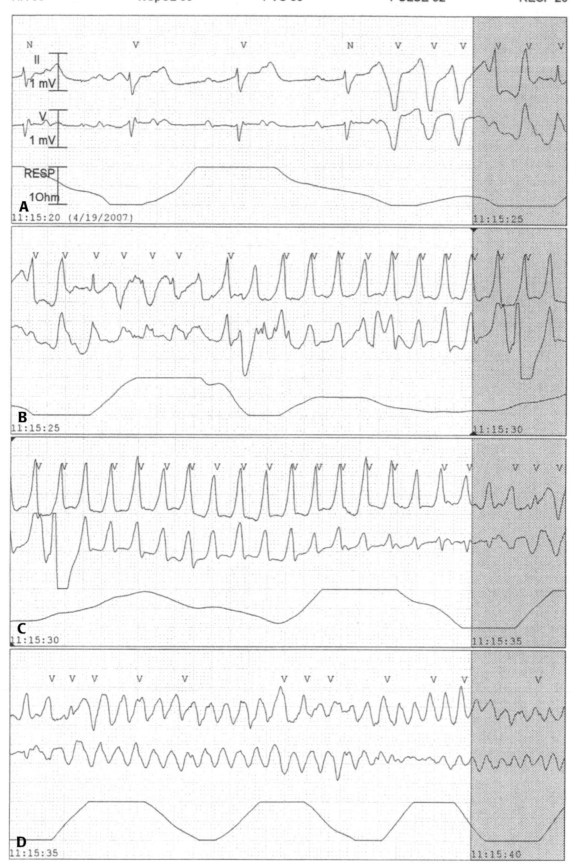

Figure 19.2 Continuous rhythm strip from a 74-year-old female after turning off temporary pacing wire (panel A, third-degree AV block converting to wide complex QRS tachycardia; panel B, conversion to monomorphic ventricular tachycardia (VT); panel C, monomorphic VT degenerating to *torsades de pointes*; panel D, *torsades de pointes*).

REFERENCES

[1] Rogers RL, Mitarai M, Mattu A. Intraventricular conduction abnormalities. *Emerg Med Clin N Am* 2006;24:41–51.

[2] Perron AD, Sweeney T. Arrhythmic complications of acute coronary syndromes. *Emerg Med Clin N Am* 2005;23:1065–82.

[3] Miller JM, Zipes DP. Therapy for cardiac arrhythmias. In: Libby P, Bonow RO, Mann DL, et al. (eds). *Braunwald's Heart Disease: A Textbook of Cardiovascular Medicine*, 8th ed. Philadelphia: Saunders, 2008;788–9.

[4] Levine MD, Brown DFM. Heart block, third degree. eMedicine Website. Available at http://www.emedicine.com/emerg/topic235.htm. Accessed June 19, 2008.

Chest pain for 12 hours in a 75-year-old female

HISTORY OF PRESENT ILLNESS

A 75-year-old female with a medical history significant for hypertension presented to the ED complaining of substernal chest pressure radiating to the left chest that started 12 hours earlier. The pressure was constant, rated at a level of 7 (on a scale of 0 to 10), and had not abated. The patient denied associated nausea, vomiting, shortness of breath or diaphoresis, and had not experienced similar symptoms in the past. The patient did not smoke or drink and denied a family history of coronary artery disease. Her only medications were lisinopril and atenolol.

PHYSICAL EXAMINATION

GENERAL APPEARANCE: The patient appeared well nourished, well hydrated and in no acute distress.

VITAL SIGNS

Temperature	98.5°F (36.9°C)
Pulse	128 beats/minute
Blood pressure	139/70 mmHg
Respirations	18 breaths/minute
Oxygen saturation	98% on room air

HEENT: Unremarkable.

NECK: Supple, no jugular venous distension.

CARDIOVASCULAR: Tachycardic rate, regular rhythm without rubs, murmurs or gallops.

LUNGS: Clear to auscultation bilaterally.

ABDOMEN: Soft, nontender, nondistended.

RECTAL: Brown stool, hemoccult negative.

EXTREMITIES: No clubbing, cyanosis or edema.

NEUROLOGIC: Nonfocal.

The patient was placed on the cardiac monitor, a stat 12-lead ECG was obtained (Figure 20.1) and a peripheral intravenous line was placed, with blood drawn and sent for laboratory testing.

What is your diagnosis?

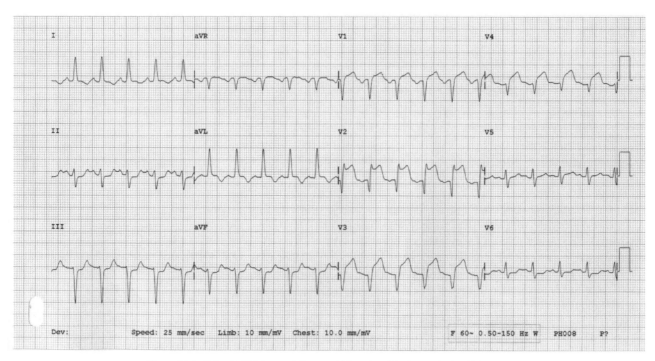

Figure 20.1 12-lead ECG from a 75-year-old female with chest pain for 12 hours.

ANSWER

The diagnosis is acute anterior myocardial infarction (MI). The patient's ECG showed sinus tachycardia, rate 128, with ST-segment elevation in leads V_1 to V_4, with reciprocal ST-segment depression in leads II, III and V_6. The patient received aspirin orally, sublingual nitroglycerin, intravenous metoprolol, intravenous heparin and Integrilin (glycoprotein IIb/IIIa inhibitor). The patient was taken for emergent percutaneous transluminal coronary angioplasty (PTCA), which revealed a 99% stenosis of her left anterior descending (LAD) coronary artery. The LAD was stented and the patient was admitted to the ICU, where she continued to improve with resolution of her ST-segment elevations (Figure 20.2, ECG obtained two weeks post-angioplasty).

Anterior myocardial infarction

In MI of the anterior wall, ST-segment elevation in leads V_1, V_2 and V_3 indicates occlusion of the left anterior descending coronary artery.[1] ST-segment elevation in these three leads and in lead aVL in association with ST-segment depression of more than 1 mm in lead aVF indicates proximal occlusion of the LAD artery. In this case, the ST-segment vector is directed upward, toward leads V_1, aVL and aVR, and away from the inferior leads. ST-segment elevation in leads V_1, V_2 and V_3 without significant inferior ST-segment depression suggests occlusion of the LAD artery after the origin of the first diagonal branch.

ST-segment elevation in leads V_1, V_2 and V_3 with elevation in the inferior leads suggests occlusion of the LAD artery distal to the origin of the first diagonal branch in a vessel that wraps around to supply the inferoapical region of the left ventricle.[1] New right bundle-branch block with a Q wave preceding the R wave in lead V_1 is a specific but insensitive marker of proximal occlusion of the LAD artery in association with anteroseptal MI.

Coronary artery disease is the leading cause of death in the United States. In 2006, approximately 1.2 million Americans sustained a MI.[2] Of these, one-quarter to one-third had an ST-segment elevation MI (STEMI). Of all patients having an MI, 25–35% will die before receiving medical attention, most often from ventricular fibrillation. For those who reach a medical facility, the prognosis is considerably better and has improved over the years: in-hospital mortality rates fell from 11.2% in 1990 to 9.4% in 1999.[2] Most of this decline is due to decreasing mortality rates among patients with STEMI as a consequence of improvements in initial therapy, including fibrinolysis and primary percutaneous coronary intervention (PCI). In an analysis by the National Registry of Myocardial Infarction (NRMI), the rate of in-hospital mortality was 5.7% among those receiving reperfusion therapy, compared to 14.8% among those who were eligible for but did not receive such therapy.[2]

In comparison with conservative medical management, fibrinolytic therapy leads to improved left ventricular systolic function and survival in patients with MI associated with either ST-segment elevation or left bundle-branch block (LBBB).[2] However, fibrinolytic therapy has several limitations, including patients with contraindications to fibrinolysis (27% in one report), failure of thrombolytic therapy to open occluded vessels (15% of patients given thrombolytics) and

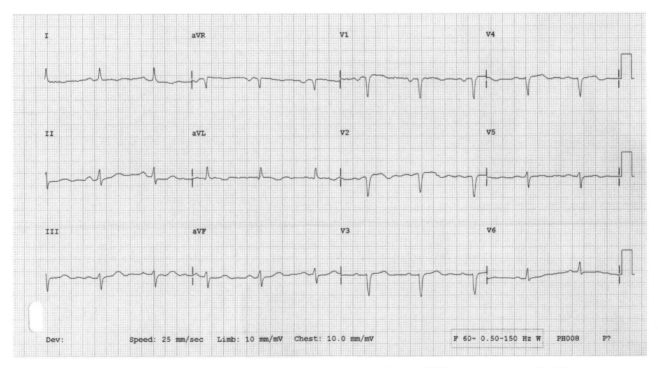

Figure 20.2 12-lead ECG from a 75-year-old female two weeks following PTCA for an acute anterior MI, demonstrating resolution of significant ST-segment elevation in anterior leads.

reocclusion of the infarct-related artery within three months after MI in patients receiving thrombolytic therapy (25% of patients).[2]

Primary PCI consists of urgent balloon angioplasty (with or without stenting) with platelet glycoprotein IIb/IIIa inhibitors but not fibrinolytic therapy to open the infarct-related artery during an acute STEMI. After identifying the site of recent thrombotic occlusion on coronary angiography, a metal wire is advanced past the thrombus over which a balloon catheter (with or without a stent) is positioned at the site of the occlusion and inflated, thereby mechanically restoring antegrade flow. Primary PCI restores angiographically normal flow in the previously occluded artery in more than 90% of patients, whereas fibrinolytic therapy is reported to do so in only 50–60% of such patients.[2]

In a meta-analysis of 23 randomized, controlled comparisons of PCI (involving 3872 patients) and fibrinolytic therapy (3867 patients), the rate of death four to six weeks after treatment was significantly lower among those who underwent primary PCI (7% versus 9%).[3] Rates of nonfatal reinfarction and stroke were also significantly reduced. Most of these trials were performed in high-volume interventional centers by experienced operators with minimal delay after the patient's arrival. If primary PCI is performed at low-volume centers by less-experienced operators with longer delays between arrival and treatment, such superior outcomes may not be seen.

One of the indications for thrombolysis is ongoing symptoms for less than 12 hours. One nonsystematic review found that the earlier thrombolytic treatment was given after the onset of symptoms, the greater the absolute benefit of treatment.[4] For each hour of delay in thrombolytic treatment, the absolute risk reduction (ARR) of death decreased by 0.16% (ARR for death if given within 6 hours of symptoms = 3%; ARR for death if given 7–12 hours after onset of symptoms = 2%).[4] Too few people in the review received treatment more than 12 hours after the onset of symptoms to determine whether the benefits of thrombolytic treatment given after 12 hours would outweigh the risks.

Schomig and colleagues conducted a study to assess whether an invasive strategy based on PCI with stenting is associated with reduction of infarct size in patients with acute STEMI presenting greater than 12 hours after the symptom onset, compared to conventional conservative treatment strategy.[5] Conducted from May 2001 to December 2004, the study included 365 patients aged 18–80 years without persistent heart attack symptoms admitted with the diagnosis of acute STEMI between 12–48 hours from symptom onset. Patients were randomized to receive either an invasive strategy ($n = 182$), based predominantly on coronary stenting plus intravenous abciximab (a glycoprotein IIb/IIIa inhibitor), or conventional conservative treatment strategy ($n = 183$), which included an intravenous infusion of heparin. The researchers found that the final left ventricular infarct size was significantly smaller in patients assigned to the invasive group (median = 8%) versus those assigned to the conservative group (median = 13%).[5] The average difference in final left ventricular infarct size between the invasive and conservative groups was 5%. The outcomes of death, recurrent MI or stroke at 30 days occurred in 8 patients in the invasive group (4.4%) and 12 patients in the conservative group (6.6%), a 33% lower risk of these outcomes for patients in the invasive group. The researchers concluded that this finding increased the evidence supporting the invasive strategy and deserves consideration when current treatment guidelines for this category of patients is reassessed.

KEY TEACHING POINTS

1. An ECG demonstrating ST-segment elevation in leads V_1, V_2 and V_3 is consistent with an anterior wall myocardial infarction (MI) and indicates occlusion of the left anterior descending (LAD) artery.
2. In comparison with conservative management, fibrinolytic therapy leads to improved left ventricular systolic function and survival in patients with ST-segment elevation myocardial infarction (STEMI) or left bundle-branch block (LBBB).
3. Primary percutaneous coronary intervention (PCI) restores angiographically normal flow in previously occluded artery in more than 90% of patients, whereas fibrinolytic therapy does so only in 50–60% of such patients.

REFERENCES

[1] Zimetbaum PJ, Josephson ME. Current concepts: use of the electrocardiogram in acute myocardial infarction. *N Engl J Med* 2003;348:933–40.
[2] Keeley EC, Hillis LD. Primary PCI for myocardial infarction with ST-segment elevation. *N Engl J Med* 2007;356:47–54.
[3] Keeley EC, Boura JA, Grines CL. Primary angioplasty versus intravenous thrombolytic therapy for acute myocardial infarction: a quantitative review of 23 randomised trials. Lancet 2003;361:13–20.
[4] Fibrinolytic Therapy Trialists' (FTT) Collaborative Group. Indications for fibrinolytic therapy in suspected acute myocardial infarction: collaborative overview of early mortality and major morbidity results of all randomized trials of more than 1000 patients. *Lancet* 1994;343:311–22.
[5] Schömig A, Mehilli J, Antoniucci D, et al. Mechanical reperfusion in patients with acute myocardial infarction presenting more than 12 hours from symptom onset. A randomized controlled trial. *JAMA* 2005;293:2865–72.

21

Shortness of breath and cough in an 80-year-old female

HISTORY OF PRESENT ILLNESS

An 80-year-old female with a medical history significant for chronic obstructive pulmonary disease, hypertension, hyperlipidemia and chronic upper back pain presented to the ED complaining of two weeks of increasing shortness of breath, cough, wheezing and dyspnea on exertion. Her symptoms had acutely worsened over the past two days, and were not relieved with her ipratropium inhaler. She was seen by her primary care provider nine days previously and started clarithromycin for bronchitis. The patient denied fever or chills, chest pain, leg swelling, focal weakness, numbness or tingling. She reported chronic back pain, which had not worsened.

PHYSICAL EXAMINATION

GENERAL APPEARANCE: The patient was breathing rapidly, appeared dyspneic and spoke only four- or five-word sentences.

VITAL SIGNS

Temperature	98.3°F (36.8°C)
Pulse	95 beats/minute
Blood pressure	106/71 mmHg
Respirations	32 breaths/minute
Oxygen saturation	87% on room air
	93% on 2 liters oxygen by nasal canula

HEENT: PERRL, EOMI, oropharynx dry.

NECK: Supple, no jugular venous distension.

CARDIOVASCULAR: Distant heart sounds, regular rate and rhythm without rubs, murmurs or gallops, palpable radial and dorsalis pedis pulses bilaterally.

LUNGS: Diminished breath sounds throughout, diffuse wheezing, scattered rhonchi, prolonged expiratory phase.

ABDOMEN: Soft, nontender, nondistended.

RECTAL: Normal tone, brown stool, hemoccult negative.

EXTREMITIES: No clubbing, cyanosis or edema.

NEUROLOGIC: Nonfocal.

A peripheral intravenous line was placed, blood was drawn and sent for laboratory testing, and a 12-lead ECG and portable chest radiograph were obtained (Figures 21.1 and 21.2, respectively). The patient received multiple bronchodilator treatments (nebulized albuterol and ipratropium bromide) and prednisone 60 mg orally with minimal improvement of her symptoms. Laboratory tests revealed a leukocyte count of 12.7 K/μL (normal 3.5–12.5 K/μL) with 87% neutrophils (normal 50–70%), hematocrit of 32% (normal 34–46%), brain natriuretic peptide (BNP) of 384 pg/mL (normal <100 pg/mL), D-dimer positive, troponin I less than 0.02 ng/mL (normal 0.00–0.09 ng/mL); the remainder of the patient's laboratory tests (electrolytes, creatinine and glucose) were within normal limits.

What is your diagnosis?

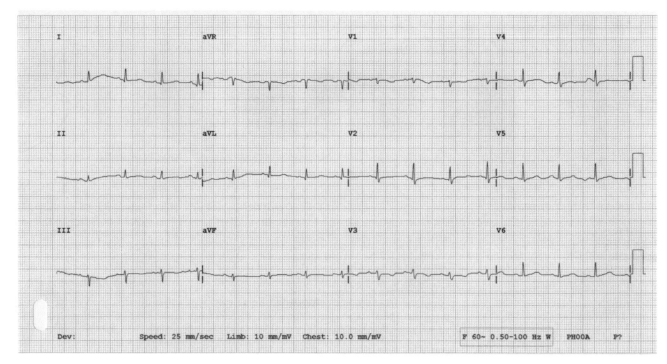

Figure 21.1 12-lead ECG from an 80-year-old female with cough and shortness of breath.

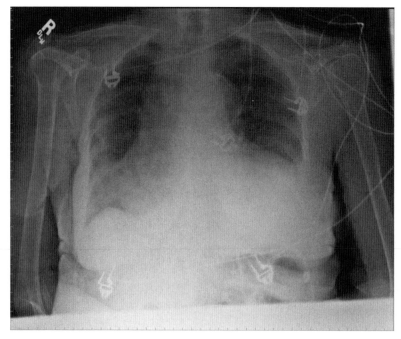

Figure 21.2 Portable chest radiograph from an 80-year-old female with cough and shortness of breath.

ANSWER

The diagnosis is Stanford type A aortic dissection. The ECG demonstrates a regular sinus rhythm, rate 93, with diffuse T-wave flattening. The portable chest radiograph shows a left base infiltrate or effusion, as well as an interstitial radiopacity in the right lower lung zone, cardiomegaly, and mediastinal widening. A CT angiogram of the chest was obtained to rule out pulmonary embolism (positive D-dimer), which subsequently demonstrated an aortic dissection extending from the aortic root into the ascending arch (Stanford type A), as well as a small pericardial effusion and bilateral pleural effusions (Figure 21.3). Dilatation of the ascending aorta was noted to be 5 cm maximally; the dissection flap did not definitively extend into the supra-arch vessels. The aortic arch caliber was noted to be 3 cm. The patient was admitted to the cardiothoracic surgery service for emergent repair of her aortic dissection. Intraoperative diagnosis was subacute Stanford type A aortic dissection with early cardiac tamponade.

Aortic dissection

Acute aortic dissection (AAD) is a cardiovascular emergency that requires prompt diagnosis and treatment. AAD usually occurs in the presence of hypertension. The condition arises as an intimal tear of the aorta; blood later dissects into the aortic media to form a false and true lumen.[1] Systemic hypertension is thought to be the most important predisposing factor.[2] Other acquired predisposing conditions include direct trauma, iatrogenic retrograde dissection from catheter-related aortic intimal injury and previous valvular, coronary bypass or aortic surgery. Cocaine use also predisposes to aortic dissection by the sudden increase in aortic wall stress created by catecholamine surge.[2] An unexplained relationship may exist between aortic dissection and pregnancy, with about half of all dissections in young women occurring

during pregnancy. In younger patients, inherited conditions such as Marfan syndrome, Ehlers-Danlos syndrome, bicuspid aortic valve, coarctation of the aorta and Turner syndrome predispose to AAD.[2] Depending on the study population, the incidence of AAD ranges from 5–30 cases per 1 million population per year.[3]

Aortic dissections are classified by the portion of the aorta involved. In the Stanford system, type A dissection involves the ascending aorta, either alone or with the descending aorta. Type B dissection is confined to the descending aorta.[4] In the DeBakey classification, type I dissection involves the entire aorta, type II dissection involves only the ascending aorta, and type III dissection involves only the descending aorta, sparing the ascending aorta and the arch.[2] Classification by site is important because it carries both therapeutic and prognostic significance. Dissections are also classified temporally as acute (present less than two weeks) and chronic (present longer than two weeks).[4] The majority of aortic dissections are acute.

The classic description of pain in AAD is the instantaneous onset of chest pain that is maximal at its onset and described as knife-like, ripping or tearing.[3] This presentation is often the exception rather than the rule. Sharp, knife-like or tearing pain is reported only in approximately 50% of patients.[3] Patients with dissections of the descending aorta more commonly report back pain rather than chest pain; patients with descending AADs are also more likely to report radiation of pain to the hips and legs. More than one-third of patients present with symptoms attributable to secondary organ involvement (e.g., neurologic symptoms, syncope, abdominal pain, gastrointestinal bleeding, dysphagia and hoarseness).[3]

In patients presenting with symptoms concerning for AAD, an ECG should be obtained to assess for cardiac ischemia. Although normal in only 30% of aortic dissections, there are no ECG findings pathognomonic for AAD.[4] The chest radiograph is abnormal in 85–90% of patients, with

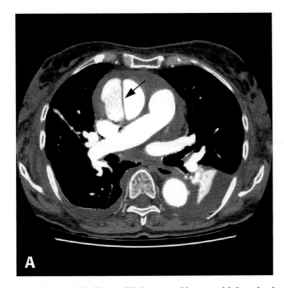
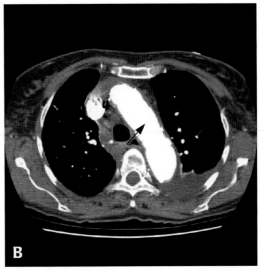

Figure 21.3 Chest CT from an 80-year-old female demonstrating Stanford type A aortic dissection (arrow, panel A) and dilated aortic arch (arrow, panel B).

mediastinal widening larger than 8 cm being the most common finding (occurs in 63% of type A dissections and 56% of type B dissections).[4] At most centers, helical CT has become the emergency imaging modality of choice, with diagnostic accuracy in the detection of AAD approaching 100%.[1,3] Although the sensitivity and specificity of MRI ranges from 95–100%, technical limitations (long study times, restricted patient access, restricted monitoring) limit its use in the emergent setting. Transesophageal echocardiography is an acceptable modality for diagnosing AAD (its reported sensitivity approaches 98%), particularly in unstable patients.[1,3]

The initial management of all patients with aortic dissection is medical, with aggressive heart rate and blood pressure control. In hypertensive patients, therapy begins with a betablocker (esmolol or metoprolol) with the goal of lowering the heart rate to 60 beats/minute. This is followed by the addition of a potent IV vasodilator such as nitroprusside, which is titrated to achieve a systolic pressure of 100–120 mmHg.[4] Proximal dissections (Stanford type A) are a surgical emergency, whereas type B dissections are usually managed nonoperatively.

von Kodolitsch et al. evaluated 250 patients in a prospective, observational study with acute chest pain, back pain or both and clinical suspicion of AAD in an attempt to identify independent predictors of AAD.[5] Aortic pain with immediate onset, a tearing or ripping character or both; mediastinal widening, aortic widening or both on chest radiography; and pulse differentials, blood pressure differentials or both ($p < 0.001$ for all) were identified as independent predictors of AAD. Probability of aortic dissection was low with absence of all three variables (7%), intermediate with isolated findings of aortic pain or mediastinal widening (31% and 39%, respectively), and high with isolated pulse or blood pressure differentials or any combination of the three variables ($\geq 83\%$). In this study, 4% of all aortic dissections were assigned to the low-probability group, 19% to the intermediate-probability group, and 77% to the high probability group.

Park et al. evaluated the clinical characteristics and outcomes of patients with painless AAD in a retrospective case record study.[6] Of 977 patients in the International Registry of Acute Aortic Dissection (IRAAD) database from 1997 to 2001, 63 (6.4%) had painless AAD (group 1) and 914 (93.6%) had painful AAD (group 2). Patients in group 1 were older than those in group 2 (mean age 66 vs. 61 years). Type A dissection was more frequent in group 1 (74.6% vs. 60.9%). Syn-cope (33.9% vs. 11.7%), congestive heart failure (19.7% vs. 3.9%), and stroke (11.3% vs. 4.7%) were more frequent presenting signs in group 1. Diabetes (10.2% vs. 4.0%), aortic aneurysm (29.5% vs. 13.1%), and prior cardiovascular surgery (48.1% vs. 19.7%) were also more common in group 1. In-hospital mortality was greater in group 1 (33.3% vs. 23.2%), especially due to type B dissection (43.8% vs. 10.4%), and the prevalence of aortic rupture was greater among patients with type B dissection in group 1 (18.8% vs. 5.9%).

KEY TEACHING POINTS

1. Acute aortic dissection is a vascular emergency that arises as an intimal tear of the aorta. Blood later dissects into the aortic media to form a false and true lumen.
2. In the Stanford classification system, type A dissection involves the ascending aorta, either alone or with the descending aorta; type B dissection is confined to the descending aorta.
3. Sharp, knife-like or tearing pain is reported only in approximately 50% of patients with AAD; other findings include abnormal chest radiography and pulse or blood pressure differentials between upper extremities.
4. Helical CT (in stable patients) and transesophageal echocardiography (in unstable patients) are the imaging modalities of choice for diagnosing aortic dissection.
5. Type A dissections are surgical emergencies, whereas type B dissections are generally managed nonoperatively (medical management with strict blood pressure control).

REFERENCES

[1] Jeudy J, Waite S, White CS. Nontraumatic thoracic emergencies. *Radiol Clin N Am* 2006;44:273–93.
[2] Kamalakannan D, Rosman HS, Eagle KA. Acute aortic dissection. *Crit Care Clin* 2007;44:779–800.
[3] Winters ME, Kluetz P, Zilberstein J. Back pain emergencies. *Med Clin N Am* 2006;90:505–23.
[4] Gupta R, Kaufman S. Cardiovascular emergencies in the elderly. *Emerg Med Clin N Am* 2006;24:339–70.
[5] von Kodolitsch Y, Schwartz AG, Nienaber CA. Clinical prediction rule of acute aortic dissection. *Arch Intern Med* 2000;160:2977–82.
[6] Park SW, Hutchinson S, Mehta RH, et al. Association of painless acute aortic dissection with increased mortality. *Mayo Clin Proc* 2004;79:1252–7.

22

Weakness, fatigue and shortness of breath in an 88-year-old male

HISTORY OF PRESENT ILLNESS

An 88-year-old male with a medical history significant for diabetes, hyperlipidemia, chronic kidney disease and hypothyroidism was brought to the ED by ambulance complaining for two weeks of worsening shortness of breath, fatigue and general body weakness. He denied chest pain, cough, fevers, abdominal pain, lightheadedness or dizziness. The patient reported a 10 lb (4.5 kg) weight gain over the last several months, and had noted some swelling of both legs during this period. The patient's medications included metformin, terazosin, lisinopril/hydrochlorothiazide, glipizide, levothyroxine and lovastatin. The patient denied tobacco or alcohol use.

PHYSICAL EXAMINATION

GENERAL APPEARANCE: The patient was sitting upright in no acute distress; he was noted to be slightly breathless while speaking, unable to complete full sentences.

VITAL SIGNS

Temperature	98.5°F (36.9°C)
Pulse	38 beats/minute
Blood pressure	182/90 mmHg
Respirations	20 breaths/minute
Oxygen saturation	94% on room air

HEENT: Unremarkable.

NECK: No jugular venous distension.

CARDIOVASCULAR: Regular, bradycardic rate without rubs, murmurs or gallops.

LUNGS: Bilateral rales at the bases without wheezes or rhonchi.

ABDOMEN: Soft, nontender, nondistended.

EXTREMITIES: 2+ pitting edema bilaterally.

NEUROLOGIC: Nonfocal.

A rhythm strip obtained from the paramedics was reviewed (Figure 22.1), and a 12-lead ECG was obtained (Figure 22.2). Laboratory test results included a troponin I of 0.08 ng/mL (normal 0.0–0.09 ng/mL), a brain natriuretic peptide (BNP) level of 560 pg/mL (normal <100 pg/mL), a creatinine of 1.5 mg/dL (normal <1.3 mg/dL), and a potassium of 5.6 mEq/L (normal 3.5–5.3 mEq/L). A chest radiograph was obtained (Figure 22.3).

What is your diagnosis?

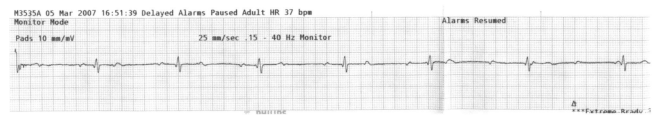

Figure 22.1 Rhythm strip from an 88-year-old male with weakness, fatigue and shortness of breath.

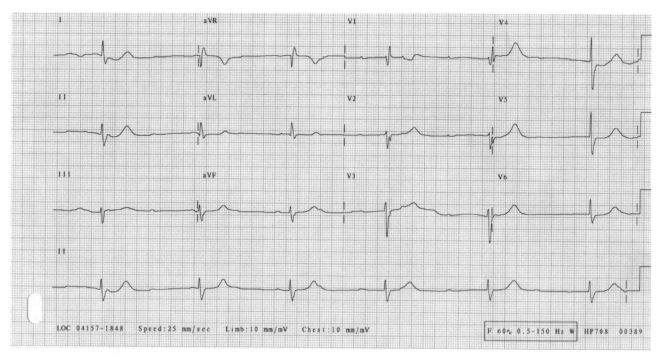

Figure 22.2 12-lead ECG from an 88-year-old male with weakness, fatigue and shortness of breath.

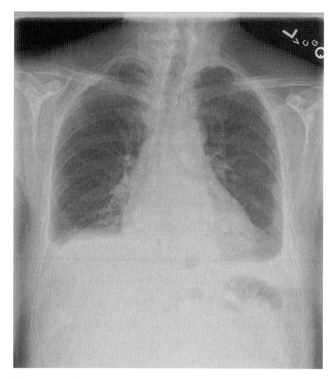

Figure 22.3 Chest radiograph of an 88-year-old male with weakness, fatigue and shortness of breath.

The diagnosis is third-degree heart block with congestive heart failure exacerbation. The rhythm strip and ECG show complete atrioventricular (AV) dissociation, whereas the chest radiograph demonstrates small bilateral pleural effusions with minimal pulmonary vascular congestion. Pacer pads were applied to the chest, and a cardiology consult was obtained in the ED. The patient was admitted to the medicine service for urgent placement of a permanent transvenous pacemaker.

Third-degree atrioventricular block

In third-degree heart block, also known as complete heart block, no atrial impulses reach the ventricle through the atrioventricular (AV) conduction system.[1,2] Therefore, the atria and ventricles are controlled by different pacemaker sites and function independently. The atrial pacemaker can be either sinus or ectopic. The ventricular escape rhythm can also have varying pacemaker sites, resulting in differing rates. Rarely, the ventricular escape rhythm is absent and the patient presents in asystole. More often, the site of escape is just below the level of the AV block.

The atrial rate is usually greater than the ventricular rate in patients with third-degree AV block. There is no meaningful relationship between the P waves and the QRS complexes. The P waves appear in a regular rhythm and "march" through the rhythm strip at a specific rate.[1,2] The QRS complexes should appear in a regular fashion, and generally also "march" through the rhythm strip. The duration of the QRS complex and the ventricular rate depend on the site of the block. When the ventricular escape rhythm is located near the His bundle, the rate is greater than 40 beats/minute and the QRS complexes tend to be narrow.[1,3] When the site of escape is distal to the His bundle, the rate tends to be less than 40 beats/minute and the QRS complexes tend to be wide.

Emergency management for patients in third-degree heart block should include special attention to the ABCs (airway, breathing and circulation), including supplemental oxygen, initiation of an intravenous line, frequent monitoring of blood pressure and continuous cardiac monitoring. AV-nodal blocking agents should be withheld, and transcutaneous pacing pads should be applied and tested when needed.[4] Patients in whom capture cannot be obtained with a transcutaneous pacemaker need urgent placement of a transvenous pacemaker, even if the patient is asymptomatic. Hemodynamically stable patients in whom transcutaneous pacing can be successfully performed can go to a telemetry bed or ICU at the discretion of the treating cardiologist. These patients, as with all patients in third-degree heart block, require placement of a permanent pacemaker.[5]

Hemodynamically unstable patients may be treated with atropine. However, if the rhythm is a wide complex escape rhythm, atropine is likely to be unsuccessful.[4] In addition, caution should be taken when administering atropine to a patient with a suspected acute MI, as the resulting vagolysis may lead to unopposed sympathetic stimulation. This can cause increased ventricular irritability and potentially dangerous ventricular dysrhythmias. Similarly, isoproterenol may accelerate a ventricular escape rhythm but has a low probability for efficacy. Hemodynamically unstable patients for whom timely cardiologic consultation is unavailable should undergo temporary transvenous pacemaker insertion in the ED if transcutaneous pacing or pharmacologic therapy are unsuccessful.

KEY TEACHING POINTS

1. In third-degree (complete) heart block, atrial impulses do not reach the ventricles through the AV conduction system.
2. Emergency management for patients in third-degree heart block includes special attention to the ABCs.
3. Patients in whom capture cannot be obtained with a transcutaneous pacemaker require urgent placement of a transvenous pacemaker, even if the patient is asymptomatic.
4. Hemodynamically unstable patients should be given atropine, dopamine, or possibly isoproterenol to increase the heart rate while a transcutaneous pacemaker is being initiated for pacing.
5. If a transcutaneous pacemaker does not capture and improve the hemodynamic status of unstable patients, a transvenous pacemaker should be emergently inserted in the ED.

REFERENCES

[1] Ufberg JW, Clark JS. Bradydysrhythmias and atrioventricular conduction blocks. *Emerg Med Clin N Am* 2006;24:1–9.

[2] Brady, WJ, Harrigan, RA. Atrioventricular block. In: Chan TC, Brady WJ, Harrigan RA, et al. (eds). *ECG in Emergency Medicine and Acute Care*. Philadelphia: Elsevier, 2005;86–8.

[3] Mangrum JM, DiMarco JP. The evaluation and management of bradycardia. *N Engl J Med* 2000;342:703–9.

[4] Levine, MD. Heart block, third degree. eMedicine Website. Available at http://www.emedicine.com/emerg/topic235.htm. Accessed June 30, 2008.

[5] Kusumoto, FM, Goldschlager, N. Medical progress: cardiac pacing. *N Engl J Med* 1996;334:89–98.

23

Sudden onset of back pain in a 91-year-old male

HISTORY OF PRESENT ILLNESS

A 91-year-old male with a medical history significant for borderline hypertension presented to the ED complaining of the sudden onset of severe back pain beginning one hour prior to arrival. He described the pain as sharp and radiating throughout his entire back, from his upper thoracic area to his lumbar region. The patient denied chest pain, dyspnea, focal weakness or numbness. He did not take any medications. The patient was active, participating in many sports and had been a Senior Olympic gold medalist in swimming. He did not smoke or drink alcohol.

PHYSICAL EXAMINATION

GENERAL APPEARANCE: The patient was an athletic, well-hydrated male who appeared to be in moderate discomfort.

VITAL SIGNS

Temperature	98.0°F (36.6°C)
Pulse	60 beats/minute
Blood pressure	220/110 mmHg
Respirations	22 breaths/minute
Oxygen saturation	98% on room air

HEENT: Unremarkable.

NECK: Supple, no jugular venous distension.

CARDIOVASCULAR: Regular rate and rhythm without rubs, murmurs or gallops.

LUNGS: Bibasilar rales, no wheezes or rhonchi.

ABDOMEN: Soft, nontender, nondistended, without pulsatile masses.

EXTREMITIES: No clubbing, cyanosis or edema; strong radial, femoral and dorsalis pedis pulses bilaterally.

NEUROLOGIC: Nonfocal.

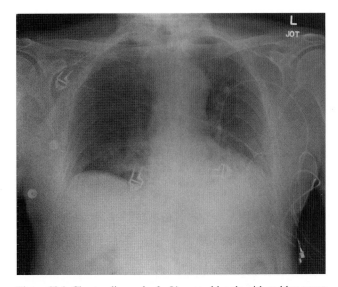

Figure 23.1 Chest radiograph of a 91-year-old male with sudden onset of sharp back pain.

The patient was placed on the cardiac monitor, a peripheral intravenous line was placed, and blood was drawn and sent for laboratory testing. Laboratory tests (including a complete blood count, electrolytes, creatinine, glucose and troponin I) were all within normal limits. A 12-lead ECG demonstrated a normal sinus rhythm, rate 55 beats/minute, without any acute ST-T wave changes. A portable chest radiograph was obtained (Figure 23.1).

What is your diagnosis?

ANSWER

The diagnosis is a descending thoracic aortic intramural hema-toma (Stanford type B). The chest radiograph demonstrates a widened mediastinum. A CT angiogram of the chest and abdomen was obtained, which demonstrated a hematoma of the arch and descending portion of the thoracic aorta, extend-ing into the abdominal aorta (Figure 23.2). No obvious dis-section or intimal flap was identified. A nitroglycerin drip for blood pressure control was started, which brought his blood pressure down to 130/60, and the patient was admitted to the ICU by cardiothoracic surgery for observation and close mon-itoring. The patient was pain-free upon admission to the ICU. He was discharged on hospital day #6 with continued medical management of his thoracic aortic intramural hematoma.

Aortic intramural hematomas

Intramural hematoma (IMH) of the aorta constitute 10–20% of acute aortic syndromes, with arterial hypertension the most frequent predisposing factor.[1] IMH is classified as Stanford type A (involving the ascending aorta or ascending and descending aorta) or Stanford type B (involving only the descending aorta), analogous to aortic dissection.[2] IMH of the aorta is considered a variant of acute aortic dissection, with hemorrhage within the wall of the aorta but lacking an intimal tear or visible flap.[2,3] This lack of an intimal tear suggests that the bleeding within the aortic wall likely comes from tearing of the small penetrating blood vessels (the vaso vasorum) of the aortic wall. Because there are no tears in the aortic lining, this localized hematoma has no Doppler flow seen on echocardio-gram and no enhancement with contrast administration on CT scan. However, in some cases IMH can rupture into the aortic lumen, creating an aortic dissection. IMH can also progress by rupturing outward into the adventitia or through the entire aortic wall, leading to aortic rupture.[3]

Chest radiography is of limited value for diagnosing acute aortic syndrome (aortic dissection, nondissecting aneurysm, intramural hematoma). In one study, board-certified radio-logists who were blinded to results from other diagnostic procedures re-evaluated the admission chest radiograph for patients admitted with aortic disease.[4] They evaluated each

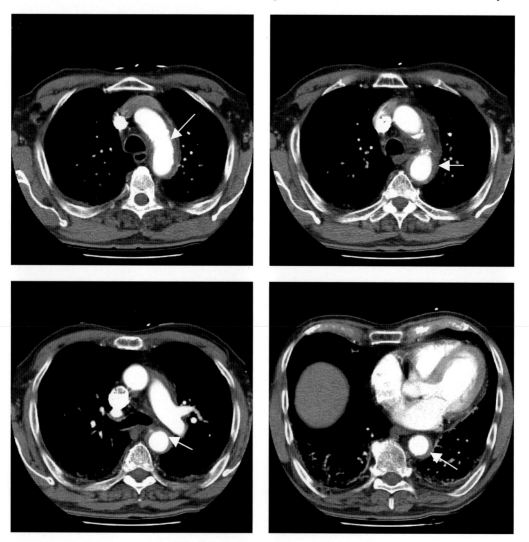

Figure 23.2 CT angiogram of the chest demonstrating IMH in the arch and descending thoracic aorta (arrows) in a 91-year-old male with sudden onset of sharp back pain.

radiograph for the presence or absence of seven radiographic features of aortic disease: continuous or hump-like widening of the aortic contour; widening of the mediastinal shadow; tracheal shift to the right or distortion of the left mainstem bronchus; displacement of intimal calcification greater than 6 mm into the aortic shadow; kinking or tortuosity of the aorta; opacification of the pulmonary window between the aortic knob and the left pulmonary artery; and blurring or double density of the aortic contour. Chest radiography had a sensitivity of 64% and a specificity of 86% for aortic disease. Sensitivity was 67% for overt aortic dissection, 61% for nondissecting aneurysm, and 63% for intramural hemorrhage or penetrating ulcer. Sensitivity was lower for pathology confined to the proximal aorta (47%) than for disease involving distal aortic segments (77%).[4]

On unenhanced chest CT, IMH is visible as a crescent of high-attenuation material within the aortic wall.[5] This rim of high attenuation represents acute bleeding into the aortic wall, occasionally involving the entire circumference of the aorta. Features reported as predictors that IMH will progress to overt dissection include the presence of penetrating atherosclerotic ulcer, greater maximum thickness of the hematoma, flattening of the true lumen so that the short-axis diameter is less than 75% of the long-axis diameter, involvement of the ascending aorta, and the presence of either pericardial or pleural effusions.[5] MRI allows detection of the age of the IMH, and may be useful to monitor IMH over time.

Emergency management of patients diagnosed with aortic IMH involves strict blood pressure control, pain management and urgent cardiothoracic surgery consultation. If surgery is not urgently indicated, these patients should be admitted to the ICU for close monitoring. Long-term management for aortic IMHs is similar to that for aortic dissection: surgical repair for type A hematomas and medical management for type B hematomas.[2] Although some authors have recommended medical management for type A IMHs, von Kodilitsch et al. found in a multicenter observational trial that early mortality was 8% in patients with type A hematoma who underwent prompt surgery versus 55% in those patients not receiving surgery.[6]

KEY TEACHING POINTS

1. Intramural hematoma (IMH) of the aorta constitutes 10–20% of acute aortic syndromes, with arterial hypertension the most frequent predisposing factor.
2. In some cases, IMH can rupture into the aortic lumen, creating an aortic dissection.
3. The diagnostic test of choice for diagnosing IMH is contrast-enhanced CT; MRI is useful to establish the age of the hematoma and to monitor IMH over time.
4. Emergency treatment of IMH involves analgesia, strict blood pressure control and urgent cardiothoracic surgical consultation.
5. Management for aortic IMH is similar to that for aortic dissection: surgical repair for type A hematomas and medical management for type B hematomas.

REFERENCES

[1] Tatli S, Yucel EK, Lipton, MJ. CT and MR images of the thoracic aorta: current techniques and clinical applications. *Radiol Clin N Am* 2004;42:565–85.

[2] Saborio DV, Sadeghi A, Burack JH, et al. Management of intramural hematoma of the ascending aorta and aortic arch: the risks of limited surgery (case report). *Tex Heart Inst J* 2003;30:325–7.

[3] Haro LH, Krajicek M, Lobl JK. Challenges, controversies, and advances in aortic catastrophes. *Emerg Med Clin N Am* 2005;23:1159–77.

[4] von Kodolitsch Y, Neinaber CA, Dieckmann C, et al. Chest radiography for the diagnosis of acute aortic syndrome. *Am J Med* 2004;116:73–7.

[5] Chiles C, Carr JJ. Vascular diseases of the thorax: evaluation with multidetector CT. *Radiol Clin N Am* 2005;43:543–69.

[6] von Kodolitsch Y, Csosz SK, Koschyk DH, et al. Intramural hematoma of the aorta: predictors of progression to dissection and rupture. *Circulation* 2003;107:1158–63.

PART III

PULMONOLOGY

24

Pleuritic chest pain in a 27-year-old male

HISTORY OF PRESENT ILLNESS

A 27-year-old male presented to the ED complaining of four days of worsening right-sided chest pain, described as sharp and worse on inspiration. The pain began suddenly four days prior following a severe coughing spell. He also described increased dyspnea but denied fevers, bloody sputum or recent trauma.

PHYSICAL EXAMINATION

GENERAL APPEARANCE: The patient was a moderately obese male in no acute distress, speaking full sentences.

VITAL SIGNS

Temperature	98.1°F (36.1°C)
Pulse	88 beats/minute
Blood pressure	120/80 mmHg
Respirations	24 breaths/minute
Oxygen saturation	96% on room air

HEENT: Unremarkable

NECK: Supple, no jugular venous distension, trachea midline.

CARDIOVASCULAR: Regular rate and rhythm without rubs, murmurs or gallops.

LUNGS: Absent breath sounds in the right lung field, breath sounds clear to auscultation in the left lung field.

ABDOMEN: Soft, nontender, nondistended.

EXTREMITIES: No clubbing, cyanosis or edema.

NEUROLOGIC: Nonfocal.

The patient was placed on a cardiac monitor, supplemental oxygen by nasal canula was administered and a peripheral intravenous line was placed. A chest radiograph was obtained (Figure 24.1), which demonstrated a complete right-sided

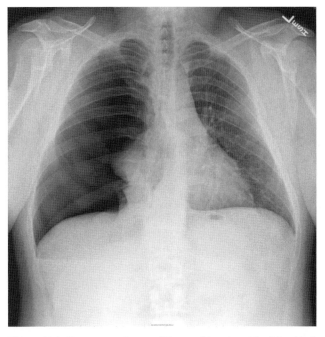

Figure 24.1 Chest x-ray from a 27-year-old male with right-sided, pleuritic chest pain, demonstrating complete right-sided pneumothorax.

pneumothorax. A Thoravent® (thoracic vent and Heimlich valve) was placed in the right anterior chest, which resulted in a large, rapid rush of air escaping the catheter. After approximately 20 minutes, the patient described a "wave-like" sensation running through his right chest and became acutely dyspneic, tachypneic and diaphoretic, with oxygen saturations dropping to 87% on 2 liters oxygen by nasal canula. A repeat portable chest radiograph was obtained (Figure 24.2).

What is your diagnosis?

ANSWER

The diagnosis is re-expansion pulmonary edema. The chest radiograph in Figure 24.2 demonstrates complete re-expansion of the collapsed right lung, with a fluffy opacity in the right lung field consistent with pulmonary edema. The patient was placed on high-flow oxygen by face mask, received IV furosemide and was admitted to the telemetry unit for observation and repeat chest radiograph the following morning. The patient had good diuresis from the Lasix® with improvement in his respiratory symptoms; his repeat chest radiograph demonstrated substantial clearing of the pulmonary edema without evidence of residual pneumothorax. He was discharged home much improved with the Thoravent® in place and instructions to follow up with thoracic surgery in five days. Repeat chest radiograph at that time showed no evidence of pneumothorax, and the Thoravent® was removed.

Re-expansion pulmonary edema

Re-expansion pulmonary edema (RPE) may develop in certain patients whose lung has been rapidly re-inflated after a period of collapse, such as from a pneumothorax or a pleural effusion.[1] Patients with RPE have various degrees of hypoxia and hypotension. The reported incidence of RPE ranges from 1–14%.[2] On rare occasions, the pulmonary edema is bilateral and the patient requires intubation and mechanical ventilation. Even more rarely, RPE can be fatal.

The risk factors for developing RPE include collapse of the affected lung for more than three days, large pneumothorax, negative pleural pressure suction of greater than 20 cm H_2O and rapid re-expansion.[2] The pathogenesis of RPE involves two main entities: alteration of capillary permeability and increased hydrostatic pressure.[3] Inflammatory mediators, such as neutrophils, IL-8 and leukotrienes, may play a role in the development of RPE. Similarly, re-oxygenation of the collapsed hypoxic lung may contribute to RPE through oxygen free-radical generation and leukocyte influx during re-expansion or re-oxygenation of the collapsed lung.[4]

Patients with RPE typically have coughing spells or chest tightness during or immediately after tube thoracostomy or thoracentesis. The symptoms usually progress for 12–24 hours and serial chest radiographs reveal progressive ipsilateral pulmonary edema, which may progress to involve the contralateral lung.[1] If the patient does not die within the first 48 hours, recovery is usually complete. Treatment is primarily supportive, with the administration of supplemental oxygen and diuretics; intubation and mechanical ventilation may be necessary.[1,3]

Measures to prevent development of RPE include slow evacuation of the pneumothorax with intermittent clamping.[2] An alternative to this may be simple repetitive aspiration of less than 1000 mL air and the avoidance of negative pressure suction. Routine supplemental oxygen and hydration

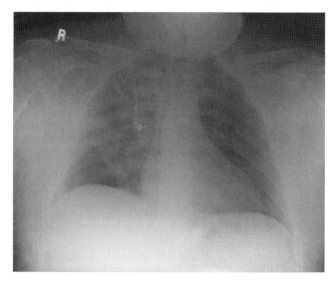

Figure 24.2 Chest x-ray from a 27-year-old male shortly after right chest wall Thoravent® placement for right-sided pneumothorax.

before chest tube thoracostomy should be performed for large pneumothoraces.[2] Finally, chest tube thoracostomy or thoracentesis should be terminated if the patient develops tightness of the chest or experiences coughing, as these symptoms may indicate the development of RPE.[1,3]

KEY TEACHING POINTS

1. Re-expansion pulmonary edema (RPE) can occur in patients whose lung has been rapidly re-inflated after a period of collapse (usually more than 72 hours) secondary to a pneumothorax or pleural effusion.
2. The risk factors for developing RPE include collapse of the affected lung for more than three days, large pneumothorax, negative pleural pressure suction of greater than 20 cm H_2O and rapid lung re-expansion.
3. Patients with RPE typically have coughing spells or chest tightness during or immediately after tube thoracostomy or thoracentesis.
4. The symptoms of RPE usually progress for 12–24 hours; serial chest radiographs reveal progressive ipsilateral pulmonary edema, which may progress to involve the contralateral lung.
5. Treatment of RPE is primarily supportive with the administration of supplemental oxygen and diuretics, and intubation and mechanical ventilation when necessary.

REFERENCES

[1] Light RW, Lee YCG. Pneumothorax, chylothorax, hemothorax, and fibrothorax. In: Mason RJ, Murray JF, Broaddus VC, et al. (eds). *Murray and Nadel's Textbook of Respiratory Medicine*, 4th ed. Philadelphia: Elsevier, 2005:1507–8.

[2] Beng ST, Mahadevan M. An uncommon life-threatening complication after chest tube drainage of pneumothorax in the ED. *Am J Emerg Med* 2004;22:615–9.

[3] Genofre EH, Vargas FS, Teixeira LR, et al. Reexpansion pulmonary edema. *J Pneumol* 2003;29:101–6.

[4] Her C, Mandy S. Acute respiratory distress syndrome of the contralateral lung after reexpansion pulmonary edema of a collapsed lung. *J Clin Anesth* 2004;16:244–50.

25

Acute onset of shortness of breath in a 30-year-old female

HISTORY OF PRESENT ILLNESS

A 30-year-old female presented to the ED complaining of acute onset shortness of breath and a sensation of her heart pounding approximately five hours prior to presentation. The patient was seen in the orthopedics clinic earlier in the day for a right knee injury she sustained playing soccer two weeks previously. Shortly after the injury, she was placed in a right knee brace, which she had been wearing for the past two weeks. The patient was discharged from the clinic with the diagnosis of possible right anterior cruciate ligament tear, and was instructed to continue wearing her brace until her scheduled return to the clinic one week following an outpatient MRI.

The patient reported that upon leaving the orthopedic clinic, she began to experience difficulty breathing, made worse with exertion, as well as the sensation of her heart pounding. She denied chest pain, recent cough, fevers or abdominal pain. She did feel lightheaded, and experienced nausea and vomited three times. She had noted significant swelling to her right knee that had not dissipated since the injury, as well as some swelling to her shin and calf. The patient had no significant medical issues; her only medication was oral contraceptives. She drank alcohol and smoked cigarettes on occasion, and denied any illicit drug use.

PHYSICAL EXAMINATION

GENERAL APPEARANCE: The patient appeared short of breath, diaphoretic and somewhat anxious.

VITAL SIGNS

Temperature	97.4°F (36.3°C)
Pulse	120 beats/minute
Blood pressure	146/54 mmHg
Respirations	24 breaths/minute
Oxygen saturation	96% on room air

HEENT: Unremarkable.

NECK: Supple, no jugular venous distension.

CARDIOVASCULAR: Tachycardic rate, regular rhythm without rubs, murmurs or gallops.

LUNGS: Clear to auscultation bilaterally without rales, rhonchi or wheezes.

ABDOMEN: Soft, nontender, nondistended.

RECTAL: Normal tone, brown stool, hemoccult negative.

RIGHT LOWER EXTREMITY: Swelling and moderate effusion of the knee, as well as mild swelling of the anterior shin and calf; tenderness to the anterior knee just below patella, anterior drawer sign noted, no popliteal mass. Dorsalis pedis pulse palpable.

NEUROLOGIC: Nonfocal.

The patient was placed on the cardiac monitor, 2 liters oxygen by nasal cannula was administered, a peripheral intravenous line was placed, and blood was drawn and sent for laboratory testing. A 12-lead ECG (Figure 25.1) and portable AP chest radiograph (Figure 25.2) were obtained. Laboratory tests revealed a troponin I of 2.15 ng/mL (normal 0.00–0.09 ng/mL), leukocyte count of 16.3 K/µL (normal 3.5–12.5 K/µL) with 88% neutrophils (normal 50–70%), and hematocrit of 45%. The serum pregnancy test was negative, the glucose returned at 193 mg/dL (normal 60–159 mg/dL) and the remainder of the electrolytes and creatinine were within normal limits.

Shortly after beginning the ED evaluation, the patient began complaining of sharp, substernal chest pain, made worse by deep inspiration. Her respiratory rate increased to 32 breaths/minute and her oxygen saturation declined to 92% on 2 liters nasal cannula, at which time she was placed on a 100% non-rebreather mask. Approximately one and a half hours after arrival in the ED, her blood pressure dropped to 88/54 mmHg despite receiving a 1-liter normal saline bolus intravenously.

What is your diagnosis?

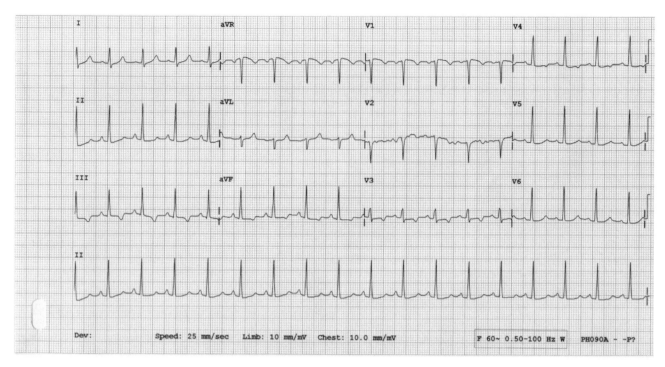

Figure 25.1 12-lead ECG from a 30-year-old female with acute onset shortness of breath.

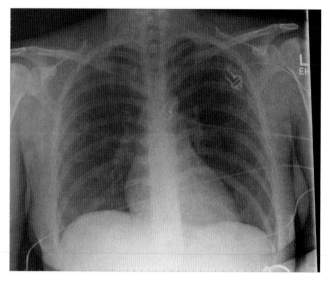

Figure 25.2 Anteroposterior chest radiograph from a 30-year-old female with acute onset shortness of breath.

ANSWER

The diagnosis is bilateral pulmonary emboli. The ECG in Figure 25.1 demonstrates sinus tachycardia, rate 110 beats/minute, with inverted T waves in leads III, aVF, V_3 and V_4. The chest radiograph in Figure 25.2 is normal. A CT angiogram (CTA) of the chest was ordered along with the initial laboratory tests as the patient was determined to be at high risk for pulmonary embolism. The patient initially received enoxaparin 1 mg/kg subcutaneously around the time her blood pressure began to drop, and a second peripheral IV was obtained. At the same time, as her blood pressure failed to improve following a second liter NS bolus, a dopamine infusion was started at 5 μg/kg/min, titrated to 10 μg/kg/min with improvement of her blood pressure to 104/68 (pulse 112 beats/minute). Once the patient's hemodynamic status improved slightly, she was transported to the CT scanner with a nurse, emergency physician and intubation equipment.

The resulting CTA demonstrated large bilateral pulmonary emboli (Figure 25.3). Upon return from the CT scanner, the intensivist was consulted and a decision was made to discontinue the dopamine drip and begin Levophed® at 2 μg/min, titrating to maintain systolic blood pressure at 90–100 mmHg. An arterial blood gas obtained on a 100% non-rebreather mask revealed a pH of 7.27 (normal 7.35–7.45), pCO_2 of 35 mmHg (normal 35–45 mmHg), pO_2 of 60 mmHg (normal 80–95 mmHg) and bicarbonate of 16.2 mmol/L (normal 23–28 mmol/L). A decision was made to administer thrombolytics, and an infusion of tissue plasminogen activator (t-PA) was given at 50 mg/hour IV over 2 hours (total 100 mg t-PA). At the completion of the t-PA infusion, the patient's vital signs demonstrated a pulse of 79 beats/minute, blood pressure of 110/76 and respirations of 26 breaths/minute, with an oxygen saturation of 100% on 15 L oxygen by non-rebreather mask. The Levophed® drip was discontinued and the patient was transferred to the ICU.

A repeat 12-lead ECG performed the following morning in the ICU demonstrated resolution of the T-wave inversions noted on the initial ECG (Figure 25.4). Doppler ultrasound of the right leg on hospital day #2 revealed a noncompressible, occlusive thrombus in the distal right superficial femoral vein with extension into the popliteal vein.

Pulmonary embolism

INCIDENCE AND ETIOLOGY: Although the exact incidence of pulmonary embolism (PE) is uncertain, it is estimated that 600,000 episodes occur each year in the United States, resulting in 100,000 to 200,000 deaths.[1] When the diagnosis of PE is confirmed and effective therapy is initiated, recurrence of PE is rare and death is uncommon – with the exception of patients who initially present with hemodynamic impairment, among whom the mortality approaches 30%.[1] The majority of preventable deaths associated with PE can be ascribed to a missed diagnosis rather than to a failure of existing therapies.

Most PEs arise from deep veins of the leg. Although deep vein thrombosis (DVT) starts in calf veins, it has already propagated above the knee in 87% of symptomatic patients before the diagnosis is made.[2] Thrombosis in the veins is triggered by venostasis, hypercoagulability and vessel wall inflammation, known as Virchow's triad.[2] All known clinical risk factors for DVT and PE have their basis in one or more elements of this triad. These risk factors include previous DVT or PE, recent surgery, prolonged immobilization, inherited forms of hypercoagulability (e.g., antiphospholipid syndrome, Factor V Leiden deficiency), advanced age, malignancy, pregnancy, congestive heart failure, use of contraceptives/hormone replacement therapy, and long air (or land) travel.[3,4]

PE ranges from incidental, clinically unimportant thromboembolism to massive embolism with sudden death. As thrombi form in the deep veins of the leg, pelvis or arms, they may dislodge and embolize to the pulmonary arteries

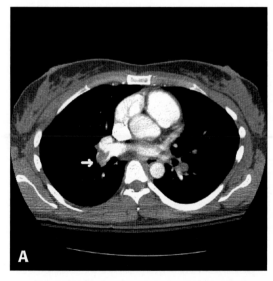
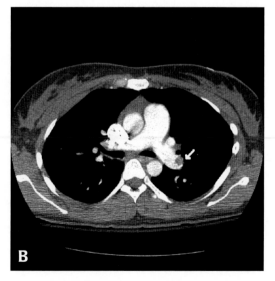

Figure 25.3 CTA from a 30-year-old female with acute dyspnea, demonstrating large right (arrow, panel A) and left (arrow, panel B) pulmonary emboli.

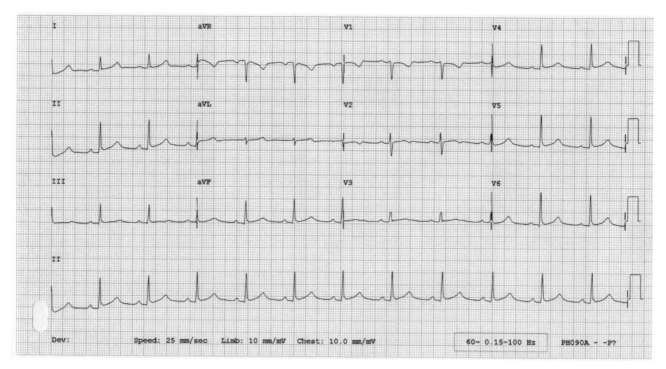

Figure 25.4 12-lead ECG obtained from a 30-year-old female following treatment with t-PA for bilateral pulmonary emboli.

with potentially serious consequences.[5] Pulmonary arterial obstruction and the release by platelets of vasoactive agents such as serotonin elevate pulmonary vascular resistance. The resulting increase in alveolar dead space and redistribution of blood flow (which creates areas of decreased ventilation to perfusion) impair gas exchange; stimulation of irritant receptors causes alveolar hyperventilation.[2] Reflex bronchoconstriction augments airway resistance. As right ventricular afterload increases, tension rises in the right ventricular wall and may lead to dilatation, dysfunction and ischemia of the right ventricle.[2]

SIGNS AND SYMPTOMS: Symptoms that should invoke suspicion of PE include chest pain, shortness of breath, chest wall tenderness, back pain, shoulder pain, upper abdominal pain, syncope, hemoptysis, painful respirations, new onset wheezing, any new cardiac dysrhythmia or other unexplained symptom referable to the thorax.[2] Apprehension or anxiety are also common symptoms in patients with PE. The classic findings of hemoptysis, dyspnea and chest pain are neither sensitive nor specific for the diagnosis of PE; fewer than 20% of patients with documented PE have this "classic triad."[3] Chest pain from noninfarcting PE can be highly variable and vague; as high as 30% of patients with definite PE deny any perception of chest pain.[6] Patients presenting with PE frequently complain of dyspnea. Physical signs that should raise the clinical suspicion of PE include tachypnea, tachycardia, rales, fever, lower extremity edema, a cardiac murmur, S3 or S4, cyanosis, hypotension and neck vein distention.[2,3]

Despite its shortcomings as a single diagnostic step, the presence of hypoxemia (pulse oximetry less than 95% breathing room air) that cannot be explained by a known disease process increases the probability of PE.[6] Conversely, lack of hypoxemia can be used with other criteria to justify not pursuing further evaluation for PE. Additionally, when PE is diagnosed the severity of hypoxemia represents a powerful independent predictor of patient outcome.[6]

Wells et al. have published, refined and internally validated a clinical decision rule for pre-test probability of PE.[7–10] Wells Criteria for pre-test probability of PE consist of seven weighted criteria (Table 25.1). Summation of these point values can be trichotomized into low (less than 2 points), moderate (2–6 points) or high (more than 6 points) pre-test probabilities, with prevalences for PE of 2–4%, 19–21% and 50–67%, respectively. Alternatively, a total score can be dichotomized

TABLE 25.1 Wells clinical prediction rule for pulmonary embolism

Clinical feature	Points
Clinical symptoms of DVT	3
Other diagnosis less likely than PE	3
Pulse >100 beats/minute	1.5
Immobilization or surgery within previous 4 weeks	1.5
Previous DVT or PE	1.5
Hemoptysis	1
Malignancy treated within past 6 months or palliative	1

into a PE-unlikely (less than or equal to 4 points) or PE-likely (more than 4 points) pre-test probabilities, with prevalences for PE of 5–8% and 39–41%, respectively.[7,8,10]

DIAGNOSTIC TESTS: ECG, chest radiography and arterial blood gas (ABG) analysis have limited roles in the evaluation of PE. The primary utility of ECG is its ability to point to an alternate diagnosis, such as acute coronary syndrome or pericarditis.[3] Sinus tachycardia is a common ECG finding in patients with PE. The most frequent electrocardiographic abnormality is T-wave inversion in the anterior leads, especially leads V_1 to V_4 (found in 68% of patients with PE).[3,5] The classic finding of $S_1Q_3T_3$ lacks sensitivity and specificity (54% and 62%, respectively).[3] New right-bundle branch block or atrial fibrillation may be seen but is uncommon.[5]

Chest radiography seldom provides specific information, but may be useful to suggest alternative diagnoses such as pneumonia, congestive heart failure or pneumothorax.[6] Unilateral basilar atelectasis increases the probability of PE. If symptoms have been present three days or more, pulmonary infarction sometimes shows an apex-central, pleural-based, wedge-shaped area of infiltrate ("Hampton's hump").[6] Unilateral lung oligemia (Westermark's sign) is a rare radiographic manifestation of a large PE. ABG analysis has a limited role in the evaluation of PE. The pO_2 on ABG analysis has a zero or even negative predictive value in a typical population of patients in whom PE is suspected.[2] It is a relatively invasive procedure that lacks the sensitivity or specificity to rule in or out disease.[3]

The measurement of the degradation products of cross-linked fibrin (D-dimer) circulating in plasma is a highly sensitive but nonspecific screening test for suspected venous thromboembolism (VTE).[1] Specificity is known to be low secondary to false-positive results from numerous causes, such as trauma, postoperative state, sepsis and myocardial infarction.[3] It is also less likely to be helpful in elderly patients or patients with significant co-morbid disease. The role of D-dimer generally has been reserved for ruling out PE or VTE in low-risk patients.[3,5] Wells et al. found that patients with a low clinical probability of VTE and a negative D-dimer assay could be discharged safely without further workup for PE, with only 0.4% found to have VTE on follow-up examination.[11]

Troponin I levels may be useful in predicting in-hospital mortality in acute PE. La Vecchia et al. carried out a prospective clinical trial to assess the prevalence of cTnI positivity at various cut-off concentrations, and to evaluate the impact of increases on prognosis in a cohort of patients without known coronary artery disease.[12] Their data indicated that an increased cTnI concentration is associated with increased disease severity. Increases were also associated with significantly more extensive and proximal involvement of the pulmonary vasculature as assessed by spiral CT; many of the clinical parameters of these patients (oxygen saturation, blood pressure, heart rate, echocardiographic right ventricular abnormalities and estimated pulmonary artery pressure elevations)

also suggested a more severe clinical profile. According to the authors, these findings support a link between the degree of troponin increase and the severity of clinical presentation.[12]

Most pulmonary emboli arise from the deep veins of the legs. Ultrasonography is positive in 10–20% of patients without leg symptoms or signs who undergo evaluation, and in approximately 50% of patients with proven PE.[1,13] Therefore, the possibility of PE cannot be ruled out on the basis of negative ultrasonography.[1] Moreover, positive ultrasonographic findings in patients without symptoms or signs referable to the legs should be interpreted with caution. Because ultrasonographic studies may be falsely positive or may detect residual abnormalities related to previous VTE, only positive studies with appropriate clinical circumstances should serve as the basis for initiating therapy.

Ventilation-perfusion (V/Q) scanning is a valuable tool in diagnosing PE when the results are definitive.[1] A normal V/Q scan essentially rules out PE, and a high-probability scan for PE is strongly associated with its presence. Whereas normal results or results indicating a high probability of disease are extremely helpful, nondiagnostic results are difficult to interpret and much more common.[5] Rarely does the ventilation scanning clarify the interpretation of perfusion lung scans. Furthermore, in the presence of a high index of clinical suspicion, results of lung scanning indicating a low probability of PE may inadvertently steer clinicians away from the correct diagnosis. Such results should instead be interpreted as nondiagnostic.[5]

Most hospitals now employ CT angiography (CTA) as the primary method for evaluating PE.[6] Images can be obtained in a few seconds, so the time required for the test primarily depends upon scanner availability, transport time and radiologist interpretation time. For the most part, the radiologist indicates the test is positive or negative, similar to results of conventional catheter-based pulmonary angiography.[6] This binary output makes CTA easier to interpret and integrate into medical decision-making, compared with the "probability" result of V/Q scanning. In the case of CTA, the legs can also be scanned (CT venogram, or CTV), which allows evaluation for DVT. More recently, multidetector CTA-CTV has been shown to have a higher diagnostic sensitivity than CTA alone (90% vs. 83%, respectively), with a similar specificity (95% vs. 96%, respectively).[13]

In hemodynamically unstable patients with large pulmonary emboli, echocardiography (ECHO) is useful because it is noninvasive, can be performed at the bedside, can assist in the recognition and differentiation of PE and is capable of assessing the severity of the PE and the patient's response to therapy.[14] Although predominantly employed to characterize the presence and the extent of right ventricular pressure overload, transthoracic ECHO (TTE) or transesophageal ECHO (TEE) may detect emboli in transit or may provide alternative diagnoses, such as aortic dissection, pericardial disease, hypovolemia, myocardial dysfunction or infarction, and valvular insufficiency. ECHO also may be helpful in identifying

PE patients with a patent foramen ovale (PFO), which has been associated with increased mortality, ischemic stroke and a complicated course.[14]

Ryu et al. provide a diagnostic algorithm for suspected PE that incorporates clinical suspicion, D-dimer level and radiologic testing.[15,16] If the suspicion for PE is low, a normal D-dimer level can exclude the diagnosis. If clinical suspicion is moderate to high (or the D-dimer is positive), the authors suggest CTA is an appropriate diagnostic approach. When contrast is contraindicated, V/Q scanning and sonography of the lower extremities are options. Pulmonary angiography should be considered if the results of the CTA are inadequate and the suspicion for PE remains high.[15,16]

TREATMENT OF PULMONARY EMBOLISM: Traditionally, the treatment of both PE and DVT had been anticoagulation with unfractionated heparin and initiation of long-term oral anticoagulation with Vitamin K antagonists, such as warfarin. However, data published over the last decade indicates that treatment with low-molecular-weight heparin (LMWH) is superior to treatment with unfractionated heparin.[4,17,18] Treatment with Vitamin K antagonists should be initiated concurrently with LMWH and continued until the International Normalized Ratio (INR) is stable (between 2.0 and 3.0).[4] In patients who have severe chronic kidney disease, LMWH should not be used because of its renal clearance and the potential for bleeding complications. More recently, fondaparinux (Arixtra®) has been approved for the treatment of PE. Fondaparinux is a synthetic antithrombotic agent with specific anti-factor Xa activity. Its pharmacologic properties allow for a simple, fixed-dose, once daily regimen of subcutaneous injection without the need for monitoring.[19] Fondaparinux has been shown to be at least as effective and safe as intravenous unfractionated heparin in the treatment of hemodynamically stable patients with PE.[19] For hemodynamically unstable patients with PE, thrombolytic therapy is uniformly acknowledged as the treatment of choice.[14]

THROMBOLYSIS FOR MASSIVE PULMONARY EMBOLISM: The principal criterion to characterize acute PE as massive is systemic arterial hypotension.[20] Despite anticoagulation, the mortality rate doubles for submassive PE patients with preserved systemic arterial pressure and right ventricular dysfunction. The mortality rate is even greater in patients who present with profound hypotension due to massive PE.[20] Primary therapy with fibrinolysis or embolectomy is generally considered for patients presenting with either massive or submassive PE.[21] The U.S. Food and Drug Administration has approved t-PA (alteplase) 100 mg administered as a continuous infusion over two hours for the fibrinolysis of massive PE.[21] Every patient being considered for fibrinolysis requires meticulous screening for contraindications because the risk of intracranial hemorrhage (ICH) may be as high as 3%. Although fibrinolysis is generally considered to be a lifesaving intervention in patients with massive PE, the extent of the clinical benefit remains unclear.[20] In a recent analysis of

the International Cooperative Pulmonary Embolism Registry (ICOPER) data, fibrinolytics did not reduce the rate of mortality or recurrent PE at 90 days.[20] In submassive PE, the Management Strategies and Prognosis of Pulmonary Embolism-3 Trial (MAPPET-3) demonstrated a reduction in the need for escalation of therapy among patients receiving alteplase.[22]

The management of patients with acute massive PE who do not respond to fibrinolytic therapy remains unclear. In the setting of PE, the recovery of right ventricular function is an early marker of thrombolysis efficacy, as well as a predictor of in-hospital course.[23] Furthermore, residual pulmonary vascular obstruction (more than 30% at 10 days) after thrombolytic therapy is associated with adverse outcomes and increased long-term mortality.[24] Meneveau et al. compared rescue surgical embolectomy and repeat thrombolysis in patients who did not respond to thrombolysis for massive PE.[23] In 40 nonresponders, rescue surgical embolectomy led to a better in-hospital course when compared with repeat thrombolysis in patients with massive PE.[23]

KEY TEACHING POINTS

1. The classic findings of hemoptysis, dyspnea and chest pain are neither sensitive nor specific for a diagnosis of PE; fewer than 20% present with this "classic" triad.

2. Thirty percent of patients with definite PE deny any perception of chest pain.

3. Wells Criteria for determining the pre-test probability of PE are useful in stratifying patients into low, medium or high-risk likelihoods of PE.

4. ECG, chest radiography and ABG analysis each have limited roles in the evaluation of PE.

5. D-dimer is a useful test to rule out PE in low-risk patients.

6. Most hospitals employ CTA as the primary method of evaluation for PE, with multidetector CTA-CTV demonstrating even greater sensitivity than conventional CTA for diagnosing PE.

7. Stable patients with PE should be treated with either low-molecular-weight heparin or fondaparinux (Arixtra®) while warfarin is initiated and reaching therapeutic levels.

8. Unstable patients with major pulmonary emboli should be treated with thrombolytic therapy (t-PA, 100 mg intravenous infusion over two hours) and admitted to the ICU.

REFERENCES

[1] Fedullo PF, Tapson VF. The evaluation of suspected pulmonary embolism. *N Engl J Med* 2003;349:1247–56.

[2] Feied C, Handler JA. Pulmonary embolism. eMedicine Website. Available at http://www.emedicine.com/emerg/topic490.htm. Accessed on June 25, 2008.

[3] Laack TA, Goyal DG. Pulmonary embolism: an unsuspected killer. *Emerg Med Clin N Am* 2004;22:961–83.

[4] Rogers RL. Venous thromboembolic disease in the elderly patient: atypical, subtle, and enigmatic. *Clin Geriatr Med* 2007;23:413–23.

[5]   Goldhaber SZ. Medical progress: pulmonary embolism. *N Engl J Med* 1998;339:93–104.

[6]   Kline JA, Runyon MS. Pulmonary embolism and deep vein thrombosis. In: Marx JA, Hockberger RS, Walls RM, et al. (eds). *Rosen's Emergency Medicine: Concepts and Clinical Practice*, 6th ed. Philadelphia: Mosby, 2006:1371–81.

[7]   Wells PS, Ginsberg JS, Anderson DR, et al. Use of a clinical model for safe management of patients with suspected pulmonary embolism. *Ann Intern Med* 1998;129:997–1005.

[8]   Wells PS, Anderson DR, Rodger M, et al. Derivation of a simple clinical model to categorize patients' probability of pulmonary embolism: increasing the model's utility with the SimpliRED D-dimer. *Thromb Haemost* 2000;83:416–20.

[9]   Wells PS, Anderson DR, Rodger M, et al. Excluding pulmonary embolism at the bedside without diagnostic imaging: management of patients with suspected pulmonary embolism presenting to the emergency department by using a simple clinical model and D-dimer. *Ann Intern Med* 2001;135:98–107.

[10] Wolf SJ, McCubbin TR, Feldhaus KM, et al. Prospective validation of Wells criteria in the evaluation of patients with suspected pulmonary embolism. *Ann Emerg Med* 2004;44:503–10.

[11] Wells PS, Anderson DR, Rodger M, et al. Evaluation of D-dimer in the diagnosis of suspected deep-vein thrombosis. *N Engl J Med* 2003;349:1227–35.

[12] La Vecchia L, Ottani F, Favero L, et al. Increased cardiac troponin I on admission predicts in-hospital mortality in acute pulmonary embolism. *Heart* 2004;90:633–7.

[13] Stein PD, Fowler SE, Goodman LR, et al. Multidetector tomography for acute pulmonary embolism. *N Engl J Med* 2006;354:2317–27.

[14] Wood KE. Major pulmonary embolism: review of a pathophysiologic approach to the golden hour of hemodynamically significant pulmonary embolism. *Chest* 2002;121:877–905.

[15] Ryu JH, Swensen SJ, Olson EJ, et al. Diagnosis of pulmonary embolism with use of computed tomographic angiography. *Mayo Clin Proc* 2001;76:59–65.

[16] Makkar S. Tips from other journals: diagnostic approaches to possible pulmonary embolism. *Am Fam Physician* 2001; 64:841.

[17] van Dongen CJJ, Van Den Belt AGM, Prins MH, et al. Fixed dose subcutaneous low molecular weight heparins versus adjusted dose unfractionated heparin for venous thromboembolism. *Cochrane Database Syst Rev* 2004;4:CD001100. DOI:10.1002/14651858.

[18] Quinlan D, McQuillan A, Eikelboom J. Low-molecular-weight heparin compared with intravenous unfractionated heparin for treatment of pulmonary embolism: a meta-analysis of randomized, controlled trials. *Ann Intern Med* 2004;140:175–83.

[19] Buller HR, Davidson BL, Decousus H, et al. Subcutaneous fondaparinux versus intravenous unfractionated heparin in the initial treatment of pulmonary embolism. *N Engl J Med* 2003;349:1695–702.

[20] Kucher N, Rossi E, De Rosa M, et al. Massive pulmonary embolism. *Circulation* 2006;113:577–82.

[21] Piazza G, Goldhaber SZ. Acute pulmonary embolism. Part II: Treatment and prophylaxis. *Circulation* 2006;114:e42–7.

[22] Konstantinides S, Geibel A, Heusel G, et al. Heparin plus alteplase compared with heparin alone in patients with submassive pulmonary embolism. *N Engl J Med* 2002;347:1143–50.

[23] Meneveau N, Seronde MF, Blonde MC, et al. Management of unsuccessful thrombolysis in acute massive pulmonary embolism. *Chest* 2006;129:1043–50.

[24] Meneveau N, Ming LP, Seronde MF, et al. In-hospital and long-term outcome after sub-massive and massive pulmonary embolism submitted to thrombolytic therapy. *Eur Heart J* 2003;24:1447–54.

26

Recurrent pneumonias in a 37-year-old male

HISTORY OF PRESENT ILLNESS

A 37-year-old male a with medical history significant for sleep apnea and hydrocephalus (diagnosed as a child with placement of a ventriculoatrial shunt) presented to the ED complaining of nausea, vomiting, diarrhea and fevers for one day. He denied chest pain, shortness of breath or cough. He was initially seen in a medical clinic and received IV hydration and promethazine with improvement of his symptoms. However, he remained tachycardic and his oxygen saturation on room air was 93% while lying flat, improving to 97% on sitting upright. He was transferred to the ED for further evaluation and treatment.

PHYSICAL EXAMINATION

GENERAL APPEARANCE: The patient appeared well nourished, well hydrated and in no acute respiratory distress.

VITAL SIGNS

Temperature	99°F (37.2°C)
Pulse	108 beats/minute
Blood pressure	110/70 mmHg
Respirations	26 breaths/minute
Oxygen saturation	96% on room air

HEENT: Unremarkable.

NECK: Supple, no jugular venous distension.

CARDIOVASCULAR: Tachycardic rate, regular rhythm without rubs, murmurs or gallops.

LUNGS: Scattered rhonchi, no rales or wheezes.

ABDOMEN: Soft, nontender, nondistended.

EXTREMITIES: No clubbing, cyanosis or edema.

NEUROLOGIC: Nonfocal.

In the ED, the patient received an albuterol nebulizer treatment, a 1-liter normal saline IV bolus and an additional dose of promethazine. A chest radiograph was obtained (Figure 26.1). Following treatment, his heart rate improved to 95 beats/minute with oxygen saturation on room air improving to 97%. At time of ED discharge, he was able to tolerate fluids and ambulate without problems. His presumptive discharge diagnosis was acute gastroenteritis.

The patient returned to the ED 24 hours later with persistent vomiting, shortness of breath, dry cough, fevers and fatigue. A repeat chest radiograph demonstrated an opacification at the right lung base as well as a small, right-sided pleural effusion (Figure 26.2). The patient was given IV antibiotics (moxifloxacin) and admitted for pneumonia. His blood cultures were negative during this hospitalization. The patient was re-admitted to the hospital on two more occasions over two consecutive months, with the diagnosis of unresolving versus recurrent pneumonias. During the second hospitalization, his blood cultures grew out *Serratia marcescens*.

What is your diagnosis?

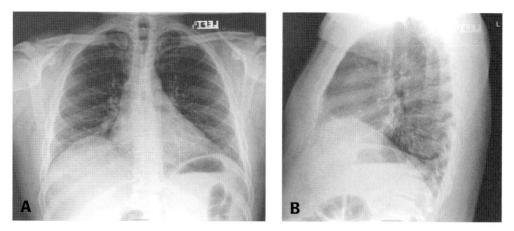

Figure 26.1 Posteroanterior (panel A) and lateral (panel B) chest radiograph from a 37-year-old male with nausea, vomiting, diarrhea and fevers for one day.

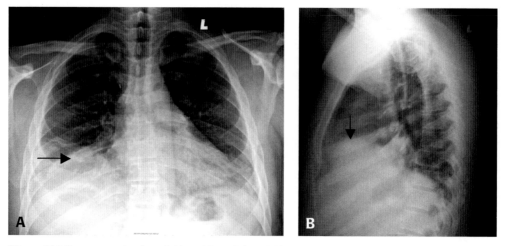

Figure 26.2 Posteroanterior (panel A) and lateral (panel B) chest radiograph from a 37-year-old male on return to ED one day following his initial visit for presumed gastroenteritis, demonstrating a right lower lobe infiltrate (arrows).

ANSWER

The diagnosis is recurrent pneumonias resulting from septic emboli and *Serratia* bacteremia arising from the fragmented ventriculoatrial shunt catheter. A transthoracic echocardiogram was obtained that showed a linear density transversing from the right atrium to the right ventricle across the tricuspid valve, likely the catheter (Figure 26.3). At the distal portion of the linear density, a fluffy nodule consistent with either possible thrombus or vegetation was seen. It was concluded that the shunt catheter had dislodged from the original ventriculoatrial shunt and was likely the source of recurrent septic emboli to the lungs. The patient was admitted to the thoracic surgery service and underwent successful surgical removal of the catheter tip from the right side of the heart, with subsequent resolution of his recurrent pneumonias.

Infections associated with ventriculoatrial shunts

The frequency of long-term prosthetic device infection varies with the type of implant, as do mortality rates associated with these devices. Mortality rates are particularly high when infection is associated with cardiovascular implants.[1] Such prostheses allow organisms to adhere to their surface and, in some cases, produce a biofilm. This biofilm is an extracellular polysaccharide matrix that protects the bacteria via physiologic as well as mechanical factors.[2] In general, rates of infection are greater after revision of a device than following primary device implantation procedures.[1] Approximately 25,000 cerebrospinal fluid shunt operations are performed each year in the United States, 18,000 of which are initial shunt placements.[1] Approximately 85% of individuals with cerebrospinal fluid shunts undergo at least two shunt revisions. Ventriculoperitoneal (VP) shunts are the most common neurosurgical shunts used, and are associated with less severe complications than ventriculoatrial (VA) shunts.[3]

The incidence of VA shunt infection in recent years has averaged less than 10%.[4] Clinical manifestations of VA shunt infection vary and depend on many factors, including the site of shunt infection, whether or not the infection site is proximal or distal, intraluminal or extraluminal, the virulence of infecting pathogens, and the presence or absence of shunt malfunction.[4] Intraluminal infection can result in bacteremia and sepsis; severe sepsis and septic shock are unusual. Right-sided infective endocarditis and septic pulmonary emboli have been described.[4]

Blood cultures are usually positive when an intraluminal infection is present and are important in diagnosing a VA shunt infection. The list of pathogens associated with cerebrospinal fluid shunts includes (but is not limited to) coagulase-negative staphylococci (e.g., *S. aureus*), Gram-negative bacilli (e.g., *E. coli*, *Proteus mirabilis*, *P. aeruginosa*, *Klebsiella pneumoniae*, *H. influenzae*), streptococci (e.g., group G and B), *S. pneumoniae*, and *Propionibacterium acnes*.[1] Imaging is an important tool used for the detection of

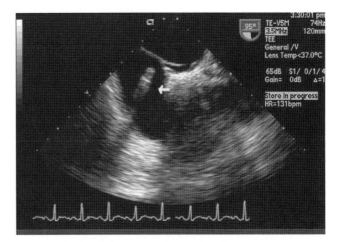

Figure 26.3 Transthoracic echocardiogram image demonstrating VA catheter tip (arrow) extending into the right ventricle in a 37-year-old male with recurrent pneumonias.

device-related infection. When suspecting endocarditis associated with prosthetic valves, electrocardiac devices, or VA shunts, transthoracic or transesophageal echocardiography should be used, with the transesophageal technique yielding greater sensitivity.[1]

As with other types of cardiovascular device-related infections, foreign body removal of the VA shunt with antimicrobial therapy is the preferred treatment option.[4] Infected ventricular shunts are surgically managed in two stages. The infected shunt is removed and an external ventricular catheter is inserted to drain cerebrospinal fluid and monitor intracranial pressure.[5] The external ventricular catheter is usually replaced every 5–10 days to prevent ventriculitis, and systemic antibiotics are administered for 10–14 days. Repeat analysis of cerebrospinal fluid is performed to ensure sterility before a new ventricular shunt is inserted, preferably on the contralateral side, typically within two weeks of the initial surgery.[5]

KEY TEACHING POINTS

1. Prosthetic indwelling device infections account for about half of the two million cases of nosocomial infection that occur in the United States each year.
2. Ventriculoperitoneal (VP) shunts are the most common neurosurgical shunts used and are associated with less severe complications than ventriculoatrial (VA) shunts.
3. Intraluminal infection of VA shunts can result in bacteremia and sepsis, right-sided infective endocarditis, septic pulmonary emboli and recurrent pneumonias.
4. Blood cultures and transthoracic or transesophageal echocardiography are essential diagnostic tools in evaluating for VA shunt-related infections.
5. Treatment for VA shunt infections involves prompt antimicrobial therapy and shunt removal.

REFERENCES

[1] Sampedro MF, Patel R. Infections associated with long-term prosthetic devices. *Infect Dis Clin N Am* 2007;21:785–819.

[2] Schlossberg D. Clinical approach to antibiotic failure. *Med Clin N Am* 2006;90:1265–77.

[3] Lam CH, Villemure JG. Comparison between ventriculo-atrial and ventriculoperitoneal shunting in the adult population. *Br J Neurosurg* 1997;11:43–8.

[4] Baddour LM, Wilson WR. Infections of prosthetic valves and other cardiovascular devices. In: Mandell GL, Bennett JE, Dolin R (eds.). *Principles of Infectious Disease*, 6th ed. Philadelphia: Elselvier, 2005:1024–32.

[5] Darouiche RO. Current Concepts: treatment of infections associated with surgical implants. *N Engl J Med* 2004;350:1422–9.

27

Hemoptysis in a 47-year-old male

HISTORY OF PRESENT ILLNESS

A 47-year-old male presented to the ED complaining of three episodes of coughing up 1–2 tablespoons of bright red blood earlier that day. He denied fevers, chills, night sweats, shortness of breath, malaise, weight loss, abdominal pain, nausea or vomiting; he also denied recent nosebleeds. His medical history included open angle glaucoma, osteoarthritis and a previous lung infection diagnosed some years ago for which he was prescribed antibiotics for six months, the name of which he could not recall. He did not smoke cigarettes and denied personal or family history of cancer. He had not traveled outside the area recently but as a child grew up in Malaysia, and one year ago moved to Northern California from Arizona, where he had spent most of his adult life.

PHYSICAL EXAMINATION

GENERAL APPEARANCE: The patient was a well-nourished, well-hydrated male who appeared comfortable and in no acute discomfort.

VITAL SIGNS

Temperature	97.7°F (36.5°C)
Pulse	87 beats/minute
Blood pressure	165/100 mmHg
Respirations	18 breaths/minute
Oxygen saturation	98% on room air

HEENT: PERRL, EOMI, oropharynx pink and moist, no lesions, mucosal ulcers or bleeding. Nares pink and moist without evidence of bleeding.

NECK: Supple, no cervical lymphadenopathy.

CARDIOVASCULAR: Regular rate and rhythm without rubs, murmurs or gallops.

LUNGS: Clear to auscultation bilaterally without rales, rhonchi or wheezes.

ABDOMEN: Soft, nontender, nondistended.

EXTREMITIES: No clubbing, cyanosis or edema.

SKIN: Warm and dry without pallor, no rashes or lesions.

NEUROLOGIC: Nonfocal.

A chest radiograph (posteroanterior and lateral views) was obtained (Figure 27.1).

What is your diagnosis?

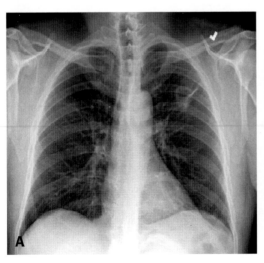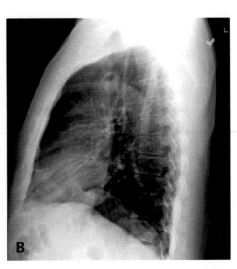

Figure 27.1 Posteroanterior (panel A) and lateral (panel B) views of chest radiograph from a 47-year-old male with hemoptysis.

ANSWER

The diagnosis is bacterial infection of a cavitary lesion from previous coccidioidomycosis infection. The chest radiograph demonstrates a 2.5-cm cavitary lesion in the apex of the left lung (arrows, Figure 27.2). Upon further investigation, the patient's previous lung infection turned out to be coccidioidomycosis, for which he was prescribed fluconazole for six months. Following the chest radiograph, the patient underwent a CT scan of the chest with intravenous contrast, which also demonstrated a 2-cm spherical, thick-walled cavitary lesion in the anterior left upper lobe (Figure 27.3). The patient was admitted to the medical service and treated with intravenous ampicillin/sulbactam for possible bacterial infection of this cavitary lesion. Coccidioidomycosis IgG antibody serologies returned positive, whereas acid-fast bacilli tests of the sputum were negative. The patient's hemoptysis resolved, and he was discharged on hospital day #2 with follow up arranged with a pulmonologist.

Coccidioidomycosis

Coccidioidomycosis is an infection caused by inhalation of arthroconidia of dimorphic fungi of the genus *Coccidioides*.[1] Two species of this genus, *C. immitis* (isolated from California) and *C. posadasii* (isolated outside of California) produce identical diseases.[1] These soil-dwelling fungi have an endemic range that encompasses semi-arid to arid life zones, principally in the southwestern United States and northern Mexico. *Coccidioides* is also found in parts of Argentina, Brazil, Columbia, Guatemala, Honduras, Nicaragua, Paraguay and Venezuela.[1] Hyperendemic areas include Kern, Tulare and Fresno counties in the San Joaquin Valley of California, and Pima, Pinal and Maricopa counties in Arizona. There are approximately 150,000 infections per year in the United States.[1]

Coccidioidomycosis is not a contagious disease. Patients with coccidioidomycosis do not require isolation if hospitalized, although care must be taken in disposing of materials contaminated with secretions.[2]

Sixty percent of people infected with *C. immitis* have no symptoms or have an illness indistinguishable from an upper respiratory infection.[2] In others, symptoms develop one to three weeks after exposure. The typical presentation is a lower respiratory infection accompanied by systemic symptoms, such as fever, sweating, anorexia, weakness, arthralgias, cough, sputum production and chest pain.[2] Erythema nodosum or erythema multiforme may develop. The mainstays of diagnosis are sputum culture and serologic testing. Chest radiographic findings may include infiltrates, pleural effusion and hilar adenopathy.[2] The acute infection almost always resolves without specific therapy, although the illness may last several weeks. Disseminated disease occurs in approximately 1% of infected persons.[3] Dissemination occurs more frequently in the very young or very old, certain racial or ethnic groups, individuals with AIDS or other immunosuppressive disorders, and during the second half of pregnancy or postpartum.[4] Aside from pulmonary involvement, tissues most commonly involved are skin, bone, joints and meninges; tenosynovitis and sinus tract formation have been reported.[4] In patients with severe primary infection or disseminated disease, therapy with amphotericin B (intravenous) or one of the azoles (e.g., itraconazole, fluconazole) is recommended, with treatment for six months.[1-4]

Several types of pulmonary disease can develop after initial infection. These include the formation of pulmonary nodules (coccidioidomas), cavitary disease and progressive pneumonia.[4] The nodules are typically solitary, measuring 2–3 cm in diameter, representing areas of granulomatous organization of coccidioidal pneumonia and raising concern for lung cancer. Thin-walled cavities are seen in approximately 0.1%

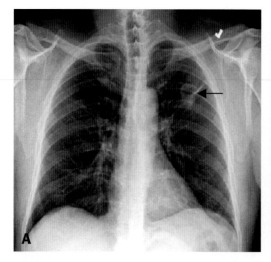
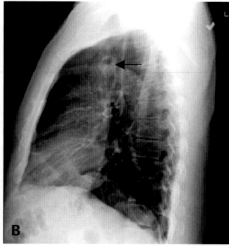

Figure 27.2 Posteroanterior (panel A) and lateral (panel B) views of chest radiograph from a 47-year-old male with cavitary lesion (arrows) from previous coccidioidomycosis infection.

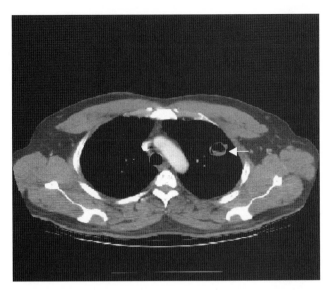

Figure 27.3 Chest CT from a 47-year-old male with hemoptysis, demonstrating a cavitary lesion in the left upper lung field (arrow).

of all patients, which often spontaneously resolve within two years.[4] Thick-walled cavities are more likely to remain present for prolonged periods. Chronic fibrocavitary infection with progressive fibrosis similar to that seen with histoplasmosis may also be seen in coccidioidomycosis, occurring primarily in those with underlying emphysema.[4]

Hemoptysis occurs in one-third of cases of cavitary coccidioidomycosis, usually not life-threatening.[5] When the cavity is in the periphery of the lung, it may rupture into the pleural space causing a hydropneumothorax. Ninety percent of the cavities are solitary, 70% are in the upper lung field, and about 60% are 2–4 cm in diameter.[5] Once a cavity has formed, further spread of the infection is unlikely, presumably because cell-mediated immunity is well established. Symptoms in patients with cavitation are due to complications, such as hemoptysis and secondary infection, which can be bacterial or fungal; aspergillus mycetoma is the most common.[5] However, *C. immitis* itself can proliferate in its mycelial form, producing a similar mycetoma. Pulmonary resection has a role in managing severe hemoptysis or cavities that enlarge or rupture during chemotherapy.[2] Surgery is also indicated to drain empyemas, close persistent bronchopleural fistulas or expand lungs that are restricted by residual disease.

KEY TEACHING POINTS

1. Coccidioidomycosis is caused by inhalation of soil-dwelling fungi of the *Coccidioides* genus; it is endemic to the San Joaquin Valley, California and several counties in Arizona.

2. There are approximately 150,000 cases of coccidioidomycosis per year in the United States; the typical presentation of significant *Coccidioides* infection is a lower respiratory infection accompanied by systemic symptoms, such as fever, sweating, anorexia, weakness, arthralgias, cough, sputum production and chest pain.

3. Several types of pulmonary disease can develop after the initial infection, including the formation of pulmonary nodules (coccidioidomas), cavitary disease and progressive pneumonia.

4. Hemoptysis occurs in one-third of cases of cavitary coccidioidomycosis, usually caused by a secondary bacterial or fungal infection.

5. In patients with severe primary infection or disseminated disease, IV therapy with amphotericin B or one of the azoles is recommended for six months.

6. Pulmonary resection may play a role in managing severe hemoptysis or cavities that enlarge or rupture during pharmacologic therapy.

REFERENCES

[1] Anstead GM, Graybill JR. Coccidioidomycosis. *Infect Dis Clin N Am* 2006;20:621–43.

[2] Stevens DA. Current concepts: coccidioidomycosis. *N Engl J Med* 1995;332:1077–82.

[3] Spinello IM, Johnson RH. A 19-year-old pregnant woman with a skin lesion and respiratory failure. *Chest* 2006;130: 611–5.

[4] Wheat LJ. Endemic mycosis. In: Cohen J, Powderly WG, Berkley SF, et al. (eds.). *Cohen & Powderly: Infectious Diseases*, 2nd ed. Philadelphia: Mosby, 2004:434–6.

[5] Nardell EA, Kucyj G. Case 21-1994: a 20-year-old Mexican immigrant with recurrent hemoptysis and a pulmonary cavitary lesion. *N Engl J Med* 1994;330:1516–22.

28

Cough, fever and shortness of breath in a 62-year-old male

HISTORY OF PRESENT ILLNESS

A 62-year-old male with a medical history significant for chronic alcohol abuse presented to the ED complaining of persistent cough productive of green sputum, fevers to 104°F (40°C), chills and rigors, shortness of breath, and sharp chest pain with cough and deep inspiration for three days. He reported nausea and vomiting but denied abdominal pain or diarrhea. He also denied recent travel, leg swelling or tobacco use. His last alcoholic drink was 24 hours prior to presentation.

PHYSICAL EXAMINATION

GENERAL APPEARANCE: The patient looked older than his stated age. He was a cachectic and ill-appearing male, in moderate respiratory distress, speaking only three- or four-word sentences.

VITAL SIGNS

Temperature	104°F (40°C)
Pulse	120 beats/minute
Blood pressure	110/65 mmHg
Respirations	30 breaths/minute
Oxygen saturation	96% on room air

HEENT: PERRL, EOMI, sclera anicteric, oropharynx dry.

NECK: Supple, no jugular venous distension.

CARDIOVASCULAR: Tachycardic rate, regular rhythm without rubs, murmurs or gallops.

LUNGS: Mild expiratory wheezes throughout all lung fields, scattered rhonchi, crackles and egophony at the right lower and mid-lung fields.

ABDOMEN: Soft, nontender, nondistended.

EXTREMITIES: No clubbing, cyanosis or edema; no calf swelling.

NEUROLOGIC: Nonfocal.

The patient was placed on the cardiac monitor with continuous pulse oximetry and supplemental oxygen (2 liters by nasal cannula), which increased his oxygen saturation to 98%. A

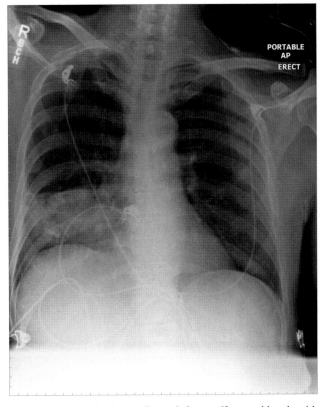

Figure 28.1 Portable chest radiograph from a 62-year-old male with cough, fever and shortness of breath for three days.

peripheral intravenous line was placed, and blood was drawn and sent for cultures and laboratory testing. A 12-lead ECG demonstrated sinus tachycardia, rate 120 without acute ST-T wave changes. A 1-liter bolus of normal saline was administered IV, as well as acetaminophen orally for the fever; a portable chest radiograph was obtained (Figure 28.1). Laboratory tests were significant for a leukocyte count of 20 K/μL (normal 3.5–12.5 K/μL), with 35% immature bands (presence of bands abnormal) and sodium of 125 mEq/L (normal 137–145 mEq/L).

What is your diagnosis?

ANSWER

The diagnosis is community-acquired pneumonia (CAP). The chest radiograph demonstrated a right middle lobe infiltrate (arrow, Figure 28.2). The patient's calculated Pneumonia Severity Index (PSI) score was 117 (62 points for male age, 10 points for respiratory rate greater than 29, 15 points for temperature greater than or equal to 40°C and 20 points for sodium less than 130 mEq/L), which placed him in Risk Class IV. This estimated his 30-day mortality risk at 9.3%. The patient received moxifloxacin 400 mg IV, albuterol nebulized treatments and was admitted to the medicine service. Intravenous antibiotics were continued, and the patient's symptoms improved by hospital day #3, at which time he was afebrile with a room air oxygen saturation of 98%. He was discharged on hospital day #4 to complete a ten-day course of oral moxifloxacin, with close follow up arranged with his primary care provider. He was encouraged to stop drinking, and was given resources to assist him.

Community-acquired pneumonia

Pneumonia is an important cause of morbidity and mortality in adults; more than 5 million cases occur annually in the United States.[1] Patients with CAP are most often managed in an outpatient setting. The mortality rate in this patient population is low (less than 1%), in contrast to patients who require hospitalization (mortality rate approximates 15%).[2] CAP is usually acquired by inhalation or aspiration of pulmonary pathogenic organisms into a lung segment or lobe.[3] Less commonly, CAP may result from secondary bacteremia from a distant source, such as an *Escherichia coli* urinary tract infection or bacteremia. CAP due to aspiration or oropharyngeal contents is the only form of CAP that typically has multiple pathogens.[3] *Streptococcus pneumoniae* is the most commonly diagnosed etiology of CAP among hospitalized patients.[1] Common bacterial etiologies of CAP and their associated severities are listed in Table 28.1.

Cough is a common presenting complaint of patients diagnosed with pneumonia; however, only a small fraction of patients who present with cough are diagnosed with pneumonia (4% in one large series).[2,4] Patients with respiratory complaints should be screened at triage with pulse oximetry because hypoxia is an important diagnostic clue to the presence of pneumonia.[2] Typically, patients with bacterial CAP present with variable degrees of fever, usually with productive cough, and often with pleuritic chest pain.[3] The clinical presentation of patients with CAP due to atypical pathogens (e.g., *M. pneumoniae*, *C. pneumoniae*, *L. pneumophila*) is usually less acute than the presentation of typical bacterial pathogens (e.g., *S. pneumoniae*, *H. influenzae*).[3] With typical bacterial CAP, abnormal physical findings are generally confined to the chest. Rales on auscultation of the chest over the involved lobe or segment are common. If consolidation is present, increased tactile fremitus, bronchial breathing and "E-to-A" changes may be present.[3] Purulent sputum is characteristic of pneumonia caused by typical bacterial pathogens, and is not

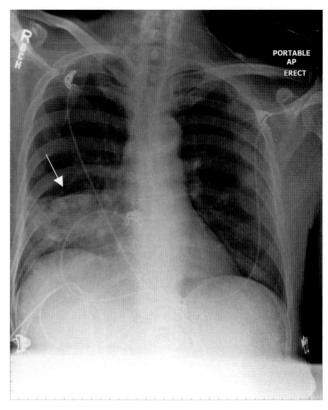

Figure 28.2 Portable chest radiograph from a 62-year-old male with a right middle lobe infiltrate consistent with pneumonia (arrow).

usually a feature of atypical pathogens with the exception of Legionnaires' disease (caused by *L. pneumophila*).[3]

Chest radiography is typically the most important test for establishing the diagnosis of pneumonia. Routine chest radiography is not necessary for all patients who present with cough. It can be reserved for patients without a history of asthma who have findings suggestive of pneumonia (e.g., fever, tachycardia, decreased oxygen saturation or focal abnormality on lung examination).[2] Among patients suspected of having pneumonia, these clinical findings have been prospectively validated and better predict the presence of an infiltrate than physician judgment.[5] Patients with serious underlying disease or severe sepsis/septic shock for whom hospitalization is considered should have a chest radiograph performed.[2]

Laboratory studies are of limited use to establish the diagnosis and specific cause of pneumonia. For the patient with mild disease who is to be treated at home, little or no laboratory data is needed.[1] Although a white blood cell (WBC) count greater than 15,000/mm[3] increases the probability that the pneumonia is bacterial rather than viral or atypical in origin, leukocytosis is neither sensitive or specific enough to aid in therapeutic decisions.[2] A WBC count may be helpful if it reveals evidence of neutropenia or lymphopenia, which might occur in immunosuppression. In sicker patients who require admission, electrolytes, blood urea nitrogen, serum glucose and a complete blood count (CBC) should be obtained. Serum lactate levels are useful in identifying septic patients and

TABLE 28.1 Bacterial etiologies of CAP[1]		
Mild (Outpatient)	Moderate (Medical ward)	Severe (ICU)
Mycoplasma pneumoniae	Streptococcus pneumoniae	Streptococcus pneumoniae
Chlamydia pneumoniae	Mycoplasma pneumoniae	Legionella pneumophila
Streptococcus pneumoniae	Chlamydia pneumoniae	Staphylococcus aureus
Haemophilus influenzae	Haemophilus influenzae	Gram-negative bacilli
	Legionella pneumophila	
	Anaerobes	

their response to therapy, as well as evaluating for possible *Pneumocystis carinii* pneumonia (PCP) in patients known or suspected to have HIV infection.

Gram stain and culture of the sputum is not routinely done in the ED. This is controversial because of the time it takes to induce a good sample, as well as the possibility of ED patients presenting with cough having TB. Furthermore, uncontaminated specimens with a single etiologic agent are rare. If obtained, these should be reserved for the subset of patients with serious illness (e.g., requiring ICU admission) in whom the bacteriologic diagnosis is highly uncertain or an unusual pathogen is suspected, and for those in whom the outcome may depend on optimal antimicrobial therapy.[2] The need for routine blood cultures among patients admitted for pneumonia is also controversial.[6,7] Routine blood cultures for patients admitted with pneumonia have shown mixed results in terms of improved diagnostic accuracy or ability to guide therapy.[8] It is considered best practice to obtain blood cultures in seriously ill patients before antibiotics are initiatiated.[2] Bacteremia occurs in approximately 25–30% of hospitalized pneumococcal pneumonia cases but the diagnosis and therapy are usually well established before blood culture results are available.[2]

Outpatients diagnosed with CAP who are otherwise healthy can be treated with a macrolide (erythromycin, azithromycin or clarithromycin) or doxycycline as monotherapy.[9] Those who have had recent antibiotic exposure may be offered a fluoroquinolone alone (levofloxacin, moxifloxacin or gatifloxacin), amoxicillin-clavulanate, or the combination of azithromycin or clarithromycin plus high-dose amoxicillin. Although the fluoroquinolones offer convenient once-daily dosing, increasing resistance among isolates to this class of agents has been recently demonstrated.[9] Inpatients requiring treatment of CAP but who are not admitted to the ICU should be offered azithromycin or clarithromycin plus a β-lactam agent or a third-generation cephalosporin (e.g., ceftriaxone). Respiratory fluoroquinolones may be offered as monotherapy. For ICU patients with a concern for pseudomonas infection, an antipseudomonal agent plus ciprofloxacin, or antipseudomonal agents with an aminoglycoside plus a respiratory fluoroquinolone or a macrolide are recommended.[9]

Between 30–50% of patients hospitalized with pneumonia are placed in low-risk categories, many of whom could potentially be managed at home.[10] The decision regarding hospitalization should be based on the stability of the patient's clinical condition, the risk of death and complications, the presence or absence of other active medical problems, and the

patient's psychosocial characteristics.[10] Disease-specific prediction rules are available that can be used to assess the initial severity of pneumonia and predict the risk of death. The most widely used and rigorously studied prediction rule – the Pneumonia Severity Index (PSI) – has been validated in more than 50,000 patients from a variety of inpatient and outpatient populations.[11,12] The PSI is based on data commonly available upon presentation (Table 28.2), and stratifies patients into five risk classes in which 30-day mortality rates range from 0.1–27.0%. The greater the PSI score, the greater the risk of death,

TABLE 28.2 Pneumonia severity index for CAP[11]	
Characteristic	Points assigned
Demographic Factor	
Age (in years)	
Men	Age
Women	Age − 10
Nursing home resident	+10
Coexisting illnesses	
Neoplastic disease	+30
Liver disease	+20
Congestive heart failure	+10
Cerebrovascular disease	+10
Renal disease	+10
Findings on Physical Examination	
Altered mental status	+20
Respiratory rate $\geq$30/min	+20
Systolic blood pressure <90 mmHg	+20
Temperature <35°C or $\geq$40°C	+15
Pulse $\geq$125 beats/min	+10
Laboratory and X-ray Findings	
Arterial pH <7.35	+30
Blood urea nitrogen $\geq$30 mg/dL	+20
Sodium <130 mmol/liter	+20
Glucose $\geq$250 mg/dL	+10
Hematocrit <30%	+10
Partial pressure of arterial oxygen	
<60 mmHg or O_2 saturation <90%	+10
Pleural effusion	+10

PSI Class	30-day mortality
I*	0.10%
II (less than 70 points)	0.60%
III (71–90 points)	0.90%
IV (91–130 points)	9.30%
V (more than 130 points)	27%

* For class I, age less than 50 years; no cancer, congestive heart failure, cerebrovascular, renal or liver disease; normal vital signs/examination.

admission to the ICU, readmission and the longer the length of hospitalization.

Mortality is sufficiently low in PSI classes I–III (less than 1%) that outpatient management is appropriate in the absence of extenuating circumstances. Some low-risk patients, especially those who are elderly or PSI class III, may look sick or be reluctant to be treated at home. Many of these patients may be appropriate candidates for a short hospitalization or 23 hours of observation.[10] Mortality increases to 9–27% in PSI classes IV–V, suggesting that these higher-risk patients should be hospitalized.

A similar tool to the PSI that is easier to use is the CURB-65 rule.[13] This rule uses only five criteria to determine patients at lower risk for adverse events: confusion, uremia (blood urea nitrogen greater than or equal to 20 mg/dL), respiratory rate greater than or equal to 30 breaths/minute, blood pressure less than 90 mmHg systolic or 60 mmHg diastolic, and age greater than or equal to 65. The risk of 30-day mortality increases with a greater number of these factors present: 0.7% with no factors, 9.2% with two factors and 57% with five factors. It is suggested that patients with zero to one feature may receive treatment as an outpatient, patients with two features be admitted, and ICU-level care be considered for patients with three or more factors.[2,13]

KEY TEACHING POINTS

1. Patients with community-acquired pneumonia (CAP) appropriate for the outpatient setting have a low mortality (less than 1%) compared to hospitalized patients, who have a mortality rate of approximately 15%.
2. *Streptococcus pneumoniae* is the most commonly diagnosed etiology of CAP among hospitalized patients.
3. Typically, patients with bacterial CAP present with variable degrees of fever, productive cough and pleuritic chest pain.
4. Laboratory tests have little use in outpatient management of patients with CAP, whereas tests obtained on admitted patients should include electrolytes, blood urea nitrogen, serum glucose and complete blood count (CBC).
5. Blood cultures should be obtained in seriously ill and admitted patients with CAP, preferably before the initiation of antibiotics.
6. Disease-specific prediction rules (e.g., Pneumonia Severity Index and CURB-65) can be used to assess the initial

severity of pneumonia, predict the risk of death and aid in deciding which patients diagnosed with CAP require hospital admission.

REFERENCES

[1] Plouffe JF, Martin DR. Pneumonia in the emergency department. *Emerg Med Clin N Am* 2008;26:389–411.

[2] Moran GJ, Talan DA, Abrahamain FM. Diagnosis and management of pneumonia in the emergency department. *Infect Dis Clin N Am* 2008;22:53–72.

[3] Cunha BA. Pneumonia, community-acquired. eMedicine Website. Available at http://www.emedicine.com/med/topic3162.htm. Accessed August 19, 2008.

[4] Metley JP, Stafford RS, Singer DE. National trends in the use of antibiotics by primary care physicians for adult patients with cough. *Arch Intern Med* 1998;158:1813–8.

[5] Emerman CL, Dawson N, Speroff T, et al. Comparison of physician judgment and decision aids for ordering chest radiographs for pneumonia in outpatients. *Ann Emerg Med* 1991;20:1215–9.

[6] Moran GJ, Abrahamian FM. Blood cultures for pneumonia: can we hit the target without a shotgun? *Ann Intern Med* 2005;46:407–8.

[7] Walls RM, Resnick J. The Joint Commission on Accreditation of Healthcare Organizations and Center for Medicare and Medicaid Services community-acquired pneumonia initiative: what went wrong? *Ann Emerg Med* 2005;46: 409–11.

[8] Kennedy M, Bates DW, Wright SB, et al. Do emergency department blood cultures change practice in patients with pneumonia? *Ann Emerg Med* 2005;46:393–400.

[9] Patel SM, Saravolatz LD. Monotherapy versus combination therapy. *Med Clin N Am* 2006;90:1183–95.

[10] Halm EA, Teirstein AS. Clinical practice: management of community-acquired pneumonia. *N Engl J Med* 2002;347: 2039–45.

[11] Fine MJ, Auble TE, Yealy DM, et al. A prediction rule to identify low-risk patients with community-acquired pneumonia. *N Engl J Med* 1997;336:243–50.

[12] Auble TE, Yealy DM, Fine MJ. Assessing prognosis and selecting an initial site of care for adults with community-acquired pneumonia. *Infect Dis Clin North Am* 1998;12:741–59.

[13] Lim WS, Van Der Eerden MM, Liang R, et al. Defining community-acquired pneumonia severity on presentation to hospital: an international derivation and validation study. *Thorax* 2003;58:377–82.

PART IV

GASTROENTEROLOGY

29

Abdominal pain and dysuria in a 16-year-old male

HISTORY OF PRESENT ILLNESS

A 16-year-old male presented to the ED complaining of suprapubic pain radiating to the right testicle, dysuria, urgency and frequency for eight days. The patient was seen one week prior to his ED visit by his primary care provider (PCP), at which time he described the previous complaints as well as subjective fevers. At that time, the patient's temperature was 99.2°F (37.3°C). He was noted to be well appearing and in no acute discomfort. The abdominal examination revealed mild suprapubic tenderness to palpation without the presence of rebound or guarding, no costovertebral angle tenderness (CVAT) was noted and his genitourinary (GU) examination was normal. A urinalysis was negative for infection and the patient was diagnosed with a viral syndrome.

Three days prior to his ED presentation, the patient reported a temperature of 103°F (39.4°C) and severe suprapubic pain. The following day, the intensity of his pain diminished somewhat and his fever resolved. In the ED, the patient continued to complain of crampy abdominal pain at a level of 6 (on a scale of 0 to 10), with associated dysuria, urgency and frequency. He denied nausea, vomiting, diarrhea, constipation or penile discharge, and was tolerating oral liquids.

PHYSICAL EXAMINATION

GENERAL APPEARANCE: The patient was lying supine on the gurney, appeared comfortable and in no acute discomfort.

VITAL SIGNS

Temperature	98.7°F (37.1°C)
Pulse	88 beats/minute
Blood pressure	120/80 mmHg
Respirations	20 breaths/minute
Oxygen saturation	100% on room air

HEENT: Unremarkable.

NECK: Supple.

CARDIOVASCULAR: Regular rate and rhythm without rubs, murmurs or gallops.

LUNGS: Clear to auscultation bilaterally.

ABDOMEN: Soft, nondistended; suprapubic, periumbilical and right lower quadrant tenderness to palpation without rebound or guarding (maximal point of tenderness over suprapubic area). No CVAT.

RECTAL: Normal tone, brown stool, hemoccult negative.

GENITOURINARY: Circumcised, no penile discharge, testes descended bilaterally, no testicular swelling or tenderness, no hernias.

EXTREMITIES: No clubbing, cyanosis or edema.

NEUROLOGIC: Nonfocal.

A peripheral intravenous line was placed, and blood was drawn and sent for laboratory testing. Laboratory tests revealed a leukocyte count of 16 K/μL (normal 3.5–12.5 K/μL) with 84% neutrophils (normal 50–70%); electrolytes, creatinine, glucose and urinalysis were within normal limits.

What is your diagnosis?

ANSWER

The diagnosis is intra-abdominal abscess from perforated appendicitis. The patient underwent a CT scan of the abdomen and pelvis with oral and intravenous contrast, which demonstrated a 7 cm × 4 cm intra-abdominal abscess in the right lower quadrant (Figure 29.1), resulting from a perforated appendix. The patient was admitted to the surgery service, received intravenous ciprofloxacin and metronidazole, and subsequently underwent percutaneous drainage of the abscess by interventional radiology on hospital day #2. The patient was discharged on hospital day #4 with instructions to continue his oral antibiotics for two weeks. The patient underwent successful interval appendectomy approximately four months following percutaneous abscess drainage.

Appendicitis

Appendicitis occurs when a fecalith, fecal matter or lymphoid hyperplasia obstructs the appendix.[1] Obstruction leads to inflammation, rising intraluminal pressures, and ultimately ischemia. Subsequently, the appendix enlarges and incites inflammatory changes in the surrounding tissues, such as in the pericecal fat and peritoneal cavity. If untreated, the inflamed appendix may eventually perforate.[1] Appendectomy is the most common emergent operation in the world.[2] More than 250,000 appendicitis-related admissions occur annually in the United States, totaling nearly $3 billion in hospital charges.[2] The current incidence of appendicitis is 86 per 100,000 patients per year, with a lifetime risk of 6.7% for females and 8.6% for males.[1,2]

The anatomic location of the appendix affects the clinical presentation as well as the subsequent risk of developing appendicitis. In a study of 10,000 autopsies, the appendix was located behind the cecum in the retrocecal fossa in 65% of cases, and in the pelvis in 31% of cases.[3] This ratio is reversed in patients who undergo an operation for appendicitis. A retrocecal location of the appendix is less likely to become obstructed due to the position of its lumen.[3]

Symptoms of appendicitis usually begin with abdominal pain, often in the periumbilical area. Classically, the pain migrates to McBurney's point (two-thirds the distance from the umbilicus along a straight line toward the anterior superior iliac spine of the pelvis), 6–18 hours from onset.[4] The pain steadily worsens until the appendix perforates if not diagnosed in a timely manner. At the time of perforation, localized pain may decrease but the more generalized pain of peritonitis predominates. Anorexia is the next most common symptom after pain, occurring in about 95% of patients. Nausea is seen in approximately 75% of cases, whereas vomiting is seen in 60–70% of cases. Diarrhea, or more accurately tenesmus, may occur but is usually seen late in the clinical course of appendicitis, when the sigmoid colon becomes irritated by a severely inflamed or perforated appendix.[4] About 75% of patients have a low-grade fever, but a higher fever or the absence of fever does not eliminate the diagnosis.[5]

The most common finding on physical examination is localized abdominal tenderness, usually in the right lower quadrant. Pain may be noted over McBurney's point; however, because only 35% of patients have the base of their appendix within 5 cm of this point, the pain of appendicitis can be localized over other areas of the abdomen.[3] Direct rebound tenderness is a response to the inflamed appendix and its proximity to the peritoneal surface.[2] This localized peritoneal irritation may also be demonstrated by indirect referred tenderness in the right lower quadrant elicited during left lower quadrant palpation (i.e., Rovsing's sign). Involuntary guarding refers to muscle contraction in response to the inflamed parietal peritoneum. This finding, along with rebound tenderness, are independent predictors of appendicitis.[6] A positive psoas sign occurs when a patient experiences pain while on their left side and an examiner slowly extends the right thigh. Pain occurs as the iliopsoas is irritated by the inflamed appendix.[2] The obturator sign may be elicited when an examiner internally rotates the flexed right thigh while the patient is supine. This brings the obturator internus muscle in contact with an irritated pelvis, which produces hypogastric pain. The patient's temperature is a poor predictor of appendicitis; however, when

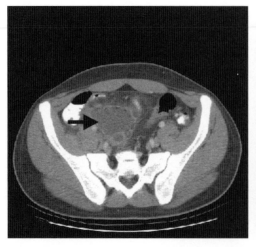 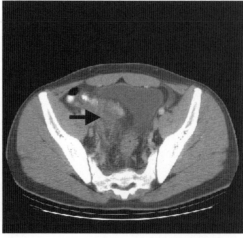

Figure 29.1 CT of the pelvis from a 16-year-old male with suprapubic pain, demonstrating abscess in the right lower quadrant (arrows) resulting from a perforated appendix.

high and accompanied by tachycardia a ruptured appendix with intra-abdominal abscess should be suspected.[2,7]

About 80–90% of patients with acute appendicitis have an elevated white blood cell (WBC) count above 10,000/mm^3 (this percentage is slightly lower in elderly and very young patients). Unfortunately, the WBC count is nonspecific and often elevated with other etiologies of abdominal pain.[3] The sensitivity of C-reactive protein (CRP) varies from 40–99%, depending on the study. A urinalysis is helpful in differentiating urinary tract disease from acute appendicitis; mild sterile pyuria may be seen in patients with appendicitis due to irritation of the ureter by the appendix. However, significant pyuria (more than 20 WBC per high-power field) suggests urinary tract pathology.[3] All women of childbearing age with abdominal pain should be tested for pregnancy, as a positive test expands the differential diagnosis of right lower quadrant pain.

In patients where the history, physical examination and laboratory findings do not clearly suggest the diagnosis of appendicitis, imaging studies are indicated. A plain film radiograph of the abdomen may reveal a fecalith; however, a fecalith is present in only 10% of the cases of appendicitis.[4] Graded compression ultrasonography has been prospectively demonstrated to improve the clinical accuracy of the diagnosis of acute appendicitis.[3] It may be particularly helpful in women of childbearing age, in whom pelvic conditions can mimic appendicitis. It is often advocated as the initial imaging modality in children and pregnant patients to spare them radiation exposure. The sensitivity and specificity of ultrasonography for acute appendicitis in most studies is 75–90% and 85–95%, respectively.[3]

Abdominal CT has become the most important imaging study in the evaluation of patients with atypical presentations of appendicitis.[8] Studies have demonstrated a decreased negative laparotomy rate and appendiceal perforation rate when pelvic CT was used in selected patients with suspected appendicitis. Advantages of CT scanning include its superior sensitivity and accuracy compared to other imaging techniques, availability, lack of invasiveness and potential to reveal alternative diagnoses. Disadvantages include radiation exposure, potential for anaphylactic reaction if intravenous contrast is used, lengthy acquisition time if oral contrast is used and patient discomfort if rectal contrast is used.[8]

Appendiceal rupture puts patients at risk for serious sequelae, including peritonitis, sepsis and even death. It remains a persistent problem. Increased time between symptom onset and surgical treatment may be a risk factor for ruptured appendicitis. Bickell et al. demonstrated that the risk of rupture after 36 hours of untreated symptoms is approximately 5%, which increases by 5% for each ensuing 12-hour period after 36 hours.[9] They concluded that physicians should be cautious about delaying surgery beyond 36 hours from symptom onset in patients with appendicitis.[9] The perforation rate in cases of appendicitis has varied from 10–85% depending upon age, gender and whether or not the institution where the patient is evaluated is located in the inner city.[4] In most major hospital centers, the incidence of perforation in the general pediatric population ranges from 20–40%.[4] These patients often present dehydrated and toxic-appearing, with obvious physical signs of peritonitis; they should immediately be fluid resuscitated and treated with antibiotics before taken to the operating room.

There is a small subgroup of patients with appendiceal perforations in whom the diagnosis is missed or who do not present for medical evaluation until late in the course of their illness. Many of these patients may have been ill for 7–10 days; CT often reveals a walled-off abscess or phlegmon in the right lower quadrant.[4] These patients can often be treated medically and have their abscesses drained percutaneously by an interventional radiologist. After stabilization and recovery, patients who have undergone successful percutaneous drainage are discharged home. These patients should be followed closely, complete a course of antibiotics and be scheduled to return for interval appendectomy.[2]

KEY TEACHING POINTS

1. The current incidence of appendicitis is 86 per 100,000 patients per year, with a lifetime risk of 6.7% for females and 8.6% for males.
2. Classic signs and symptoms of acute appendicitis include periumbilical pain migrating to the right lower quadrant, anorexia, nausea, vomiting and fever.
3. The most common finding on physical examination is localized abdominal tenderness, usually in the right lower quadrant; additional findings may include rebound tenderness, as well as the presence of a Rovsing's, obturator or psoas signs.
4. In patients where the history, physical examination and laboratory findings are not consistent with the diagnosis of appendicitis, imaging studies (abdominal CT or ultrasound) are indicated.
5. A small subgroup of patients with appendiceal rupture may present late in the disease process, and may have a walled-off phlegmon or abscess.

REFERENCES

[1] Rybkin AV, Thoeni RF. Current concepts in imaging of appendicitis. *Radiol Clin N Am* 2007;45:411–22.
[2] Dominguez EP, Sweeney JF, Choi YU. Diagnosis and management of diverticulitis and appendicitis. *Gastroenterol Clin N Am* 2006;35:367–91.
[3] Wolfe JM, Henneman PL. Acute appendicitis. In: Marx JA, Hockberger RS, Walls RM, et al. (eds.). *Rosen's Emergency Medicine: Concepts and Clinical Practice*, 6th ed. Philadelphia: Mosby, 2006:1451–8.
[4] Halter JM, Baesl T, Nicolette L, et al. Common gastrointestinal problems and emergencies in neonates and children. *Clin Fam Pract* 2004;6:731–54.
[5] Pearl RH, Hale DA, Molloy M, et al. Pediatric appendectomy. *J Ped Surg* 1995;30:173–81.
[6] Andersson RE, Hugander AP, Ghazi SH, et al. Diagnostic value of disease history, clinical presentation, and

inflammatory parameters of appendicitis. *World J Surg* 1999;23:133–40.

[7] Cardall T, Glasser J, Guss DA. Clinical value of the total white blood cell count and temperature in the evaluation of patients with suspected appendicitis. *Acad Emerg Med* 2004;11:1021–7.

[8] Craig S. Appendicitis, acute. eMedicine Website. Available at http://www.emedicine.com/emerg/topic41.htm. Accessed June 24, 2008.

[9] Bickell NA, Aufses AH, Rojas M, et al. How time affects the risk of rupture in appendicitis. *J Am Coll Surg* 2006;202: 401–6.

30

Left upper quadrant abdominal pain in an 18-year-old male

HISTORY OF PRESENT ILLNESS

An 18-year-old male presented to the ED with a one-day history of severe left upper quadrant abdominal pain. The pain came on suddenly while sitting and was described as sharp, constant and radiating to the back. The pain worsened on inspiration, and was rated at a level of 8 (on a scale of 0 to 10). He denied nausea or vomiting, fevers, diarrhea, constipation or dysuria, as well as recent trauma. Six weeks prior to these current symptoms, the patient developed fevers, a sore throat, generalized malaise and mild, diffuse abdominal pain. These symptoms gradually resolved with rest, fluids and acetaminophen. A throat swab for group A strep at that time was negative.

PHYSICAL EXAMINATION

GENERAL APPEARANCE: The patient appeared well nourished, well hydrated and in no acute discomfort.

VITAL SIGNS

Temperature	98°F (36.6°C)
Pulse	90 beats/minute
Blood pressure	117/78 mmHg
Respirations	20 breaths/minute
Oxygen saturation	100% on room air

HEENT: PERRL, EOMI, sclera anicteric, oropharynx pink and moist without exudates.

NECK: Supple, no jugular venous distension.

CARDIOVASCULAR: Regular rate and rhythm without rubs, murmurs or gallops.

LUNGS: Clear to auscultation bilaterally.

ABDOMEN: Soft, nondistended, active bowel sounds present. Palpable spleen with left upper quadrant tenderness to deep palpation; no rebound or guarding noted.

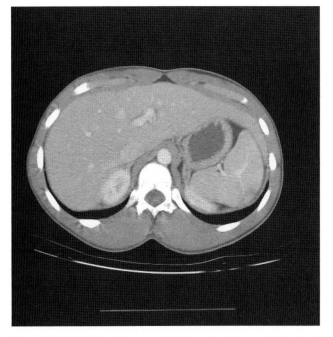

Figure 30.1 CT of the abdomen with IV contrast from an 18-year-old male with left upper quadrant abdominal pain.

EXTREMITIES: No clubbing, cyanosis or edema.

SKIN: No rashes.

A peripheral intravenous line was placed, morphine sulfate IV was administered for pain, and blood was drawn and sent for laboratory testing. Laboratory tests, including a complete blood count, creatinine, PT, aPTT and INR, were within normal limits. A CT scan of the abdomen with intravenous contrast was obtained (Figure 30.1).

What is your diagnosis?

ANSWER

The diagnosis is a grade I spontaneous splenic laceration secondary to infectious mononucleosis. The CT scan demonstrated some irregular, band-shaped areas of nonenhancing splenic parenchyma at the posterior and lateral aspects of the spleen, compatible with splenic laceration (arrow, Figure 30.2). During the patient's initial illness eight weeks prior, his laboratory results demonstrated a complete blood count with 16% atypical lymphocytes and a positive monospot test. Following the diagnosis of grade I splenic laceration, the patient was admitted to the surgical service for close observation and nonoperative management (serial examinations and hematocrit testing). The patient's hematocrit and vital signs remained stable, his pain improved and he was discharged on hospital day #3 with instructions to avoid strenuous physical activity and contact sports for a minimum of three weeks.

Infectious mononucleosis and splenic injury

Infectious mononucleosis (IM), a common entity caused by the Epstein-Barr virus (EBV), is a self-limiting viral illness most common in children and young adults. It is characterized by a triad of fever, pharyngitis and lymphadenopathy associated with atypical lymphocytes and heterophil antibodies, as well as myalgias and reversible splenomegaly.[1,2] More than 90% of adults eventually acquire EBV, establishing a latent infection of B-lymphocytes, thereby acquiring a lifelong infection typical of members of the herpes virus family.[3] EBV is probably acquired during childhood by salivary contact as a consequence of intermittent, asymptomatic shedding of the virus into oropharyngeal secretions among family members. The individual immune response to EBV is highly variable, and likely determines its severity or whether EBV causes symptomatic disease.[4] This depends on the proliferation and activation of T cells in response to infection. For reasons that remain unexplained, infection acquired during childhood is usually asymptomatic or yields nonspecific symptoms. In developed societies, primary EBV infection is shifted to later ages, in which 50–74% of individuals develop symptoms consistent with IM.[3] The risk of developing symptomatic infection drops 100-fold by age 35 or older.[5]

Serious complications of IM usually come after the illness. The rare deaths that occur are mostly attributed to neurologic sequelae and splenic rupture.[3] EBV infection results in the proliferation of mononuclear cells, which collect in the reservoirs of lymphoid tissue, including the spleen. As a result, the spleen becomes congested and enlarged, causing thinning of the splenic capsule; splenomegaly occurs in 50% of patients with IM.[2] Although relatively rare, complaints of significant left upper quadrant abdominal pain in IM should invoke consideration of spontaneous splenic laceration or rupture, which occurs in 0.1–0.5% of patients.[3,6] Presence of severe left shoulder pain, known as Kehr's sign, indicates splenic injury with blood irritating diaphragmatic nerves.[3]

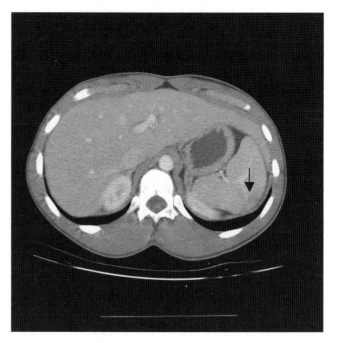

Figure 30.2 Grade I splenic laceration (arrow) in an 18-year-old male with spontaneous onset of sharp, left upper quadrant abdominal pain.

Patients with spontaneous splenic laceration or rupture secondary to IM often present with acute onset of severe abdominal pain that may be diffuse or localized to the left side. Splenomegaly alone (without splenic rupture) rarely causes pain.[2] Abdominal symptoms of spontaneous splenic laceration or rupture secondary to IM may be accompanied by pallor, tachycardia, hypotension, oliguria, orthostasis and syncope. Abnormal laboratory studies include low hematocrit and leukocytosis with or without the presence of atypical lymphocytes. Up to 90% of patients may also have abnormally elevated liver function studies.[2] Ultrasound is an effective bedside tool for visualizing the spleen and any free fluid in the abdomen. CT scan is confirmatory and allows for grading the severity of splenic damage. Splenomegaly, splenic lacerations, subcapsular hematomas and hemoperitoneum are readily visualized with contrast-enhanced CT.[2] The presence of acute bleeding may also be seen in some instances.

There is debate over surgical versus conservative treatment for splenic lacerations/rupture in IM.[1–3] Patients who are hemodynamically compromised warrant early surgical intervention with total splenectomy. More recent recommendations state that splenic laceration/rupture may be managed conservatively if bleeding is not profuse (defined by some as requiring less than two units of transfused blood).[3] Nonoperative percutaneous drainage may be an alternative to laparotomy in some cases. Spleen preservation will avoid the potential for long-term complications of asplenia, including the risk of severe sepsis due to encapsulated bacteria.[2,3] Finally, an enlarged spleen in IM may remain susceptible to delayed rupture for several weeks, although the exact period is unknown. Therefore, a patient considered for conservative treatment should be advised to avoid physical activities for a considerable time, at least until the spleen has returned to normal size (e.g., four to six weeks).[2]

KEY TEACHING POINTS

1. Spontaneous splenic laceration/rupture is a rare but serious sequelae of infectious mononucleosis (IM), affecting less than 1% of patients.
2. Symptoms and signs of spontaneous splenic laceration/rupture may include diffuse or left upper quadrant abdominal pain, left shoulder pain, pallor, tachycardia, hypotension, orthostasis and syncope.
3. Laboratory abnormalities seen with spontaneous splenic rupture associated with IM may include leukocytosis, presence of atypical lymphocytes, low hematocrit and abnormal liver function tests.
4. Bedside ultrasound is useful in identifying free fluid in the abdomen associated with spontaneous splenic rupture. Abdominal CT scan is confirmatory and useful in grading the severity of splenic damage in hemodynamically stable patients.
5. Patients with splenic injury secondary to IM should be admitted to the surgical service for either conservative management or splenectomy based on hemodynamic stability, type and grade of injury, and numerous other factors.

REFERENCES

[1] Rothwell S, McAuley D. Case report: Spontaneous splenic rupture in infectious mononucleosis. *Emerg Med* 2001;13: 364–6.
[2] Brichkov I, Cummings L, Fazylov R, et al. Nonoperative management of spontaneous splenic rupture in infectious mononucleosis: the role of emerging diagnostic and treatment modalities. *Am Surg* 2006;72:401–4.
[3] Auwaerter PG. Infectious mononucleosis: return to play. *Clin Sports Med* 2004;23:485–97.
[4] Baumgarten E, Herbst H, Schmitt M, et al. Life-threatening infectious mononucleosis: is it correlated with virus-induced T cell proliferation? *Clin Infect Dis* 1994;19:152–6.
[5] Auwaerter PG. Infectious mononucleosis in middle age [clinical conference]. *JAMA* 1999;281:454–9.
[6] Farley DR, Zietlow SP, Bannon MP, et al. Spontaneous rupture of the spleen due to infectious mononucleosis. *Mayo Clin Proc* 1992;67:846–53.

31

Abdominal pain and vomiting in a 29-year-old female

HISTORY OF PRESENT ILLNESS

A 29-year-old female presented to the ED with several days of mild, diffuse abdominal pain, nausea and vomiting. Eight days prior to presentation she had undergone a lower abdominal cesarean section. The patient denied diarrhea or constipation, dysuria, fevers, chills, chest pain or shortness of breath. She described her pain as crampy and constant, rated at a level of 4 (on a scale of 0 to 10), which was not relieved with acetaminophen. On examination she was afebrile, with normal pulse and blood pressure. She appeared to be in no acute distress. Abdominal examination revealed a soft, slightly distended abdomen with mild, diffuse tenderness to palpation without associated rebound or guarding. Her incision was healing well without associated erythema or discharge. A peripheral intravenous line was placed, blood was drawn and sent for laboratory testing, and intravenous fluids were administered along with an antiemetic. An abdominal radiograph (kidney, ureter, and bladder, or KUB) was obtained (Figure 31.1).

The radiograph demonstrated a nonspecific bowel gas pattern without the presence of free air or air-fluid levels. Laboratory tests, including a complete blood count, electrolytes, creatinine, glucose, liver function tests, amylase and urinalysis, were normal. The patient's symptoms improved after IV hydration and antiemetics. She was discharged home with precautions to return for worsening symptoms.

Three days later, the patient returned to the ED complaining of persistent nausea, vomiting and worsening abdominal pain. She denied fevers or diarrhea but reported no flatus for the past 24 hours.

PHYSICAL EXAMINATION

GENERAL APPEARANCE: The patient appeared well nourished, slightly dehydrated and in mild discomfort.

VITAL SIGNS

Temperature	98.6°F (37°C)
Pulse	90 beats/minute
Blood pressure	130/90 mmHg
Respirations	18 breaths/minute
Oxygen saturation	98% on room air

HEENT: Unremarkable.

NECK: Supple.

CARDIOVASCULAR: Regular rate and rhythm without rubs, murmurs or gallops.

LUNGS: Clear to auscultation bilaterally.

ABDOMEN: Soft, mildly distended, with diffuse tenderness to palpation without associated rebound or guarding. Bowel sounds were absent. The surgical incision was healing well without erythema or discharge.

RECTAL: Normal tone, paucity of stool, hemoccult negative.

EXTREMITIES: No clubbing, cyanosis or edema.

NEUROLOGIC: Nonfocal.

Laboratory tests on this repeat visit revealed a leukocyte count of 13.1 K/μL (normal 3.5–12.5 K/μL) with 77% neutrophils (normal 50–70%) and a creatinine of 1.7 mg/dL (increased from 0.8 mg/dL on the previous visit). Intravenous fluids and antiemetics were administered, and a CT scan of the abdomen and pelvis with oral and intravenous contrast was obtained (Figure 31.2).

What is your diagnosis?

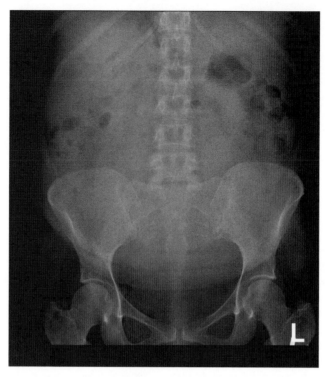

Figure 31.1 Abdominal radiograph (KUB) from a 29-year-old female with abdominal pain, nausea and vomiting following a cesarean section.

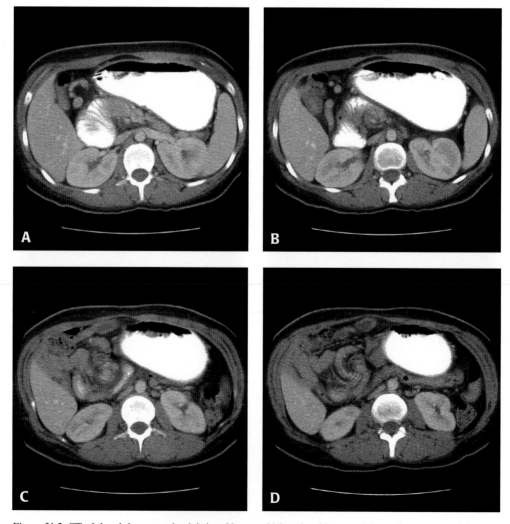

Figure 31.2 CT of the abdomen and pelvis in a 29-year-old female with several days of nausea, vomiting and abdominal pain (panels A–D from superior to inferior transverse images).

The diagnosis is malrotation of the midgut. The CT scan revealed moderate dilatation of the proximal duodenum, a distended stomach, and mesenteric swirling in the right upper abdomen (arrows, Figure 31.3). These findings were significant for a partial obstruction secondary to an internal hernia or mesenteric volvulus. The patient was taken to the operating room and underwent an exploratory laparotomy with a Ladd's procedure (division of Ladd's band with appendectomy). Intraoperative findings included a significant band from the cecum and right colon crossing over the malrotated duodenum, which was divided; the duodenum was freed without evidence of volvulus. The bowel was healthy without evidence of ischemia. The patient was discharged home on postoperative day #3 with an uneventful recovery.

Malrotation of the midgut

Malrotation of the midgut is a term used to describe abnormal rotation of the fetal intestines around the axis of the superior mesenteric artery.[1] These congenital anomalies include nonrotation, incomplete rotation, reversed rotation, and fixation abnormalities of the mesentery.[1,2] Rotational anomalies may become symptomatic at any age, including late in adult life. However, 80% of patients who become symptomatic do so in the first month of life.[2] The true incidence of malrotation is unknown. Estimates in the literature range from 1 in 200 to 1 in 6000 live births.[3] Autopsy studies suggest that some form of malrotation may exist in 0.5–1% of the population.[2,3] The most feared complication associated with anomalies of intestinal rotation is ischemic necrosis of the intestines with midgut volvulus.[2]

Not all patients with malrotation present with symptoms.[4] Many live without any complaints, with the anomaly discovered incidentally at autopsy. Some may present with chronic and unexplained abdominal discomfort, and even fewer may report acute episodes of agonizing abdominal pain.[4] Symptoms may arise from acute or chronic intestinal obstruction caused by the presence of abnormal peritoneal bands (e.g., Ladd's bands) or a volvulus. The presence of Ladd's bands in patients with anomalies of intestinal rotation can lead to vomiting due to compression of the duodenum by these peritoneal bands between the abnormally positioned cecum and the right retroperitoneum.[2] Patients with Ladd's bands and anomalies of intestinal rotation frequently present with a history of chronic vomiting (often bilious) associated with failure to gain weight.[2]

The diagnosis of rotational anomaly can be identified from radiographic studies. In the absence of volvulus, a plain radiograph of the abdomen is of little diagnostic value.[4] The absent cecal gas shadow or the localization of small intestinal loops predominantly on the right side should arouse suspicion of malrotation.[4] The accuracy of the upper gastrointestinal series (UGI) is reported to be over 80%.[5] The finding on UGI of a right-sided duodenojejunal junction or proximal jejunal loops is highly suggestive of malrotation.[5] CT scan of the abdomen is the radiographic test of choice for diagnosing malrotation. Malrotation can be diagnosed on CT by the anatomic location of a right-sided small bowel, a left-sided colon, an abnormal relationship of the superior mesenteric vessels, and aplasia of the pancreatic uncinate process.[4] Ultrasonography can be used to diagnose malrotation with midgut volvulus by detecting the superior mesenteric vein (SMV) rotated around the superior mesenteric artery (SMA). This sonographic sign, known as the whirlpool sign, corresponds to a clockwise wrapping of the SMV and mesentery around the SMA.[6] The appearance of this characteristic sign can facilitate the preoperative diagnosis of midgut volvulus and malrotation. The disadvantage of ultrasonography is that it is operator-dependent.[6]

The classic treatment for incomplete intestinal rotation is the Ladd's procedure, which involves immobilization of the right colon, division of Ladd's bands and mobilization

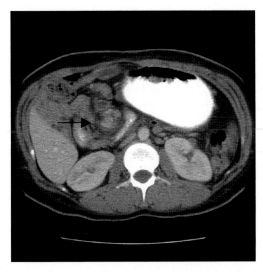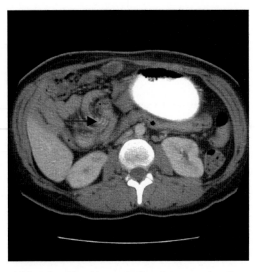

Figure 31.3 CT of the abdomen and pelvis in a 29-year-old female with midgut volvulus, demonstrating distended stomach with mesenteric swirling in the right upper abdomen (mesenteric swirling, arrows).

of the duodenum, division of adhesions around the SMA to broaden the mesenteric base, and appendectomy.[4] Generally, symptomatic patients with malrotation require surgical intervention. Treatment for patients discovered to have malrotation (e.g., incidental radiologic finding) who are asymptomatic is more controversial, although some surgeons recommend that all patients with malrotation receive laparotomy.[4] Intestinal rotation abnormalities without the presence of volvulus have been successfully managed using laparoscopic surgical techniques.[7]

KEY TEACHING POINTS

1. Midgut malrotation, an anomaly of fetal intestinal rotation usually presenting in the first month of life, may present in adulthood.
2. Symptomatic patients present either acutely, with symptoms of bowel obstruction and intestinal ischemia from midgut or cecal volvulus, or more chronically, with vague abdominal pain with or without vomiting.
3. Patients with compression of the duodenum by Ladd's bands may present with bilious emesis and abdominal pain, even in the absence of midgut volvulus.
4. Radiographic diagnosis of midgut malrotation can be made by upper gastrointestinal series (UGI), CT scan of the abdomen or ultrasonography. CT scan of the abdomen is the radiographic test of choice.
5. The classic treatment for incomplete intestinal rotation is the Ladd's procedure, which involves immobilization of the right colon, division of Ladd's bands and mobilization of the duodenum, division of adhesions around the SMA, and appendectomy.

REFERENCES

[1] Wai C-T, Cheah W-K. Gastrointestinal: midgut malrotation in an adult. *J Gastroent Hepatol* 2006;21:917.
[2] Gosche JR, Vick L, Boulanger SC, et al. Midgut abnormalities. *Surg Clin N Am* 2006;86:285–99.
[3] Kapfer SA, Rappold JF. Intestinal malrotation – not just the pediatric surgeon's problem. *J Am Coll Surg* 2004;199:628–35.
[4] Gamblin TC, Stephens RE, Johnson RK, et al. Adult malrotation: a case report and review of the literature. *Curr Surg* 2003;60:517–20.
[5] Kanazawa T, Kasugai K, Miyata M, et al. Case report: midgut malrotation in adulthood. *Intern Med* 200;39:626–31.
[6] Chin L-W, Wang H-P. Ultrasonographic diagnosis of elderly midgut volvulus in the ED. *Am J Emerg Med* 2006;24:900–2.
[7] Mazziotti MV, Stasberg SM, Langer JC. Intestinal rotation abnormalities without volvulus: the role of laparoscopy. *J Am Coll Surg* 1997;185:172–6.

32

Right lower quadrant abdominal pain and fever in a 36-year-old male

HISTORY OF PRESENT ILLNESS

A 36-year-old male with a medical history significant for polycystic kidney disease and a known right inguinal hernia presented to the ED complaining of one day of fever and right lower quadrant abdominal pain. The patient described the pain as cramping and constant, with radiation to the right groin. He reported nausea without vomiting, and denied diarrhea, constipation, dysuria, hematuria or anorexia. He reported that his right inguinal hernia had been present for many years with swelling into the right scrotum, which was unchanged. He denied any redness to the skin overlying the hernia.

PHYSICAL EXAMINATION

GENERAL APPEARANCE: The patient appeared well hydrated and well developed but in moderate discomfort.

VITAL SIGNS

Temperature	100.9°F (38.3°C)
Pulse	87 beats per minute
Blood pressure	148/100 mmHg
Respirations	18 breaths per minute
Oxygen saturation	98% on room air

HEENT: Unremarkable.

NECK: Supple.

CARDIOVASCULAR: Regular rate and rhythm without rubs, murmurs or gallops.

LUNGS: Clear to auscultation bilaterally.

ABDOMEN: Soft, nondistended, active bowel sounds present. Tenderness noted in the right lower quadrant and suprapubic regions, with voluntary guarding but no rebound tenderness. No masses present.

GENITOURINARY: A large hernia sac was present in the right scrotum; the area was mildly tender but easily reducible. There was neither erythema nor increased warmth over the sac.

EXTREMITIES: No clubbing, cyanosis or edema.

NEUROLOGIC: Nonfocal.

A peripheral intravenous line was placed, blood was drawn and sent for laboratory testing, and morphine sulfate and Zofran® were administered IV for pain and nausea, respectively. A 1-liter bolus of normal saline was also given. Laboratory tests were significant for a leukocyte count of 11.8 K/μL (normal 3.5–12.5 K/μL) with 82% neutrophils (normal 50–70%); the electrolytes, creatinine glucose, liver function tests and urinalysis were all within normal limits. A CT scan of the abdomen and pelvis with intravenous and oral contrast was obtained (Figure 32.1).

The CT scan interpreted by the radiologist demonstrated a normal appendix and presence of a right inguinal hernia with small bowel extending within it, without evidence of strangulation or localized inflammation. Because the patient was still having discomfort despite pain medication, a surgical consultation was obtained in the ED. The hernia was noted to be reducible and no acute surgical issue was determined to be present. The patient was therefore discharged from the ED with a prescription for hydrocodone and an outpatient surgery clinic referral to evaluate for elective right inguinal herniorrhaphy.

Approximately 36 hours after discharge, the patient returned to the ED complaining of worsening lower abdominal pain not controlled with hydrocodone. The patient was afebrile with normal vital signs and appeared in moderate distress. Abdominal examination demonstrated bilateral lower abdominal tenderness, right greater than left, with guarding and rebound tenderness. Laboratory tests were essentially unchanged from his prior visit. A second CT scan of the abdomen and pelvis with intravenous and oral contrast was obtained (Figure 32.2).

What is your diagnosis?

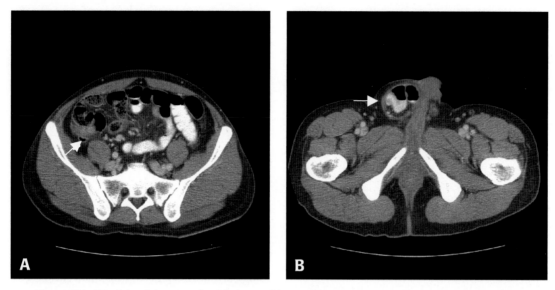

Figure 32.1 CT of the abdomen and pelvis from a 36-year-old male with one day of right lower quadrant abdominal pain, demonstrating a normal air-filled appendix (arrow, panel A) and a large right inguinal hernia sac (arrow, panel B).

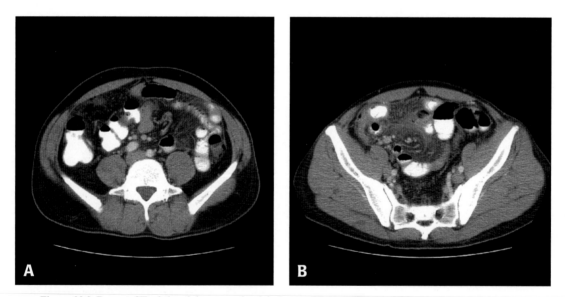

Figure 32.2 Repeat CT of the abdomen and pelvis from a 36-year-old male with two days of right lower quadrant abdominal pain.

The diagnosis is perforated Meckel's diverticulitis. The repeat CT scan demonstrated bowel wall thickening in the right lower quadrant, with one segment of bowel wall appearing to represent the appendix. Stranding and infiltration of adjacent fat was noted, along with the presence of small amounts of pneumoperitoneum (Figure 32.3). The bowel loops within the hernia did not show inflammation or thickening. The findings were suspicious for ruptured appendicitis. Intravenous antibiotics were given and the patient was taken to the OR. A laparotomy was performed; upon surgical exploration of the right lower quadrant, a Meckel's diverticulum that had perforated into the small bowel mesentery was discovered. Although the appendix itself appeared normal, periappendiceal changes were noted. A small bowel resection to remove the perforated Meckel's diverticulum was performed, as well as an appendectomy. The patient's recovery was uneventful.

Meckel's diverticulum

Meckel's diverticulum is the most common congenital anomaly of the GI tract (1–3% of the population), resulting from failure of the omphalomesenteric duct to become obliterated.[1] As a congenital variant, Meckel's diverticula are often found in children and are much less common in the adult population. Anatomically, this structure is located within 75 cm of the ileocecal valve in 75% of cases.[2] The vascular supply to a Meckel's diverticulum is a vestige of the vitelline artery and arises directly from the mesentery. There is ectopic gastric and pancreatic mucosa found in a Meckel's diverticulum in 95% of resected specimens for gastrointestinal bleeding and in 30–65% of asymptomatic patients.[2] A commonly quoted "rule of 2s" applies to Meckel's diverticula: 2% of the population have the anomaly, it is approximately 2 inches in length, it is usually found within 2 feet of the ileocecal valve, it is often found in children under 2 years of age, and it affects males twice as often as females.[3]

A person with Meckel's diverticulum has a 4–6% lifetime risk of developing a complication.[4] The major complications are hemorrhage, obstruction, intussusception, diverticulitis and perforation. Bleeding is the most common complication occurring in childhood, whereas most adults present with obstruction, diverticulitis or both.[4] Although rare, Meckel's diverticulum can be part of a hernia's contents.

Various imaging techniques have been used to diagnose Meckel's diverticulum. Plain films are of limited value; however, they may show enteroliths, bowel obstruction, or the presence of gas or a gas-fluid level in the diverticulum.[5] Meckel's diverticulum is not often seen on routine barium studies because of its small ostium, it is often filled with intestinal contents, and peristalsis results in rapid emptying. Meticulous examination with enteroclysis has been reported to be more sensitive.[5] Although of limited value, sonography has been used for the investigation of Meckel's diverticulum.[6] High-resolution sonography usually shows a fluid-filled structure in the right lower quadrant having the appearance of a blind-ending, thick-walled loop of bowel, with the typical gut signature and a clear connection to a peristaltic, normal small bowel loop.

On CT, Meckel's diverticulum is difficult to distinguish from normal small bowel in uncomplicated cases.[5] However, a blind-ending fluid- or gas-filled structure in continuity with the small bowel may be seen. CT may also show enteroliths, intussusception, diverticulitis or small bowel obstruction. CT enteroclysis (CTE) combines the advantages of CT and barium enteroclysis, and has resulted in better visualization of the small bowel and higher sensitivity in the diagnosis of Meckel's diverticulum.[7] CTE combines the improved spatial and temporal resolution of multidetector CT with large volumes of

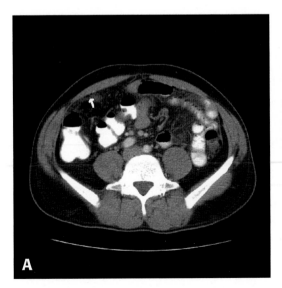 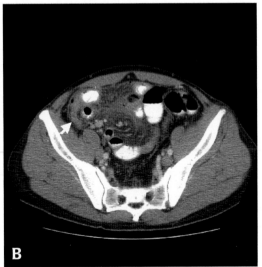

Figure 32.3 Repeat CT of the abdomen and pelvis from a 36-year-old male with right lower quadrant abdominal pain, demonstrating small areas of pneumoperitoneum (arrow, panel A) and appendix with stranding and infiltration of adjacent fat (arrow, panel B).

ingested neutral enteric contrast material to permit visualization of the small bowel wall.[7] The potential drawbacks to using CTE in the ED include requiring placement of a nasogastric tube for enteral contrast infusion as well as fluoroscopy to determine the placement of the nasogastric tube prior to contrast infusion and CT.

Scintigraphy with ^{99m}Tc-Na-pertechnetate has only minor diagnostic value and a limited sensitivity (60%) in diagnosing Meckel's diverticulum.[5] However, it aids in the diagnosis of diverticula with ectopic gastric mucosa. Pertechnetate is taken up by mucin-secreting cells of the gastric mucosa and ectopic gastric tissue. Higher sensitivity in pediatric (85–90%) than adult (60%) patients occurs, possibly due to earlier symptoms (such as hemorrhage) in patients with ectopic gastric mucosa.[5]

Meckel's diverticulitis may mimic appendicitis. The correct diagnosis is usually established at laparotomy or laparoscopy. No clinical features are pathognomonic, and the diagnosis is rarely made preoperatively.[8] Routine laboratory studies, such as leukocyte and erythrocyte counts, serum electrolytes, blood glucose, serum creatinine and coagulation screen, are helpful. CT and ultrasonography have been used for the diagnosis of Meckel's diverticulitis; despite the availability of these modern imaging techniques, the diagnosis remains challenging. Rangarajan et al. described a case similar to this in which the clinical diagnosis was appendicular perforation, whereas laparoscopy revealed a perforated Meckel's diverticulum.[8] Meckel's diverticulitis should be kept in mind in the differential diagnosis of an acute abdomen.

KEY TEACHING POINTS

1. Meckel's diverticulum, the most common congenital anomaly of the GI tract, is best described by the "rule of 2s."
2. A person with Meckel's diverticulum has a 4–6% lifetime risk of developing a complication such as hemorrhage, obstruction, intussusception, diverticulitis or perforation.
3. CT enteroclysis (CTE) combines the advantages of CT and barium enteroclysis, resulting in better visualization of the small bowel and higher sensitivity in the diagnosis of Meckel's diverticulum.
4. Meckel's diverticulitis may mimic appendicitis; the correct diagnosis is usually established at laparotomy or laparoscopy.
5. Complications from a Meckel's diverticulum should be considered as one of the differential diagnoses of an acute abdomen in patients of any age.

REFERENCES

[1] Kaltenback T, Nguyen C, Lau J, et al. Multidetector CT enteroclysis localized a Meckel's diverticulum in a case of obscure GI bleeding. *Gastrointest Endosc* 2006;64:441–2.

[2] Gosche JR, Vick L, Boulanger SC, et al. Midgut abnormalities. *Surg Clin N Am* 2006;86:285–99.

[3] Dumper J, Mackenzie S, Mitchell P, et al. Complications of Meckel's diverticula in adults. *Can J Surg* 2006;49:353–7.

[4] Zacharakis E, Papadopoulos V, Athanasiou T, et al. An unusual presentation of Meckel diverticulum as strangulated femoral hernia. *South Med J* 2008;101:96–8.

[5] Elsayes KM, Menias CO, Harvin HJ, et al. Imaging manifestations of Meckel's diverticulum. *Am J Roentgenol* 2007;189:81–8.

[6] Mostbeck GH, Liskutin J, Dorffner R, et al. Ultrasonographic diagnosis of a bleeding Meckel's diverticulum. *Pediatr Radiol* 2000;30:382.

[7] Maglinte DDT, Sandrasegaran K, Lappas JC. CT enteroclysis: techniques and applications. *Radiol Clin N Am* 2007; 45:289–301.

[8] Rangarajan M, Palanivelu C, Senthilkumar R, et al. Laparoscopic surgery for perforation of Meckel's diverticulum. *Singapore Med J* 2007;48:e102–5.

33

Abdominal pain and diarrhea in a 64-year-old female

HISTORY OF PRESENT ILLNESS

A 64-year-old female with a remote surgical history significant for a total abdominal hysterectomy presented to the ED complaining of four days of diffuse abdominal pain and multiple episodes of watery diarrhea. She described her pain initially as intermittent and crampy, becoming constant on the day of presentation. She rated the pain at a level of 7 (on a scale of 0 to 10). She denied fevers or chills but reported significant nausea without vomiting. She also reported at least 10 episodes of nonbloody diarrhea per day beginning four days ago. Her diarrhea stopped on the day of presentation, and she was not passing gas.

PHYSICAL EXAMINATION

GENERAL APPEARANCE: The patient appeared well nourished, somewhat dehydrated and in moderate discomfort.

VITAL SIGNS

Temperature	97.8°F (36.5°C)
Pulse	95 beats/minute
Blood pressure	165/90 mmHg
Respirations	20 breaths/minute
Oxygen saturation	98% on room air

HEENT: Unremarkable.

NECK: Supple, no jugular venous distension.

CARDIOVASCULAR: Regular rate and rhythm without rubs, murmurs or gallops.

LUNGS: Clear to auscultation bilaterally.

ABDOMEN: A low, horizontal scar was noted; the abdomen was moderately distended with hypoactive bowel sounds. Palpation demonstrated diffuse tenderness with both rebound and guarding.

RECTAL: Normal tone, brown stool, hemoccult negative.

EXTREMITIES: No clubbing, cyanosis or edema.

NEUROLOGIC: Nonfocal.

A peripheral intravenous line was placed, blood was drawn and sent for laboratory testing, and the patient was given morphine sulfate and Phenergan® IV for pain and nausea, respectively. She also received a 500 mL normal saline IV fluid bolus. Laboratory tests revealed a leukocyte count of 8.3 K/μL (normal 3.5–12.5 K/μL) with 83% neutrophils (normal 50–70%), hematocrit of 47% (normal 34–46%), BUN of 24 mg/dL (normal 7–17 mg/dL) and creatinine of 1.2 mg/dL (normal <1.3 mg/dL). An abdominal radiograph series was obtained (Figure 33.1).

What is your diagnosis?

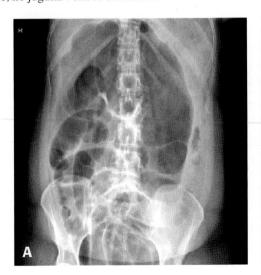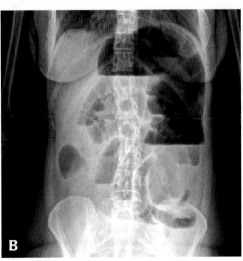

Figure 33.1 Supine (panel A) and upright (panel B) abdominal radiographs from a 64-year-old female with four days of diffuse abdominal pain and diarrhea.

ANSWER

The diagnosis is bowel obstruction with perforated viscus secondary to cecal volvulus. The abdominal radiograph series demonstrates multiple dilated small bowel loops in the mid-to-upper abdomen, as well as a dilated large bowel loop in the left upper abdomen (upright view, panel B, Figure 33.1). No free air was identified on the plain films. A CT of the abdomen and pelvis with oral and intravenous contrast (Figure 33.2) revealed the presence of a markedly dilated cecum positioned in the left upper abdomen, associated dilatation of the small bowel to 3 cm, several foci of free air, and a swirling pattern in the mesentery. These findings were consistent with a perforated cecal volvulus. The patient was taken to the OR and upon laparotomy, a massively distended cecum was identified as well as tears in the bowel wall taenia, with a small perforation site. No adhesions from her previous hysterectomy were identified. The patient underwent a right hemicolectomy with side-to-side anastomosis between the ileum and the distal ascending colon. Her recovery was uneventful.

Cecal volvulus

Cecal volvulus is an axial twist of the cecum, ascending colon and terminal ileum around a mesenteric pedicle.[1] Cecal volvulus is relatively uncommon, with an incidence of 2.8–7.1 per 1 million people per year. It accounts for approximately 1% of acute intestinal obstruction in British, Western European and American series.[1] It also causes proximal colonic obstruction and secondary small bowel dilatation. Recognition of the distended cecum on imaging studies is the key to differentiating volvulus from an isolated small bowel obstruction.[2]

Patients with cecal volvulus are usually in the sixth decade of life; many have underlying congenital or acquired abnormalities that lead to increased cecal mobility.[3] Cecal volvulus typically presents with acute onset of pain, nausea and vomiting.[4] On abdominal plain films, cecal volvulus usually shows a dilated loop of bowel with a "coffee bean" appearance in the left upper quadrant, although this characteristic finding is not always seen on plain radiographs.[4,5]

CT reveals the presence and location of the volvulus and has the added benefit of allowing early identification of potentially fatal complications, such as ischemia or perforation.[6] A CT sign specific for volvulus is the "whirl," which has been described as volvulus of the midgut, cecum and sigmoid colon.[6] The "whirl" is composed of spiral loops of collapsed cecum and sigmoid colon. Low-attenuating fatty mesentery with enhancing engorged vessels radiate from the twisted bowel. In the central eye of the "whirl," a soft-tissue density pinpoints the source of the twist. The degree of cecal rotation can even be predicted by the "whirl's" tightness.[6]

Emergency management of patients with cecal volvulus includes pain control, aggressive intravenous hydration with normal saline, nasogastric suctioning and prompt surgical consultation. The rates of reduction in cecal volvulus achieved through colonoscopy are much lower than those achieved in sigmoid volvulus. Furthermore, in patients with cecal volvulus the recurrence rate exceeds 50%.[6] Although successful reduction by barium enema has been reported, high rates of perforation may occur; therefore, the standard of care for treatment of cecal volvulus is almost always operative, with either cecopexy or right-sided hemicolectomy.[5]

KEY TEACHING POINTS

1. Cecal volvulus involves an axial twist of the cecum, ascending colon and terminal ileum around a mesenteric pedicle, leading to large bowel obstruction.
2. Cecal volvulus usually occurs in the sixth decade of life and typically presents with acute onset of abdominal pain, nausea and vomiting.
3. In cases of cecal volvulus, plain abdominal radiographs may show the characteristic "coffee bean" appearance of the dilated large bowel.

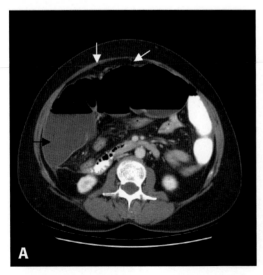
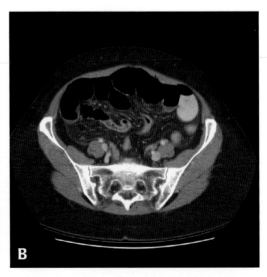

Figure 33.2 CT of the abdomen and pelvis from a 64-year-old female with cecal volvulus, demonstrating a massively distended cecum (dark arrow, panel A) with several small foci of free air (white arrows, panel A), as well as dilated loops of small bowel and a swirling pattern of the mesentery (panel B).

4. Management of patients with cecal volvulus should include pain control, intravenous hydration, nasogastric suctioning and prompt surgical consultation.

5. Definitive treatment of cecal volvulus is predominantly surgical, with either cecopexy or right-sided hemicolectomy; attempts at reduction by colonoscopy or contrast enemas lead to low success rates and the potential for perforation.

REFERENCES

[1] Majeski J. Operative therapy for cecal volvulus combining resection with colopexy. *Am J Surg* 2005;189:211–3.

[2] Qalbani A, Paushter D, Dachman AH. Multidetector row CT of small bowel obstruction. *Radiol Clin N Am* 2007; 45:499–512.

[3] Kahi CJ, Rex DK. Bowel obstruction and pseudo-obstruction. *Gastroenterol Clin N Am* 2003;32:1229–47.

[4] Martinez JP, Mattu A. Abdominal pain in the elderly. *Emerg Med Clin N Am* 2006;24:371–88.

[5] Hsia R, Chiao A, Law-Courter J. Images in emergency medicine. *Ann Emerg Med* 2007;49:272, 281.

[6] Moore CJ, Corl FM, Fishman EK. Pictorial essay. CT of cecal volvulus: unraveling the image. *Am J Roentgen* 2001;177:95–8.

34

Rectal and abdominal pain in a 70-year-old male

HISTORY OF PRESENT ILLNESS

A 70-year-old male with a history of anemia presented to the ED complaining of several hours of lower abdominal and rectal pain. The pain started suddenly, was described as severe and localized to the lower abdomen, and was associated with nausea. The patient could not have a bowel movement since the onset of the pain. He denied previous abdominal surgeries, associated urinary symptoms, fevers or chills.

PHYSICAL EXAMINATION

GENERAL APPEARANCE: The patient appeared in acute pain, unable to find a comfortable position on the gurney.

VITAL SIGNS

Temperature	98.8°F (37.1°C)
Pulse	79 beats/minute
Blood pressure	137/81 mmHg
Respirations	22 breaths/minute
Oxygen saturation	100% on room air

HEENT: Unremarkable.

NECK: Unremarkable.

CARDIOVASCULAR: Regular rate and rhythm without rubs, murmurs or gallops.

LUNGS: Clear to auscultation bilaterally.

ABDOMEN: Distended, hypoactive bowel sounds, presence of a firm and tender mass in the peri- and infraumbilical region; no rebound or guarding noted.

RECTAL: Normal rectal tone, presence of a firm mass without blood.

A peripheral intravenous line was placed, blood was drawn and sent for laboratory testing, and morphine sulfate was

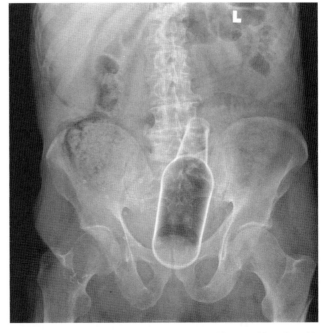

Figure 34.1 Abdominal radiograph from a 70-year-old male with sudden onset of abdominal and rectal pain.

administered intravenously for pain. Laboratory results revealed a leukocyte count of 12.2 K/μL (normal 3.5–12.5 K/μL) with 86% neutrophils (normal 50–70%), hematocrit of 32% (normal 39–51%), with the remainder of the laboratory tests (electrolytes, BUN, creatinine and glucose) within normal limits. An abdominal radiograph was obtained (Figure 34.1).

What is your diagnosis?

The diagnosis is rectal foreign body. The abdominal radiograph demonstrates an opacity that has the appearance of a bottle projecting over the pelvis, measuring 20 cm in length by 7 cm in diameter. These findings are compatible with a bottle within the patient's rectum. An upright chest radiograph did not demonstrate free air under the diaphragm. Manual attempts to remove the foreign body in the ED were unsuccessful. The patient was admitted to the surgical service, and the bottle was manually removed in the OR under general anesthesia. The patient had an uneventful recovery.

Rectal foreign bodies

Colorectal foreign body insertion is most commonly performed for sexual stimulation (60–78%) but has also been associated with sexual assault (10–40%).[1] Objects placed as a result of assault, trauma or eroticism include sex toys, tools and instruments, bottles, cans and jars, poles, pipes and tubing, fruits and vegetables, stones, balls, balloons, umbrellas, light bulbs and flashlights.[2] Up to 20% of cases of traumatic rectal injury seen in the ED result from rectal foreign body insertion.[1] Patients presenting with a rectal foreign body are predominately male, usually in their fourth or fifth decades of life, and present between 6–48 hours after insertion.[3] They usually present to the ED because of pain, often after multiple attempts to remove the object.[4] Presentation is often delayed because of embarrassment. The keys to appropriate care for these patients are respect for their privacy, evaluation of the type and location of the foreign body, determination if removal can safely be performed in the ED or if operative referral is needed, and the use of appropriate techniques for removal.[4] Mortality from retained rectal foreign bodies is rare and results from bleeding, rectal perforation or laceration, and infectious complications.[4]

Diagnosis of rectal foreign body can usually be made from the history. Therefore, the physical examination should concentrate on excluding anorectal or intestinal perforation and determining which objects will be accessible in the ED.[5] Rectal foreign bodies can be classified as high-lying or low-lying, depending on their location relative to the rectosigmoid junction.[2–4] Objects that are above the sacral curve and rectosigmoid junction are difficult to visualize and remove, and are often unreachable by rigid proctosigmoidoscope. Digital rectal examination is useful to identify blood (indicates possible laceration or perforation), as well as objects that are low-lying or palpable. It may also identify candidates (and objects) appropriate for ED removal.[2,5] Plain radiographs of the abdomen should be obtained, as these will assist in delineating the shape, position and number of objects, as well as evaluating for pneumoperitoneum.[3,5] If a foreign body with a sharp edge is suspected from the history, the clinician should not perform the digital rectal examination until radiographs are obtained.

The majority of rectal foreign bodies are easily removed in the ED.[2] Relaxation of the anal sphincter is essential, so sedation is often necessary to retrieve these foreign bodies. Foreign body removal in the ED is contraindicated in patients who have severe abdominal pain or signs of perforation, a nonpalpable foreign body or broken glass in the rectum; in these cases, a general surgeon should be consulted.[5] Other situations precluding ED removal include a foreign body that is unusually difficult to remove, or when there is insufficient experience or equipment to perform the procedure. The usual treatment of these patients by surgery includes attempted visualization and removal under general anesthesia using flexible rectosigmoidoscopy.[1] In rare cases, laparotomy may be necessary to remove the foreign body.

Chen et al. reported a case series of 10 male patients (mean age 57 years) with 12 presentations of retained rectal foreign bodies.[6] Glass bottles and vibrators were the most common objects encountered. The majority of the objects were extracted by nonsurgical methods using either anoscopy ($n = 4$), rigid sigmoidoscopy ($n = 2$) or colonoscopy ($n = 1$). Obstetric forceps were used to remove an incarcerated bowling pin. Emergent laparotomies were performed in cases with overt peritonitis ($n = 2$), pelvic sepsis ($n = 1$), and an impacted high-lying glass bottle. Minor complications, such as mucosal abrasions or superficial tears, were found in 62.5% of the nonsurgically treated cases. Delayed bleeding occurred in two of the cases. There was no mortality in this small series.

KEY TEACHING POINTS

1. Patients with a rectal foreign body may present with rectal pain, abdominal pain or rectal bleeding.
2. The type of object, length of time since insertion, presence of rectal or abdominal pain, fever or bleeding are important historical elements in patients with rectal foreign bodies.
3. Digital rectal examination is useful to identify blood as well as objects that are low-lying or palpable, and possible candidates for ED removal.
4. Plain radiographs of the abdomen should be obtained to assist in delineating the shape, position, and number of objects, as well as evaluating for pneumoperitoneum.
5. Although the majority of rectal foreign bodies are easily removed in the ED, foreign body removal is contraindicated in patients who have severe abdominal pain or signs of perforation, a nonpalpable foreign body or broken glass in the rectum.

REFERENCES

[1] Yacov Y, Tsivian A, Sidi AA. Emergent and surgical interventions for injuries associated with eroticism: a review. *J Trauma* 2007;62:1522–30.
[2] Hellinger MD. Anal trauma and foreign bodies. *Surg Clin N Am* 2002;82:1253–60.

[3] Singaporewalla RM, Tan DEL, Tan TK. Use of endoscopic snare to extract a large rectosigmoid foreign body with review of literature. *Surg Laparosc Endosc Percutan Tech* 2007;17:145–8.

[4] Munter DW. Foreign bodies, rectum. eMedicine Website. Available at http://www.emedicine.com/emerg/topic933.htm. Accessed July 8, 2008.

[5] Strear CM, Coates WC. Anorectal procedures. In: Roberts JR, Hedges JR, Chanmugam AS, et al. (eds.). *Clinical Procedures in Emergency Medicine*, 4th ed. Philadelphia: Elsevier, 2004:868–80.

[6] Huang W-C, Jiang J-K, Wang H-S, et al. Retained rectal foreign bodies. *J Chin Med Assoc* 2003;66:606–11.

35

Abdominal pain in a 75-year-old male

HISTORY OF PRESENT ILLNESS

A 75-year-old male with a surgical history significant for a remote right hemicolectomy presented to the ED complaining of several months of intermittent epigastric and right upper quadrant abdominal pain. In the ED, the patient reported a dull, constant pain localized to his epigastrium and right upper quadrant, which he rated at a level of 3 (on a scale of 0 to 10). The patient denied fevers, nausea, vomiting, diarrhea, constipation, dysuria, chest pain or shortness of breath.

PHYSICAL EXAMINATION

GENERAL APPEARANCE: The patient was a well-developed, well-hydrated elderly male in no acute discomfort.

VITAL SIGNS

Temperature	98.6°F (37°C)
Pulse	77 beats/minute
Blood pressure	145/90 mmHg
Respirations	20 breaths/minute
Oxygen saturation	99% on room air

HEENT: Unremarkable.

NECK: Supple, no jugular venous distension.

CARDIOVASCULAR: Regular rate and rhythm without rubs, murmurs or gallops.

LUNGS: Clear to auscultation bilaterally.

ABDOMEN: Midline vertical scar present in lower abdomen (previous hemicolectomy). Soft, nondistended, active bowel sounds present. Tenderness to palpation noted in the epigastrium and right upper quadrant without presence of a Murphy's sign. No pulsatile masses were appreciated. Femoral pulses were present and equal bilaterally.

RECTAL: Normal tone, brown stool, hemoccult negative.

EXTREMITIES: No clubbing, cyanosis or edema.

NEUROLOGIC: Nonfocal.

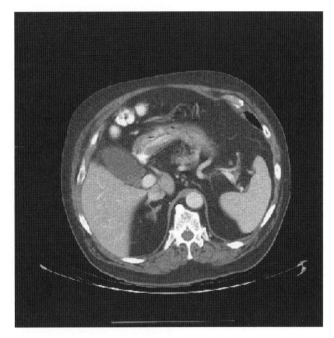

Figure 35.1 CT of the abdomen from a 75-year-old male with epigastric and right upper quadrant pain.

A peripheral intravenous line was placed, blood was drawn and sent for laboratory testing, and the patient was given a GI cocktail (Maalox® 30 mL and viscous lidocaine 10 mL orally) with initial improvement of his symptoms. Laboratory tests revealed a leukocyte count of 10.9 K/μL (normal 3.5–12.5 K/μL) with a differential demonstrating 87% neutrophils (normal 50–70%); liver function tests, amylase, electrolytes, glucose and serum creatinine were all within normal limits. The patient's pain returned to its previous level, and a CT scan of the abdomen and pelvis with oral and intravenous contrast (Figure 35.1) followed by an ultrasound of the right upper quadrant (Figure 35.2) were subsequently obtained.

What is your diagnosis?

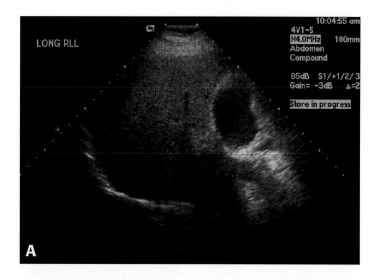

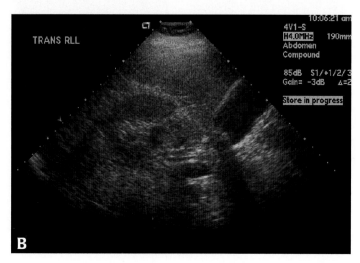

Figure 35.2 Long (panel A) and transverse (panel B) ultrasound images of right upper quadrant from a 75-year-old male with epigastric and right upper quadrant pain.

ANSWER

The diagnosis is acute, gangrenous cholecystitis. The CT scan image in Figure 35.1 demonstrates gallbladder sludge without pericholecystic fluid. The right upper quadrant ultrasound demonstrates the presence of gallstones with gallbladder wall thickening (arrows, Figure 35.3). The patient received cefotetan 2 gm IV preoperatively and was taken to the OR for a laparoscopic cholecystectomy. At surgery, the patient was found to have a gangrenous gallbladder adherent to the liver. It was removed laparoscopically, although with difficulty. The patient underwent an uneventful postoperative course.

Abdominal pain in the elderly

Abdominal pain is the fourth most common ED complaint in older patients. It accounts for approximately 3–4% of all ED visits in the group 65 years and older.[1] Morbidity and mortality among older patients with abdominal pain are high; evaluation and management often requires admission to the hospital and surgical consultation.[2] In retrospective studies, more than half of older patients presenting to the ED with acute abdominal pain required hospital admission, and 20–33% required immediate surgery.[2,3] Surgical intervention occurs twice as often in older patients when compared to a younger population.[2] Overall mortality rates from retrospective series vary between 2–13%.[2,4]

Making the correct diagnosis of abdominal pain in elderly patients is difficult due to multiple factors. These include difficulty in obtaining history from the patient, lack of consistent physiologic response (including fever and leukocytosis), and confusing clinical presentations due to comorbid conditions.[5] The patient's ability to provide a history is frequently compromised by an altered ability to communicate, resulting from hearing and vision loss, cerebrovascular accidents leading to receptive or expressive aphasia, Alzheimer's disease and other age-related dementias.[5] Other barriers to obtaining an adequate history include the patient's fear of loss of independence

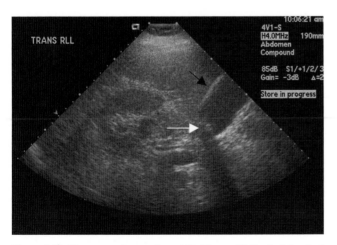

Figure 35.3 Transverse image (panel B, Figure 35.2) of abdominal ultrasound demonstrating gallbladder wall thickening (dark arrow) and gallstones with acoustic shadowing (white arrow).

and stoicism. Altered pain perception in the elderly may influence the patient's ability to adequately describe pain.[5]

Medication use in the elderly may mask or create abdominal pathology. Acetaminophen and NSAIDs may reduce the likelihood of fever, whereas corticosteroids may alter the serum leukocyte count and blunt the inflammatory response, preventing peritoneal signs from developing.[6] Chronic narcotic use may blunt pain that normally accompanies an abdominal catastrophe. Antibiotics may cause abdominal pain, vomiting and diarrhea. This is important to consider when evaluating an elderly patient on multiple medications.[6] The physical examination in elderly patients with abdominal pain can be misleadingly benign, secondary to a lower likelihood of localized tenderness despite a focal surgical condition, reduced rebound and guarding from decreased abdominal wall musculature, and suppressed tachycardia from medications (such as beta- or calcium-channel blockers) or intrinsic cardiac disease.[2]

Many laboratory tests for abdominal pain in the elderly are nonspecific and may give a false sense of security when normal.[5] For example, the total leukocyte count may be normal in the face of appendicitis or cholecystitis. Specific testing may be helpful in certain diagnoses, such as pancreatitis (lipase) or mesenteric ischemia (lactate), or in select circumstances such as a prothrombin time for a patient taking warfarin.[5] Liberal use of radiologic studies in elderly patients with abdominal pain is frequently warranted, ranging from plain abdominal radiographs (demonstrating free intraperitoneal air or air-fluid levels) to ultrasound (useful in imaging the biliary tract and the abdominal aorta) to computed tomography. CT use has been shown to be highly prevalent among older ED patients with acute abdominal pain, with the results often diagnostic, especially for patients with emergent conditions.[1]

Causes of abdominal pain in the elderly include biliary tract disease (cholelithiasis, cholecystitis, cholangitis), small and large bowel obstruction, appendicitis, acute pancreatitis, peptic ulcer disease and perforation, diverticular disease, abdominal aortic aneurysm, mesenteric ischemia, and atypical causes (e.g., urinary tract infections, pyelonephritis, myocardial infarction, pneumonia, congestive heart failure, constipation). Constipation is common in the elderly population and may be a side-effect of certain opiate-containing pain medications, as well as resulting from decreased fluid intake. Symptoms from serious intra-abdominal pathology may be incorrectly attributed to constipation.

Biliary disease remains the leading reason for acute abdominal surgery in the elderly population.[6] The likelihood of cholelithiasis increases with age, and the severity of gallstone disease is much higher in the elderly population. The prevalence of gallbladder perforation, gangrene, emphysematous cholecystitis, ascending cholangitis, gallstone ileus, choledocholithiasis and gallstone-induced pancreatitis are all greater in this population.[6] Elderly patients tend to have typical right upper quadrant or epigastric pain but more than half of elderly patients with acute cholecystitis do not have nausea and vomiting, and a significant proportion do not have fever.[5,6] Leukocytosis is absent in 30–40% and a significant percentage have normal liver function tests.[6] Ultrasound is the study of choice for diagnosing cholecystitis and is as sensitive in the elderly as in younger patients.[6] If no gallstones are found and clinical suspicion for gallbladder disease remains high, radionuclide scanning (cholescintigraphy) should be performed, as elderly patients have an increased likelihood of acalculous cholecystitis.[5,6]

The incidence of complications caused by biliary disease increases markedly in elderly patients. When the diagnosis of biliary disease is made, broad-spectrum antibiotics, specifically covering Gram-negative and anaerobic organisms, should be started immediately and prompt surgical evaluation initiated. Delayed surgical treatment in this population is associated with increased morbidity and mortality.

KEY TEACHING POINTS

1. Morbidity and mortality rates among older patients with abdominal pain are high; evaluation and management often requires admission to the hospital and prompt surgical consultation.

2. Difficulty in obtaining an accurate history, lack of consistent physiologic responses, confusing clinical presentations due to comorbid conditions, and medications that may mask clinical features of disease lead to diagnostic delays in determining the cause of abdominal pain in elderly patients.

3. Many laboratory tests (e.g., leukocyte count, liver function tests) may be normal in the presence of significant disease in elderly patients with abdominal pain.

4. Liberal use of radiologic studies, particularly ultrasound and CT, is recommended in elderly patients with abdominal pain in which the diagnosis remains unclear.

5. Biliary tract disease remains the leading reason for acute abdominal surgery in the elderly population. Once the diagnosis is made, broad-spectrum antibiotics should be started immediately and prompt surgical evaluation initiated.

REFERENCES

[1] Hustey FM, Meldon SW, Banet GA, et al. The use of abdominal computed tomography in older patients with acute abdominal pain. *Am J Emerg Med* 2005;23:259–65.

[2] Lyon C, Clark DC. Diagnosis of acute abdominal pain in older patients. *Am Fam Physician* 2006;74:1537–44.

[3] Bugliosi TF, Meloy TD, Vukov LF. Acute abdominal pain in the elderly. *Ann Emerg Med* 1990;19:1383–6.

[4] Abi-Hanna P, Gleckman R. Acute abdominal pain: a medical emergency in older patients. *Geriatrics* 1997;52:72–4.

[5] Yeh EL, McNamara RM. Abdominal pain. *Clin Geriatr Med* 2007;23:255–70.

[6] Martinez JP, Mattu A. Abdominal pain in the elderly. *Emerg Med Clin N Am* 2006;24:371–88.

36

Abdominal pain and anorexia in a 77-year-old female

HISTORY OF PRESENT ILLNESS

A 77-year-old female with a medical history significant for prior cerebrovascular accident with residual left-sided hemiplegia, hypertension, coronary artery disease and seizure disorder presented to the ED by ambulance complaining of several days of worsening abdominal pain, weakness, nausea and decreased oral intake. The patient was bedridden, communicative and oriented. On presentation, she described her abdominal pain as moderate to severe. The family reported that for three days prior to presentation, she was able to eat only very small amounts because eating caused her to feel "bloated and full." She denied fevers or chills, black stools or blood in her stool. She did experience one episode of coffee-ground emesis just prior to presentation. The patient denied chest pain but reported shortness of breath at rest. The patient's medications include hydrochlorothiazide, phenytoin, lisinopril, omeprazole, Nifedical® and lovastatin.

PHYSICAL EXAMINATION

GENERAL APPEARANCE: The patient appeared pale, dehydrated and in moderate discomfort.

VITAL SIGNS

Temperature	99°F (37.2°C)
Pulse	90 beats/minute
Blood pressure	100/60 mmHg
Respirations	24 breaths/minute
Oxygen saturation	99% on room air

HEENT: PERRL, EOMI, dry mucous membranes.

NECK: Supple, no jugular venous distension.

CARDIOVASCULAR: Regular rate and rhythm without rubs, murmurs or gallops.

LUNGS: Crackles at the bases bilaterally, no rhonchi or wheezes.

ABDOMEN: Soft, moderately distended abdomen with diffuse, mild tenderness to palpation without rebound or guarding.

RECTAL: Normal tone, brown stool, trace hemoccult positive.

EXTREMITIES: Cool, pale with delayed capillary refill; no clubbing, cyanosis or edema.

NEUROLOGIC: Alert and oriented to person, place and time; residual-left sided hemiplegia noted.

Intravenous fluids (normal saline) were started after blood was drawn and sent for laboratory testing, as well as blood type and antibody screen. A complete blood count revealed a leukocyte count of 7.9 K/μL (normal 3.5–12.5 K/μL) with 46% immature bands (presence of bands is abnormal) and hematocrit of 31% (normal 39–51%). A chemistry panel revealed a creatinine of 2.0 mg/dL (normal <1.5 mg/dL), potassium of 5.6 mEq/L (normal 3.5–5.3 mEq/L), CO_2 of 18 mEq/L (normal 22–30 mEq/L), with an anion gap of 19 mEq/L (normal 5–16 mEq/L). A serum lactate level returned elevated at 6.7 mmol/L (normal 0.7–2.1 mmol/L). Liver function tests and amylase were mildly elevated. A troponin I returned at 0.08 ng/mL (normal 0.0–0.09 ng/mL), and a urinalysis showed no evidence of infection.

During the ED evaluation, the patient's blood pressure dropped precipitously to 60/40 mmHg and she developed worsening dyspnea. Her blood pressure remained low despite intravenous fluid boluses, and a norepinephrine infusion was initiated. The patient's respiratory status continued to worsen, thus she was endotracheally intubated using rapid sequence induction. A nasogastric tube was placed and 1 liter of dark brown gastric contents returned upon saline lavage. An arterial blood gas performed post-intubation with the patient on 100% oxygen revealed pH 7.17 (normal 7.35–7.45), pCO_2 47 mmHg (normal 35–45 mmHg), pO_2 147 mmHg (normal 80–95 mmHg) and bicarbonate 15 mmol/L (normal 23–28 mmol/L), with a base excess of −11 mmol/L (normal −2.4 to 2.3 mmol/L).

What is your diagnosis?

The diagnosis is acute mesenteric ischemia. A CT scan of the abdomen and pelvis with intravenous contrast was obtained, which demonstrated attenuation and diminished flow through the celiac trunk, as well as occlusion of the superior mesenteric artery (Figure 36.1). An intraluminal filling defect of the superior mesenteric vein was also noted, as well as mild dilatation of small bowel loops with pneumatosis intestinalis. These findings are consistent with ischemic bowel disease (mesenteric ischemia). Additionally, portal venous gas was noted in the left hepatic lobe with mild low-attenuation, compatible with a hepatic infarct. The decision was made by the family to withdraw support, and the patient expired a short time later.

Acute mesenteric ischemia

Acute mesenteric ischemia is the result of interruption of intestinal blood flow by embolism, thrombosis or a low-flow state.[1] It leads to mediator release, inflammation, and ultimately infarction. The early detection of acute mesenteric ischemia is crucial for the preservation of bowel viability; emergency physicians must maintain a high index of suspicion to identify mesenteric ischemia when there is a paucity of physical examination findings.[2] Recognition of acute mesenteric ischemia can be difficult, as most patients present with nonspecific symptoms. Abdominal pain is the most common complaint. Classically, the pain is out of proportion to physical findings. However, signs of an acute abdomen with distension, guarding, rigidity and hypotension may also occur, particularly when the diagnosis has been delayed.[3] Fever, diarrhea, nausea and anorexia are commonly reported; melena or hematochezia occurs in 15% of cases, and occult blood is detected in at least half of patients.[3]

Embolic occlusion of the superior mesenteric artery (SMA) is the cause of mesenteric ischemia in more than half of all cases.[3] Most emboli originate in the heart, potentiated by cardiac dysrhythmias or depressed systolic function due to

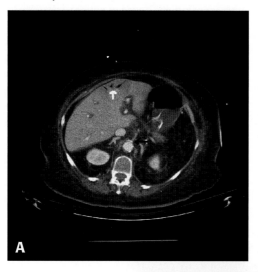
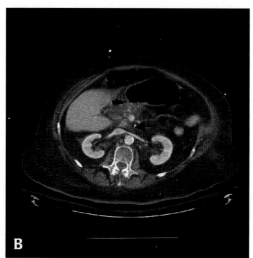
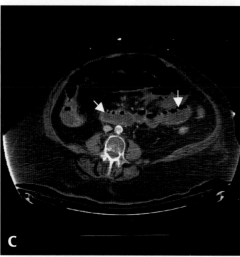

Figure 36.1 CT of the abdomen from a 77-year-old female with mesenteric ischemia demonstrating attenuation of celiac trunk caliber with diminished blood flow (dark arrow, panel A) and portal venous gas (white arrow, panel A), occlusion of the SMA (dark arrow, panel B), and pneumatosis intestinalis in small bowel loops (white arrows, panel C).

ischemic heart disease. In 25% of cases, thrombosis of pre-existing atherosclerotic lesions occurs. Many of these patients report chronic symptoms consistent with previous transient mesenteric ischemia. Nonocclusive mesenteric ischemia, which accounts for 20–30% of all cases, presents similarly but occurs with patent mesenteric arteries. Microvascular vasoconstriction is the underlying process in nonocclusive mesenteric ischemia, precipitated by splanchnic hypoperfusion due to depressed cardiac output or renal or hepatic disease.[3]

A complete blood count with differential, electrolyte panel, coagulation studies, liver function tests, and an amylase or lipase level should be drawn in any patient with suspected acute mesenteric ischemia. The most common laboratory abnormalities are hemoconcentration, leukocytosis, and metabolic acidosis with high anion gap and lactate concentrations.[4] High levels of serum amylase, aspartate aminotransferase, lactate dehydrogenase and creatine phosphokinase are frequently observed on presentation, but none is sufficiently sensitive or specific to be diagnostic. Hyperphosphatemia and hyperkalemia are usually late findings and are frequently associated with bowel infarction.[4]

Plain abdominal films may exclude other causes of abdominal pain, such as obstruction or perforation, but are not helpful in the early diagnosis of mesenteric ischemia.[5] Mesenteric angiography has been the gold standard for diagnosis of arterial causes of acute mesenteric ischemia. However, abdominal CT scans are valuable to exclude other causes of abdominal pain from the differential diagnosis, as well as to distinguish between possible causes of acute mesenteric ischemia. Kirkpatrick et al. prospectively evaluated 62 patients with suspected acute mesenteric ischemia using biphasic CT, including CT angiography.[6] They found that any one of many conditions – pneumatosis intestinalis, venous gas, SMA occlusion, celiac or inferior mesenteric artery occlusion with distal SMA disease, arterial embolism or, alternatively, bowel-wall thickening plus focal lack of bowel-wall enhancement, solid-organ infarction or venous thrombosis – had a sensitivity and specificity for acute mesenteric ischemia of 96% and 94%, respectively.

Treatment for acute mesenteric ischemia initially includes aggressive resuscitation (IV fluids, airway stabilization), stabilization of cardiac function and initiation of broad-spectrum antibiotic coverage.[5] Medications with vasoconstrictive effects should be discontinued. If evidence of peritonitis exists, surgical consultation and laparotomy are indicated. Resection of infarcted bowel as well as embolectomy can be accomplished during surgical exploration.[3] For SMA emboli, treatment options to restore intestinal blood flow include surgical revascularization, intra-arterial thrombolysis, intra-arterial vasodilatation or systemic anticoagulation.

KEY TEACHING POINTS

1. The early detection of acute mesenteric ischemia is crucial for the preservation of bowel viability; emergency physicians must maintain a high index of suspicion, especially if a paucity of physical findings exists.
2. Classically, abdominal pain is out of proportion to physical examination findings. However, signs of acute abdomen with distension, guarding, rigidity and hypotension may also occur, particularly when the diagnosis has been delayed.
3. The most common laboratory abnormalities of acute mesenteric ischemia include hemoconcentration, leukocytosis, and metabolic acidosis with a high anion gap and elevated lactate concentrations.
4. Mesenteric angiography is the gold standard for the diagnosis of arterial causes of acute mesenteric ischemia. However, abdominal CT is valuable to exclude other causes of abdominal pain, as well as to identify possible causes of acute mesenteric ischemia.
5. Treatment for acute mesenteric ischemia involves aggressive resuscitation, stabilization of cardiac function, initiation of broad-spectrum antibiotic coverage, and surgical or interventional radiology consultation.

REFERENCES

[1] Acute mesenteric ischemia: acute abdomen and surgical gastroenterology. Merck Manual Professional Website. Available at http://www.merck.com/mmpe/sec02/ch011/ch011c.html. Accessed June 30, 2008.

[2] Sharieff GQ, Shad JA, Garmel G. An unusual case of mesenteric ischemia in a patient with new-onset diabetes mellitus. *Am J Emerg Med* 1997;15:282–4.

[3] Sreenarasimhaiah J. Clinical review: diagnosis and management of intestinal ischaemic disorders. *BMJ* 2003;326: 1372–6.

[4] Oldenburg WA, Lau LL, Rodenberg TJ, et al. Acute mesenteric ischemia: a clinical review. *Arch Intern Med* 2004;164:1054–62.

[5] Tessler D, Fogel R. GI consult: mesenteric ischemia syndromes (website). Available at http://www.emedmag.com/html/pre/gic/consults/121502.asp. Accessed June 30, 2008.

[6] Kirkpatrick IDC, Kroeker MA, Greenberg HM. Biphasic CT with mesenteric CT angiography in the evaluation of acute mesenteric ischemia: initial experience. *Radiology* 2003; 229:91–8.

37

Sudden onset of back pain in an 84-year-old male

HISTORY OF PRESENT ILLNESS

An 84-year-old male with a medical history significant for hypertension, chronic obstructive pulmonary disease and a 40 pack/year history of tobacco use was brought to the ED by paramedics complaining of the sudden onset of severe back pain radiating to his abdomen. He denied chest pain or shortness of breath but reported numbness and pain in both legs.

PHYSICAL EXAMINATION

GENERAL APPEARANCE: The patient was somnolent but arousable and appeared to be in significant distress.

VITAL SIGNS

Temperature	97.5°F (36.4°C)
Pulse	100 beats/minute
Blood pressure	135/70 mmHg
Respirations	24 breaths/minute
Oxygen saturation	98% on room air

HEENT: Unremarkable.

NECK: Supple, no jugular venous distension.

CARDIOVASCULAR: Tachycardic rate, regular rhythm, no rubs, murmurs or gallops, weak femoral pulses bilaterally.

LUNGS: Minimal expiratory wheezes bilaterally, no rales or rhonchi.

ABDOMEN: Distended, hypoactive bowel sounds, diffuse tenderness to palpation without rebound or guarding, no pulsatile masses.

RECTAL: Normal tone, soft brown stool, hemoccult negative.

EXTREMITIES: Bilateral lower extremities appeared mottled, cool to touch, with delayed capillary refill.

NEUROLOGIC: Somnolent, arousable, otherwise nonfocal.

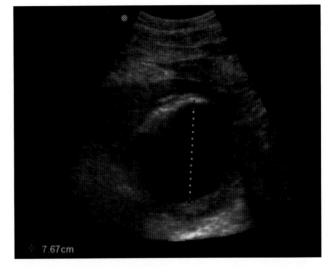

7.67cm

Figure 37.1 Bedside abdominal ultrasound from an 84-year-old male with sudden onset of back pain.

The patient was placed on the cardiac monitor, and a rapid bedside abdominal ultrasound was obtained (Figure 37.1). Two large-bore intravenous lines were placed, and blood was drawn and sent for laboratory testing. His hematocrit returned at 34% (normal 39–51%).

What is your diagnosis?

ANSWER

The diagnosis is ruptured abdominal aortic aneurysm (AAA). The bedside ultrasound demonstrated an AAA with maximal diameter of 7.7 cm. Vascular surgery was consulted emergently, and the patient was typed and crossmatched for 10 units of packed red blood cells. At the request of the vascular surgery service, a stat CT of the abdomen and pelvis to evaluate the AAA for rupture was obtained. The CT scan demonstrated the presence of a ruptured AAA, approximately 10 cm in diameter, with active extravasation and a large hematoma (Figure 37.2).

The patient was taken directly from the CT scanner to the OR by the vascular surgeon. A stent was placed endovascularly into the aneurysm, after which the patient's abdomen was noted to be more tense. A laparotomy was subsequently performed secondary to concern for the development of abdominal compartment syndrome. Upon entering the peritoneum, significant bleeding was noted from several areas of the aorta and iliac arteries. Attempts to control the bleeding were unsuccessful, and the patient expired in the OR shortly thereafter.

Abdominal aortic aneurysms

An aortic aneurysm is a true aneurysm of the aorta in which all three layers of the aortic wall become dilated.[1] An abdominal aortic aneurysm (AAA) is defined as an abdominal aortic diameter 1.5 times the diameter at the level of the renal arteries. A diameter greater than 3 cm is considered aneurysmal in most patients.[1] The incidence of AAA is 36 cases per 100,000 person-years, and is increasing.[1] The incidence increases exponentially with age. Present in only 1% of men between the ages of 55 and 64, clinically significant aneurysms (more than 4 cm) increase in frequency by 3–4% per decade thereafter.[1] Tobacco use, hypertension, a family history of AAA, and male gender are clinical risk factors for the development of an AAA.[2] Ruptured AAA is the 13th leading cause of death in the United States.[3]

The most important factor determining risk of rupture is the size of the aneurysm. The rupture risk increases dramatically with increased size, with most ruptured AAAs having a diameter greater than 5 cm.[4] However, no aneurysm is completely "safe." Any aneurysm can rupture and may be the source of the symptoms causing the patient's presentation. Rupture of an AAA usually occurs into the retroperitoneum, where hemorrhage may be temporarily limited by clotting and tamponade at the rupture site. Of patients with ruptured AAAs, 10–30% have free intraperitoneal rupture, which is often rapidly fatal.[4] Occasionally, rupture occurs into the gastrointestinal tract or the inferior vena cava. Complications may also arise from intact AAAs. The walls of AAAs are often lined with clot and atheromatous material, which can embolize and occlude distal vessels. Aortic thrombosis may occur rarely. Patients may also have complications caused by impingement of the aneurysm on adjacent structures.[4]

Most unruptured AAAs are asymptomatic and are diagnosed incidentally on tests performed for other indications. Some unruptured aortic aneurysms may cause back, flank or abdominal pain, especially if they are increasing rapidly in size.[1] Symptomatic aneurysms are at increased risk of rupture. A review summarizing the utility of the physical examination suggests that the only maneuver of demonstrated value is abdominal palpation to detect a widened aortic pulsation.[5] Pooled data reveal that the sensitivity of abdominal palpation increases from 29% for small AAAs (less than 4 cm) to 50% for AAAs between 4–5 cm, to 76% for AAAs of more than 5 cm in diameter.[5] Obesity decreases this sensitivity. Findings such as bruits, thrills, quality of pulsation, and quality and discrepancy of femoral pulses proved inaccurate in the diagnosis.[1,5]

The classic presentation of a ruptured AAA includes the triad of hypotension, abdominal or back pain, and a pulsatile abdominal mass.[2] Rupture is often the first manifestation of

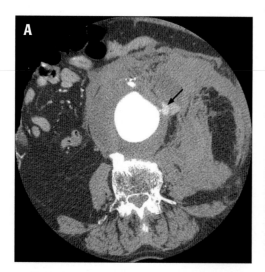
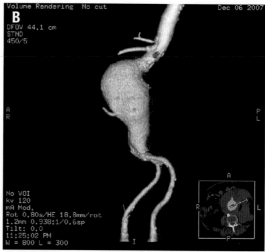

Figure 37.2 CT of the abdomen and pelvis from an 84-year-old male with sudden onset of back pain demonstrating AAA with active extravasation (panel A, arrow indicates extravasation); three-dimensional CT reconstruction of AAA (panel B).

an AAA. Most patients with ruptured AAA experience pain in the abdomen, back or flank.[4] Pain is usually acute, severe and constant, and can radiate to the chest, thigh, inguinal area or scrotum. Rupture of an AAA may be accompanied by nausea and vomiting, and sudden hemorrhage can cause syncope or near-syncope. Hypotension is the least consistent part of the triad, occurring in only one-half to two-thirds of patients, and is often a late finding.[4] In some patients, rupture is initially contained within the retroperitoneum, blood loss is small, and the presentation is delayed or less dramatic. The patient with a ruptured AAA occasionally has symptoms for several days or weeks before seeking medical attention; the duration of symptoms therefore does not exclude the diagnosis of a ruptured AAA.[4]

Numerous studies have determined ultrasound to be a significant advance in the timely diagnosis of ruptured AAA. Ultrasonography is virtually 100% sensitive in detecting AAAs and, when performed by emergency physicians with training, is a fast and accurate test. It should be the first line of imaging in patients for whom this diagnosis is suspected.[6] It can significantly expedite transfer to the operating room, therefore reducing morbidity and mortality. Although ultrasound is ideal for identifying AAAs, it is typically poor for identifying the presence of leaking.[6] In unstable patients, hemodynamic instability plus identification of AAA by ultrasound (or a known AAA) is an indication for immediate laparotomy. However, in stable patients further imaging may be necessary to determine if the finding of AAA is causal or incidental. CT findings in patients with ruptured AAAs include retroperitoneal hematoma, focal discontinuity in circumferential calcification, high-attenuating peripheral crescent, indistinct aortic wall, and contrast medium extravasation.[6] In addition to better identification of a leak, a CT scan aids in the operative planning for repair and may diagnose additional intra-abdominal pathology.

A ruptured, leaking or symptomatic AAA must be managed aggressively. When the diagnosis is suspected, continuous monitoring, two large-bore IVs and saline resuscitation should be initiated immediately.[1] The patient should be typed and crossmatched for at least 10 units of blood. Resuscitation with saline and blood products should continue to a level that maintains cerebral and end-organ perfusion – a systolic blood pressure of 90–100 mmHg is the goal in most patients.[1] Overly aggressive elevation of blood pressure can lead to rupture of a contained hematoma. A vascular surgeon should be notified early and be actively involved throughout the evaluation. Definitive management is immediate surgical repair; surgery should not be delayed for additional (and unnecessary) testing.

The diagnostic strategy employed to confirm AAA depends on the patient's condition. Hypotensive patients need bedside ultrasonography. The finding of a normal aortic diameter effectively excludes the diagnosis, whereas the finding of an AAA in a hemodynamically unstable patient virtually confirms the diagnosis and mandates immediate surgery.[1] Patients without hypotension should get an expedited CT scan to confirm AAA with or without leak or rupture.[1,4] Appropriate staff and equipment should accompany the patient to the CT scanner, if this test is required. Emergent surgery that reveals an intact, symptomatic aneurysm carries a much higher mortality than elective repair.[1]

The two primary methods of AAA repair are open and endovascular. Traditional open AAA repair involves direct access to the aorta and iliac arteries.[2] This method is well established as definitive, requiring essentially no follow up radiologic studies. The majority of patients undergoing open AAA repair remain without significant graft-related complications for the rest of their lives.[2] One feared complication is aortoenteric fistula with massive GI bleed. Endovascular repair of an AAA involves gaining access to the lumen of the aorta, usually via small incisions over the femoral vessels. An Endograft, typically cloth with a stent exoskeleton, is placed within the lumen of the AAA extending distally into the iliac arteries. Close follow up is required after endovascular repair, with CT scans performed at 1, 6 and 12 months, then yearly to ensure that the graft is accomplishing its intended goals (e.g., asymptomatic patient, decreasing AAA size, structurally intact Endograft, and neither fixation site problems nor significant graft migration).[2]

KEY TEACHING POINTS

1. Abdominal aortic aneurysm (AAA) rupture is the 13th leading cause of death in the United States.
2. The most important factor determining risk of rupture is the size of the aneurysm, with most ruptured AAAs having a diameter greater than 5 cm.
3. The classic presentation of a ruptured AAA includes the triad of abdominal or back pain, a pulsatile abdominal mass, and hypotension.
4. Bedside ultrasound should be used to diagnose ruptured AAA in unstable patients, whereas a CT scan can be used in stable patients in whom the diagnosis is unclear.
5. Management of a ruptured AAA includes hemodynamic monitoring, aggressive fluid resuscitation, type and crossmatching for 10 units of packed red blood cells and urgent vascular surgery consultation for definitive repair.

REFERENCES

[1] Gupta R, Kaufman S. Cardiovascular emergencies in the elderly. *Emerg Med Clin N Am* 2006;24:339–70.
[2] Upchurch GR, Schaub TA. Abdominal aortic aneurysm. *Am Fam Physician* 2006;73:1198–206.
[3] Martinez JP, Mattu A. Abdominal pain in the elderly. *Emerg Med Clin N Am* 2006;24:371–88.
[4] Bessen HA. Abdominal aortic aneurysm. In: Marx JA, Hockberger RS, Walls RM, et al. (eds.). *Rosen's Emergency Medicine: Concepts and Clinical Practice*, 6th ed. Philadelphia: Mosby, 2006:1330–40.
[5] Lederle FA, Simel DL. Does this patient have abdominal aortic aneurysm? *JAMA* 1999;281:77–82.
[6] Haro LH, Krajicek M, Lobl JK. Challenges, controversies, and advances in aortic catastrophes. *Emerg Med Clin N Am* 2005;23:1159–77.

38

Intermittent abdominal pain for one day in an 86-year-old female

HISTORY OF PRESENT ILLNESS

An 86-year-old female with a medical history significant for coronary artery disease, remote history of coronary bypass surgery, and successful endovascular stent placement for abdominal aortic aneurysm (AAA) three months earlier presented to the ED complaining of one day of intermittent, diffuse abdominal pain. The patient denied associated nausea or vomiting, fevers, dysuria, chest pain or shortness of breath. She reported a normal bowel movement earlier in the day without blood or black stool. Her episodes of abdominal pain were reported to occur approximately every 20 minutes, with complete resolution of her pain between episodes. The patient had undergone an abdominal CT one month earlier, which demonstrated a stable AAA with stent in place.

PHYSICAL EXAMINATION

GENERAL APPEARANCE: The patient was an elderly female who appeared well hydrated and in no acute discomfort.

VITAL SIGNS

Temperature	98.1°F (36.7°C)
Pulse	76 beats per minute
Blood pressure	128/60 mmHg
Respirations	16 breaths per minute
Oxygen saturation	97% on room air

HEENT: PERRL, EOMI, no scleral icterus, oropharynx pink and moist.

NECK: Supple, no jugular venous distension.

CARDIOVASCULAR: Regular rate and rhythm without rubs, murmurs or gallops.

LUNGS: Clear to auscultation bilaterally.

ABDOMEN: Soft, mildly distended with increased tympany and hypoactive bowel sounds present. Nontender without a pulsatile mass.

RECTAL: Normal tone, soft, brown stool, hemoccult negative.

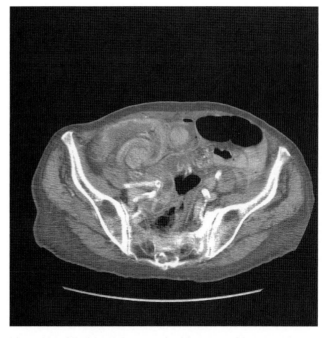

Figure 38.1 CT of the abdomen and pelvis from an 86-year-old female with intermittent abdominal pain for one day.

EXTREMITIES: Well perfused without clubbing, cyanosis or edema.

NEUROLOGIC: Nonfocal.

A peripheral intravenous line was placed, and blood was drawn and sent for laboratory testing. Laboratory tests, including a complete blood count, electrolytes, creatinine, glucose, serum lactate and urinalysis, were all within normal limits. During the patient's ED stay, she was observed to have several intermittent bouts of severe abdominal pain, occurring approximately every 30 minutes. A CT scan of the abdomen and pelvis with oral and intravenous contrast was obtained (Figure 38.1).

What is your diagnosis?

ANSWER

The diagnosis is ileocecal intussusception due to tumor at the ileocecal valve, with small bowel perforation and free intraperitoneal air. The CT scan demonstrated abnormal loops of small and large bowel in the right lower quadrant with a low-attenuation "ring" surrounding the loop of bowel, suggesting either intussusception or internal herniation (arrow, Figure 38.2). Small collections of free air were also noted in this area. Intravenous antibiotics were administered and the patient was taken to the OR, where an ileocecal intussusception secondary to a 6-cm tumor as lead point at the ileocecal valve was discovered. A right hemicolectomy was performed with removal of the intussusception, followed by an end-to-end ileocolic anastomosis.

Intussusception in adults

Intussusception occurs when a segment of bowel plus the adjacent mesentery, the intussusceptum, prolapses into the lumen of the contiguous distal bowel, called the intussuscipiens.[1] It is thought that any abnormality of the intestinal wall or its lumen that alters or unbalances the peristaltic activity may initiate the invagination process. A lead point has been said to be present in up to 90% of symptomatic cases, although lower figures have been reported.[1] Intussusception in adults occurs infrequently, differing from childhood intussusception in its presentation, cause and treatment.[2] Intussusception remains a rare condition in adults, representing 1% of bowel obstructions and 0.003–0.02% of all hospital admissions.[3] Adults

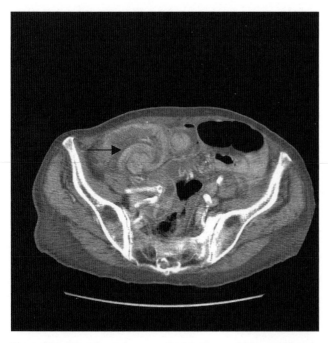

Figure 38.2 CT of the abdomen and pelvis from an 86-year-old female demonstrating abnormal loops of small and large bowel in the right lower quadrant, with a low-attenuation "ring" surrounding the loop of bowel (arrow), suggestive of intussusception.

present with a variety of symptoms that can be acute, intermittent or chronic; intussusception in adults rarely presents with the classic triad of vomiting, abdominal pain and passage of blood per rectum, making the diagnosis difficult.[2,3]

In adults, intussusception is almost always associated with pathological lead points, such as neoplasms, inflammatory lesions or a Meckel's diverticulum.[4] Malignant neoplasms cause most adult intussusceptions, except in the case of enteroenteric intussusceptions (involving mesenteric small bowel), which are usually associated with benign lesions such as lipomas, adenomatous polyps, lymphoid hyperplasia or stromal cell tumors.[4] Asymptomatic enteroenteric intussusceptions that involve more benign etiologies and lack a lead point are generally self-limiting if the intussusception length is less than 3.5 cm.[1,4]

Intussusception is easily diagnosed by means of CT or MRI.[5] The appearance of bowel-within-bowel configuration with or without contained fat and mesenteric vessels is pathognomonic.[5] Other diagnostic modalities for intussusception include contrast enemas and Doppler ultrasound.[4] Persistent, symptomatic intussusception in adults is nearly always treated surgically, largely because of the high proportion of cases with structural causes and the relatively high incidence of malignancy, particularly in the colon.[6] Appropriate therapy for cases of enteroenteric intussusception is more controversial because of the lower prevalence of malignancy in small bowel intussusception. Surgical resection or intervention is not warranted in cases of transient intussusception in the setting of a known benign cause, such as celiac sprue.[6] A transient, short, nonobstructing intussusception detected incidentally by CT in a relatively asymptomatic patient may not require intervention. Fixed or symptomatic intussusceptions of the small bowel, although more likely benign in etiology than colonic intussusceptions, may be malignant in a significant proportion of cases. In these cases, resection without reduction is generally recommended unless preservation of bowel length is necessary.[6]

KEY TEACHING POINTS

1. Intussusception remains a rare condition in adults, representing 1% of bowel obstructions and 0.003–0.02% of all hospital admissions.
2. Intussusception in adults rarely presents with the classic triad of vomiting, abdominal pain and passage of blood per rectum, making the diagnosis challenging.
3. CT is the most useful imaging tool in making the diagnosis of intussusception in adults.
4. Persistent, symptomatic intussusception in adults is nearly always treated surgically, largely because of the high proportion of cases with structural causes and the relatively high incidence of malignancy, particularly in the colon.
5. Enteroenteric intussusceptions less then 3.5 cm long, without a lead point or other underlying cause in an asymptomatic patient, is typically self-limiting and of little clinical significance.

REFERENCES

[1] Jain P, Heap SW. Intussusception of the small bowel discovered incidentally by computed tomography. *Australas Radiol* 2006;50:171–4.

[2] Croome KP, Colquhoun PHD. Intussusception in adults. *Can J Surg* 2007;50:E13–4.

[3] Azar T, Berger D. Adult intussusception. *Ann Surg* 1997; 226:134–8.

[4] Lin H-H, Chan D-C, Yu C-Y, et al. Is this a lipoma? *Am J Med* 2008;121:21–3.

[5] Warshauer DM, Lee JKT. Adult intussusception detected at CT or MR imaging: clinical-imaging correlation. *Radiol* 1999;212:853–60.

[6] Huang BY, Warshauer DM. Adult intussusception: diagnosis and clinical relevance. *Radiol Clin N Am* 2003;41:1137–51.

PART V

GENITOURINARY AND GYNECOLOGY

39

Right flank pain in a 20-year-old female

HISTORY OF PRESENT ILLNESS

A 20-year-old gravida 1, para 1 female presented to the ED complaining of severe right-sided flank pain that began suddenly four hours prior to arrival. Her pain was sharp and constant, radiating to the right lower abdomen with associated nausea and one episode of vomiting. She denied fevers or chills, dysuria, hematuria, constipation or diarrhea. She was currently on her normal menstrual cycle. She denied recent trauma or any personal or family history of kidney stones. She had not previously experienced similar pain.

PHYSICAL EXAMINATION

GENERAL APPEARANCE: The patient was a well-nourished, well-hydrated female in moderate discomfort.

VITAL SIGNS

Temperature	98°F (36.6°C)
Pulse	96 beats/minute
Blood pressure	109/79 mmHg
Respirations	20 breaths/minute
Oxygen saturation	98% on room air

HEENT: PERRL, EOMI, oropharynx clear with moist mucous membranes.

NECK: Supple.

CARDIOVASCULAR: Regular rate and rhythm without rubs, murmurs or gallops.

LUNGS: Clear to auscultation bilaterally.

ABDOMEN: Soft, nontender, nondistended. No costovertebral angle tenderness.

PELVIC: No discharge or bleeding, normal-sized, nontender uterus, os closed, right adnexal mass palpable with mild tenderness.

NEUROLOGIC: Nonfocal.

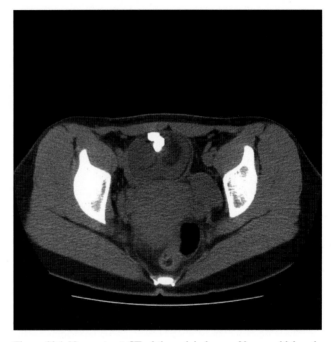

Figure 39.1 Noncontrast CT of the pelvis from a 20-year-old female with right flank pain.

A peripheral intravenous line was placed, blood was drawn and sent for laboratory testing, and morphine sulfate, ketorolac, and Zofran® were administered intravenously for pain and nausea, respectively. A urine pregnancy test was negative. A clean catch urinalysis demonstrated a large amount of blood but was otherwise normal. Her creatinine was within the normal range. A noncontrast CT of the abdomen and pelvis was obtained (Figure 39.1).

What is your diagnosis?

The diagnosis is right ovarian (adnexal) torsion due to a 6-cm dermoid cyst. The noncontrast CT scan of the abdomen and pelvis demonstrated a 6.8 cm × 5.1 cm heterogenous mass lesion with components of soft tissue, calcium and fat in the right para-midline anterior pelvis, suggestive of a dermoid cyst (Figure 39.2). The pelvic organs appeared otherwise unremarkable. The gynecology service was consulted, and the patient was taken to the OR. During laparoscopy, a 6-cm dermoid cyst was discovered, causing torsion of the right ovary. The ovary was detorsed and the dermoid cyst was excised from the ovary. The ovary was viable, and the ovarian bed was subsequently cauterized with excellent hemostasis. The patient recovered uneventfully. Pathology identified the cyst as a mature cystic teratoma.

Ovarian torsion resulting from a dermoid cyst

A dermoid (cystic teratoma) is a benign, cystic lesion containing tissue from all three embryonic layers: endoderm, mesoderm and ectoderm. Ovarian dermoids constitute 10–15% of ovarian tumors. They tend to occur in young women during their reproductive years, although they have been reported in prepubertal and elderly patients.[1] Ovarian dermoids present with discomfort, pain or pressure symptoms, or when a complication occurs. Torsion is the most common complication of dermoid cysts, occurring in approximately 3.5% of cases.[1] Cases of dermoid tumors with ovarian torsion presenting as appendicitis or renal colic have been described.[2,3] Less than 1% of dermoid cysts are malignant. Although ovarian dermoids can be detected by ultrasound, CT or MRI, CT is the best imaging procedure for identifying cystic teratomas of the ovary.[4]

Torsion of the uterine adnexa is a gynecologic emergency, requiring prompt diagnosis and emergency surgical treatment. It can involve the fallopian tube, the ovary or other adnexal structures. Risk factors for ovarian torsion include ovarian enlargement, adnexal masses (including tumors), pregnancy, ovulation induction, and previous pelvic surgery.[5] The most common risk factor associated with torsion is the presence of a dermoid cyst (32%).[5] Torsion may also occur in a normal ovary. Although adnexal torsion is generally viewed as uncommon, studies suggest that adnexal torsion is the fifth most common gynecological emergency, representing 2–3% of acute surgical emergencies.[6]

Ovarian torsion results from partial or complete rotation of the ovarian pedicle on its long axis, potentially compromising venous and lymphatic drainage. If the rotation is partial or intermittent, venous and lymphatic congestion and its associated symptoms may subside quickly.[6] If rotation of the ovarian pedicle is complete and prolonged, venous and arterial thrombosis may occur, resulting in adnexal infarction. The pain is proportional to the degree of circulatory compromise from torsion. If torsion is complete, the pain is acute and severe, typically accompanied by nausea and

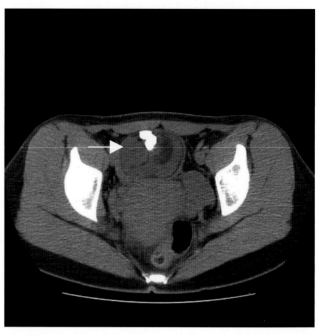

Figure 39.2 Noncontrast CT of the pelvis from a 20-year-old female demonstrating a 6.8 × 5.1 cm heterogenous mass lesion in the right paramidline anterior pelvis (arrow) consistent with a dermoid cyst.

vomiting.[5] However, spontaneous detorsion may occur and the pain will subside. Adnexal torsion is rarely bilateral and is more common on the right side. It is more common in young women, with the greatest incidence in the 20- to 30-year age group.[6]

Physical findings and characteristics of pain in ovarian torsion are variable. The "classic" history of ovarian torsion is the abrupt onset of colicky pain in a lower quadrant, with radiation to the flank or groin, mimicking renal colic.[7] However, only 44% of patients diagnosed with ovarian torsion in one study had such crampy or colicky pain.[7] Additionally, 51% of patients in the same study had radiation of pain to the flank, back or groin. Fifty-nine percent of patients had abrupt onset of pain, whereas 43% of patients had prior episodes of this pain. The majority of patients in this study had nausea and vomiting (70%) and lower quadrant pain (90%), but these findings mimic many other causes of abdominal pain and are not specific to ovarian torsion.[7]

On physical examination, the most consistent finding of ovarian torsion is a palpable mass felt 50–80% of the time during pelvic examination.[5] Laboratory tests should include a urine or serum β-hCG to rule out ectopic pregnancy and a urinalysis to evaluate for infection or stone. Studies have demonstrated elevated white blood cell counts in 16–38% of cases of ovarian torsion but this finding is nonspecific.[6] In cases of suspected ovarian torsion, immediate ultrasound is the investigation of choice; greater than 93% of patients with torsion will have abnormal ultrasound findings.[6] Ultrasonographic findings depend on the duration of torsion and the degree of ovarian ischemia; the most common finding is ovarian enlargement.[8] In the early stages of ovarian torsion, the ovary is enlarged with prominent peripheral follicles. With pro-longed and complete torsion, infarction may appear as cystic, clotted areas on the ovary. Abnormal flow on color Doppler sonography increases the likelihood of identifying torsion, but torsion may occur with incomplete vascular obstruction; therefore, evidence of vascular flow does not rule out torsion with certainty.[6,8]

Treatment of a torsed ovary with a dermoid cyst or other abnormality requires detorsion of the ovary and removal of the cyst if the ovary is viable; a nonviable ovary must be removed.[5] The procedure can be done by laparoscopy or laparotomy. In the past, oophorectomy was considered the standard of care because of concern that untwisting of the adnexa might precipitate pulmonary embolism from a thrombosed vein.[6] Several studies have shown that in the absence of a grossly necrotic ovary, untwisting of the adnexa can be performed and the ovary salvaged without significant risk of thromboembolism.[9,10] Conversely, hemorrhagic infarction or a gangrenous adnexal structure requires surgical removal without attempts at detorsion.[6]

KEY TEACHING POINTS

1. Ovarian torsion is a gynecologic emergency requiring prompt diagnosis and emergency surgical treatment.
2. Torsion is the most common complication of dermoid cysts, occurring in approximately 3.5% of cases.
3. The pain of ovarian torsion is proportional to the degree of circulatory compromise; if torsion is complete, the pain is acute and severe, typically accompanied by nausea and vomiting.
4. On physical examination, the most consistent finding in patients with ovarian torsion is a palpable mass.

5. Abnormal flow on color Doppler sonography increases the likelihood of identifying torsion, but torsion may occur with incomplete vascular obstruction; therefore, evidence of vascular flow does not rule out torsion with certainty.
6. Treatment of a torsed ovary with a dermoid cyst or other abnormality requires detorsion of the ovary and removal of the cyst if the ovary is viable; a nonviable ovary requires removal.

REFERENCES

[1] Williams KM, Bain CJ, Kelly MD. Laparoscopic resection of a torted ovarian dermoid cyst. *World J Emerg Surg* 2007;2:12.
[2] Torbati SS, Krishel SJ. Dermoid tumor with ovarian torsion masking as appendicitis. *J Emerg Med* 2000;18:103.
[3] Huang C-YC, Chen C-C, Lee Y-K, et al. Ovarian torsion caused by teratoma masquerading as renal colic. *Emerg Med J* 2008;25:182.
[4] Buy J-N, Ghossain MA, Moss AA, et al. Cystic teratoma of the ovary: CT detection. *Radiology* 1989;171:697–701.
[5] Schwartz G. Radiological case of the month: Torsed ovary with a dermoid cyst. *Arch Pediatr Adolesc Med* 1998;152:503–4.
[6] Martin C, Magee K. Ovarian torsion in a 20-year-old patient. *Can J Emerg Med* 2006;8:126–9.
[7] Houry D, Abbott JT. Ovarian torsion: a fifteen-year review. *Ann Emerg Med* 2001;38:156–9.
[8] Albayram F, Hamper UM. Ovarian and adnexal torsion: spectrum of sonographic findings with pathologic correlation. *J Ultrasound Med* 2001;20:1083–9.
[9] Cohen SB. Laparoscopic detorsion allows sparing of the twisted ischemic adnexa. *J Am Assoc Gynecol Laparosc* 1999;6:139–43.
[10] Zweizig S, Perron J, Grubb D, et al. Conservative management of adnexal torsion. *Am J Obstet Gynecol* 1993;168:1791–5.

40

Right lower quadrant abdominal pain in a 28-year-old female

HISTORY OF PRESENT ILLNESS

A 28-year-old gravida 0, para 0 female whose last reported menstrual period was two weeks earlier presented to the ED complaining of right-sided abdominal pain that began on the morning of presentation. She described her pain as sharp and constant, rated at a level of 8 (on a scale of 0 to 10), and localized to the right lower quadrant. The patient reported three episodes of nausea and vomiting as well as loose stools, but denied vaginal bleeding or discharge. She reported fevers to 102°F (38.9°C) with associated chills and loss of appetite over the past several days. She had no prior history of abdominal surgeries and denied sexual activity.

PHYSICAL EXAMINATION

GENERAL APPEARANCE: The patient was a moderately obese, well-hydrated female in moderate discomfort.

VITAL SIGNS

Temperature	102°F (38.9°C)
Pulse	121 beats/minute
Blood pressure	154/87 mmHg
Respirations	22 breaths/minute
Oxygen saturation	99% on room air

HEENT: Unremarkable.

NECK: Supple.

CARDIOVASCULAR: Tachycardic rate, regular rhythm without rubs, murmurs or gallops.

LUNGS: Clear to auscultation bilaterally.

ABDOMEN: Soft, nondistended, active bowel sounds present. Tenderness to palpation in both the right upper and right lower quadrants, with maximal point tenderness in the right lower quadrant. Neither a Murphy's sign nor Rovsing's sign was present. Right-sided costovertebral tenderness was noted.

RECTAL: Normal tone, no masses, brown stool, hemoccult negative.

PELVIC: No cervical motion or adnexal tenderness on bimanual examination, no blood or discharge from the cervix.

EXTREMITIES: No clubbing, cyanosis or edema.

NEUROLOGIC: Nonfocal

A peripheral intravenous line was placed, blood was drawn and sent for laboratory testing, and Dilaudid® and Phenergan® were administered intravenously to control pain and nausea, respectively. Laboratory tests were significant for a leukocyte count of 18 K/μL (normal 3.5–12.5 K/μL) with 90% neutrophils (normal 50–70%). A urinalysis obtained by midstream clean catch revealed large blood with the absence of nitrites or leukocyte esterase; the urine microscopic examination showed 11–25 red blood cells, 11–25 white blood cells, many bacteria and more than 50 squamous cells. The urine pregnancy test was negative. The serum creatinine was within normal limits. The patient was given 2 liters normal saline intravenously, and a CT scan of the abdomen and pelvis with oral and intravenous contrast was obtained (Figure 40.1).

What is your diagnosis?

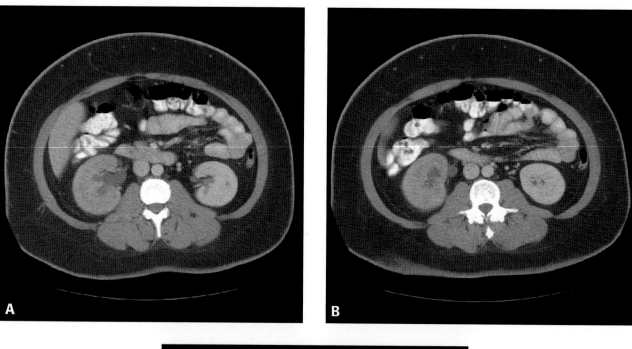

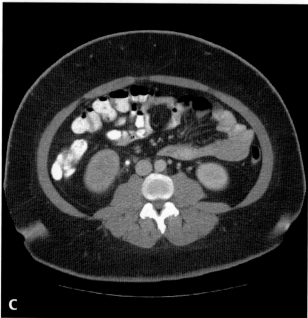

Figure 40.1 CT of the abdomen from a 28-year-old female with right lower quadrant abdominal pain for one day (panel A, most superior image).

ANSWER

The diagnosis is an obstructing right ureteral stone with upper urinary tract infection, possible urosepsis. The CT scan of the abdomen and pelvis demonstrates a 5-mm calculus in the right proximal ureter (arrow, image C, Figure 40.2), causing mild right hydronephrosis (panels A and B, Figure 40.1); the appendix was normal. The patient was given ciprofloxacin 400 mg IV in the ED. Urology was consulted and the patient was taken to the OR, where a 6 French double J stent was placed in the right ureter, bypassing the stone. The patient's clinic condition improved by hospital day #2, and the patient was discharged with instructions to complete 14 days of ciprofloxacin, with follow up arranged in the urology clinic in one week. The urine culture from the initial midstream urine obtained in the ED grew out only 10–25,000 CFU/mL Gram-negative rods, most likely contaminant.

Ureteral colic and infected ureteral stones

Up to 12% of the population will have a urinary tract stone during their lifetime, with recurrence rates approaching 50%.[1] Fifty-five percent of individuals with recurrent stones have a family history of urolithiasis; having such a history increases the risk of stones by a factor of three.[1] The classic presentation of a renal stone is acute, colicky flank pain radiating to the groin. As the stone descends in the ureter, the pain may localize in the abdominal area overlying the stone and radiate to the testicle or ovary. Peritoneal signs are typically absent. As the stone approaches the ureterovesical junction, lower quadrant pain radiating to the tip of the ureter, urinary urgency and frequency, and dysuria are characteristic, mimicking the

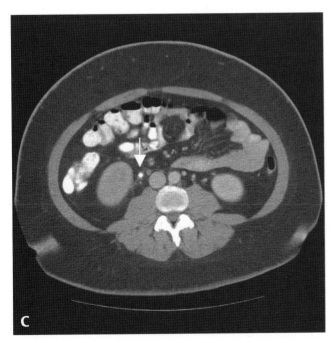

Figure 40.2 CT of the abdomen from a 28-year-old female demonstrating a 5-mm ureteral stone in the proximal right ureter (arrow).

symptoms of bacterial cystitis.[1] Physical examination typically demonstrates a patient trying to find a comfortable position. Tenderness over the costovertebral angle or lower quadrant may be present. Gross or microscopic hematuria occurs in approximately 90% of patients; however, the absence of hematuria does not preclude the presence of stones.[2]

The preferred imaging study to confirm the diagnosis of a urinary tract stone in a patient with acute flank pain is an unenhanced, helical CT of the abdomen and pelvis.[1,3] In one study, the sensitivity of CT was 96%, as compared to 87% for urography, and the respective specificities were 100% and 94% ($p < 0.001$ for both comparisons).[3] Positive and negative predictive values were 100% and 91%, respectively, for CT, compared with 97% and 74%, respectively, for urography. CT scans that were negative for stone disease revealed other abnormalities in 57% of patients, including appendicitis, pelvic inflammatory disease, diverticulitis, abdominal aortic aneurysm and bladder cancer.[3] If CT is unavailable, plain abdominal radiography should be performed because 75–90% of urinary calculi are radioopaque.[1] Although ultrasonography has high specificity (greater than 90%), its sensitivity is much lower than that of CT, typically in the range of 11–24%.[1] Thus, ultrasonography is not routinely used but is an appropriate initial imaging test when ureteral colic occurs during pregnancy.[4]

Urgent intervention is indicated in a patient with an obstructed, infected urinary tract, impending renal deterioration, intractable pain or vomiting, anuria, or high-grade obstruction of a solitary or transplanted kidney.[1] Obstructive pyelonephritis is one of the most serious complications of renal calculus disease. The most severe manifestation of this syndrome, pyonephrosis, is associated with a high mortality and the risk of renal loss.[5] Gram-negative sepsis, which may accompany pyelonephritis, also carries substantial risk. Fear of these complications has led to the clinical dogma that obstructing stones with suspected infection should be managed with emergency decompression of the collecting system, either by percutaneous nephrostomy or retrograde ureteral catheterization with stenting.[5] Finally, midstream urine culture and sensitivity (C&S) alone have low sensitivities and specificities (30.2% and 73%, respectively) to detect infected urine proximal to a ureteral obstruction.[6] In patients with ureteral obstructions, pelvic urine C&S (obtained by ureteral catheterization during ureteroscopy) is a more appropriate and sensitive indicator of a potentially dangerous infection.[6]

KEY TEACHING POINTS

1. In cases of ureteral stones, gross or microscopic hematuria occurs in approximately 90% of patients; however, the absence of hematuria does not preclude the presence of nephrolithiasis.

2. The preferred imaging study to confirm the diagnosis of a urinary tract stone in a patient with acute flank pain is an unenhanced, helical CT of the abdomen and pelvis.

3. Urgent urologic intervention is indicated in a patient with an obstructed, infected upper urinary tract, impending renal deterioration, intractable pain or vomiting, anuria, or high-grade obstruction of a solitary or transplanted kidney.

4. Obstructing stones with suspected infection should be managed with emergency decompression of the collecting system.

REFERENCES

[1] Teichman JMH. Acute renal colic from ureteral calculus. *N Engl J Med* 2004;350:684–93.

[2] Bove P, Kaplan D, Dalrympl N, et al. Reexamining the value of hematuria testing in patients with acute flank pain. *J Urol* 1999;162:685–7.

[3] Vieweg J, Chu T, Freed K, et al. Unenhanced helical computerized tomography for the evaluation of patients with acute flank pain. *J Urol* 1998;160:679–84.

[4] Shokeir AA, Mahran MR, Abdulmaaboud M. Renal colic in pregnant women: role of renal resistive index. *Urology* 2000;55:344–7.

[5] Pearle MS, Pierce HL, Miller GL, et al. Optimal method of urgent decompression of the collecting system for obstruction and infection due to ureteral calculi. *J Urol* 1998;160: 1260–4.

[6] Mariappan P, Loong CW. Midstream urine culture and sensitivity test is a poor predictor of infected urine proximal to the obstructing ureteral stone or infected stones: a prospective clinical study. *J Urol* 2004;171:2142–5.

41

Abdominal pain and vaginal bleeding in a 33-year-old female

HISTORY OF PRESENT ILLNESS

A 33-year-old gravida 0, para 0 female whose last reported menstrual period was eight weeks ago presented to the ED complaining of two days of right lower quadrant pain and vaginal bleeding. She reported her pain as crampy, constant, non-radiating and rated it at a level of 8 (on a scale of 0 to 10). The patient also reported mild vaginal bleeding, using one pad every four hours. She reported associated nausea, light-headedness, fatigue and shortness of breath with exertion but denied chest pain, diarrhea or constipation, fevers, vaginal discharge or dysuria.

PHYSICAL EXAMINATION

GENERAL APPEARANCE: The patient was a pale, ill-appearing female in no acute distress.

VITAL SIGNS

Temperature	98°F (36.6°C)
Pulse	110 beats/minute
Blood pressure	90/60 mmHg
Respirations	22 breaths/minute
Oxygen saturation	99% on room air

HEENT: Unremarkable.

NECK: Supple, no jugular venous distension.

CARDIOVASCULAR: Tachycardic rate, regular rhythm without rubs, murmurs or gallops.

LUNGS: Clear to auscultation bilaterally.

ABDOMEN: Nondistended, diffuse tenderness to palpation with rebound and guarding in the right lower quadrant.

PELVIC: Scant blood in the vaginal vault, os closed, no cervical motion tenderness, right adnexal tenderness.

EXTREMITIES: No clubbing, cyanosis or edema.

NEUROLOGIC: Nonfocal.

Two peripheral intravenous lines were placed, and blood was drawn and sent for laboratory testing. A bedside Focused Assessment with Sonography for Trauma (FAST) exam was obtained (Figure 41.1).

What is your diagnosis?

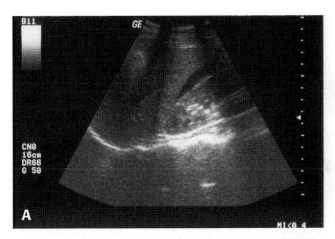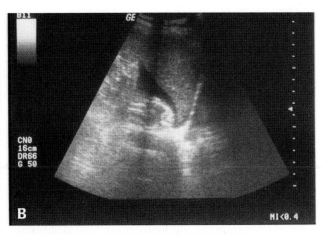

Figure 41.1 Abdominal ultrasound images (FAST) from a 33-year-old female with abdominal pain and vaginal bleeding (panel A, right upper quadrant; panel B, left upper quadrant).

ANSWER

The diagnosis is ruptured ectopic pregnancy. The ultrasound images show free fluid in the right upper quadrant in Morrison's pouch (the hepatorenal recess, Figure 41.2, panel A) and the left upper quadrant (the splenorenal recess, Figure 41.2, panel B) consistent with bleeding from a ruptured ectopic pregnancy. The serum pregnancy test was positive, and the initial hematocrit was 36% (normal 34–46%). The obstetrics/gynecology service was emergently consulted before the laboratory tests returned, and the patient was crossmatched for 6 units of packed red blood cells. She was taken emergently to the OR, where a ruptured ectopic pregnancy was discovered in the right fallopian tube with blood and clots in the abdominal cavity. The ruptured tube was surgically repaired, the abdominal cavity was copiously irrigated, and all blood and blood clots were removed. A repeat hematocrit (three hours after the initial hematocrit) dropped to 26%. The patient had an uneventful postoperative course and recovered fully without requiring a blood transfusion.

Ectopic pregnancy

Ectopic pregnancy is defined as any pregnancy implanted outside the uterine cavity. It remains the leading cause of pregnancy-related first-trimester death among women in the United States.[1] Ectopic pregnancy is a high-risk condition that occurs in 1.9% of reported pregnancies.[2] Approximately 97% of ectopic pregnancies are tubal in location.[1,2] Although the incidence of ectopic pregnancy has increased, the case fatality rate has dropped from 69% in 1876 to 0.35% in 1970, and to 0.05% in 1986.[1] With documented intrauterine pregnancy, the risk of coexisting ectopic (heterotopic pregnancy) is approximately 1 in 10,000–30,000 patients.[1] The risk increases to approximately 1 in 100 patients if the woman is being treated for infertility.

Risk factors for ectopic pregnancy include a history of pelvic inflammatory disease (PID), previous ectopic, tubal or uterine surgery or instrumentation, uterine or tubal anomalies, fertility drugs, and cigarette smoking.[3] Intrauterine devices (IUD) have not been shown to be a risk factor for ectopic pregnancy or pelvic inflammatory disease; however, ectopic pregnancy must be ruled out in a pregnant female with an IUD. A woman with a history of one ectopic pregnancy has a recurrence rate of 15–20%, that increases to 32% with two previous ectopic pregnancies.[3] Ectopic pregnancy is more frequently diagnosed in women over 35 and in non-Caucasian women.

Ectopic pregnancy is usually an acute presentation of pelvic or lower quadrant abdominal pain in a woman of reproductive age who presents to the ED. Although the clinical triad of lower abdominal pain, vaginal bleeding and amenorrhea is considered specific for ectopic pregnancy, women generally do not present with all three symptoms.[4] The presentation of any component of this triad should prompt further investigation to exclude ectopic pregnancy. Abdominal pain is the most common presenting symptom of ectopic pregnancy; abdominal tenderness is the most common physical sign.[4] Considering the high potential mortality of this condition, any woman of reproductive age presenting to the ED with abdominal symptoms should have a beta-human chorionic gonadotropin (β-hCG) blood or urine test to exclude the possibility of ectopic pregnancy.

Diagnostic tests for ectopic pregnancy include a urine pregnancy test, ultrasonography, β-hCG measurements, serum progesterone levels and, on occasion, diagnostic curettage or culdocentesis.[2] The first step in the diagnosis of an ectopic pregnancy is to evaluate for an intrauterine pregnancy. Transvaginal ultrasound (TVUS) can identify intrauterine pregnancy at a gestational age of 5.5 menstrual weeks at nearly 100% accuracy.[1] Confirmation of an intrauterine pregnancy almost definitively rules out an ectopic pregnancy. In the absence of a

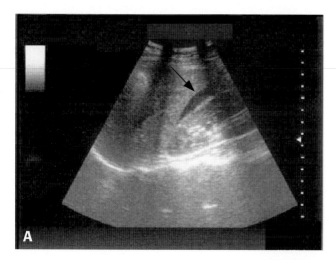 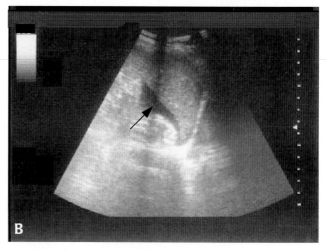

Figure 41.2 Abdominal ultrasound (FAST) from a 33-year-old female with abdominal pain and vaginal bleeding, demonstrating free fluid in Morrison's pouch (arrow, panel A) and in the splenorenal recess (arrow, panel B).

reliable last menstrual period, the β-hCG level is instrumental in the evaluation of ectopic pregnancy. The concept of a discriminatory zone (defined as the level of β-hCG at which an intrauterine pregnancy should be visualized) should be used to help facilitate ultrasound findings.[1] With abdominal ultrasound, most radiologists use a β-hCG level of 6500 mIU/mL. This has been further refined with the use of TVUS, reducing the discriminatory zone to 1500–2500 mIU/mL.[1–3] When the β-hCG level has reached the discriminatory zone and an intrauterine pregnancy cannot be diagnosed, an extrauterine pregnancy should be highly suspected.

Measurement of serum progesterone has been proposed as both a screening tool for ectopic pregnancy and to determine the pregnancy's viability.[5] Serum progesterone levels of at least 25 ng/mL are rarely associated with an ectopic pregnancy (1–2% of cases).[5] Serum progesterone levels of less than 5 ng/mL are associated with a viable pregnancy in only 0.16% of cases; the finding of a low serum progesterone level in association with an abnormally rising β-hCG level is essentially 100% predictive of a nonviable pregnancy.[5] In one prospective study of 718 symptomatic first-trimester ED patients, no patient with an ectopic pregnancy had a progesterone level greater than 22 ng/mL, lending further support to progesterone levels as helpful in ruling out the diagnosis of ectopic pregnancy.[6]

Diagnostic uterine curettage may detect chorionic villi. If chorionic villi are not detected, ectopic pregnancy should be suspected.[2] Curettage should only be considered when β-hCG levels are falling or when levels are elevated and ultrasonography does not show intrauterine pregnancy.[2] Diagnostic uterine curettage could terminate a desired pregnancy, so its use should be reserved for possibly undesired pregnancies. Culdocentesis is not commonly used in stable patients with suspected ectopic pregnancy given the advent of ultrasonography.[5] Culdocentesis is less sensitive and specific than ultrasonography for detecting hemoperitoneum, and several series report nondiagnostic ("dry") taps in about one-quarter of patients.[5] However, culdocentesis could be considered to verify hemoperitoneum in the unstable patient who cannot tolerate the time required for ultrasonography, or when emergency transfer for gynecologic consultation and definitive care is being considered.

Treatment for ectopic pregnancy has evolved over time and depends on the stability of the patient.[3] Approximately 68–77% of ectopic pregnancies resolve spontaneously.[3] Expectant or medical management may be considered in a hemodynamically stable and compliant patient. Noninvasive therapies are preferred over surgery to prevent scarring of the fallopian tubes, which increases the risk of subsequent ectopic pregnancies. Expectant management is most effective if the ectopic pregnancy is less than 3.5 cm in diameter with declining β-hCG levels.[3] For medical management, methotrexate is the drug used most commonly to treat early ectopic pregnancy. It causes destruction of rapidly-dividing fetal cells and involution of the pregnancy.[5] Medical treatment is most often used for patients with a tubal mass less than 4 cm in diameter and no sonographic evidence of rupture. Medical therapies are associated with an 85% success rate.[5] Pelvic pain is common (60%) in patients receiving methotrexate, even when successful. Indications of methotrexate failure and the need for rescue surgery include decreasing hemoglobin levels, significant pelvic fluid or unstable vital signs. All patients receiving methotrexate require close follow up until the β-hCG level reaches zero, which may take two to three months.[5] Although abdominal pain is a common adverse effect of methotrexate therapy, rupture of a known ectopic pregnancy must be considered.

Classically, approximately 20% of women with ectopic pregnancies manifest signs and symptoms warranting immediate intervention.[5] These include significant hypovolemia, large amounts of peritoneal fluid or an open cervical os. For patients with significant signs of hypovolemia, rapid volume resuscitation should be instituted with intravenous fluids and blood products as necessary, and a baseline hemoglobin level and type and crossmatch should be obtained.[5] A dilatation and curettage or evacuation procedure with examination of endometrial contents for products of conception can be performed urgently in the unstable patient with an open cervical os. If the patient remains unstable, immediate surgery is the preferred management.

Laparoscopic conservative surgery (tube-sparing salpingostomy) is the mainstay in managing ectopic pregnancy, and has nearly replaced laparotomy and salpingectomy.[4] Laparoscopy has similar tubal patency and future fertility rates as medical management.[2] Laparoscopy may be indicated for patients who are hemodynamically stable after volume replacement, for those who are hemodynamically stable but exhibit significant peritoneal signs, and for those in whom ultrasonography is diagnostic or suggestive of ectopic pregnancy.[5] All patients with ectopic pregnancy who are Rh-negative should be given Rh immunoglobulin 50 μg intramuscularly.

KEY TEACHING POINTS

1. Ectopic pregnancy is the leading cause of pregnancy-related first-trimester death among women in the United States.

2. Risk factors for ectopic pregnancy include a history of PID, previous ectopic, tubal or uterine surgery or instrumentation, uterine or tubal anomalies, use of fertility drugs, and cigarette smoking.

3. Any woman of reproductive age presenting to the ED with abdominal pain should have a β-HCG blood or urine test, as ectopic pregnancy must be considered if the tests are positive.

4. Diagnostic tests for ectopic pregnancy include a urine pregnancy test, ultrasonography, β-hCG measurements, serum progesterone level and, on occasion, diagnostic curettage or culdocentesis.

5. Expectant or medical management with methotrexate may be used in a hemodynamically stable, compliant patient

with a small tubal mass, no evidence of rupture, and close follow up.

6. Surgery (laparoscopy or laparotomy) is the mainstay of treatment for the hemodynamically unstable patient presenting with ectopic pregnancy.

REFERENCES

[1] Mukul LV, Teal SB. Current management of ectopic pregnancy. *Obstet Gynecol Clin N Am* 2007;34:403–19.

[2] Lozeau A-M, Potter B. Diagnosis and management of ectopic pregnancy. *Am Fam Physician* 2005;72:1707–14, 1719–20.

[3] Ferentz KS, Nesbitt LS. Common problems and emergencies in the obstetric patient. *Prim Care Clin Office Pract* 2006;33:727–50.

[4] Bhatt S, Ghazele H, Dogra VS. Sonographic evaluation of ectopic pregnancy. *Radiol Clin N Am* 2007;45:549–60.

[5] Lipscomb GH, Stovall TG, Ling FW. Nonsurgical treatment of ectopic pregnancy. *N Engl J Med* 2000;343:1325–9.

[6] Buckley RG, King KJ, Disney JD, et al. Serum progesterone testing to predict ectopic pregnancy in symptomatic first-trimester patients. *Ann Emerg Med* 2000;36:95–100.

42

Genital trauma in a 34-year-old male

HISTORY OF PRESENT ILLNESS

A 34-year-old male with a history of intravenous drug abuse was brought to the ED by paramedics with the chief complaint of severe penile pain. He reported that 18 hours earlier his girlfriend had placed a metal ring at the base of his penis. The patient was unable to remove the ring, where it remained overnight. The patient complained of severe pain and swelling to his penis, as well as suprapubic pain. He denied nausea or vomiting and had been unable to urinate for the past several hours. He denied similar episodes.

PHYSICAL EXAMINATION

GENERAL APPEARANCE: The patient was lying supine on the gurney in significant discomfort, unable to find a comfortable position.

VITAL SIGNS

Temperature	98.6°F (37°C)
Pulse	110 beats/minute
Blood pressure	140/90 mmHg
Respirations	24 breaths/minute

ABDOMEN: Soft, mild suprapubic tenderness with distended bladder, no rebound or guarding.

GENITOURINARY: A 1.3-cm wide by 0.5-cm thick metallic ring present at the base of the patient's penis, located at the penile-scrotal junction. The ring could not be removed manually. Distal to this ring, the penis was red, swollen, tense and tender to palpation (Figure 42.1); sensation to the penile shaft and meatus was intact. The circumference of the penis distal to the ring measured 18 cm. The testes were descended bilaterally and nontender.

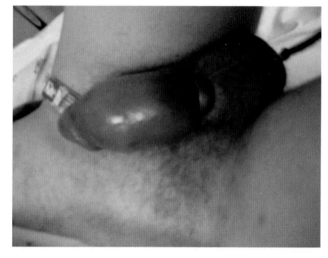

Figure 42.1 Photograph of a 34-year-old male with severe penile pain following placement of a metal ring.

A peripheral intravenous line was placed, blood was drawn and sent for laboratory testing, and morphine sulfate IV was administered for pain control.

What is your diagnosis?

ANSWER

The diagnosis is penile incarceration from a constricting metal ring. An unsuccessful attempt was made in the ED to cut the ring with standard ring cutters. The urologist was urgently consulted and the patient was taken to the operating room. A suprapubic catheter was placed, with drainage of 1 liter of clear urine. After two hours using 10 diamond-embedded circular drill bits attached to a hand-held drill, the ring was successfully divided at two points 180° apart and removed. Upon removal, relief of venous congestion and "pinking up" of the penile tissue was achieved. Urethroscopy revealed pink mucosa of the urethra, and the patient was admitted to the urology service for observation. By hospital day #4, the patient was able to urinate through his urethra. The suprapubic tube was removed and the patient was discharged on hospital day #5. At follow up with the urologist one month later, the patient reported normal functioning of his penis.

Penile incarceration from constricting devices

Constricting devices placed on the penis, either to enhance sexual performance or serve autoerotic intentions, can be made of all materials.[1] Although most reported devices causing penile incarceration are metal rings, higher-grade penile injuries are more frequently sustained by nonmetallic objects.[2] Wearing constricting rings on a flaccid or semi-erect penis might result in the inability to remove the device once erection has been achieved because detumescence cannot take place due to impaired venous outflow; thus, these men often present to the ED.[1] Symptoms and diagnosis of constricting devices are clear-cut, and depend on the nature of the foreign body and the length of time it has been attached to the organ.

Evaluation of patients with penile incarceration should include the assessment of color, temperature, sensation of the organ, ability to void and the presence of pulses (by Doppler flowmeter).[1] If the patient seeks help within approximately two hours, it is likely that the patient will require removal of the device by some improvised means, followed by conservative management to facilitate free blood flow and micturation.[3] However, a long-standing constriction (i.e., more than two hours) can lead to necrosis of the penile tissue and urethral injury.[4] Several clinical syndromes can result from penile incarceration, ranging from mild, nonsignificant vascular obstruction that resolves after decompression to gangrene of the penis accompanied with impaired renal function.[5]

Initial management of penile incarceration from constricting devices involves attempts at manual removal of the ring by the emergency physician, employing equipment ordinarily available in the hospital (e.g., ring cutters, bolt cutters, motorized rotary tools). Care should be taken to protect the penile skin and tissue from the cutting device. The ring may require being cut at two opposite points to facilitate removal. If unsuccessful, pain control with parenteral opioid analgesics should be provided and the urologist consulted for further attempts at removal employing larger equipment (e.g., heavy-duty air grinder, circular disc or saber saw, portable dental drills).[1] Blood aspiration may be helpful to reduce the diameter of the organ and facilitate removal of the device. If the constricting device cannot be removed in a timely manner, if the patient is unable to urinate after removal or urethral trauma is suspected, a suprapubic catheter may be needed.

KEY TEACHING POINTS

1. Constricting rings on a flaccid or semi-erect penis can result in the inability to remove the device once erection has been achieved because detumescence cannot take place due to impairment of venous outflow.
2. Evaluation of patients with penile incarceration should include the assessment of color, temperature, sensation of the organ, ability to void and the presence of pulses.
3. Several clinical syndromes can result from penile incarceration, ranging from nonsignificant vascular obstruction that resolves after decompression to gangrene of the penis.
4. Initial management of penile incarceration from constricting devices involves prompt attempts at manual removal of the ring by the emergency physician. If unsuccessful, IV pain medications should be administered and a urologist urgently consulted for removal of the constricting device.

REFERENCES

[1] Yacobi Y, Tsivian A, Sidi A. Emergent and surgical interventions for injuries associated with eroticism: a review. *J Trauma* 2007;62:1522–30.

[2] Silberstein J, Grabowski J, Lakin C. Penile constriction devices: case report, review of literature, and recommendations for extrication. *J Sex Med* 2008. E-pub ahead of print.

[3] Perabo FG, Steiner G, Albers P, et al. Treatment of penile strangulation caused by constricting devices. *Urology* 2002; 59:137.

[4] Van Ophoven A, de Kernion JB. Clinical management of foreign bodies of the genitourinary tract [review]. *J Urol* 2000;164:274–87.

[5] Ivanovski O, Stankov O, Kuzmanoski M, et al. Penile strangulation: two case reports and review of the literature. *J Sex Med* 2007;4:1775–80.

43

Recurrent vaginal bleeding after miscarriage in a 39-year-old female

HISTORY OF PRESENT ILLNESS

A 39-year-old gravida 14, para 4, spontaneous abortion 2, therapeutic abortion 8 (G14, P4, AB 10) female presented to the ED with vaginal bleeding beginning earlier in the day. The patient had a spontaneous abortion one month prior to presentation; this was her third visit to the ED for vaginal bleeding since that time. Her bleeding had resolved spontaneously on the two previous visits, her hematocrits were stable and she was discharged home. On the last visit, the OB/GYN service was consulted and the patient received oral Methergine® prior to discharge. On this visit, the patient reported the sudden onset of vaginal bleeding five hours prior to arrival. She reported soaking five pads and had passed several small clots during this time. By the time the patient arrived at the ED, the bleeding had slowed considerably.

PHYSICAL EXAMINATION

GENERAL APPEARANCE: The patient appeared well nourished, well hydrated and in no acute discomfort.

VITAL SIGNS

Temperature	98°F (36.6°C)
Pulse	71 beats/minute
Blood pressure	108/60 mmHg
Respirations	20 breaths/minute
Oxygen saturation	100% on room air

HEENT: Unremarkable.

NECK: Supple.

CARDIOVASCULAR: Regular rate and rhythm without rubs, murmurs or gallops.

LUNGS: Clear to auscultation bilaterally.

ABDOMEN: Soft, nondistended, mild suprapubic tenderness without rebound or guarding.

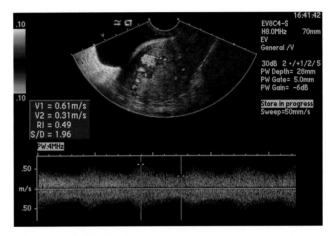

Figure 43.1 Doppler pelvic ultrasound image from a 39-year-old female with recurrent vaginal bleeding one month following spontaneous miscarriage.

PELVIC: Moderate amount of blood with small clots in the vaginal vault, slow trickle of blood from a closed os. A firm, approximately eight-week-size uterus with mild tenderness to palpation was noted. No adnexal tenderness or abnormal masses.

EXTREMITIES: No clubbing, cyanosis or edema.

NEUROLOGIC: Nonfocal.

SKIN: Warm, well-perfused, no rashes or pallor.

A peripheral intravenous line was placed, and blood was drawn and sent for laboratory testing. A hematocrit returned at 36% (decreased from 41% at an ED visit six days earlier), and a serum β-hCG was 6 mIU/mL (11 mIU/mL on her previous ED visit). A pelvic ultrasound was obtained (Figure 43.1).

What is your diagnosis?

The diagnosis is bleeding from a uterine arteriovenous malformation. The Doppler ultrasound demonstrated significant vascularity within the endometrial canal involving the uterus. Peak systolic velocity of the blood flow within this vascularity was found to be 61 cm/sec with relatively low resistance indices. All findings were consistent with an acquired uterine arteriovenous malformation. The OB/GYN service was consulted; no bleeding was noted from the cervix upon repeat speculum examination. The option of surgery was discussed with the patient, including hysterectomy, and the patient chose to defer to a later date. The patient was discharged home with bleeding precautions and expectant management, with close follow up arranged with the gynecologist.

Uterine arteriovenous malformations

Uterine arteriovenous malformation (AVM) is a rare but potentially life-threatening condition. It may result in profuse or irregular bleeding from the abnormal connections between artery and vein. Uterine AVMs must be considered whenever there is unexpected, excessive, intermittent vaginal bleeding, particularly after delivery or surgical procedures of the uterus.[1] Prompt diagnosis and treatment are required.

The true incidence of uterine AVMs is unknown.[2] To date, only case reports or small case series exist, making it impossible to estimate a true incidence. It is known that AVMs are more common in females and have a predilection for pelvic blood vessels, although they rarely involve the uterus.[2] In general, AVMs are either congenital or acquired.[1–3] Acquired etiologies include trauma, surgery, neoplasm and infection.[3] Histologically, the lesions consist of arteries and veins of various sizes communicating directly to form a fistula. The vessels are ambiguous with thickened intima and some elastin in the walls, making the distinction between artery and vein difficult.[3] The mechanism for the formation of acquired AVMs remains unclear but is probably due to local trauma or subinvolution of a placental site. Given this patient's history of multiple therapeutic abortions, a traumatic etiology was most likely.

Although symptoms may vary, bleeding is typically intermittent and torrential, suggestive of arterial hemorrhage.[1] AVMs may present as a secondary or late postpartum hemorrhage. Abnormal bleeding after miscarriage is rarely caused by uterine AVMs, whereas post-procedural bleeding is typical of uterine AVMs.[1] Doppler ultrasound is helpful in the detection of these lesions (because it demonstrates their vascular nature) and in following their resolution.[3] Endovaginal ultrasonography (EVUS) with color Doppler demonstrates a tangle of vessels with multidirectional flow, creating a mosaic pattern.[4] The diagnosis is confirmed by the spectral Doppler finding of high-velocity, high-diastolic turbulent arterial flow within the AVM. Peak systolic velocity recorded within the AVM is usually high, in the range of 40–100 cm/sec.[5] Three-dimensional power Doppler sonography provides additional assistance in the evaluation of uterine vascular AVMs by depicting a clearer view of the orientation of its tortuous vessels. Doppler ultrasound is used to monitor AVMs for response or recurrence after embolization.[5]

Acute treatment of uterine AVMs consists of stabilization and management of active bleeding. A Foley balloon inserted into the uterus may tamponade the site of active bleeding.[2] Intravenous estrogen has been suggested and may provide an endometrial covering over the AVM.[2] In the past, ultimate treatment of uterine AVMs has been contingent on whether the patient desires fertility; hysterectomy was the treatment of choice for a symptomatic AVM if the patient no longer desires fertility.[2] However, with increased experience with embolization of the uterine arteries, this method is currently recommended as the first choice for treatment in women of all age groups, not only those desiring future fertility.[1]

Long-term medical management has also been described, and may be appropriate for patients without heavy bleeding.[1] The successful use of the combined oral contraceptive pill (estrogen/progesterone) has been reported at three months in a patient by ultrasound demonstrating regression of the lesion.[6] Treatment with intramuscular followed by oral methylergonovine maleate has been associated with resolution of an AVM diagnosed and followed by ultrasound, although the authors of this report stress that noninvasive therapy should only be attempted in patients with close clinical follow up.[3] Finally, in the stable patient without heavy bleeding, expectant management may have a role provided close clinical follow up is available.[1]

KEY TEACHING POINTS

1. Uterine arteriovenous malformation (AVM) is a rare but potentially life-threatening condition, and should be considered whenever there is unexpected, excessive, intermittent vaginal bleeding, particularly after delivery or after surgical procedures (e.g., therapeutic abortion, dilatation and curettage).
2. Transvaginal ultrasound with Doppler is the imaging modality of choice for diagnosing uterine AVMs.
3. Initial treatment of uterine AVMs that present with heavy bleeding includes patient stabilization, control of bleeding with Foley balloon tamponade and intravenous estrogens, intravenous fluid and blood transfusion as needed.
4. Ultimate treatment of uterine AVMs may involve embolization of the uterine arteries or hysterectomy. Medical or expectant management may be considered in stable patients with close clinical follow up only in the absence of heavy bleeding.

REFERENCES

[1] Grivell RM, Reid KM, Mellor A. Uterine arteriovenous malformations: a review of the current literature. *Obstet Gynecol Surv* 2005;60:761–7.

[2] Hoffman MK, Meilstrup JW, Shackelford DP, et al. Arterio-venous malformations of the uterus: an uncommon cause of vaginal bleeding. *Obstet Gynecol Surv* 1997;52:736–40.

[3] Flynn MK, Levins D. The noninvasive diagnosis and man-agement of a uterine arteriovenous malformation. *Obstet Gynecol* 1996;88:650–2.

[4] Sheth S, Macura K. Sonography of the uterine myometrium: myomas and beyond. *Ultrasound Clin* 2007;2:267–95.

[5] Bhatt S, Dogra VS. Doppler imaging of the uterus and adnexae. *Ultrasound Clin* 2006;1:201–21.

[6] Khatree MHD, Titiz H. Medical treatment of uterine arteri-ovenous malformation. *Aust N Z J Obstet Gynaecol* 1999;39: 378–80.

44

Scrotal pain and swelling in a 75-year-old male

HISTORY OF PRESENT ILLNESS

A 75-year-old male recently diagnosed with prostate cancer having received multiple rounds of radiation therapy presented to the ED complaining of several days of worsening scrotal pain, redness and swelling. The patient had been diagnosed with bilateral epididymitis three weeks earlier, and had completed a 10-day course of oral ciprofloxacin one week prior to the development of his current symptoms. He reported low-grade fevers and mild lower abdominal pain. He denied nausea, vomiting, diarrhea or dysuria. He currently rated his pain at a level of 5 (on a scale of 0 to 10) at rest but his pain increased to 10 with movement or palpation.

PHYSICAL EXAMINATION

GENERAL APPEARANCE: The patient was an elderly, moderately obese male in no acute discomfort.

VITAL SIGNS

Temperature	99.4°F (37.4°C)
Pulse	105 beats/minute
Blood pressure	109/57 mmHg
Respirations	16 breaths/minute
Oxygen saturation	97% on room air

HEENT: PERRL, EOMI, oropharynx dry.

NECK: Supple, no jugular venous distension.

CARDIOVASCULAR: Tachycardic rate, regular rhythm without rubs, murmurs or gallops.

LUNGS: Clear to auscultation bilaterally.

ABDOMEN: Soft, mild lower abdominal tenderness bilaterally, no rebound or guarding.

GENITOURINARY: Small pockets of pus as well as areas of necrosis were evident on visual inspection of the scrotum, which was diffusely edematous and erythematous (Figure 44.1). The

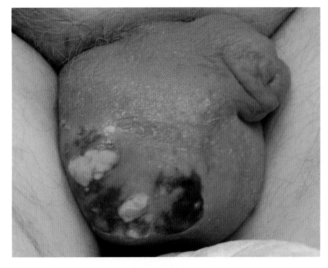

Figure 44.1 Scrotum of a 75-year-old male with several days of scrotal pain and swelling.

scrotum was warm and markedly tender to palpation without crepitus. The testes were not palpable due to significant edema and tenderness.

A peripheral intravenous line was placed, and blood was drawn and sent for cultures and laboratory testing. A 1-liter normal saline IV bolus and morphine sulfate IV were administered. Laboratory tests were remarkable for a leukocyte count of 16 K/μL (normal 3.5–12.5 K/μL) with 95% neutrophils (normal 50–70%) and hematocrit of 28% (normal 39–51%). The electrolytes, BUN, creatinine and glucose were within normal limits.

What is your diagnosis?

ANSWER

The diagnosis is bilateral necrotizing epididymo-orchitis with scrotal and testicular abscesses. Urology was consulted emergently, and a CT of the abdomen and pelvis demonstrated severe, diffuse scrotal skin thickening and inflammatory changes, as well as small, bilateral high-density hydroceles with extensive irregular enhancement and inflammation, consistent with scrotal abscesses and infected hydroceles (Figure 44.2). The patient received piperacillin/tazobactam IV and was taken to the OR by urology for scrotal exploration. Upon exploration, the patient was found to have bilateral testicular abscesses with necrosis and significantly reduced blood flow to both testicles. Bilateral inflamed, fibrotic and necrotic epididymides, as well as bilateral scrotal abscesses with skin necrosis and ischemia were also present. The patient underwent excision of necrotic tissue from the skin and dartos and a bilateral orchiectomy, and was discharged markedly improved on hospital day #4 with a Foley catheter and to continue oral antibiotics (cephalexin).

Epididymo-orchitis, testicular abscess and Fournier's gangrene

By definition, orchitis is inflammation of the testis; acute orchitis represents sudden occurrence of pain and swelling of the testis associated with acute inflammation of that testis.[1] Epididymitis is defined as inflammation of the epididymis. Acute epididymitis represents sudden occurrence of pain and swelling of the epididymis associated with acute inflammation.

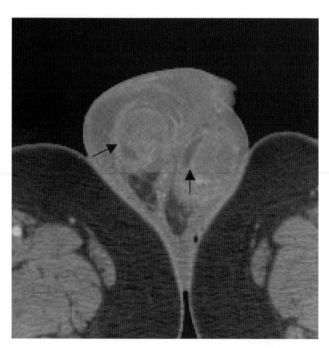

Figure 44.2 CT of the scrotum from a 75-year-old male with scrotal pain and swelling, demonstrating bilateral scrotal abscesses and infected hydroceles (arrows).

Most cases of orchitis, especially bacterial, occur secondary to local spread of ipsilateral epididymitis (termed epididymo-orchitis). Urinary tract infections (UTI) are usually the underlying cause in boys and elderly men.[1] In young, sexually-active men, sexually transmitted illnesses (STI) are often responsible. Because bacterial orchitis is usually associated with epididymitis, it is often caused by urinary pathogens, including E. coli and Pseudomonas. Less commonly, Staphylococcus or Streptococcus species are responsible. The most common sexually-transmitted organisms responsible are Neisseria gonorrhoeae, C. trachomatis and Treponema pallidum.

Patients with epididymo-orchitis usually present with unilateral testicular pain, as well as fever, dysuria and painful scrotal enlargement.[2] Tenderness to palpation on the affected side is present, as well as palpable swelling of the epididymis. Urethral discharge, hydrocele, erythema or edema of the scrotum on the affected side may also be present.[3] Laboratory tests to assist in the diagnosis include urinalysis, urine microscopy and urine culture.[1] For a patient in whom an STI is suspected, urethral swab should be obtained for culture. The most important differential diagnosis in young men and boys is testicular torsion.[1,3] Testicular torsion is often difficult to differentiate from an acute inflammatory condition. Scrotal ultrasound (using Doppler imaging to determine testicular blood flow) is especially helpful in differentiating torsion from acute inflammatory conditions such as epididymo-orchitis.[1]

Treatment for epididymo-orchitis includes bed rest, scrotal elevation and support, analgesics and oral antibiotics.[3] Empiric therapy should be given to all patients with epididymo-orchitis before culture results are available. The antibiotic regimen should be based on the results of tests immediately available, as well as age, sexual history, recent instrumentation or catheterization, and any known urinary tract abnormalities the patient may have.[3] Males younger than 35 years need empiric coverage for C. trachomatis and N. gonorrhoeae, usually with a combination of ceftriaxone and either doxycycline or azithromycin.[4] Prepubertal patients and males older than 35 years require empiric coverage for coliform bacteria (enteric Gram-negative bacilli and Pseudomonas). Both of these patient populations may be treated with trimethoprim-sulfamethoxazole (TMP-SMX); a fluoroquinolone (e.g., ciprofloxacin) may be prescribed in patients older than 35 years.

If a patient with epididymo-orchitis does not receive appropriate treatment, complications include pyocele, testicular infarction, testicular abscess, scrotal abscess and fulminant necrotizing fasciitis (Fournier's gangrene).[2] Formation of an intratesticular abscess is usually secondary to epididymo-orchitis, but other causes include mumps, trauma and testicular infarction.[5] Sonographic features of intratesticular abscesses include shaggy irregular walls, an intratesticular location of the abscess, low-level internal echoes and occasional hypervascular margins.[5] Abscess formation is rare but if it occurs, percutaneous or open drainage is necessary.

Fournier's gangrene is a necrotizing fasciitis of the perineal, genital or perianal regions.[6] The infective process leads to thrombosis of subcutaneous blood vessels, resulting in gangrene of the overlying skin. These pathologic processes may also affect other areas of the body. Historically, Fournier's gangrene portended a dismal prognosis, with mortality rates as high as 67%.[7] The natural course of this necrotizing fasciitis is rapid progression, ultimately resulting in the patient's demise. Those with the disease are almost always recognized to have an underlying systemic disorder. The most common associations are diabetes (present in 40–60% of patients) and chronic alcoholism (25–50% of cases).[6] Immunosuppression, either after organ transplantation, caused by chemotherapy or malignant disease, or from HIV infection, is also associated with an increased risk of Fournier's gangrene.[6]

Fournier's gangrene commonly begins with local discomfort, itching and swelling of the scrotum and perineum.[7] At presentation, edema and crepitus may be noted, with systemic symptoms of fever, leukocytosis, anemia and electrolyte abnormalities. The precise etiology of Fournier's gangrene remains unclear. Trauma to the perineum, ascending infection from a perirectal site, microvascular disease, UTIs, urethral strictures, periurethral diverticulae, testicular pathology and epididymal disease have all been implicated as initiating factors.[7]

Aggressive resuscitation with intravenous fluids, empiric antibiotics that cover Gram-positive, Gram-negative and anaerobic bacteria, and correction of electrolyte disturbances should be started as soon as the diagnosis of Fournier's gangrene is considered.[8] Polymicrobial culture of aerobic and anaerobic commensal organisms is recommended. Several causative organisms have been described, including *Clostridium*, *Klebsiella*, *Streptococcus*, *Corynebacterium*, *Staphylococcus* and *Bacteroides* species, as well as coliform bacteria.[8] Urgent surgical debridement remains the cornerstone of treatment. The patient and surgical team must be prepared for potentially major surgery. The testes are rarely affected due to the abdominal source of their blood supply.[8] Adjuvant hyperbaric oxygen therapy has proved beneficial in some studies, although its role remains controversial.[8,9] Once the risk of sepsis has been eradicated, and the patient is clinically improved, the focus may shift to reconstruction of the affected area.[8]

KEY TEACHING POINTS

1. Patients with epididymo-orchitis generally present with unilateral testicular pain, fever, dysuria and painful scrotal enlargement.
2. Treatment for epididymo-orchitis includes bed rest, scrotal elevation and support, analgesics and oral antibiotics, with close follow up.
3. Epididymo-orchitis can progress to testicular and scrotal abscesses, as well as Fournier's gangrene, if left untreated.
4. Fournier's gangrene is an aggressive necrotizing fasciitis of the perineal, genital or perianal regions, and represents a true urological emergency.
5. The four main principles in the management of Fournier's gangrene are resuscitation, antibiotics, debridement and, when appropriate, reconstruction.

REFERENCES

[1] Nickle JC. Inflammatory conditions of the male genitourinary tract: prostatitis and related conditions, orchitis, and epididymitis. In: Wein AJ, et al. (eds.). *Campbell-Walsh Urology*, 9th ed. Philadelphia: Saunders, 2007:327–9.

[2] Muttarak M, Chiangmai WN, Kitirattrakarn P. Necrotizing epididymo-orchitis with scrotal abscess. *Biomed Imaging Interv J* 2005;1:e11. Available at http://www.biij.org/2005/2/e11. Accessed June 23, 2008.

[3] Walker P, Wilson J. National guideline for the management of epididymo-orchitis (UK). *Sex Transm Infect* 1999;75:515–35.

[4] Brooks MB. Epididymitis. eMedicine Website. Available at http://www.emedicine.com/emerg/topic166.htm. Accessed June 23, 2008.

[1] Dogra V, Bhatt S. Acute painful scrotum. *Radiol Clin N Am* 2004;42:349–63.

[5] Smith GL, Bunker CB, Dinneen MD. Fournier's gangrene. *Br J Urol* 1998;81:347–55.

[6] Corman JM, Moody JA, Aronson WJ. Fournier's gangrene in a modern surgical setting: improved survival and aggressive management. *BJU International* 1999;84:85–8.

[7] Aho T, Canal A, Neal DE. Fournier's gangrene. *Nature Clin Pract Urol* 2006;3:54–7.

[8] Chang I-J, Lee C-C, Chen S-Y. Fulminant gangrenous and crepitating scrotum. *Arch Dermatol* 2006;142:797–8.

PART VI

NEUROLOGY/NEUROSURGERY

45

Left-sided weakness in a 13-year-old male

HISTORY OF PRESENT ILLNESS

A 13-year-old male with no significant medical history presented to the ED two hours after developing left-sided weakness and some confusion while doing his homework, according to his parents. No seizure activity was reported. By the time the patient was evaluated in the ED, his symptoms had completely resolved. He denied headaches, visual changes, dizziness, fevers or neck stiffness. He had not experienced any similar episodes previously.

PHYSICAL EXAMINATION

GENERAL APPEARANCE: The patient was well appearing and in no acute discomfort.

VITAL SIGNS

Temperature	98.5°F (37°C)
Pulse	90 beats/minute
Blood pressure	110/70 mmHg
Respirations	20 breaths/minute
Oxygen saturation	100% on room air

HEENT: PERRL, EOMI, no facial asymmetry.

NECK: Supple, no meningeal signs.

CARDIOVASCULAR: Regular rate and rhythm without rubs, murmurs or gallops.

LUNGS: Clear to auscultation bilaterally.

ABDOMEN: Soft, nontender, nondistended.

EXTREMITIES: No clubbing, cyanosis or edema.

NEUROLOGIC: Alert and oriented to person, place and time; cranial nerves II–XII grossly intact; upper extremity and lower extremity strength 5/5 bilaterally, proximally and distally; no pronator drift, no dysmetria, normal gait.

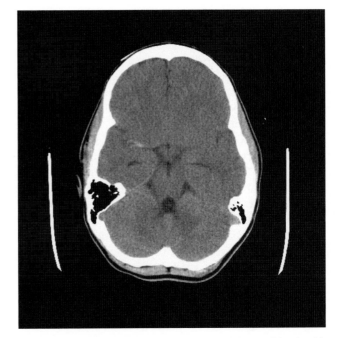

Figure 45.1 Noncontrast CT of the brain from a 13-year-old male with transient left-sided weakness.

A peripheral intravenous line was placed, and blood was drawn and sent for laboratory testing. Laboratory tests, including a complete blood count, electrolytes, creatinine and random glucose, were within normal limits. A noncontrast CT of the brain was obtained (Figure 45.1). While the patient was still in the ED, his left-sided weakness returned approximately three hours after his initial symptoms (left arm and leg strength noted to be 3/5 on repeat examination).

What is your diagnosis?

ANSWER

The final diagnosis is acute cerebrovascular accident (CVA) secondary to partial occlusion of the right middle cerebral artery (MCA). The initial head CT demonstrated a thrombus in the right MCA (hyperdense MCA sign). When the patient's symptoms returned, neurology was immediately consulted; it was decided not to give thrombolytics (t-PA) based on limited data of thrombolytics in children and the finding that the patient's symptoms improved shortly after the onset of symptoms. A CT angiogram of the brain was obtained, which demonstrated a filling defect in the proximal right MCA consistent with a thrombus (Figure 45.2).

Unfractionated heparin was administered with an initial intravenous bolus and a maintenance drip of 20 units/kg/hour. The patient was admitted to the pediatric ICU. The patient's symptoms continued to improve during his hospital course. On hospital day #5, a magnetic resonance angiogram (MRA) of the brain demonstrated evidence of acute infarct involving the right lentiform nucleus, right caudate head, and a portion of the caudate body and external capsule (Figure 45.3). Slight local mass effect was seen without midline shift.

A work-up to identify hypercoagulability proved negative, and an echocardiogram was normal. The patient was transitioned to low-molecular-weight heparin (enoxaparin) administered subcutaneously on hospital day #4, and he was discharged on hospital day #6 with nearly complete resolution of his symptoms. He was instructed to continue enoxaparin twice per day as an outpatient, which he continues five months after his stroke.

Stroke in children

Stroke is a heterogeneous disorder and an important cause of mortality and chronic morbidity in children. The estimated incidence of cerebrovascular disease in children is approximately 25 per 100,000 in neonates and 1.3–13 per 100,000

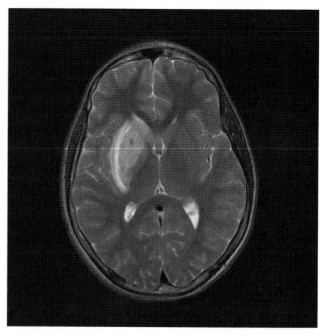

Figure 45.3 MRA of the brain from a 13-year-old male with left-sided weakness, demonstrating acute infarct involving the right lentiform nuclei, right caudate head and a portion of the caudate body, as well as the external capsule.

per year in children aged 1–18 years; half of these are due to ischemia.[1] Ischemic stroke is currently defined as a focal neurologic deficit lasting more than 24 hours with no etiology other than vascular. Transient ischemic attacks (TIAs), currently defined as neurologic deficits lasting less than 24 hours, are commonly associated with infarction in children; many series in children have included these patients.[1]

Several factors increase the risk of ischemic stroke in children. Congenital heart disease remains an important risk factor.[2] Other risk factors include atherosclerotic and non-atherosclerotic vasculopathies, hemoglobinopathies such as sickle cell disease, cerebral and meningeal infections, prothrombotic states, dehydration, sepsis and brain trauma.[2,3] In children with acute ischemic stroke (AIS), prothrombotic disorders have been identified in one-third to one-half of patients.[3] However, stroke occurs with no identifiable disorder in nearly 50% of children.[3]

The clinical presentation of AIS is related to the age of the child and the size and location of the stroke.[4] In the first year of life, infants with AIS typically present with seizures, hypotonia, apnea or decreased levels of consciousness. Older children with AIS may present with hemiplegia, aphasia, seizures or other focal neurologic deficits.[4] Signs and symptoms of AIS are often misinterpreted as other systemic or neurological disorders in children. The lack of specific symptoms of AIS and similarities with more common disorders often leads to delays in hospital presentation and diagnosis.

CT scan of the brain is the initial imaging test of choice when considering AIS in children, as it is the preferred imaging study to identify acute hemorrhage. Work-up should also

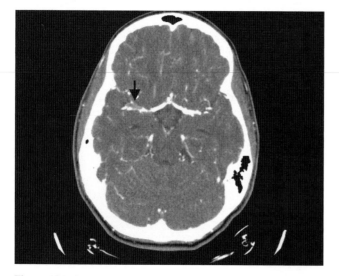

Figure 45.2 CT angiogram of the brain demonstrating right MCA thrombus (arrow) in a 13-year-old male with left-sided weakness.

include MRI, MRA, and conventional four-vessel angiography in selected cases, especially when a clear risk factor for hemorrhage cannot be established or in patients with multiple risk factors.[2] In addition to complete blood count, electrolyte panel, serum glucose and coagulation studies, a comprehensive coagulation work-up should be performed, particularly if a family history of thrombosis or hemorrhage exists.

Initial treatment of children with AIS includes prompt recognition and immediate stabilization, with particular attention to the airway, breathing and circulation. Although several cases describing the successful use of thrombolytic agents in pediatric patients presenting with AIS have been reported, intravascular thrombolysis is controversial and efficacy has not been established in this patient population.[5–8] Tissue plasminogen activator (t-PA) is clot-selective, has a shorter half-life than other thrombolytic agents (i.e., urokinase or streptokinase) and produces lower levels of fibrinogen degradation products; however, no trial to date has demonstrated acceptable safety in the pediatric stroke population.[2] The delay in diagnosis that often occurs in children with AIS reduces the likelihood that a child will be evaluated early enough to benefit from thrombolytic agents.[2] Thrombolytic therapy has been recommended for childhood AIS in special situations but should only be considered at institutions able to support its complications with neurology, radiology, and pediatric neurosurgical support.[4]

The use of antiplatelet and antithrombotic therapies is primarily based on adult studies and expert opinion.[4] Consensus guidelines for the treatment of AIS in children have been published.[9,10] Treatment guidelines from the Seventh Conference of American College of Chest Physicians on Antithrombotic and Thrombolytic Therapy include the following: children with non-sickle cell-related AIS should be treated with anticoagulation (low-molecular-weight heparin or unfractionated heparin) for five to seven days and then switched to aspirin (3–5 mg/kg/day); children with sickle cell-related AIS should receive emergent exchange transfusion; and children with carotid or vertebral artery dissection-related or cardioembolic AIS should be treated with anticoagulation (low-molecular-weight heparin or unfractionated heparin) for three to six months and then switched to aspirin (3–5 mg/kg/day).[4,10]

KEY TEACHING POINTS

1. Acute ischemic stroke (AIS) in children is more common than previously thought, and must be included in the differential diagnosis for any child presenting to the ED with acute, focal weakness or other stroke-like symptoms.

2. Risk factors for AIS in children include congenital heart disease, atherosclerotic and nonatherosclerotic vasculopathies, hemoglobinopathies (such as sickle cell disease), cerebral and meningeal infections, prothrombotic states, dehydration, sepsis and brain trauma.

3. In the first year of life, infants with AIS typically present with seizures, hypotonia, apnea or decreased levels of consciousness, whereas older children with AIS may present with hemiplegia, aphasia, seizures or other focal neurologic deficits.

4. Intravascular thrombolysis in children presenting with AIS is controversial; currently, efficacy has not been established in this patient population.

5. Treatment of children presenting with AIS includes anticoagulation with unfractionated or low-molecular-weight heparin and use of antiplatelet agents (e.g., aspirin). Emergent exchange transfusion is recommended in patients with sickle cell disease.

REFERENCES

[1] Nowak-Gottl U, Gunther G, Kurnik K, et al. Arterial ischemic stroke in neonates, infants, and children: an overview of underlying conditions, imaging methods, and treatment modalities. *Semin Thrombos Hemost* 2003;29:405–14.

[2] Carvalho KS, Garg BP. Arterial strokes in children. *Neurol Clin N Am* 2002;20:1079–100.

[3] DeVeber G. Arterial ischemic strokes in infants and children: overview of current approaches. *Semin Thrombos Hemost* 2003;29:567–73.

[4] Lynch JK, Han CJ. Pediatric stroke: what do we know and what do we need to know? *Semin Neurol* 2005;25:410–23.

[5] Thirumalai SS, Shubin RA. Successful treatment for stroke in a child using recombinant tissue plasminogen activator. *J Child Neurol* 2000;15:558.

[6] Carlson MD, Leber S, Deveikis J, et al. Successful use of rt-PA in pediatric stroke. *Neurology* 2001;57:157–8.

[7] Shuayto MI, Lopez JI, Greiner F. Administration of intravenous tissue plasminogen activator in a pediatric patient with acute ischemic stroke. *J Child Neurol* 2006;21:604–6.

[8] Cannon BC, Kertesz NJ, Friedman RA, et al. Use of tissue plasminogen activator in a stroke after radiofrequency ablation of a left-sided accessory pathway. *J Cardiovasc Electrophysiol* 2001;12:723–5.

[9] Paediatric Stroke Working Group. Stroke in Childhood: Clinical Guidelines for Diagnosis, Management and Rehabilitation. London: Royal College of Physicians, 2004.

[10] Monagle P, Chan A, Massicotte P, et al. Antithrombotic therapy in children: the Seventh ACCP Conference on Antithrombotic and Thrombolytic Therapy. *Chest* 2004;126: 645S–87S.

46

Worst headache of life in a 23-year-old female

HISTORY OF PRESENT ILLNESS

A 23-year-old female with no significant medical history presented to the ED with a severe headache, described as the worst headache of her life. The headache came on suddenly three hours earlier while sitting, involved her entire head, and was rated at a level of 10 (on a scale of 0 to 10). She reported associated nausea, vomiting and sensitivity to light, but denied neck stiffness, fevers or chills, visual changes, focal weakness, numbness or trauma. She had not experienced such headaches in the past and denied illicit drug use. Her only medication was oral contraceptives. Her last normal period was two weeks earlier.

PHYSICAL EXAMINATION

GENERAL APPEARANCE: The patient appeared well nourished, well hydrated, lethargic and in acute discomfort.

VITAL SIGNS

Temperature	97.9°F (36.6°C)
Pulse	94 beats/minute
Blood pressure	118/69 mmHg
Respirations	18 breaths/minute
Oxygen saturation	100% on room air

HEENT: PERRL, EOMI, no nystagmus, moderate photophobia.

NECK: Supple, no meningeal signs.

CARDIOVASCULAR: Regular rate and rhythm without rubs, murmurs or gallops.

LUNGS: Clear to auscultation bilaterally.

ABDOMEN: Soft, nontender, nondistended.

EXTREMITIES: No clubbing, cyanosis or edema.

NEUROLOGIC: Somnolent but easily arousable, oriented to person, place and time. Cranial nerves II–XII grossly intact; upper and lower extremity strength 5/5 bilaterally, proximal and distal. Sensation grossly intact, no pronator drift, no dysmetria on finger-to-nose testing.

A peripheral intravenous line was placed, blood was sent for laboratory testing, and a noncontrast CT of the brain was obtained (Figure 46.1). The patient was given morphine sulfate and Zofran® IV for pain and nausea, respectively. Laboratory tests, including a complete blood count, electrolytes, creatinine, glucose and coagulation studies, were within normal limits. A serum pregnancy test was negative.

What is your diagnosis?

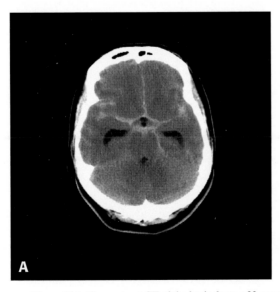
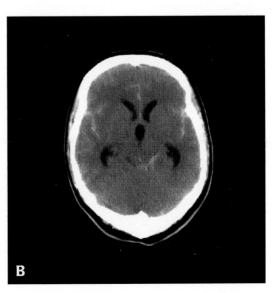

Figure 46.1 Noncontrast CT of the brain from a 23-year-old female with the sudden onset of a severe headache.

ANSWER

The diagnosis is spontaneous subarachnoid hemorrhage (SAH). The noncontrast CT of the brain demonstrated diffuse SAH as well as hydrocephalus and effacement of the basal cisterns, findings concerning for transtentorial herniation (Figure 46.2). The patient's mental status continued to deteriorate and she was emergently intubated for airway protection using rapid sequence induction and modest hyperventilation to decrease cerebral edema. The patient was transferred to the neurosurgical service and emergently underwent a right frontal ventriculostomy to relieve the hydrocephalus and prevent further herniation. Approximately five hours following the diagnostic CT, a cerebral angiogram was performed that demonstrated an aneurysm arising at the bifurcation of the right middle cerebral artery (panel A, Figure 46.3). Endovascular coiling with embolization of the aneurysm was successfully performed (panel B, Figure 46.3). The patient was extubated on hospital day #3 with continued neurological improvement.

Subarachnoid hemorrhage

Nontraumatic (spontaneous) subarachnoid hemorrhage (SAH) is a neurologic emergency characterized by the extravasation of blood into the spaces covering the central nervous system that are filled with cerebrospinal fluid.[1] The leading cause of nontraumatic SAH is rupture of an intracranial aneurysm, which accounts for 80% of cases and has a high rate of complications and death.[1] Nonaneurysmal SAH, including isolated perimesencephalic subarachnoid hemorrhage, occurs in about 20% of cases and carries a good prognosis; neurologic complications are uncommon. According to Edlow et al., 1 in 100 headache patients presenting to EDs have SAH.[2] Of

patients with severe, abrupt-onset headache and normal neurologic examinations, about 10% have SAH. The incidence of aneurysmal SAH is 6–10 per 100,000 persons in the United States each year (approximately 30,000 annually).[3,4]

SAH is more common in African-Americans and Hispanics than Caucasians, and post-menopausal women are more frequently affected than men.[2] Important risk factors for SAH include heavy alcohol use, cigarette smoking, hypertension, a family history of SAH, cocaine use, and possibly oral contraceptive use. Other disorders associated with SAH include autosomal dominant polycystic kidney disease, Ehlers-Danlos syndrome type IV and neurofibromatosis type I.[2] Spontaneous SAHs are frequently associated with Valsalva maneuvers (e.g., during bowel movements or heavy lifting), and may occur post-coital.

SAH should always be suspected in patients with a "typical" presentation, which includes some or all of the following: sudden onset of severe headache (frequently described as the "worst ever"), associated with nausea, vomiting, neck pain, photophobia, and loss or alteration of consciousness.[1] The physical examination may show retinal hemorrhages, nuchal rigidity, restlessness, a diminished level of consciousness and focal neurologic signs.[5] In the absence of the classic signs and symptoms, SAH may be misdiagnosed. The frequency of misdiagnosis may be as high as 50% in patients presenting for their first physician visit.[1] Common incorrect diagnoses include migraine and tension-type headaches. In a Canadian study from 2002–2005, approximately 1 in 20 SAH patients were missed during an ED visit, with lower-acuity patients having a greater risk of misdiagnosis.[6]

The first test for a patient with a suspected SAH should be an unenhanced cranial CT. A recent retrospective review of 149 patients diagnosed with spontaneous SAH in an academic ED yielded an overall CT scan sensitivity of 93%.[4] Cranial

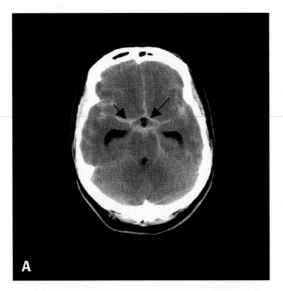
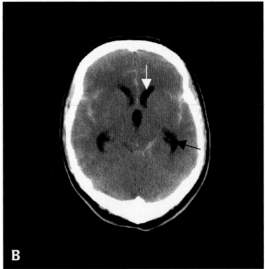

Figure 46.2 Noncontrast CT of the brain from a 23-year-old female demonstrating diffuse SAH (arrows, panel A) and hydrocephalus of the frontal horns (white arrow, panel B) and atria (dark arrow, panel B) of the lateral ventricles.

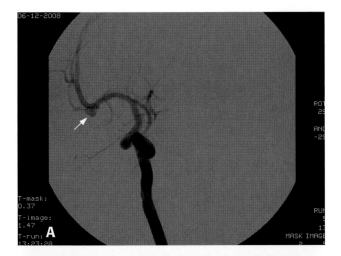

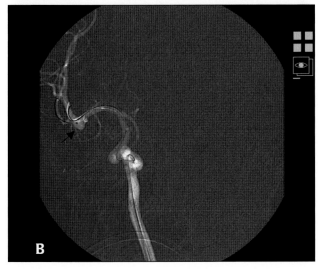

Figure 46.3 Cerebral angiogram of right internal carotid artery demonstrating aneurysm at the right middle cerebral artery bifurcation (arrow, panel A), and endovascular coiling with embolization of the aneurysm (arrow, panel B).

CT scan is highly accurate but, like all tests, has limitations.[2] One limitation is that accuracy diminishes with time due to cerebrospinal fluid (CSF) circulation and the resultant dilution and catabolism of blood.[2] A second limitation of cranial CT is "spectrum bias." In alert and awake patients (presumably with smaller volume bleeds), the cranial CT is less likely to show blood.[5] A third limitation is that intracranial blood in anemic patients (hematocrit less than 30%) may appear isodense with brain and thus more difficult to see.[2] Finally, many CT sensitivity studies relied on experienced neuroradiologists to interpret these images, whereas readings by general radiologists, neurologists and emergency physicians may be less accurate.[2,5]

For patients with an abnormal CT scan, immediate consultation with a neurologist or neurosurgeon is indicated. Until more convincing data confirm the 100% sensitivity of ultra-early or ultra-modern CT scanning in SAH, all patients

being evaluated for SAH whose CT scans are normal, technically inadequate, or nondiagnostic should undergo lumbar puncture.[1,2] CSF should be collected in four consecutive tubes, with the red blood cell (RBC) count compared in tubes 1 and 4. Findings consistent with SAH include an elevated opening pressure, an elevated RBC count that does not diminish from tube 1 to tube 4, and xanthochromia (yellow tinge of CSF caused by the enzymatic conversion of hemoglobin to bilirubin, owing to red cell breakdown and detected by spectrophotometry).[1] In patients with either equivocal or diagnostic lumbar puncture, consultation with a specialist and an imaging study (such as CT angiography of the brain or cerebral angiography) should be the next step.[1] For patients with a normal CT and lumbar puncture, symptomatic treatment of the headache, discharge and close outpatient follow up are generally considered appropriate.[5]

All patients with SAH should be evaluated and treated on an emergency basis with maintenance of airway and cardiovascular function.[1] After initial stabilization, patients should be transferred to centers with neurovascular expertise, preferably with a dedicated neurologic critical care unit. The discussion between specialists and emergency physicians should address several issues, including airway control, treatment or prevention of acute hydrocephalus, blood pressure control, seizure and vasospasm prophylaxis, appropriate analgesia and maintenance of an ideal intracranial pressure.[2] Once in the critical care setting, the main goals of treatment (including pain control) are the prevention of rebleeding, the prevention and management of vasospasm, and the treatment of other medical or neurologic complications. Currently, the main therapeutic options for definitive treatment of a ruptured aneurysm at specialized centers are microvascular neurosurgical clipping and endovascular coiling.[1]

KEY TEACHING POINTS

1. Nontraumatic subarachnoid hemorrhage (SAH) is a neurologic emergency that typically presents with the sudden onset of severe headache (frequently described as the "worst ever"), associated nausea, vomiting, neck pain, photophobia, and loss or alteration of consciousness; however, not all of these may be present.

2. Eighty percent of cases of SAH are caused by rupture of an intracranial aneurysm.

3. Evaluation of patients with suspected SAH should begin with a noncontrast cranial CT; if the CT is normal or equivocal, a lumbar puncture should be performed.

4. Patients with a normal CT and lumbar puncture can generally be discharged from the ED with close follow up arranged.

5. Emergency treatment of SAH includes close attention to the airway, breathing and circulation, pain and nausea control, efforts to prevent elevation of intracranial pressure, and prompt consultation with a neurosurgical specialist.

REFERENCES

[1] Suarez JI, Tarr RW, Selman WR. Current concepts: aneurysmal subarachnoid hemorrhage. *N Engl J Med* 2006;354:387–96.

[2] Edlow JA, Malek AM, Ogilvy CS. Aneurysmal subarachnoid hemorrhage: update for emergency physicians. *J Emerg Med* 2007;34:237–51.

[3] Edlow JA. Diagnosis of subarachnoid hemorrhage in the emergency department. *Emerg Med Clin N Am* 2003;21:73–87.

[4] Byyny RL, Mower WR, Shum N, et al. Sensitivity of non-contrast cranial computed tomography for the emergency department diagnosis of subarachnoid hemorrhage. *Ann Emerg Med* 2008;51:697–703.

[5] Edlow JA, Caplan LR. Avoiding pitfalls in the diagnosis of subarachnoid hemorrhage. *N Engl J Med* 2000;342:29–36.

[6] Vermeulen MJ, Schull MJ. Missed diagnosis of subarachnoid hemorrhage in the emergency department. *Stroke* 2007;38:1216–21.

47

Lower extremity weakness in a 26-year-old female

HISTORY OF PRESENT ILLNESS

A 26-year-old female with a medical history significant for obesity and obstructive sleep apnea presented to the ED by ambulance complaining of progressive, bilateral lower extremity weakness. She reported that on the day of presentation she could not bear weight or move her legs. She also reported numbness in both legs, as well as an inability to urinate. She had experienced cold and flu-like symptoms starting several weeks earlier, with a dry, nonproductive cough, left ear pain and tactile fevers. She was prescribed amoxicillin by her primary care provider (PCP) at this time for presumed otitis media. Four days prior to her ED presentation she again saw her PCP, complaining of pain in the right parascapular region of the thoracic spine. She was diagnosed with musculoskeletal pain and prescribed ibuprofen. Shortly after this visit, she began to experience weakness in both legs along with a "pins-and-needles" sensation from her waist down. She denied recent trauma, neck pain, upper extremity weakness or numbness, headaches, dizziness or nausea. Her only medications had been amoxicillin and ibuprofen. She smoked a half-pack of cigarettes per day, drank alcohol occasionally and denied intravenous drug use.

PHYSICAL EXAMINATION

GENERAL APPEARANCE: The patient was a well-developed, obese female lying supine on the gurney in no acute distress.

VITAL SIGNS

Temperature	100°F (37.8°C)
Pulse	95 beats/minute
Blood pressure	115/85 mmHg
Respirations	20 breaths/minute
Oxygen saturation	99% on room air

HEENT: Unremarkable.

NECK: Supple, no midline tenderness.

CARDIOVASCULAR: Regular rate and rhythm without rubs, murmurs or gallops.

LUNGS: Clear to auscultation bilaterally.

ABDOMEN: Soft, nontender, nondistended.

RECTAL: Diminished rectal tone, perianal anesthesia present, brown stool, hemoccult negative.

BACK: Tenderness to palpation over the thoracic spine.

NEUROLOGIC: Alert and oriented to person, place and time; cranial nerves II–XII grossly intact; upper extremity strength 5/5 bilaterally, proximal and distal; lower extremity strength 0/5 bilaterally, proximal and distal. Sensation grossly intact above her bra line; below this level, the patient lacked sensation to either light touch or pinprick.

A peripheral intravenous line was placed, and blood was drawn and sent for cultures and laboratory testing. Laboratory tests revealed a leukocyte count of 10.9 K/μL (normal 3.5–12.5 K/μL) with 85% neutrophils (normal 50–70%) and erythrocyte sedimentation rate (ESR) of 108 mm/hr (normal 0–20 mm/hr). Electrolytes, creatinine, glucose, PT, PTT and INR were all within normal limits. Plain radiographs of the thoracic and lumbar spine were obtained but failed to reveal abnormalities.

What is your diagnosis?

ANSWER

The diagnosis is spinal epidural abscess with spinal cord compression. An MRI was obtained, demonstrating a dorsal right paracentral epidural mass from T3 through T8 compressing the thoracic spinal cord, pushing it against the posterior aspect of the adjacent vertebral bodies (Figures 47.1–47.3). The patient received IV antibiotics (nafcillin and vancomycin), Decadron® 10 mg IV, and was taken to the operating room by a spine surgeon. A T2–T9 decompression via T3–T8 laminectomies with irrigation and debridement of the spinal canal was performed. Upon decompression of the spinal cord, gross pockets of pus were discovered. Subsequent copious irrigation and debridement of the spinal canal occurred intraoperatively. Spinal cord compression was noted, particularly in the region of T5.

Postoperatively, the patient was admitted to the ICU and IV antibiotics were continued. Blood cultures returned positive for *Staphylococcus aureus*, with sensitivities to all antibiotics tested. By hospital day #5, the patient was still unable to move her lower extremities, although some sensitivity to touch had returned. She was referred for physical and occupational therapy during her hospital course.

Spinal epidural abscess

Spinal epidural abscess (SEA) comprises 0.2–2 cases per 100,000 hospital admissions.[1] SEA is part of a continuum of infection that often develops as a result of untreated spondylodiscitis. Most patients with SEA have one or more predisposing conditions, such as an underlying disease (diabetes

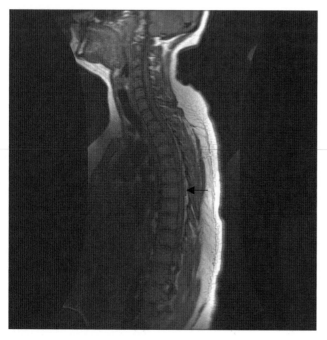

Figure 47.1 T1-weighted image of thoracic spine MRI from a 26-year-old female with lower extremity weakness, demonstrating a large dorsal epidural abscess from T3–T8 (arrow).

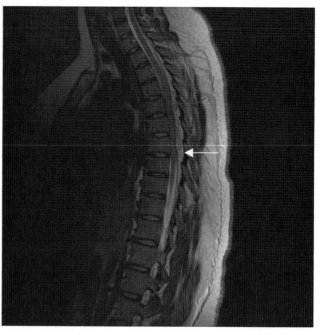

Figure 47.2 T2-weighted image of thoracic spine MRI from a 26-year-old female with spinal epidural abscess (arrow).

mellitus, alcoholism, HIV infection), a spinal abnormality or intervention (degenerative joint disease, trauma, surgery, drug injection, or placement of stimulators or catheters), or a potential local or systemic source of infection (skin and soft tissue infections, osteomyelitis, urinary tract infection, sepsis, indwelling vascular catheter, intravenous drug use, nerve acupuncture, tattooing, epidural analgesia or nerve block).[2] Patients can be affected at any age. There have been case reports of SEA in patients as young as 10 days old and as old as 87 years.[1] SEA more commonly affects the thoracic and lumbar spine but can occur at any spinal level. Furthermore, extension of the abscess is common. The average extent of an abscess spans 3–5 spinal cord segments.[1]

Almost two-thirds of all cases of SEA are caused by *Staphylococcus aureus*, with skin and soft tissue infections being the most common sites of bacterial origin.[3] The incidence of methicillin-resistant *S. aureus* (MRSA) is steadily increasing. Epidural abscesses are more common in the thoracic than in the lumbar region because of the relatively large amounts of fat within the epidural space of the thoracic spine.[3] For this same reason, these are almost always found posteriorly, as the dura is attached directly to the vertebral bodies anteriorly.

In patients with SEA, severe back pain with a radicular component is often the presenting complaint.[4] Fever is common but is not universal. Leukocytosis and elevation of the ESR are typical; in the presence of fever and back pain, the diagnosis is relatively straightforward.[4] However, only 20% of patients have the classic clinical triad of fever, back pain and neurologic deficits, so a high index of suspicion should be maintained.[1,2,4]

SEA is a progressive disease. Historically, the early stages (phases I and II) of SEA are characterized by spine pain, alone

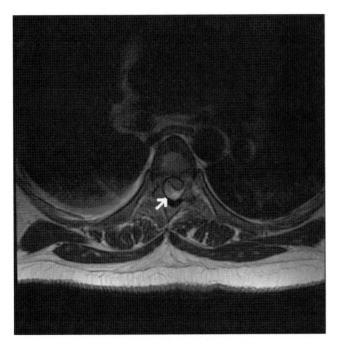

Figure 47.3 Sagittal view of T2-weighted image of thoracic spine MRI from a 26-year-old female demonstrating dorsal epidural abscess compression on the spinal cord (arrow).

or in the presence of referred or radicular pain.[5] After these "quiescent" phases, an "acute" stage of the disease is entered, often heralded by a rise in temperature and acceleration of pain. This ultimately results in weakness or paralysis (phases III and IV). This classification scheme has limited clinical utility, as the symptoms present in phases I and II are relatively nonspecific, with the diagnosis most often made in phases III and IV, which results in poor neurologic outcomes.[5]

A diagnosis of SEA should be suspected on the basis of clinical findings, and is supported by laboratory data and imaging studies. However, it can only be confirmed by surgical drainage.[2] Bacteremia causing or arising from SEA is detected in approximately 60% of patients, more commonly in those infected with *S. aureus* than with other organisms.[2] Both MRI with intravenous gadolinium and CT myelography of the spine are highly sensitive (more than 90%) in diagnosing SEA.[2] However, MRI is the imaging method of choice because it is less invasive, delineates both the longitudinal and paraspinal extension of the abscess (essential for surgical planning), and may help differentiate infection from cancer on the basis of appearance and signal intensity of the image.[2]

Paralysis from a SEA can quickly become irreversible. The immediate treatment goals are reduction of the inflammatory mass impinging on the spinal cord and eradication of the causative organism with antibiotic therapy.[3] Surgical decompression within the first 24 hours is crucial to improving long-term prognosis, and neurologic recovery after surgery is

indirectly related to the duration of the untreated neurologic deficit. Irreversible paraplegia occurs in up to 25% of patients; substantially more have residual motor weakness.[3] The use of intravenous steroids (dexamethasone) in the treatment of SEA has been sporadically reported in the literature.[6,7] Although there have been reports in which glucocorticoid therapy has been associated with adverse outcomes in patients who already had a severe case of SEA,[8] they may help reduce swelling in patients with progressive neurologic compromise awaiting surgical decompression.[2]

KEY TEACHING POINTS

1. Predisposing conditions for the development of spinal epidural abscess (SEA) include diabetes mellitus, intravenous drug use, immunocompromised state, alcoholism, spinal abnormalities or interventions, and potential local or systemic sources of infection.
2. Only 20% of patients with SEA present with the classic triad of back pain, fever and neurologic deficits.
3. Almost two-thirds of all cases of SEA are caused by *Staphylococcus aureus*, with skin and soft tissue infections being the most common sites of bacterial origin.
4. MRI with gadolinium enhancement is the imaging test of choice for diagnosing SEA.
5. The treatment of SEA is prompt surgical decompression and intravenous antibiotics; the use of intravenous dexamethasone may reduce swelling in patients with progressive neurologic compromise.

REFERENCES

[1] Winters ME, Kluetz P, Zilberstein J. Back pain emergencies. *Med Clin N Am* 2006;90:505–23.
[2] Darouiche RO. Spinal epidural abscess. *N Engl J Med* 2006;355:2012–20.
[3] Marsh EB, Chow GV, Gong GX, et al. A cut above. *Am J Med* 2007;120:1031–3.
[4] Tarulli AW, Taynor EM. Lumbosacral radiculopathy. *Neurol Clin* 2007;27:387–405.
[5] Davis DP, Wold RM, Patel RJ, et al. The clinical presentation and impact of diagnostic delays on emergency department patients with spinal epidural abscess. *J Emerg Med* 2004;26:285–91.
[6] Wessling H, de las Heras P. Cervicothoracolumbar spinal epidural abscess with tetraparesis. Good recovery after non-surgical treatment with antibiotics and dexamethasone. Case report and review of the literature. *Neurocirugia (Astur)* 2003;14:529–33.
[7] Anand S, Maini L, Agarwal A, et al. Spinal epidural abscess – a report of six cases. *Int Orthop* 1999;23:175–7.
[8] Danner RL, Hartman BJ. Update of spinal epidural abscess: 35 cases and review of the literature. *Rev Infect Dis* 1987; 9:265–74.

48

Headache, neck pain and dizziness in a 35-year-old male

HISTORY OF PRESENT ILLNESS

A 35-year-old male with no significant medical history presented to the ED complaining of right-sided neck pain for three weeks, as well as a progressively worsening right-sided headache over the past week. His neck pain had been constant, located on the right side and worse with movement, whereas the headache was described as throbbing, located on the right occipital region and radiating to the front. On the day of presentation, his headache became severe and he complained of nausea, vomiting and difficulty walking secondary to feeling "off balance." He denied visual changes, focal weakness or numbness, as well as any recent head or neck trauma.

PHYSICAL EXAMINATION

GENERAL APPEARANCE: The patient was awake and alert, and appeared to be in no acute discomfort.

VITAL SIGNS

Temperature	98.5°F (36.9°C)
Pulse	70 beats/minute
Blood pressure	175/85 mmHg
Respirations	18 breaths/minute
Oxygen saturation	100% on room air

HEENT: PERRL, EOMI, no nystagmus.

NECK: Supple, nontender, no carotid bruits.

CARDIOVASCULAR: Regular rate and rhythm without rubs, murmurs or gallops.

LUNGS: Clear to auscultation bilaterally.

ABDOMEN: Soft, nontender, nondistended.

EXTREMITIES: No clubbing, cyanosis or edema.

NEUROLOGIC: Alert and oriented to person, place and time; upper and lower extremity strength 5/5 proximal and distal; sensation grossly intact to light touch throughout. No pronator

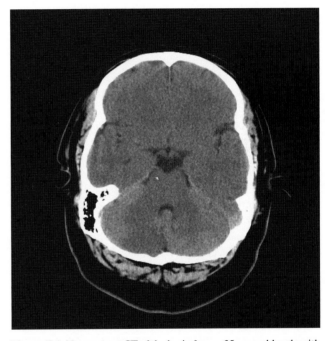

Figure 48.1 Noncontrast CT of the brain from a 35-year-old male with headache, neck pain and dizziness.

drift present; however, the patient demonstrated mild dysmetria on finger-to-nose testing bilaterally, as well as an ataxic gait upon ambulation, leaning to the left and requiring support.

A peripheral intravenous line was placed, blood was drawn and sent for laboratory testing, and a noncontrast CT scan of the brain was obtained (Figure 48.1). Laboratory tests, including a complete blood count, electrolytes, creatinine, glucose and prothrombin time, were within normal limits.

What is your diagnosis?

ANSWER

The diagnosis is acute cerebellar stroke secondary to vertebral artery dissection. The noncontrast CT scan (Figure 48.1) demonstrated a low attenuation lesion measuring 3.5 cm × 2.5 cm in the right cerebellum with minimal local mass effect. An MRI of the brain was obtained three hours following the CT, which showed an acute infarct in the right cerebellar hemisphere measuring 4 cm × 5 cm, with the infarct in the vascular distribution of the right posterior inferior cerebellar artery (Figure 48.2). An MRI and MRA of the cervical carotid and vertebral arteries demonstrated dissection of the upper right vertebral artery starting approximately 4–5 cm below the level of the origin of the basilar artery (Figure 48.3).

The patient was admitted to the internal medicine service with neurology consultation. Options regarding anticoagulation were discussed with the patient and his family, who declined heparin therapy in favor of conservative treatment with aspirin. On hospital day #3, the patient complained of a worsening headache, and a repeat noncontrast CT of the brain demonstrated evolving cerebellar infarct with mild posterior fossa mass effect, including increased effacement of the basilar cisterns with resultant mild enlargement of the lateral and third ventricles (Figure 48.4). The patient was subsequently transferred to the neurosurgical service for further observation and consideration of ventricular shunt placement. The neurosurgeon determined shunt placement at this time was not necessary. No further evolution was noted on repeat CT five days later. The patient's neurologic status was stable; he was discharged home to continue aspirin therapy.

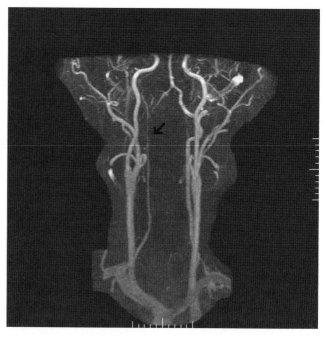

Figure 48.3 MRA of the carotid and vertebral arteries from a 35-year-old male with headache, neck pain and ataxia, demonstrating right vertebral artery dissection (dark arrow).

Cervical artery dissection

Cervical arterial dissection (CAD) results from a tear in the intimal lining of the involved vessel, occurring spontaneously or in response to major (or trivial) trauma.[1] The tear allows blood under arterial pressure to enter the wall of the artery and form an intramural hematoma, known as the false lumen.[2]

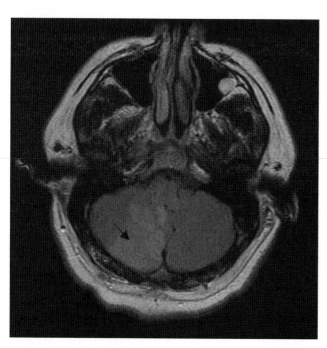

Figure 48.2 MRI of the brain from a 35-year-old male with headache, neck pain and ataxia, demonstrating acute infarct in the right cerebellar hemisphere (arrow).

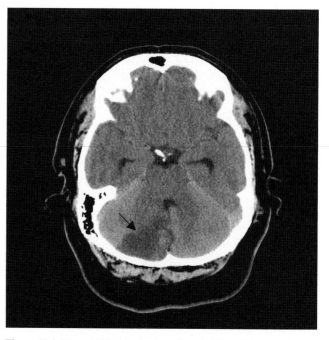

Figure 48.4 Repeat CT of the brain on hospital day #3 from a 35-year-old male with headache, neck pain and ataxia, demonstrating evolving cerebellar infarct (arrow).

Although intracranial arterial dissection is rare, dissection of the internal carotid or vertebral artery, typically occurring at the C1–C2 vertebral level, is an important cause of ischemic stroke in young and middle-aged patients. Although there is no overall gender-based predilection, women are on average about five years younger than men at the time of CAD.[2] In community-based studies in the United States and France, the annual incidence of spontaneous CAD ranged from 2.5–3.0 per 100,000 persons.[2] Given the relative frequency of dissections of the carotid and vertebral arteries in large hospital-based studies, the annual incidence of spontaneous vertebral artery dissection can be estimated at 1.0–1.5 per 100,000 persons.[2,3]

Spontaneous dissections have been described in arteries throughout the body. The extracranial segments of the carotid and vertebral arteries are much more likely to undergo dissection than either their extracranial segments or extracranial arteries of similar size, such as the coronary or renal arteries. This discrepancy may be explained by the greater mobility of the extracranial internal carotid and vertebral arteries and the potential for them to be injured by contact with bony structures, such as the cervical vertebrae or styloid processes.[2]

Patients with a spontaneous dissection of the carotid or vertebral artery are thought to have an underlying structural defect of the arterial wall, although the exact type of arteriopathy remains elusive in most cases. Foremost among the heritable connective-tissue disorders associated with an increased risk of spontaneous dissections of the carotid and vertebral arteries is Ehlers-Danlos syndrome type IV; other disorders include Marfan syndrome, autosomal dominant polycystic kidney disease and osteogenesis imperfecta.[2] A history of a minor precipitating event is frequently elicited in patients with a spontaneous dissection of the carotid or vertebral artery. Chiropractic manipulation of the neck has been associated with carotid and vertebral artery dissection; it has been estimated that as many as 1 in 20,000 spinal manipulations cause a stroke.[2] However, generalized connective-tissue disorders have been identified in one-fourth of patients with such dissections, and the initial symptoms of vertebral artery dissection commonly mimic musculoskeletal neck pain for which people go to chiropractors.[2]

Headache is the most common presenting feature of internal carotid and vertebral artery dissection, and may occur with neck pain.[1–4] Neck pain accompanies headache in 50% of patients with vertebral artery dissection and 25% of patients with carotid artery dissection.[5] In both instances, approximately 60–70% of patients present with headache that is typically, though not exclusively, in the occipital region.[4] The median time from onset of headache to onset of other neurologic symptoms has been reported to be four days with carotid dissection and 14.5 hours with vertebral dissection.[5] In cases of vertebral artery dissection, the median interval between the onset of neck pain and the appearance of other symptoms has been reported to be two weeks.[2]

The classic presentation of vertebral artery dissection is pain in the back of the neck or head, followed by ischemia of the posterior circulation. However, the initial manifestations of vertebral artery dissection are less distinct than those of carotid artery dissection, and are usually initially interpreted as musculoskeletal in nature.[2] Ischemic symptoms occur in more than 90% of patients diagnosed with vertebral artery dissection and may involve the brainstem, particularly the lateral medulla (Wallenberg syndrome), as well as the thalamus and the cerebral or cerebellar hemispheres. Isolated ischemia of the cervical spinal cord is an uncommon but increasingly recognized complication of vertebral artery dissection.[2] Transient ischemic attacks are less frequent after vertebral artery dissections than after carotid artery dissections.

Conventional angiography has long been the gold standard in the diagnosis of arterial dissections because it identifies the arterial lumen. It also allows extensive characterization of dissections of the carotid and vertebral arteries. Magnetic resonance techniques are replacing conventional angiography as the gold standard in the diagnosis of dissections of the carotid and vertebral arteries because the resolution of magnetic resonance angiography (MRA) now approaches that of conventional angiography, and MRI can show the intramural hematoma itself.[2] MRI is superior to angiography in the diagnosis of dissection without associated luminal abnormalities or in cases resulting in nonspecific occlusion. Ultrasound is useful in the initial assessment of patients who are believed to have a dissection of the carotid artery. Although the site of dissection is generally not identified, an abnormal pattern of blood flow is identified in more than 90% of patients.[2] Finally, helical CT angiography is a minimally invasive technique that can provide high-resolution images of the arterial lumen as well as the vessel wall. Results similar to those of magnetic resonance techniques have been reported for the detection and follow up of CAD, but experience with this technique remains limited.[2]

To prevent thromboembolic complications, anticoagulation with intravenous heparin followed by oral warfarin has been recommended for all patients with acute dissections of the carotid or vertebral artery, regardless of the type of symptoms, unless contraindications exist (such as intracranial extension of the dissection).[2] However, the evidence supporting such management is little more than anecdotal.[1] Progression of acute stroke, early recurrent stroke, or late recurrent stroke is rare, regardless of what (if any) treatment is administered.[1] Most dissections heal spontaneously, and anatomic resolution of CAD and associated stenosis or occlusion is common, usually occurring within three months after the dissection. Healing may be documented noninvasively by serial brain MRI, MRA or carotid duplex testing.[1,2]

In one retrospective study of 48 patients with CAD, anticoagulation was the most frequent initial medical treatment (64%).[3] Antiplatelet therapy alone (typically with aspirin) was the initial treatment in 31%. Two patients (4%) received neither anticoagulation nor antiplatelet therapy. Acute interventional therapy was attempted in four patients, with two patients receiving intravenous tissue plasminogen activator (t-PA) and two patients receiving intra-arterial thrombolytics.

The clinical outcome for the majority of patients was good (92%), with a mean follow up of 7.8 years (maximum 17.7 years).[3]

KEY TEACHING POINTS

1. Dissection of the internal carotid or vertebral artery is an important cause of ischemic stroke in young and middle-aged patients.
2. Consider vertebral artery dissection in patients presenting with neck pain and occipital headache, particularly in patients with recent neck trauma or neurologic symptoms such as ataxia, stroke or TIAs.
3. MRI followed by MRA of the cervical arteries is the imaging modality of choice in diagnosing cervical artery dissection.

4. Anticoagulation is the recommended initial treatment for cervical artery dissection, although data supporting such treatment is lacking.

REFERENCES

[1] Rothrock JF. Headaches due to vascular disorders. *Neurol Clin N Am* 2004;22:21–37.
[2] Schievinik WI. Current concepts: spontaneous dissection of the carotid and vertebral arteries. *N Engl J Med* 2001;344: 898–906.
[3] Lee VH, Brown RD, Mandrekar JN, et al. Incidence and outcome of cervical artery dissection: a population-based study. *Neurology* 2006;67:1809–12.
[4] Bogduk N. The neck and headaches. *Neurol Clin N Am* 2004; 22:151–71.
[5] Schwedt TJ, Matharu MS, Dodick DW. Thunderclap headaches. *Lancet Neurol* 2006;5:621–31.

49

Low back pain and weakness in a 37-year-old male

HISTORY OF PRESENT ILLNESS

A 37-year-old male with a medical history significant for an L3–L4 laminectomy five years earlier presented to the ED complaining of two days of progressively worsening low back pain. The patient described a markedly intensified pain starting at the low back and shooting down his legs bilaterally. He also noted decreased sensation in his legs and thighs, including his saddle area, as well as difficulty urinating. He denied fevers or chills, abdominal pain, intravenous drug use and diabetes.

PHYSICAL EXAMINATION

GENERAL APPEARANCE: The patient was a well-developed male lying supine on the gurney, in moderate discomfort.

VITAL SIGNS

Temperature	98.7°F (37°C)
Pulse	85 beats/minute
Blood pressure	150/90 mmHg
Respirations	22 breaths/minute
Oxygen saturation	100% on room air

HEENT: Unremarkable.

NECK: Supple, no midline tenderness.

CARDIOVASCULAR: Regular rate and rhythm without rubs, murmurs or gallops.

LUNGS: Clear to auscultation bilaterally.

ABDOMEN: Soft, nontender, nondistended, no pulsatile masses.

RECTAL: Saddle anesthesia to pinprick, absent rectal tone.

EXTREMITIES: No clubbing, cyanosis or edema, brisk peripheral pulses.

NEUROLOGIC: Alert and oriented to person, place and time; cranial nerves II–XII grossly intact; upper extremity strength 5/5 proximal and distal; symmetric 4/5 strength of the iliopsoas, quadriceps and hamstring muscles with a right foot drop present; bulbocavernous reflex absent, patellar reflexes 1+ on the left and absent on the right, and ankle reflexes absent bilaterally; Babinski sign absent bilaterally (great toes downgoing to plantar stimulation).

An intravenous line was placed, blood was drawn and sent for laboratory testing, and morphine sulfate was administered for pain. Laboratory tests, including a complete blood count, electrolytes and coagulation studies, were within normal limits.

What is your diagnosis?

ANSWER

The diagnosis is cauda equina syndrome. MRI of the lumbosacral spine was obtained emergently, which showed a space-occupying lesion at the L4 vertebral body (L4–L5 large disc extrusion and herniation) with mass effect upon the cauda equina (Figure 49.1). Decadron 10 mg was given IV, and the patient was transferred to the neurosurgical service. The patient underwent an L4 decompression laminectomy with L4–L5 discectomy, with complete return of strength and sensation.

Cauda equina syndrome

The adult spinal cord terminates at the level of the L1–L2 vertebrae, with the terminal bundle of lumbar and sacral nerve roots within the spinal canal forming the cauda equina below. The nerve roots then separate and exit at their specific foramina. Compression of the cauda equina is most commonly caused by herniation of a large quantity of lumbar disc material, often in association with degenerative or congenital spinal stenosis, which can result in cauda equina syndrome (CES).[1] CES is not considered a true spinal cord injury. Instead, it is an injury to the lumbosacral nerve roots within the neural canal.[2] Extremely rare causes of CES include compression by tumor, fracture, penetrating trauma, chiropractic manipulation, chemonucleolysis, postoperative hematoma, free epidural fat graft and ankylosing spondylitis.

Risk factors for disc herniation include obesity, male gender, age over 40 years, heavier lifetime lifting during occupational and leisure activities, and history of back disorders.[1] Four percent of patients with acute low back pain have a herniated disk but 95% of patients with herniation have sciatica.[3] CES complicates approximately 2% of cases of lumbar disc herniation.[4]

Clinical features of CES include perineal and other lumbosacral root sensory deficits, lower limb motor weakness, difficulty with bladder more often than bowel control, sexual dysfunction, low back pain, and unilateral or bilateral sciatica.[3–5] However, one retrospective study found that only 19% of patients diagnosed with CES over a four-year period presented with the characteristic combination of bilateral sciatica, lower limb weakness, saddle anesthesia and sphincter disturbance.[6] The strongest presenting features of CES in this study were low back pain, sacral sensory loss and urinary symptoms.

Three variations of CES have been described: acute CES that occurs suddenly in patients without previous low back problems; acute neurologic deficit in patients who have a history of back pain and sciatica; and gradual progression to CES in patients who have chronic back pain and sciatica.[1] In more than 85% of cases, signs and symptoms of CES develop in less than 24 hours.

The physical examination of a patient with low back pain and neurologic symptoms should include a thorough musculoskeletal and neurologic examination, with special focus on the low back, lower extremities and perianal area. The straight-leg-raise test, during which the examiner raises the supine patient's fully extended leg to 70°, is considered positive for disc herniation and nerve irritation when it produces radicular pain radiating down the lower limb below the knee in one or both limbs between 30° and 60° of elevation.[1] Neurologic examination should evaluate each of the spinal nerve roots. Lumbar disc herniation typically affects the nerve root inferior to the disc space. Thus, herniation of the L4–L5 intervertebral disc would typically impinge on the L5 nerve root. Sensory examination should be conducted using both light touch and pinprick (see Table 49.1 for summary of sensory, motor and reflex innervation by nerve roots L1–S5).

CES or spinal cord compression should be considered until proven otherwise in all patients who report low back pain with saddle anesthesia or bowel or bladder incontinence.[5] Bladder dysfunction is usually secondary to detrusor muscle weakness and an areflexic bladder; this dysfunction initially causes

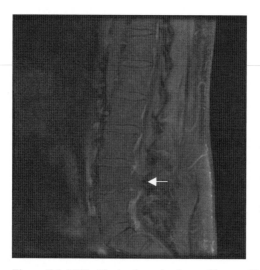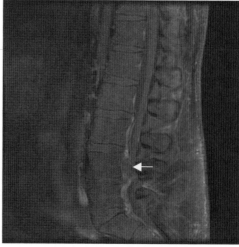

Figure 49.1 MRI of the lumbar spine from a 37-year-old male with severe low back pain, demonstrating L4–L5 large disc extrusion and herniation with mass effect on the cauda equina (arrows).

TABLE 49.1 Nerve roots with associated sensory, motor and reflex arcs

Nerve root	Sensory	Motor	Reflex
L1	Anterior aspect of thigh	Hip flexion (iliopsoas muscle)	
L2	Anterior aspect of thigh	Hip flexion Knee extension	Patellar
L3	Anterior aspect of thigh	Hip flexion Knee extension	Patellar
L4	Medial aspect of leg and and foot, great toe	Knee extension Ankle dorsiflexion and foot inversion (tibialis anterior muscle)	Patellar
L5	Lateral aspect of foot First dorsal web space	Great toe dorsiflexion Hip abduction (gluteal muscles)	
S1	Lateral aspect of foot Posterolateral aspect of calf	Foot eversion (peroneal muscles) Ankle plantar flexion	Achilles
S2	Perineum, perianal	Ankle plantar flexion Bladder and bowel control	Anal wink
S3	Perineum, perianal	Intrinsic foot muscles Bladder and bowel control	Anal wink
S4	Perineum, perianal	Intrinsic foot muscles Bladder and bowel control	Anal wink

Adapted from Ho DPE, "A case study of cauda equina syndrome," Permanente J 2003;7:15.

urinary retention followed by overflow incontinence in later stages. Patients who have back pain with urinary incontinence but have normal neurologic examinations should have a urinary post-void residual volume measured. A post-void residual volume of more than 100 mL indicates overflow incontinence and mandates further evaluation.

The anal wink reflex, elicited by gently stroking the skin lateral to the anus, normally causes reflexive constriction of the external anal sphincter. Similarly, the bulbocavernosus reflex can be elicited to check the S3–S4 nerve level. This reflex is elicited by pulling on the glans penis or clitoris (or gently pulling on an inserted Foley catheter) and noting contraction of the anal sphincter.[1] Rectal examination should be performed to assess anal sphincter tone and sensation if any characteristic signs or symptoms of CES are present.

MRI is the accepted standard to evaluate a patient with clinically significant spinal pathology, and should be emergently obtained when the diagnosis of CES is suspected. Abnormalities on MRI are commonly found in asymptomatic patients; it should therefore be used as a means of confirming a diagnosis in the presence of neurologic signs rather than as a screening tool.

Treatment with high-dose steroids may provide rapid pain relief and improved neurologic function while appropriate diagnostic studies and consultations are being obtained.[1] Dexamethasone is commonly given intravenously at doses of 4–100 mg. CES is an absolute indication for emergent surgical decompression; laminectomy followed by gentle retraction of the cauda equina (to avoid complications of increased neurologic compromise) and discectomy is the technique of choice.[1] Traditionally, patients with CES who have surgery within 24 hours of initial symptoms are believed to have

significantly improved clinical recovery. However, some studies have found no significant improvement in outcome between patients surgically treated within 24 hours compared with those surgically treated within 24–48 hours.[7]

KEY TEACHING POINTS

1. Compression of the cauda equina is most commonly caused by disc herniation, often in association with degenerative or congenital spinal stenosis, and can result in cauda equina syndrome (CES).
2. Patients with CES characteristically present with a history of low back pain, bilateral sciatica, motor and sensory disturbances including sacral and perianal anesthesia, and sphincter disturbances.
3. In more than 85% of cases, the signs and symptoms of CES develop in less than 24 hours.
4. MRI is the standard for evaluating a patient with clinically significant spinal pathology, and should be obtained emergently when CES is suspected.
5. CES requires early administration of high-dose steroids, neurosurgical consultation and emergent surgical decompression.

REFERENCES

[1] Ho DPE. A case study of cauda equina syndrome. *Permanente J* 2003;7:13–7.
[2] McKinley W, Santos K, Meade M, et al. Incidence and outcomes of spinal cord injury clinical syndromes. *J Spinal Cord Med* 2007;30:215–24.

[3]   Kinkade S. Evaluation and treatment of acute low back pain. *Am Fam Physician* 2007;75:1181–8.

[4]   Winters ME, Kluetz P, Zilberstein J. Back pain emergencies. *Med Clin N Am* 2006;90:505–23.

[5]   Bartleson JD. Spine disorder case studies. *Neurol Clin* 2006; 24:309–30.

[6]   Jalloh J, Minhas P. Delays in the treatment of cauda equina syndrome due to its variable clinical features in patients presenting to the emergency department. *Emerg Med J* 2007;24:33–4.

[7]   Ahn UM, Ahn NU, Buchowski JM. Cauda equina syndrome secondary to lumbar disc herniation. *Spine* 2000;25:1515–22.

50

Headache and left arm weakness in a 44-year-old female

HISTORY OF PRESENT ILLNESS

A 44-year-old female with a medical history significant for migraines, hypertension and menometrorrhagia presented to the ED complaining of a sudden onset left-sided headache (similar to her migraines) that had progressively worsened. The patient also developed left arm numbness and weakness. She related having increased frequency and duration of her migraines over the past week since starting oral contraceptives for dysfunctional uterine bleeding. She reported nausea but denied visual changes, neck pain, vomiting or slurred speech. Her medications included iron, Maxalt® for migraines and oral contraceptives (Levora®). The patient did not drink, smoke or use drugs.

PHYSICAL EXAMINATION

GENERAL APPEARANCE: The patient was awake and alert, and in no acute discomfort.

VITAL SIGNS

Temperature	97.5°F (36.4°C)
Pulse	79 beats/minute
Blood pressure	159/90 mmHg
Respirations	16 breaths/minute
Oxygen saturation	100% on room air

HEENT: PERRLA, EOMI without nystagmus, intact visual fields.

NECK: Supple, no meningeal signs.

CARDIOVASCULAR: Regular rate and rhythm without rubs, murmurs or gallops.

LUNGS: Clear to auscultation bilaterally.

ABDOMEN: Soft, nontender, nondistended.

RECTAL: Normal tone, brown stool, hemoccult negative.

EXTREMITIES: No clubbing, cyanosis or edema, bilateral equal pulses upper and lower extremities.

NEUROLOGIC: Alert and oriented to person, place and time; cranial nerves II–XII grossly intact; diminished sensation to light touch noted over left face and left arm; left upper extremity strength 4/5; left pronator drift present, otherwise no asymmetry or other focal abnormalities.

A peripheral intravenous line was placed, and blood was drawn and sent for laboratory testing. The patient's blood sugar in the ED was 66 mg/dL by bedside glucometery. She received one ampule of D50 intravenously without resolution of her weakness. A 12-lead electrocardiogram demonstrated a normal sinus rhythm with no acute ST-T wave changes. Laboratory tests were significant for a hematocrit of 29% (normal 34–46%); her electrolytes, creatinine, and troponin I were within normal limits. A noncontrast CT scan of the brain was obtained (Figure 50.1).

What is your diagnosis?

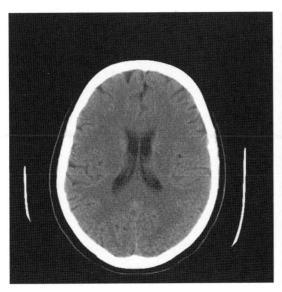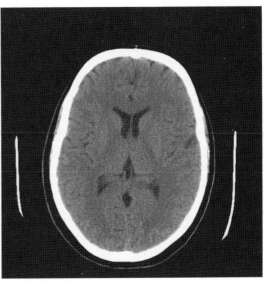

Figure 50.1 Noncontrast CT of the brain from a 44-year-old female with headache and left arm weakness.

ANSWER

The diagnosis is cerebral venous sinus thrombosis. The non-contrast CT scan of the brain did not demonstrate any intracranial hemorrhage, mass or midline shift. The patient was admitted to the medicine service and underwent an initial MRI of the brain, which demonstrated increased signal intensity at the cerebral cortex of the bilateral parietal and occipital lobes on the FLAIR and T2-weighted images with restricted diffusion, suggestive of hyperacute versus acute cortical vascular ischemia, postictal transient changes of the cerebral cortex, or encephalomyelitis (Figure 50.2).

The patient subsequently underwent a lumbar puncture to evaluate for encephalitis, the results of which were negative. The patient's hospital course was complicated by several generalized seizures, for which she was started on phenytoin. A repeat MRI with gadolinium on hospital day #3 demonstrated filling defects in the superior sagittal sinus on the post-contrast images, suggesting venous sinus thrombosis (Figure 50.3). A subsequent magnetic resonance venogram demonstrated filling defects in the superior sagittal sinus, as well as portions of the transverse sinuses, compatible with a venous sinus thrombosis (Figure 50.4). The patient was anticoagulated with enoxaparin and Coumadin®; her clinical condition and neurologic status improved gradually, with complete resolution of her neurologic deficits. She was discharged on hospital day #5 on enoxaparin, Coumadin® and phenytoin.

Cerebral venous thrombosis

Thrombosis of the cerebral veins and sinuses is a distinct cerebrovascular disorder that, unlike arterial stroke, most often

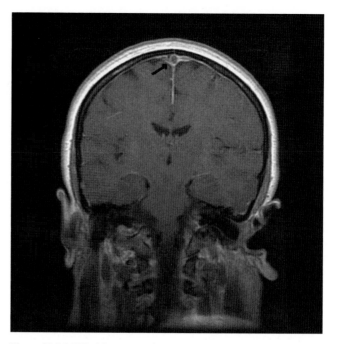

Figure 50.3 MRI with contrast demonstrating filling defect in superior sagittal sinus (arrow).

affects young adults and children. The estimated annual incidence is 3–4 cases per 1 million population, up to 7 cases per 1 million among children.[1] About 75% of the adult patients are women. Because of increased awareness of the diagnosis, improved neuroimaging techniques and more effective treatment over the past decade, more than 80% of patients now have a good neurologic outcome.[1]

A prothrombotic risk factor or a direct cause is identified in about 85% of patients with sinus thrombosis.[1] Often, a precipitating factor such as head injury or obstetrical delivery causes sinus thrombosis in a person with a genetically increased risk. During the last trimester of pregnancy and after delivery, the risk of sinus thrombosis increases. Case studies have also shown an increased risk of sinus thrombosis in women who use oral contraceptives; the risk of venous thromboembolism is increased by a factor of three or four among users of low-estrogen oral contraceptives.[1,2] Other causes of cerebral venous thrombosis include head injury, internal jugular vein catheterization, dehydration, lumbar puncture, infections (e.g., otitis and mastoiditis), malignancy and inflammatory disease (e.g., Behçet's).[1,3,4]

Cerebral venous thrombosis (CVT) presents with a remarkably wide spectrum of signs and modes of onset, thus mimicking numerous other disorders. The most common symptoms and signs are headache, seizures, focal neurological deficits, altered consciousness and papilledema, which can present in isolation or in association with other symptoms.[4] Headache is present in 80% of cases and is often the earliest indication of CVT.[3] The headache may be of the "thunderclap" type in approximately 15% of cases; aside from those instances, the headache of CVT has little distinguishing characteristics. Afflicted patients may exhibit symptoms, signs and

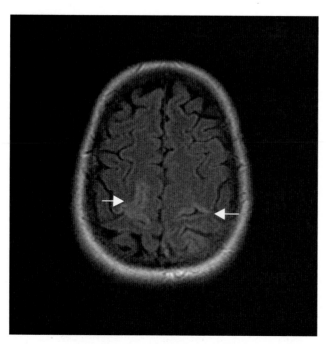

Figure 50.2 MRI of the brain demonstrating abnormal bright signal intensity of the bilateral parietal and occipital lobes (arrows).

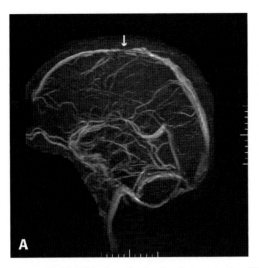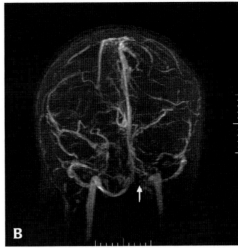

Figure 50.4 MRV of cerebral veins demonstrating filling defects in the sagittal (arrow, panel A) and right transverse (arrow, panel B) sinuses.

cerebrospinal fluid (CSF) findings characteristic of intracranial hypertension, and the associated headache may evolve over days to years.[3] Other patients experience a more fulminant, clinically devastating and potential fatal course, with progressive focal neurologic deficits and multiple seizures.

The most sensitive examination for diagnosing CVT is MRI in combination with magnetic resonance venography (MRV).[1] T_1- and T_2-weighted MRI will demonstrate a hyperintense signal from the thrombosed sinus. The characteristics of the signal depend on the age of the thrombus; these signals are isointense on T_1-weighted images during the first five days and after one month. The combination of an abnormal signal in a sinus and a corresponding absence of flow on MRV confirms the diagnosis of CVT. If MRI is not readily available, CT scanning is a useful technique for the initial examination to rule out other acute cerebral disorders and to demonstrate venous infarcts or hemorrhages. Results of CT scanning can be entirely normal.[1] CT venography is a promising new technique for creating images of the cerebral venous system. If the diagnosis remains uncertain after MRI or CT venography, cerebral angiography may be indicated. A neurologist should be consulted in cases where CVT is diagnosed, or when the diagnosis cannot be ruled out with available imaging techniques.

The goals of antithrombotic treatment in CVT are to recanalize the occluded sinus or vein, prevent the propagation of thrombus, and treat the underlying prothrombotic state. This is to prevent venous thrombosis in other parts of the body (as occurs in pulmonary embolism) and to prevent the recurrence of CVT.[4] Anticoagulants with body weight-adjusted subcutaneous low-molecular-weight heparin or dose-adjusted intravenous heparin are widely used as first-line therapy. Most neurologists now start treatment with heparin as soon as the diagnosis is confirmed, even in the presence of hemorrhagic infarcts.[1]

The optimal duration of oral anticoagulant treatment after the acute phase of CVT is unknown.[1] Recurrent sinus thrombosis occurs in 2% of patients; about 4% of patients have an extracranial thrombotic event within one year.[1,5] Usually, Vitamin K antagonists (Coumadin®) are given for six months after a first episode of sinus thrombosis (longer in the presence of predisposing factors), with a target International Normalized Ratio (INR) of 2.5.

Endovascular thrombolysis can be attempted with the administration of a thrombolytic enzyme (usually urokinase) into the sinus, sometimes in combination with mechanical thrombo-aspiration. Published reports are limited to case reports and uncontrolled studies, so it is impossible to conclude that the results associated with endovascular thrombolysis are superior to those with systemic heparin.[1,4] Until better evidence is available, endovascular thrombolysis may be performed at centers with experience in interventional neuroradiology, although this treatment should be restricted to patients with a poor prognosis.[1]

KEY TEACHING POINTS

1. Thrombosis of the cerebral veins and sinuses is a rare, distinct cerebrovascular disorder that most often affects young adults and children.

2. The most common symptoms and signs of cerebral vein thrombosis (CVT) are headache, seizures, focal neurological deficits, altered consciousness and papilledema.

3. The most sensitive imaging study for diagnosing CVT is MRI in combination with MRV.

4. Close interactions with neurology and neuroradiology (if available) are essential if CVT is considered or identified.

5. Anticoagulation with body weight-adjusted subcutaneous low-molecular-weight heparin or dose-adjusted intravenous heparin is widely considered as first-line therapy.

REFERENCES

[1] Stam J. Current concepts: thrombosis of the cerebral veins and sinuses. *N Engl J Med* 2005;352:1791–8.

[2] Petitti DB. Combination estrogen-progestin oral contraceptives. *N Engl J Med* 2003;349:1443–50.

[3] Rothrock JF. Headaches due to vascular disorders. *Neurol Clin N Am* 2004;22:21–37.

[4] Bousser MG, Ferro JM. Cerebral venous thrombosis: an update. Lancet Neurol 2007;6:162–70.

[5] Gosk-Bierska I, Wysokinski W, Brown RD, et al. Cerebral venous sinus thrombosis: incidence of venous thrombosis recurrence and survival. *Neurol* 67 2006;67:814–9.

51

Headache and seizures in a 45-year-old female

HISTORY OF PRESENT ILLNESS

A 45-year-old female with a medical history significant for a seizure disorder and migraines presented to the ED following four tonic-clonic seizures over a 30-minute period, each lasting 1–2 minutes. Between each seizure, the patient remained confused and somnolent. The seizures began while the patient was in bed; during one of the seizures, she fell onto the floor. The patient's husband called emergency services after the patient failed to recover fully following her fourth seizure. According to the husband, the patient was complaining of a migraine headache earlier in the day, for which she took sumatriptan (Imitrix®) without significant relief. Because of the headache, she did not take her antiepileptic medications that day, which included levetiracetam (Keppra®) and lamotrigine (Lamictal®). The patient smoked cigarettes but did not drink alcohol or use recreational drugs. Her recent seizure history was remarkable for one to two petite seizures per week for several years; her last tonic-clonic seizure was one month ago.

PHYSICAL EXAMINATION

GENERAL APPEARANCE: The patient appeared somnolent, minimally arousable, was able to move all extremities and withdraw from pain, but was unable to follow commands.

VITAL SIGNS

Temperature	96.7°F (35.9°C)
Pulse	110 beats/minute
Blood pressure	170/72 mmHg
Respirations	28 breaths/minute
Oxygen saturation	98% on room air

HEENT: Atraumatic, normocephalic, PERRL; roving, conjugate eye movements; oropharynx pink and moist without evidence of trauma to the tongue.

NECK: Supple, no meningeal signs.

CARDIOVASCULAR: Tachycardic rate, regular rhythm, no rubs, murmurs or gallops.

LUNGS: Clear to auscultation bilaterally.

ABDOMEN: Soft, nontender, nondistended.

EXTREMITIES: No clubbing, cyanosis or edema.

NEUROLOGIC: The patient could open her eyes to command after a delayed phase, withdrew to pain and was mumbling inappropriate words. Glasgow Coma Scale (GCS) score: eyes = 3, motor = 4, verbal = 3 for GCS = 10.

The patient was placed on a cardiac monitor with seizure precautions, an intravenous line was placed, and blood was drawn and sent for laboratory testing. Laboratory tests were significant for a leukocyte count of 34 K/μL (normal 3.5–12.5 K/μL), hematocrit of 50% (normal 34–46%), creatinine of 1.5 mg/dL (normal less than 1.1 mg/dL), glucose of 261 mg/dL (normal 60–159 mg/dL) and CO_2 of less than 5 mEq/L (normal 22–30 mEq/L). A serum pregnancy test was negative. The patient's alcohol level was less than 10 mg/dL. The patient received lorazepam (Ativan®) 2 mg IV followed by phenytoin (Dilantin®) 1 gm IV (loading dose over 1 hour). A non-contrast CT scan of the brain was obtained (Figure 51.1).

What is your diagnosis?

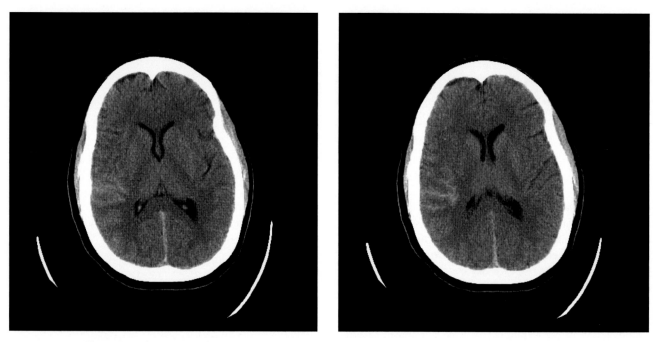

Figure 51.1 Noncontrast CT of the brain from a 45-year-old female presenting to the ED with headache and seizures.

ANSWER

The patient's diagnosis is status epilepticus (four tonic-clonic seizures over 30 minutes between which the patient did not recover) and subarachnoid hemorrhage (SAH), most likely post-traumatic. The noncontrast head CT demonstrated evidence of an acute SAH, with hemorrhage present within the right sulci, from the right occipital and temporal lobes to the upper parietal and frontal parietal junction (arrow, Figure 51.2). The ventricles and sulci were noted to be otherwise normal in size and position, with no focal mass effect or midline shift present.

The patient's neurologic status continued to improve in the ED, and she urgently received neurosurgical evaluation. A CT angiogram of the brain showed no vascular anomaly and no evidence of aneurysm. Given the patient's recent history, the CT angiogram results and the location of the subarachnoid hemorrhage, it was concluded that the hemorrhage was post-traumatic. The patient was continued on Dilantin® as well as her other antiepileptic medications; she was discharged on hospital day #5.

Status epilepticus and traumatic subarachnoid hemorrhage

Status epilepticus (SE) represents a distinct seizure phenomenon. Not simply a prolonged seizure, SE represents a reconfiguration of the excitatory and inhibitory network of the normal brain.[1] The question of exactly when a prolonged seizure or set of recurrent seizures should be considered SE continues to evolve. Based on the typical seizure duration of 1–2 minutes, SE may be considered as any seizure event

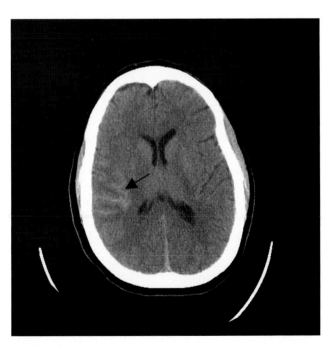

Figure 51.2 Noncontrast CT of the brain from a 45-year-old female with headache and seizures, demonstrating acute SAH within the right sulci (arrow).

greater than 5–10 minutes in length, or two or more discrete seizures between which there is incomplete recovery of consciousness.[1,2] The frequency of cases of SE in the United States is approximately 100,000–150,000 per year, with the mortality from SE estimated at approximately 20–25%.[1,2]

SE can be divided into two general types: convulsive and nonconvulsive.[3] Although the diagnosis of convulsive SE is usually obvious, the duration of seizures is often underestimated because the intensity of the jerking tends to diminish with time. The hallmark of nonconvulsive SE is altered mental status.[3] Patients demonstrate slow mentation, confusion, unresponsiveness, gross abnormal motor movements, twitches, lip smacking, mimicry or automatisms. Patients who have a first episode of SE are at substantial risk for future episodes of SE and the development of chronic epilepsy.[2]

Acute processes that cause SE include metabolic disturbances (e.g., electrolyte abnormalities, renal failure and sepsis), central nervous system infections, stroke, head trauma, drug toxicity and hypoxia.[2] Seizures caused by these acute processes are often difficult to control and are associated with a higher mortality, especially those due to hypoxia and those in older patients.[2] Chronic processes that result in SE include pre-existing epilepsy in which SE is due to breakthrough seizures or the discontinuation of antiepileptic drugs, seizures in the context of chronic ethanol abuse, and processes such as central nervous system tumors or strokes that lead to SE after a latent period.[2] In general, SE due to these processes responds well to anticonvulsant treatment, and patients often recover from the acute episode of seizures.

Initial management of a patient with SE includes prompt evaluation of the airway, breathing and circulation (ABCs), with proper assessment and control of the airway and of ventilation.[2,3] An arterial blood gas may reveal a profound metabolic acidosis (pH < 7.0) that corrects itself once seizure activity is controlled.[2] Patients should receive 100% oxygen by nonrebreather mask, and airway patency should be maintained by an oral or nasopharyngeal device while the patient remains unresponsive. Orotracheal intubation should be performed if there is clinical evidence of respiratory compromise. If neuromuscular blockade is needed to facilitate intubation, a short-acting paralytic agent (e.g., vecuronium 0.1 mg/kg) will help the physician promptly regain the ability to determine whether seizures are clinically present.[2] In cases were the diagnosis of SE is not clear, an EEG should be obtained to confirm the diagnosis, particularly when nonconvulsive SE is suspected.[3,4]

The main principle of treatment of SE is to stop the seizure as rapidly as possible and prevent recurrence.[3] Benzodiazepines (diazepam, lorazepam, midazolam) are potent, fast-acting anti-seizure drugs, and are therefore preferred as initial therapy (particularly lorazepam and diazepam). Despite the equivalence of lorazepam and diazepam as initial therapies, lorazepam has a longer duration of anti-seizure effect (12–24 hours) than diazepam (15–30 minutes), and is preferable to diazepam for the treatment of SE.[2,3] The initial dose of lorazepam in treating SE is 0.05–0.1 mg/kg IV (max 8 mg) at a rate of 2 mg/min, with onset of action in 2–3 minutes.[3] Adverse effects of intravenous benzodiazepines include respiratory depression, hypotension and impaired consciousness.

Phenytoin is useful for maintaining a prolonged anti-seizure effect after rapid termination of seizures with a benzodiazepine, as an initial therapy for terminating SE, or when benzodiazepines fail.[2] The recommended starting dose is 20 mg/kg administered intravenously at a maximal rate of 50 mg/minute. As much as 30 mg/kg may be required to stop seizures in some patients. Adverse effects of phenytoin include hypotension and cardiac dysrhythmias (bradycardia and ectopic beats). Fosphenytoin, a water-soluble prodrug of phenytoin, is converted to phenytoin by nonspecific phosphatases. Fosphenytoin offers certain pharmacokinetic advantages over phenytoin, such as: it can be infused using standard intravenous solutions, whereas phenytoin precipitates in dextrose-containing fluids; fosphenytoin can be given intramuscularly; and the rate of infusion for fosphenytoin is three times as fast as phenytoin.[5] However, fosphenytoin and phenytoin are likely to have similar time to effect in controlling SE. No clinically significant differences between the hypotensive or adverse cardiac effects of phenytoin or fosphenytoin loading have been reported, although infusion-site reactions (phlebitis and soft-tissue damage) are less common with fosphenytoin.[2]

Phenobarbital may be as effective as the combination of benzodiazepines and phenytoin for the treatment of SE.[2] However, the depressant effects of phenobarbital on respiratory drive, level of consciousness and blood pressure may complicate management, especially when phenobarbital is administered after a benzodiazepine. For these reasons, phenobarbital (20 mg/kg at a rate of 50–75 mg/minute) is recommended only when benzodiazepines and phenytoin fail.[2] Respiratory and blood pressure support must be immediately available.

SE that does not respond to a benzodiazepine, phenytoin or phenobarbital is considered refractory and requires more aggressive treatment. Continuous intravenous infusions with anesthetic doses of midazolam, propofol or barbiturates are the most useful treatments.[2] In general, the patient is placed on a continuous intravenous infusion of medication while undergoing EEG monitoring.[3] The dosage is titrated until suppression of EEG spikes or burst suppression pattern is obtained.[3] A team approach to patient care, including a neurologist or an intensivist and an anesthesiologist, is often critical because of the need for higher neurologic and cardiovascular monitoring and ventilatory support.

Traumatic SAH frequently occurs following head injury. On early CT scan, this is identified as a loss of the normal hypodensity that appears in the sulci or cisterns.[6] The sensitivity of the CT depends on the volume and hematocrit of the blood diluted in the cerebrospinal fluid, as well as the timing of the CT. Traumatic SAH generally disappears a few days following injury. CT scanning also allows classification of traumatic SAH on the basis of the amount and distribution of blood, just as it does for aneurysmal SAH. A higher incidence

of unfavorable outcomes (severe disability, persistent vegetative state and death) is associated with traumatic SAH than in patients with traumatic brain injury without subarachnoid bleeding.[6]

Emergency management of patients with SAH involves the immediate stabilization of acute life-threatening conditions and the initiation of appropriate supportive therapy. Vital signs, cardiac rhythm and oxygen saturation should be monitored, and an intravenous line should be established. The head of the bed should be elevated 30° from the horizontal to facilitate venous drainage and help reduce intracranial pressure (ICP). Patients with respiratory compromise secondary to hypoventilation, obtundation, hypoxia, hypercarbia, loss of airway protective reflexes or pulmonary edema require endotracheal intubation and assisted ventilation. Urgent consultation with a neurosurgeon should be obtained. Controlled hyperventilation with target PCO_2 levels of 25–30 mmHg is generally effective for acutely reducing elevated ICP.[7]

Administration of antihypertensive and anticonvulsant agents should be performed in consultation with a neurosurgeon. For most patients with a significant and sustained blood pressure elevation (diastolic greater than 120–130 mmHg), a titratable, short-acting agent (such as intravenous nitroprusside) should be employed. The drug should be titrated to reduce the diastolic pressure below 100–110 mmHg over 20–30 minutes. Agents such as nifedipine or hydralazine should be avoided because they cannot be titrated and may cause excessive hypotension.

Preventing seizures and concomitant increases in ICP can reduce the risk of rebleeding. Phenytoin is typically used as a prophylactic anticonvulsant. Seizures should be aggressively managed if they occur. Diazepam or lorazepam are first-line agents to treat seizures and should be followed by phenytoin loading. Phenobarbital loading is an effective alternative but its sedating effects may interfere with subsequent neurologic assessment.

Antiemetics such as ondansetron, prochlorperazine or promethazine may be necessary to control nausea and vomiting. Alert patients with significant headache or neck pain may require narcotic analgesics for pain control. Treatment with calcium-channel blockers such as nimodipine (orally or via nasogastric tube) or nicardipine (intravenously) appears to be effective in reducing the risk and severity of cerebral vasospasm; patients with relatively good neurologic status after SAH derive the most benefit.[7,8] All patients with SAH require admission to the hospital for neurologic status monitoring and evaluation for neurosurgical intervention. A neurosurgeon should be consulted immediately once the diagnosis of SAH is established; admission to a neurosurgical unit or critical care setting should be considered.

KEY TEACHING POINTS

1. Status epilepticus (SE) is defined as either a continuous seizure lasting at least five minutes or two or more discrete seizures between which there is incomplete recovery of consciousness.

2. Benzodiazepines (lorazepam, diazepam, midazolam) are first-line agents for the treatment of SE, followed by phenytoin, with phenobarbital in cases where benzodiazepines and phenytoin fail to control the seizures.

3. SE that does not respond to benzodiazepines, phenytoin, or phenobarbital is considered refractory and requires more aggressive treatment (i.e., continuous intravenous infusion with midazolam, propofol or barbiturates to induce coma).

4. A higher incidence of unfavorable outcomes is associated with traumatic SAH than in patients with traumatic brain injury without subarachnoid bleeding.

5. Emergency treatment of traumatic SAH includes airway assessment and intubation in patients with respiratory compromise, those unable to protect their airway, or those requiring modest hyperventilation to reduce ICP, as well as seizure prophylaxis with phenytoin and admission to the neurosurgical or critical care service.

REFERENCES

[1] Mirski MA, Varelas PN. Seizures and status epilepticus in the critically ill. *Crit Care Clin* 2008;24:115–47.

[2] Lowenstein DH, Allredge BK. Status epilepticus. *N Engl J Med* 1998;338:970–6.

[3] Garmel GM, Jacobs AK, Eilers MA. Tonic status epilepticus: an unusual presentation of unresponsiveness. *Ann Emerg Med* 1991;21:223–7.

[4] Rubin DH, Kornblau DH, Conway EE, et al. Neurologic disorders. In: Marx JA, Hockberger RS, Walls RM, et al. (eds.). *Rosen's Emergency Medicine: Concepts and Clinical Practice*, 6th ed. Philadelphia: Mosby, 2006:1621–2.

[5] Nandhagopal R. Generalised convulsive status epilepticus: an overview. *Postgrad Med J* 2006;82:723–32.

[6] Mattioli C, Beretta L, Gerevini, S, et al. Traumatic subarachnoid hemorrhage on the computerized tomography scan obtained at admission: a multicenter assessment of the accuracy of diagnosis and the potential impact on patient outcome. *J Neurosurg* 2003;98:37–42.

[7] Fontanarosa P, Callaway C. Subarachnoid hemorrhage. In: Harwood-Nuss A (ed.). *The Clinical Practice of Emergency Medicine*, 3rd ed. Philadelphia: Lippincott Williams & Wilkins, 2001:978–83.

[8] Harders A, Kakarieka A, Braakman R, et al. Traumatic subarachnoid hemorrhage and its treatment with nimodipine. *J Neurosurg* 1996;85:82–9.

52

Acute onset of altered consciousness in a 66-year-old male

HISTORY OF PRESENT ILLNESS

A 66-year-old male with a medical history significant for prostate cancer (including prior radiation treatment) and recent diagnosis of ocular migraines was brought to the ED by paramedics for several days of severe dizziness, vomiting, occipital headaches and the acute onset of altered consciousness. According to his sister, the patient had been experiencing intermittent occipital headaches, lightheadedness, a sensation of the room spinning with standing, and nausea with vomiting over the past several days. On the day of presentation, his symptoms worsened to the point where he could neither stand nor walk. His sister called emergency services. The patient did not drink alcohol, smoke cigarettes or use illicit drugs. His current medications included terazosin and famotidine, and he had no known drug allergies.

PHYSICAL EXAMINATION

GENERAL APPEARANCE: On initial examination, the patient was a well-developed male with spontaneous respirations, obtunded and aroused only briefly to sternal rub.

VITAL SIGNS

Temperature	98.5°F (36.9°C) rectal
Pulse	84 beats/minute
Blood pressure	123/59 mmHg
Respirations	22 breaths/minute
Oxygen saturation	99% on room air

HEENT: Atraumatic, normocephalic, pupils were small, equal and minimally reactive bilaterally. Rotatory and vertical nystagmus was present on initial examination of extraocular movements (patient was able to follow commands briefly upon arousal). The oropharynx was pink and dry.

NECK: Supple, no jugular venous distension nor meningeal signs.

CARDIOVASCULAR: Regular rate and rhythm without rubs, murmurs or gallops.

LUNGS: Clear to auscultation bilaterally.

ABDOMEN: Soft, nontender, nondistended.

RECTAL: Normal tone, brown stool, hemoccult negative.

EXTREMITIES: No clubbing, cyanosis or edema; no evidence of injection needle marks.

NEUROLOGIC: The patient would arouse briefly to sternal rub, would answer questions with one or two words, and abruptly

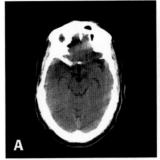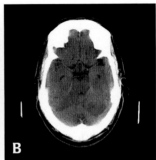

Figure 52.1 Noncontrast CT of the brain shortly after presentation (panel A) and six hours following presentation to the ED (panel B) of a 66-year-old male with acute onset of altered mental status.

become unconscious. The patient would withdraw and localize to pain, moved all extremities when aroused, but was unable to follow simple commands (e.g., could not perform pronator drift nor finger-nose-finger tests).

A peripheral intravenous line was placed, blood was drawn and sent for laboratory testing, as well as a urinalysis and urine toxicologic screen. A CT scan of the brain and chest radiograph were ordered. A bedside blood glucose test returned normal at 100 mg/dL. Twenty minutes following the initial examination, a repeat neurologic examination was performed. This time the patient remained obtunded and could not be aroused even with vigorous sternal rub; he did not withdraw to painful stimuli and a weak gag reflex was present. Both upper and lower extremities were hyperreflexic, and a Babinski reflex was present bilaterally. His vital signs remained stable (pulse 85 beats/minute, blood pressure 120/60, respirations 22 breaths/minute with oxygen saturation 99% on 2 liters nasal cannula). Narcan 0.4 mg intravenous was administered without response. The patient was subsequently intubated with etomidate and succinylcholine IV for rapid sequence induction. A noncontrast CT scan of the brain was obtained (panel A, Figure 52.1). One hour following intubation, the patient continued to be unresponsive, and pupillary examination revealed bilateral midrange, unreactive pupils. The patient was admitted to the ICU and a repeat CT of the brain was performed six hours following the initial CT (panel B, Figure 52.1).

What is your diagnosis?

ANSWER

The diagnosis is acute ischemic stroke secondary to basilar artery occlusion, involving the brainstem, midbrain and pons. The initial noncontrast CT of the brain did not demonstrate an acute intracranial process (panel A, Figure 52.1), whereas the repeat CT six hours later revealed subtle sulcal effacement in the medial aspect of the parieto-occipital regions and low-attenuation areas in the posterior fossa (panel B, Figure 52.1). These findings suggested an acute CVA in the posterior circulation. The patient remained unresponsive while intubated, and a repeat neurologic examination the following day demonstrated decerebrate posturing, hyperreflexia, bilateral Babinski reflexes, unreactive pupils and the absence of doll's eyes. Corneal reflexes remained intact. An MRI of the brain performed on hospital day #2 demonstrated an acute CVA in the bilateral cerebellum, brainstem, left thalamus/ subthalamus and posteromedial aspect of right temporal lobe,

as well as posteromedial aspect of bilateral occipital lobes with probable petechial hemorrhagic components (Figure 52.2). An MRA of the circle of Willis revealed basilar arterial thrombosis at the tip of the basilar artery extending to the proximal portions of right posterior cerebral artery, left superior cerebellar artery, and right superior cerebellar artery (Figure 52.3). With family consent, no further testing was performed, ventilatory support was withdrawn and the patient expired on hospital day #4.

Vertebrobasilar stroke and "top of the basilar" syndrome

Eighty percent of strokes are ischemic, with 20% of ischemic events involving tissue supplied by the posterior (vertebrobasilar) circulation.[1] The most common causes of vertebrobasilar ischemia are embolism, large artery atherosclerosis, penetrating small artery disease and arterial dissection.[1] Dizziness, vertigo, headache, vomiting, diplopia, loss of vision,

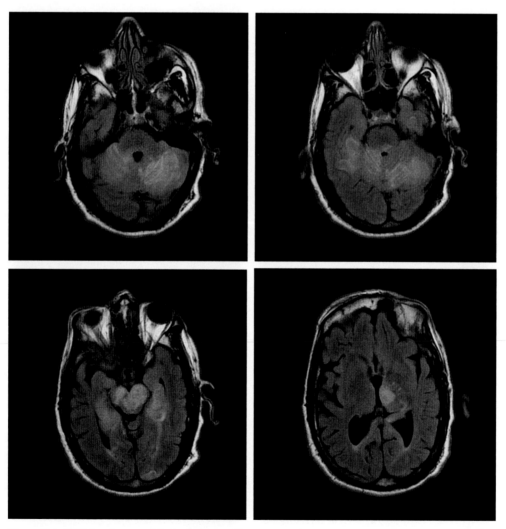

Figure 52.2 MRI flare images of the brain from a 66-year-old male with acute altered consciousness, demonstrating acute ischemic CVA (hyperintense areas) in the bilateral cerebellum, brainstem, left thalamus/ subthalamus and posteromedial aspect of right temporal lobe.

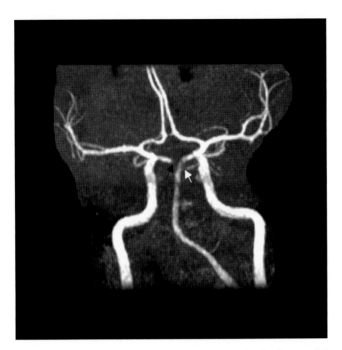

Figure 52.3 MRA of the circle of Willis demonstrating basilar arterial thrombosis at the tip extending to the proximal portions of the right posterior cerebellar artery (dark arrow) and the left superior cerebellar artery (white arrow) from a 66-year-old male with acute ischemic brainstem stroke.

ataxia, numbness and weakness involving structures on both sides of the body are frequent symptoms in patients with vertebrobasilar artery occlusive disease.

The basilar artery (BA) is the largest artery in the posterior circulation and forms the central core of this vascular territory.[2] Occlusion of the BA with progressive brainstem symptoms has a poor prognosis. The pathogenesis in younger patients is usually embolism from cardiac source or, less frequently, from vertebral artery dissection.[3] Local atherothrombosis is more commonly the cause in elderly patients.[3]

The presenting symptoms of this patient reflect the level of BA occlusion and the corresponding ischemic brainstem territory. The typical syndrome of bilateral intracranial vertebral or caudal (proximal) BA occlusion are vertigo, nausea, dysphagia and dysarthria.[3] Clinical findings with a lateral medullary infarction correspond to a Wallenberg syndrome with caudal cranial nerve findings, nystagmus, hemiataxia, a dissociated hemisensory loss (hypalgesia) and an ipsilateral Horner's syndrome. A midbasilar occlusion with a pontine infarct often causes a decreased level of consciousness, a severe hemi- or tetraparesis (occasionally with posturing of the arms), an ipsilateral VIIth nerve palsy, oculomotor signs (pinpoint pupils, internuclear ophthalmoplegia, ipsilateral gaze palsy, or one-and-a-half syndrome) and hemiataxia with superior cerebellar artery (SCA) territory involvement.[3]

"Top of the basilar" syndrome is due to infarction of the midbrain, thalamus, and portions of the temporal and occipital lobes resulting from occlusive vascular disease of the rostral (distal) BA.[4] This is often embolic in nature. Patients with

this syndrome frequently present in a coma, with midbrain ocular motor signs (skew deviation, an internal and external oculomotor palsy, and a vertical gaze palsy), severe hemiparesis and less frequently tetraparesis, or hemiataxia (with SCA territory involvement).[3] Pupillary abnormalities are also frequently present, including small and reactive pupils, large or mid-position and fixed pupils, corectopia and, occasionally, oval pupils.[4]

Based on a retrospective study, four clinical features are identifiable on patient presentation: dysarthria, pupillary disorders, bulbar symptoms and disorders of consciousness. These are significantly associated with a poor outcome in patients with stroke from basilar artery occlusion.[5] The presence of consciousness disorders alone – the most powerful factor – or the combination of the three remaining factors was associated with a poor outcome in 100% of nonautopsied cases and 87% of autopsied cases in this study. A similar study also identified decreased level of consciousness, tetraparesis and abnormal pupils as clinical predictors of poor outcome in patients with BA occlusive disease.[2]

Emergency treatment of patients with vertebrobasilar stroke syndromes involves patient stabilization with immediate attention to the ABCs (airway, breathing and circulation). A rapid blood glucose should be obtained at the bedside to rule out hypoglycemia as a treatable cause of these symptoms. Comatose patients should be intubated for airway protection. Noncontrast CT scan of the brain is the initial imaging test of choice to both rule out intracranial hemorrhage and detect early signs of ischemia. Other important imaging modalities for patients with acute stroke include CT angiography, MRI and MRA.

Intravenous administration of tissue plasminogen activator (t-PA) enhances neurologic recovery from ischemic stroke when administered within three hours of the onset of symptoms, once hemorrhage and other contraindications have been excluded.[1] Several small studies of the use of IV thrombolytic agents for vertebrobasilar disease have shown mixed results.[1] Because BA occlusions carry an increased risk of death and disability, and due to extensive experience with intra-arterial thrombolysis, several authors recommend cerebral angiography and intra-arterial thrombolysis for BA occlusion, even if it is 12–24 hours after the onset of the stroke.[1,3,6] Considering all published series, a consistent survival benefit has been predicted by revascularization of the BA (mortality 87% nonrecanalized compared with 39% recanalized; $p < 0.001$).[6] Although no large randomized studies of revascularization for acute BA occlusion have been performed, it is unlikely that endovascular efforts are inferior to the natural history of the disease; it has therefore been postulated that patients would benefit from this approach.[6]

KEY TEACHING POINTS

1. Twenty percent of ischemic strokes involve tissue supplied by the posterior (vertebrobasilar) circulation; symptoms

include dizziness, vertigo, headache, vomiting, diplopia, loss of vision, ataxia, numbness and weakness involving structures on both sides of the body.

2. "Top of the basilar" syndrome is caused by occlusion of the distal basilar artery resulting in infarction of the midbrain, thalamus, and portions of the temporal and occipital lobes.

3. Patients with "top of the basilar" syndrome frequently present with coma, midbrain oculomotor signs, severe hemiparesis (or less frequently tetraparesis) and pupillary abnormalities. The presence of coma portends a poor prognosis.

4. Initial management of patients with acute vertebrobasilar strokes includes immediate attention to the ABCs, rapid serum glucose testing and a noncontrast CT of the brain to rule out hemorrhage and evaluate for early signs of ischemia.

5. Although intravenous thrombolysis may be of some benefit in patients with vertebral artery occlusions, intra-arterial thrombolysis is recommended for basilar artery occlusion and can be performed 12–24 hours after the onset of stroke.

REFERENCES

[1] Savitz SI, Caplan LR. Current concepts: vertebrobasilar disease. *N Engl J Med* 2005;352:2618–26.

[2] Voetsch B, DeWitt D, Pessin MS, et al. Basilar artery occlusive disease in the New England Medical Center Posterior Circulation Registry. *Arch Neurol* 2004;61:496–504.

[3] Brandt T. Diagnosis and thrombolytic therapy of acute basilar artery occlusion: a review. *Clin Exp Hypertens* 2002; 24:611–22.

[4] Love BS, Billar J. Neurovascular system. In: Goetz CG (ed.). *Textbook of Clinical Neurology*, 3rd ed. Philadelphia: Saunders, 2007:424–5.

[5] Devuyst G, Bogousslavsky J, Meuli R, et al. Stroke or transient ischemic attacks with basilar artery stenosis or occlusion: clinical patterns and outcomes. *Arch Neurol* 2002;59: 567–73.

[6] Smith WS. Intra-arterial thrombolytic therapy for acute basilar occlusion: pro. *Stroke* 2007;38:701–3.

PART VII

TRAUMA

53

Left upper quadrant abdominal pain following a bicycle collision in a 13-year-old male

HISTORY OF PRESENT ILLNESS

A 13-year-old male presented to the ED complaining of abdominal pain localized to the epigastrium and left upper quadrant after running into a truck while riding his bicycle several hours prior to arrival. He reported that the handlebars were jammed into his abdomen upon collision. He described the pain as severe, worse with movement and upon deep inspiration, with radiation to the left shoulder. He denied nausea or vomiting, chest pain or shortness of breath. He was helmeted and denied head trauma, loss of consciousness or associated injuries.

PHYSICAL EXAMINATION

GENERAL APPEARANCE: The patient was lying supine on the gurney, holding his abdomen in moderate discomfort.

VITAL SIGNS

Temperature	98°F (36.6°C)
Pulse	115 beats/minute
Blood pressure	122/75 mmHg
Respirations	22 breaths/minute
Oxygen saturation	98% on room air

HEENT: Atraumatic, normocephalic, PERRL, EOMI.

NECK: Supple, no midline tenderness.

CARDIOVASCULAR: Tachycardic rate, regular rhythm without rubs, murmurs or gallops.

LUNGS: Clear to auscultation bilaterally.

ABDOMEN: Diffuse tenderness to palpation, most prominent in the left upper quadrant, with associated rebound and guarding. No ecchymosis was noted; bowel sounds were hyperactive.

EXTREMITIES: No clubbing, cyanosis or edema; no obvious deformities or swelling.

SKIN: Warm, moist, no abrasions or ecchymosis.

NEUROLOGIC: Nonfocal.

Two peripheral intravenous lines were placed, blood was drawn and sent for laboratory testing, and morphine sulfate was administered IV for pain control. Laboratory results were significant for a leukocytosis of 19 K/μL (normal 3.5–12.5 K/μL); the hematocrit was 40% (normal 39–51%). The platelet count, coagulation panel, electrolytes, liver function tests and amylase were within normal limits. A bedside ultrasound of the abdomen demonstrated free fluid in Morrison's pouch; at this time, the surgical service was urgently consulted and the decision was made to obtain a CT scan of the abdomen and pelvis with intravenous contrast (Figure 53.1). A repeat complete blood count performed four hours after the initial test revealed a hematocrit of 35%.

What is your diagnosis?

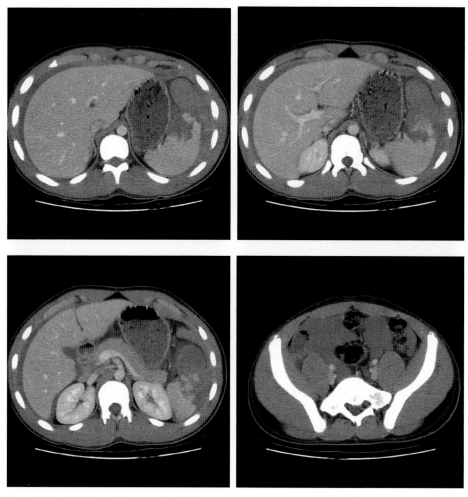

Figure 53.1 CT of the abdomen and pelvis from a 13-year-old male with left upper quadrant abdominal pain after a bicycle collision.

The diagnosis is grade 4 splenic laceration. The CT scan of the abdomen and pelvis demonstrated an extensive splenic laceration extending into the splenic hilum (arrow, Figure 53.2), associated with a large amount of intraperitoneal hemorrhage in both the abdomen and pelvis. The patient was admitted to the surgical service and serial hematocrits were followed, with the hematocrit dropping to 28% on hospital day #2 before stabilizing. The patient was managed conservatively without operative intervention and was discharged on hospital day #5. He was given strict precautions to avoid sports or any strenuous physical activity.

Pediatric intra-abdominal injury and splenic trauma

Trauma remains the leading cause of death and disability in children, with blunt trauma accounting for more than 90% of all pediatric injuries.[1] Although falls are the most common single mechanism of injury in children, injuries involving bicycles, all-terrain vehicles, motorcycles and sports occur frequently. Abdominal injuries occur in isolation or as a part of multi-system trauma. Bicycle handlebar and lap belt injuries are particularly common mechanisms that should raise the level of suspicion for a significant intra-abdominal injury (IAI), with high likelihood of requiring operative intervention.[1,2]

The spleen is the most commonly injured intra-abdominal organ in children following blunt trauma.[1,3] Traumatic splenic injury may result in hematoma, laceration, fragmentation or complete devascularization. The trauma resulting in these injuries may be relatively minor and may not be recalled by

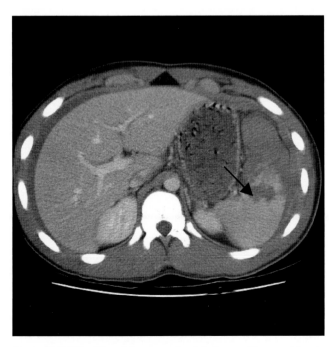

Figure 53.2 CT of the abdomen and pelvis from a 13-year-old male with left upper quadrant abdominal pain after a bicycle collision demonstrating splenic laceration (arrow).

the patient. Falling over a chair, hitting the edge of a table or colliding into a strong ocean wave are mechanisms of injury that have resulted in splenic rupture.[3]

The classic physical findings of splenic rupture are left upper quadrant pain and tenderness and left shoulder pain. Kehr's sign (left shoulder pain from irritation of the inferior border of the left diaphragm by hematoma) may be elicited by placing patients in the Trendelenburg position.[3] Associated comorbid findings or injuries can help predict which children have IAI, particularly the presence of a femur fracture or a low systolic blood pressure, which itself carries an odds ratio for IAI of 4.8.[4,5] Although any abdominal examination abnormality should be considered an indicator of IAI, a negative examination and absence of comorbid injuries do not rule out an IAI.[4]

After the history and physical examination, the next step in evaluating pediatric patients with potential IAI is considering which laboratory tests are necessary. In hypotension unresponsive to isotonic fluid boluses, the type and crossmatch for blood is the most important test to order.[4] In the stable child, laboratory tests can be used to help predict which children may have IAI. The most useful laboratory tests for this purpose include the complete blood count (CBC), liver function tests (LFT) and urinalysis (UA).[4,5] The greatest use for the hemoglobin and hematocrit is to follow serial values in known solid organ injuries. An initial hemoglobin and hematocrit are recommended in the evaluation of patients with pediatric abdominal trauma, but should not be used to decide whether to perform an additional imaging study.[4]

Focused Assessment with Sonography for Trauma (FAST) is used to detect free intraperitoneal fluid (i.e., blood) and has identified abdominal injuries in adults with a sensitivity ranging from 63–99% in published series. Several reports have shown that FAST can reliably detect intraperitoneal fluid in children with a sensitivity of 56–93% and a specificity of 79–97%.[1] However, a positive FAST in a hemodynamically stable child is of limited use because stable children with solid organ injury will likely be managed nonoperatively and will require an abdominal CT scan for diagnosis of and staging the injury. FAST may be most useful in children in two circumstances. First, in the hemodynamically unstable child with multiple injuries and several potential causes of hypotension, FAST may indicate whether intra-abdominal bleeding is the source of hypotension, therefore guiding immediate operative management. Second, FAST may serve as a screening tool, along with physical examination and laboratory evaluation, to help identify children who will benefit from abdominal CT scanning.[1]

In the hemodynamically stable patient, CT scan remains the study of choice for identification of IAI.[6] CT has become the gold standard for the diagnosis of splenic injuries after trauma.[7] As an initial diagnostic test, CT is particularly useful in diagnosing solid organ injuries, particularly to the liver, spleen and kidneys. CT allows accurate grading of these solid organ injuries, which helps guide nonoperative therapy. However, CT is less reliable for the diagnosis of intestinal and pancreatic injuries in the early post-injury period.[1] Intravenous contrast is essential in diagnosing solid organ injuries, whereas the use of oral contrast is controversial. Oral contrast may aid in the diagnosis of intestinal and pancreatic injuries through detection of extraluminal contrast and enhanced identification of the pancreas; some studies suggest that the omission of oral contrast does not delay the diagnosis of intestinal injury.[1]

Criteria for staging splenic trauma based on the American Association for the Surgery of Trauma (AAST) splenic injury scale include the following:[4]

- Grade 1: Subcapsular hematoma of less than 10% of surface area or capsular tear of less than 1 cm in depth
- Grade 2: Subcapsular hematoma of 10–50% of surface area, intraparenchymal hematoma of less than 5 cm in diameter, or laceration of 1–3 cm in depth and not involving trabecular vessels
- Grade 3: Subcapsular hematoma of more than 50% of surface area or expanding and ruptured subcapsular or parenchymal hematoma, intraparenchymal hematoma of more than 5 cm or expanding, or laceration of more than 3 cm in depth or involving trabecular vessels
- Grade 4: Laceration involving segmental or hilar vessels with devascularization of more than 25% of the spleen
- Grade 5: Shattered spleen or hilar vascular injury.

Because many of these injuries are self-limited in children, the management of splenic trauma has evolved to where stable children are managed with bed rest, frequent examinations, serial hemoglobin monitoring and close surgical supervision.[4] Splenic preservation is preferred to decrease the risk of postsplenectomy infection. The only absolute indications for performing a splenectomy in children are massive disruption and hemodynamic instability.[1,4] Patients undergoing conservative preservation management have demonstrated full recovery in 90–98% of cases.[4]

KEY TEACHING POINTS

1. The spleen is the most commonly injured intra-abdominal organ in children following blunt trauma.

2. The classic physical findings of splenic rupture are left upper quadrant abdominal pain and tenderness and left shoulder pain (Kehr's sign).

3. Laboratory tests useful in evaluating children with suspected intra-abdominal injury (IAI) include a type and crossmatch in unstable patients, a complete blood count, liver function tests and urinalysis.

4. Bedside abdominal ultrasound (FAST scan) can be useful in the hemodynamically unstable child with multiple injuries and several potential causes of hypotension to identify intra-abdominal bleeding as the source of hypotension, and to serve as a screening tool to help identify hemodynamically stable children who will benefit from abdominal CT scanning.

5. In the hemodynamically stable patient, CT scan remains the study of choice for identification of IAI and is the gold standard for the diagnosis of splenic injuries after trauma.

6. Conservative, nonoperative management of children with splenic injuries is the treatment of choice in the majority of cases, except in cases involving massive splenic disruption or hemodynamic instability.

REFERENCES

[1] Potoka DA, Saladino RA. Blunt abdominal trauma in the pediatric patient. *Clin Ped Emerg Med* 2005;6:23–31.

[2] Nadler EP, Potoka DA, Shultz BL, et al. The high morbidity associated with handlebar injuries in children. *J Trauma* 2005;58:1171–4.

[3] Sikka R. Unsuspected internal organ traumatic injuries. *Emerg Med Clin N Am* 2004;22:1067–80.

[4] Wegner S, Colletti JE, Van Wie D. Pediatric blunt abdominal trauma. *Pediatr Clin N Am* 2006;53:243–56.

[5] Holmes JF, Sokolove PE, Brant WE, et al. Identification of children with intra-abdominal injuries after blunt trauma. *Ann Emerg Med* 2002;39:500–9.

[6] Eppich WJ, Zonfrillo MR. Emergency department evaluation and management of blunt abdominal trauma in children. *Curr Opin Pediatr* 2007;19:265–9.

[7] Harbecht BG. Is anything new in adult blunt splenic trauma? *Am J Surg* 2005;190:273–8.

54

Assault with stab wounds to a 16-year-old male

HISTORY OF PRESENT ILLNESS

A 16-year-old male was brought to the ED by his mother after complaining of abdominal pain. Upon further questioning, the teenager admitted that he had been stabbed several times with a knife the prior evening, once in the abdomen and twice in the back. In the ED, he reported diffuse abdominal pain, most prominent in the left lower quadrant. He denied fevers, chills, nausea, vomiting, diarrhea or constipation. Other than the stab wounds, he denied additional injuries. His tetanus vaccination was current.

PHYSICAL EXAMINATION

GENERAL APPEARANCE: The patient was a well-developed, obese male, and in no acute discomfort.

VITAL SIGNS

Temperature	98.5°F (37°C)
Pulse	96 beats/minute
Blood pressure	100/67 mmHg
Respirations	16 breaths/minute
Oxygen saturation	98% on room air

HEENT: Atraumatic, normocephalic, PERRL, EOMI.

NECK: Supple, no midline tenderness.

CARDIOVASCULAR: Regular rate and rhythm without rubs, murmurs or gallops.

LUNGS: Clear to auscultation bilaterally.

ABDOMEN: A 2-cm vertical stab wound to left mid-abdominal wall (panel A, Figure 54.1) without bleeding, erythema or pus. The abdomen was nondistended, with diffuse tenderness to palpation, most prominent in the left mid-abdomen around the stab wound; no rebound, guarding or crepitus was noted; bowel sounds were hypoactive.

RECTAL: Normal tone; soft, brown stool, hemoccult negative.

EXTREMITIES: No clubbing, cyanosis or edema; no deformities or wounds.

LEFT FLANK: A 1.5-cm wound in the mid-left flank and a 2-cm wound in the superior left flank consistent with stab wounds were noted, without bleeding, erythema or pus (panel B, Figure 54.1); mild tenderness around the stab wounds was present without crepitus.

SKIN: No other stab wounds were appreciated on thorough skin exam with the patient completely disrobed.

NEUROLOGIC: Nonfocal.

A peripheral intravenous line was placed and blood was drawn and sent for laboratory testing. A 500-mL bolus of normal saline IV was administered, as well as morphine sulfate for pain and cefazolin 1 gm IV for infection prophylaxis. The wounds were anesthetized with lidocaine, irrigated with normal saline and packed with sterile gauze. Laboratory tests including a complete blood count, electrolytes, creatinine, glucose, liver function tests and coagulation studies were within normal limits. A chest radiograph (Figure 54.2) and CT scan of the abdomen and pelvis with oral and IV contrast (Figure 54.3) were obtained.

What is your diagnosis?

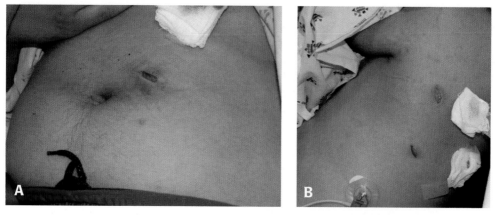

Figure 54.1 Stab wounds to the abdomen (panel A) and left flank (panel B) of a 16-year-old male.

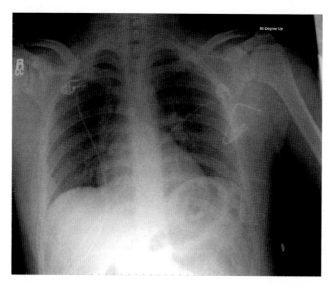

Figure 54.2 Anteroposterior chest radiograph from a 16-year-old male with multiple stab wounds (paper clips indicate location of two stab wounds on the left flank).

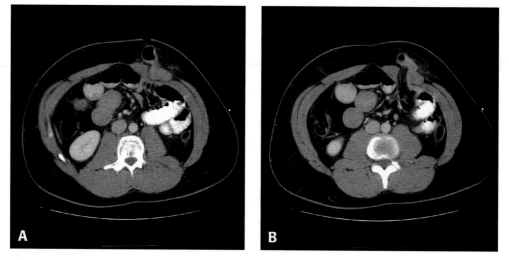

Figure 54.3 CT of the abdomen and pelvis from a 16-year-old male with multiple stab wounds.

ANSWER

The diagnosis is penetrating intra-abdominal stab wound through the left rectus abdominis muscle causing small bowel herniation into the wound with mild obstruction, as demonstrated on the CT scan (Figure 54.4). The chest radiograph did not show evidence of a pneumothorax. The surgical service was consulted, and the patient was taken to the OR for exploratory laparotomy. The herniated small bowel was reduced and the rectus abdominis muscle defect repaired. No small bowel wall injuries were identified. The stab wounds were kept open and packed with saline gauze. The patient was discharged on hospital day #3, tolerating a regular diet and with minimal pain, scheduled for close follow up in the surgery clinic.

Abdominal stab wounds

Penetrating abdominal injury implies that either a gunshot wound (GSW) or a stab wound has violated the abdominal cavity. Stab wounds are encountered three times more often then GSWs but have a lower mortality because of their lower velocity and less invasive tract.[1] However, occult injuries can be overlooked, resulting in devastating complications.[2] As a result of the greater force and extensive missile tract associated with GSWs, these account for up to 90% of the mortality associated with penetrating trauma.[1]

Stab wounds of the abdomen occur most commonly in the upper quadrants, the left more commonly than the right.[3] The liver, followed by the small bowel, is the organ most often

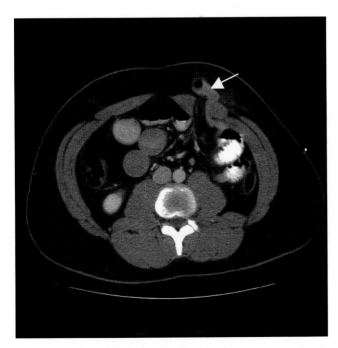

Figure 54.4 CT of the abdomen and pelvis from a 16-year-old male with a penetrating intra-abdominal stab wound demonstrating small bowel herniation into the wound (arrow) with mild obstruction.

damaged by stab wounds that penetrate the abdominal cavity. Stab wounds are multiple in 20% of cases, and involve the chest in up to 10% of cases. Anterior stab wounds penetrate the peritoneum in approximately 70% of cases but inflict injury to the viscera in only half of these.[3] Lower chest wounds are associated with coincident intraperitoneal damage approximately 15% of the time, whereas abdominal penetration from flank and back wounds have reported incidences of up to 44% and 15%, respectively.[3]

Emergency management of patients with abdominal stab wounds initially involves rapid assessment using the primary trauma survey of Advanced Trauma Life Support (ATLS): ABCDEFG (airway, breathing, circulation, disability, exposure, Foley and gastric tube). Two large-bore peripheral intravenous lines should be placed. Airway protection and ventilatory support (when required) are followed by circulatory resuscitation with fluids (normal saline or, if necessary, blood products). Following the primary survey, a careful head-to-toe secondary survey should be performed. Patients must be completely disrobed for careful inspection of all body surfaces (front, back, axilla, skin folds) for associated wounds. In addition, this may reveal unsuspected weapons. In an awake, stable patient, a brief history (events regarding the injury, medical history, medications, allergies, tetanus status, current level of pain and last meal) should be obtained. Law enforcement must be notified about all violent injuries.

Patients with evisceration of abdominal organs due to stab wounds require emergent surgical repair. In the absence of obvious evisceration, examination of the abdomen in an awake patient may identify peritoneal signs, such as pain, guarding and rebound tenderness. Abdominal distension in an unresponsive patient may be the result of active bleeding that requires emergent surgical exploration, particularly in combination with hypotension.[2] A rectal examination should be performed in all patients with penetrating abdominal injury, as blood per rectum or a high-riding prostate can indicate bowel injury and genitourinary tract injury, respectively.[2] Blood at the urethral meatus is also concerning for genitourinary tract injury; a Foley catheter should not be placed in this situation until urethral or bladder injury has been excluded.

Local wound exploration can be safely performed at the bedside in patients with abdominal stab wounds in the absence of evisceration, peritonitis or hemodynamic instability.[1] If the wound tract ends before violation of the abdominal fascia, reliable patients can be discharged home once wounds are irrigated, packed and close follow up has been arranged. If the tract is not completely visualized because of body habitus, other injuries or technical inability, further testing is necessary. Diagnostic peritoneal lavage (DPL) or diagnostic peritoneal aspiration (DPA) can be performed via a closed or open method. Aspiration of gross blood is positive for peritoneal penetration and organ injury. If gross aspiration is negative, 1 liter normal saline is infused and retrieved by gravity siphonage. The fluid is then evaluated for the presence of red blood cells (more than 10,000/mm³), white blood cells

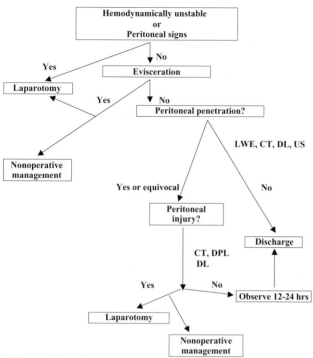

LWE – Local Wound Exploration
CT – Computed Tomography
DL – Diagnostic Laparoscopy
DPL – Diagnostic Peritoneal Lavage
US – Ultrasound

Figure 54.5 Algorithm for evaluation and management of abdominal stab wounds. From Isenhour JL, Marx J. Advances in abdominal trauma. *Emerg Med Clin N Am* 2007;25:713–33.

(more than 500/mm³), bile, fibers or particles, any of which indicate peritoneal penetration and organ injury.[2] DPL is invasive and time-consuming, and has been replaced at most institutions by focused assessment with sonography for trauma (FAST), CT scan or laparotomy.[2]

All patients with penetrating abdominal injury should undergo laboratory testing, including a complete blood count, chemistry profile, coagulation profile and urinalysis (for the presence of hematuria). Liver function tests and a serum amylase or lipase can be helpful in evaluating for hepatic or pancreatic injury, although these tests are not diagnostic. An arterial blood gas (ABG) and lactate levels provide important information regarding acid-base status and the hemodynamic stability of the patient.[2] Patients in shock should be typed and crossmatched for 4–8 units of packed red blood cells.

A chest radiograph should be obtained in all patients with abdominal stab wounds, as penetration of the chest cavity cannot be ruled out. Chest radiographs may reveal hemothoraces, pneumothoraces, or irregularities of the cardiac silhouette (which may indicate cardiac or great vessel injury).[2] Plain radiographs of the abdomen may reveal free intraperitoneal air. The FAST exam includes four views of the chest and abdomen (i.e., pericardial, right upper quadrant, left upper quadrant and pelvis). Free fluid in the abdomen is a sign of

hemorrhage secondary to liver or splenic laceration, or mesenteric injury, suggesting immediate exploratory laparotomy in unstable patients. CT is the next step in evaluating hemodynamically stable patients, as it is noninvasive, offers information about the extent of injury to visceral organs, and can help plan both operative and nonoperative management.[1,4,5] However, injuries to the bowel, diaphragm and pancreas are poorly visualized on CT (even with triple contrast), and in patients with high suspicion for injury, further diagnostic testing with laparoscopy or DPL/DPA may be warranted despite a negative abdominal CT scan.[1]

A diagnostic and therapeutic algorithm for abdominal stab wounds is summarized in Figure 54.5. In general, indications for immediate laparotomy in patients with abdominal stab wounds include hemodynamic compromise, peritoneal signs, evisceration (may be managed without laparotomy in select cases involving omental evisceration only), diaphragmatic injury, gastrointestinal hemorrhage, implements in situ (e.g., retained knife) and free intraperitoneal air. Stab wounds to the skin should not be closed due to the risk of infection, but rather irrigated and packed with sterile gauze.

KEY TEACHING POINTS

1. Abdominal stab wounds occur three times more often then GSWs but have a lower mortality.
2. Patients with stab wounds should be completely disrobed for careful inspection of all body surfaces (front, back, axilla, skin folds) for associated wounds or weapons.
3. Local wound exploration can be safely performed at the bedside in patients with abdominal stab wounds, in the absence of evisceration, peritonitis or hemodynamic instability.
4. All patients with penetrating abdominal injury should undergo a complete blood count, chemistry profile, liver function tests, coagulation profile, urinalysis (for presence of hematuria), and type and screen or crossmatch.
5. Imaging modalities useful in evaluating patients with abdominal stab wounds include plain radiographs (of the abdomen and chest), FAST and CT. DPL requires a fair amount of time to perform, and has been replaced at many institutions by DPA, ultrasound or CT.
6. Clinical indications for laparotomy in patients with abdominal stab wounds include hemodynamic compromise, peritoneal signs, evisceration, diaphragmatic injury, gastrointestinal hemorrhage, implements in situ and free intraperitoneal air.

REFERENCES

[1] Isenhour JL, Marx J. Advances in abdominal trauma. *Emerg Med Clin N Am* 2007;25:713–33.
[2] Stanton-Maxey KJ, Bjerke HS. Abdominal trauma, penetrating. eMedicine Website. Available at http://www. emedicine.com/med/topic2805.htm. Accessed July 12, 2008.

[3] Marx JA, Isenhour J. Abdominal trauma. In: Marx JA, Hockberger RS, Walls RM, et al. (eds.). *Rosen's Emergency Medicine: Concepts and Clinical Practice*, 6th ed. Philadelphia: Mosby, 2006:489–512.

[4] Chiu WC, Shanmuganathan K, Mirvis SE, et al. Determining the need for laparotomy in penetrating torso trauma; a prospective study using triple contrast enhanced abdominopelvic computed tomography. *J Trauma* 2001;51:860–9.

[5] Shanmuganathan K, Mirvis SE, Chiu WC, et al. Penetrating torso trauma: triple-contrast helical CT in peritoneal violation and organ injury – a prospective study in 200 patients. *Radiology* 2004;231:775–84.

55

Left thigh pain in an 18-year-old male

HISTORY OF PRESENT ILLNESS

An 18-year-old male presented to the ED complaining of severe left thigh pain after falling from his skateboard one day earlier, striking his left anterior thigh. He reported that his thigh had become progressively swollen and tense with the pain, currently at a level of 10 (on a scale of 0 to 10). He denied numbness or weakness to the left leg but was unable to bear weight secondary to the pain.

PHYSICAL EXAMINATION

GENERAL APPEARANCE: The patient appeared well nourished, well hydrated and in moderate discomfort.

VITAL SIGNS

Temperature	98°F (36.6°C)
Pulse	96 beats/minute
Blood pressure	135/90 mmHg
Respirations	22 breaths/minute
Oxygen saturation	99% on room air

HEENT: Unremarkable.

NECK: Supple, no midline tenderness.

CARDIOVASCULAR: Regular rate and rhythm without rubs, murmurs or gallops.

LUNGS: Clear to auscultation bilaterally.

ABDOMEN: Soft, nontender, nondistended.

LEFT LOWER EXTREMITY: Marked swelling and tenderness of the anterior thigh, with increased pain upon flexion of the left knee. The left thigh felt tense in comparison with palpation of the right thigh. Neurovascular examination of the left leg demonstrated 5/5 motor strength, normal sensation, and palpable dorsalis pedis and posterior tibialis pulses. The left hip, knee and ankle were nontender, without swelling or deformity.

NEUROLOGIC: Nonfocal.

A peripheral intravenous line was placed, blood was drawn and sent for laboratory testing, and morphine sulfate was administered for pain. Laboratory tests were significant for a leukocyte count of 13.5 K/μL (normal 3.5–12.5 K/μ) and creatine phosphokinase (CPK) of 201 U/L (normal less than 170 U/L). The remainder of the laboratory tests, including electrolytes, creatinine, hematocrit and urinalysis, were within normal limits. Radiographs of the left femur were obtained (Figure 55.1).

What is your diagnosis?

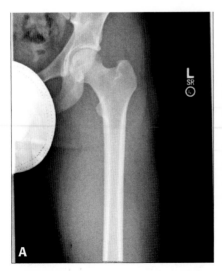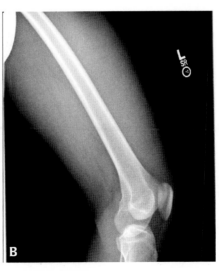

Figure 55.1 Anteroposterior (panel A) and lateral (panel B) radiographs of the left femur from an 18-year-old male with left thigh pain after falling from his skateboard.

ANSWER

The diagnosis is compartment syndrome of the anterior thigh. Orthopedics was consulted and compartment pressures were measured in the ED using a Stryker device. These were 30, 36 and 40 mmHg on three separate measurements (normal range 0–8 mmHg). The patient was taken to the OR urgently and a fasciotomy of the anterior thigh compartment was performed, which resulted in immediate bulging of the rectus femoris muscle through the anterior fasciotomy incision. At completion of the fasciotomy, the muscles of the compartment were soft and well perfused. The wound was closed with a drain in place. The drain was removed on hospital day #2, and the patient was discharged home with instructions to use crutches and weight bear as tolerated, and to avoid aspirin, NSAIDs, and strenuous physical activity for several weeks.

Compartment syndrome

Compartment syndrome (CS) is a condition in which the circulation within a closed compartment is compromised by an increase in pressure within it, causing necrosis of muscles, nerves, and eventually the skin due to excessive swelling.[1] Compartments with relatively noncompliant fascial or osseous structures are most commonly involved, such as the anterior and deep posterior compartments of the leg and the volar compartment of the forearm.[2] However, CS can develop anywhere skeletal muscle is surrounded by substantial fascia, such as in the buttock, thigh, shoulder, hand, foot, arm and lumbar paraspinous muscles.[2]

There are two types of compartment syndromes, acute and chronic. Chronic CS occurs in distance runners, resulting in exercise-related symptoms primarily in the anterolateral compartment of the leg.[3] Acute CS is a surgical emergency, in which pressure in the compartment must be relieved to avoid permanent damage to its contents. CS can occur from a variety of causes, including intravenous and intraosseous fluid infiltration, snakebites, burns, nephritic syndrome, diabetes, drug overdose or injection, and a variety of medications such as pressors, anticoagulants and platelet inhibitors.[3] However, the most common cause of acute CS is fracture of a long bone. Fractures of the tibia and forearm are particularly prone to result in CS and account for a majority of cases.[3]

Prompt recognition and surgical intervention of CS are imperative to prevent irreversible ischemic insult to muscles, nerves and vessels. In many cases, the diagnosis can be made from clinical symptoms and signs alone. The cardinal features of CS include pain out of proportion to the clinical findings; weakness and pain on passive stretch of the muscles of that compartment; hyperesthesia in the distribution of the nerves running through that compartment; and tenseness of the fascial envelope surrounding the compartment.[4] The five "P's" (pain, pallor, pulselessness, paresthesias and paralysis) associated with arterial injury are often mistakenly applied to CS.[3] Of these, the only reliable sign is pain.

If CS is suspected and adequate examination cannot be performed, compartment pressures should be measured.[2] If sophisticated equipment is not available, compartment pressure can be measured using intravenous tubing, a three-way stopcock, a syringe and a mercury manometer.[2] More accurate measuring devices include the Stryker hand-held monitor for single pressure readings, the wick monitor for continuous monitoring, and the slit catheter. Normal intracompartmental pressures range between 0–8 mmHg.[4] If compartment pressures are greater than 30 mmHg in the presence of clinical findings, immediate fasciotomy is indicated.[2] Equivocal readings require continuous monitoring and serial clinical examinations. MRI may be used to evaluate the extent of involvement but should not delay definitive intervention in emergency cases.[5] Findings consistent with CS in the acute setting include increased T2 signal with muscle enlargement, edema or both.[5]

The treatment of CS should begin with removal of any constricting bandages or cast, elevation of the affected limb, ice packs and analgesia. Once the diagnosis of CS is established, fasciotomy should be completed, ideally within six hours.[3] Fasciotomy needs to include wide incisions to completely release the constraining fascia. Acute CS of the thigh caused by hematoma formation after contusion or acute quadriceps strain has been reported.[4,6] CS of the thigh is generally rare because there is a large potential space to allow swelling, which allows an increase in interstitial pressure before endangering the circulation.[4] Furthermore, the fascial compartments of the thigh blend anatomically with the muscles of the hips, potentially allowing blood under pressure to exit the compartment.[4]

KEY TEACHING POINTS

1. Compartment syndrome (CS) is defined as an elevation of the interstitial pressure in a closed osseofascial compartment resulting in microvascular compromise.
2. The most common cause of acute CS is fracture of a long bone, particularly the tibia or forearm.
3. The cardinal features of CS are pain out of proportion to the clinical findings; weakness and pain on passive stretch of the muscles of that compartment; hyperesthesia in the distribution of the nerves running through that compartment; and tenseness of the fascial envelope surrounding the compartment.
4. The normal intracompartmental pressures range between 0–8 mmHg. If compartment pressures are greater than 30 mmHg in the presence of clinical findings, immediate fasciotomy is indicated.
5. Once the diagnosis of CS is established, fasciotomy should be performed within six hours.

REFERENCES

[1] Jobe MT. Compartment syndrome and Volkmann contracture. In: Canale ST, Daugherty K, Jones L (eds.). *Campbell's Operative Orthopedics*, 10th ed. Philadelphia: Mosby, 2003;3739–44.

[2] Azar FM. Traumatic disorders. In: Canale ST, Daugherty K, Jones L (eds.). *Campbell's Operative Orthopedics*, 10th ed. Philadelphia: Mosby, 2003:2449–57.

[3] Newton EJ. Acute complications of extremity trauma. *Emerg Med Clin N Am* 2007;25:751–61.

[4] Burns BJ, Sproule J, Smyth H. Acute compartment syndrome of the anterior thigh following quadriceps strain in a footballer. *Br J Sports Med* 2004;38:218–20.

[5] Armfield DR, Kim DH, Towers JD, et al. Sports-related muscle injury in the lower extremity. *Clin Sports Med* 2006; 25:803–42.

[6] Mithofer K, Lhowe DW, Altman GT. Delayed presentation of acute compartment syndrome after contusion of the thigh. *J Orthop Trauma* 2002;16:436–8.

56

Neck pain after a golf swing in a 26-year-old male

HISTORY OF PRESENT ILLNESS

A 26-year-old male was practicing his golf swing in his back yard when he felt a "pop" in his lower neck and the sudden onset of pain. In the ED, he denied focal weakness, numbness or tingling to his extremities. He reported his pain was worse with movement of his neck, particularly with flexion.

PHYSICAL EXAMINATION

GENERAL APPEARANCE: The patient was a well-developed male sitting upright on the gurney in no acute discomfort.

VITAL SIGNS

Temperature	98.1°F (36.7°C)
Pulse	80 beats/minute
Blood pressure	126/88 mmHg
Respirations	22 breaths/minute
Oxygen saturation	100% on room air

HEENT: Unremarkable.

NECK: Midline tenderness to palpation over the lower neck, no swelling or masses. Pain with active flexion of the neck.

CARDIOVASCULAR: Regular rate and rhythm without rubs, murmurs or gallops.

LUNGS: Clear to auscultation bilaterally.

ABDOMEN: Soft, nontender, nondistended.

EXTREMITIES: No clubbing, cyanosis or edema.

NEUROLOGIC: Alert and oriented to person, place and time; cranial nerves II–XII grossly intact; upper extremity and lower extremity strength 5/5 proximal and distal; sensation grossly intact to light touch.

A cervical spine radiograph series was obtained (Figure 56.1).

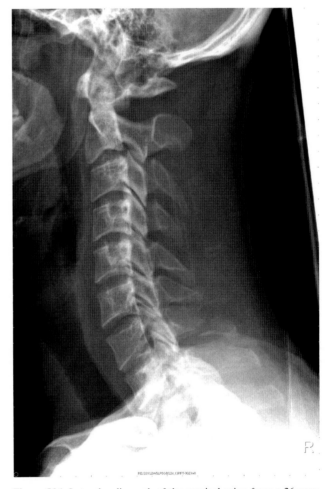

Figure 56.1 Lateral radiograph of the cervical spine from a 26-year-old male with sudden neck pain after a golf swing.

What is your diagnosis?

The diagnosis is a clay-shoveler's fracture of the C7 spinous process. The patient was placed in a cervical hard collar, prescribed Vicodin® and Valium® for pain, and referred to the orthopedic clinic as an outpatient following consultation with the spine surgeon.

Clay-shoveler's fracture

A clay-shoveler's fracture is an oblique fracture of the base of the spinous process, most commonly occurring at one of the lower cervical segments. The injury reportedly derives its name from its common occurrence in clay miners in Australia during the 1930s.[1] The most widely accepted theory for the mechanism of injury in clay-shoveler's fracture is a forceful flexion of the cervical spine, or forceful contraction of the trapezius and rhomboid muscles.[2] Today, this fracture is more commonly seen in football players and power lifters or following direct trauma to the spinous processes, such as from blows with pool cues or baseball bats.[1,2] Sudden deceleration motor vehicle crashes or direct trauma to the occiput that results in a forced flexion of the neck can also cause this type of injury.

Clay-shoveler's fracture is commonly observed in a lateral radiograph because the avulsion fragment is more readily evident (arrow, Figure 56.2).[3] As injury commonly occurs in the lower cervical vertebrae, visualization of the C7-T1 junction in the lateral view is imperative. On the lateral view, the fracture line is commonly oriented obliquely, transversing midway between the tip of the spinous process and spinolaminar junction.[4] Atypically, the fracture may extend through the spinolaminar line. Injury may also be seen in the anteroposterior view, as a vertically-slit appearance of the spinous process in the lower vertebrae (the double spinous process sign).[5] Because injury involves only the spinous process, this fracture is considered stable and is not associated with neurologic impairment. Management of this fracture involves consultation with the neurosurgeon or spine surgeon, pain control and cervical immobilization with an orthotic device for comfort. Close follow up is warranted.

KEY TEACHING POINTS

1. A clay-shoveler's fracture refers to an oblique fracture of the base of the spinous process, most commonly occurring at one of the lower cervical segments.
2. The fracture is believed to occur as a result of forceful flexion of the cervical spine, or forceful contraction of the trapezius and rhomboid muscles.
3. The injury is most commonly visualized on the lateral cervical spine radiograph, which should include the entire cervical spine and the C7-T1 junction.

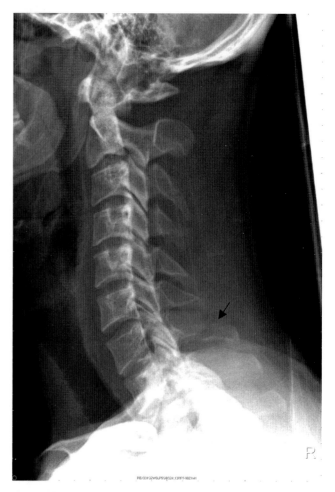

Figure 56.2 Lateral radiograph of the cervical spine from a 26-year-old male demonstrating clay-shoveler's fracture of the C7 spinous process (arrow).

4. Because the injury involves only the spinous process, this fracture is considered stable and is not associated with neurologic impairment.
5. Management involves neurosurgical or orthopedic consultation, pain control and cervical immobilization.

REFERENCES

[1] Hockberger RS, Kaji AH, Newton EJ. Spinal injuries. In: Marx JA, Hockberger RS, Walls RM, et al. (eds.). *Emergency Medicine Concepts and Clinical Practice*, 6th ed. Philadelphia: Mosby, 2006:398–439.
[2] Boden BP, Jarvis CG. Spinal injuries in sports. *Neurol Clin* 2008;26:63–78.
[3] Mueller J.B. Fractures, cervical spine. eMedicine Website. Available at http://www.emedicine.com/emerg/topic189.htm. Accessed June 30, 2008.
[4] Feldman VB, Astri F. An atypical clay shoveler's fracture: a case report. *J Can Chiropr Assoc* 2001;45:213–20.
[5] Cancelmo JJ. Clay shoveler's fracture – a helpful diagnostic sign. *Amer J Roengenol* 1972;115:540–3.

57

Cardiac arrest in a 29-year-old male

HISTORY OF PRESENT ILLNESS

An ambulance arrived to the ED with a 29-year-old male in cardiac arrest, with CPR in progress. History obtained from the paramedics indicated that the man walked into a local restaurant and had a witnessed syncopal event, at which time emergency services were called. En route to the ED, an attempt at intubation was unsuccessful; bag-valve-mask (BVM) ventilation and CPR was in progress. Three doses of epinephrine were administered through a small peripheral intravenous line.

PHYSICAL EXAMINATION

GENERAL APPEARANCE: A well-developed male lying supine on the backboard, unresponsive, with CPR and bag-valve-mask ventilation in progress.

VITAL SIGNS

Temperature	not obtainable
Pulse	120 beats/minute
Blood pressure	not obtainable
Respirations	BVM ventilation, no spontaneous respirations
Oxygen saturation	not obtainable

HEENT: Atraumatic, normocephalic, pupils fixed and dilated.

NECK: No signs of trauma.

CHEST: Good chest wall rise with BVM ventilation, coarse breath sounds bilaterally with diminished breath sounds throughout the left chest.

CARDIOVASCULAR: No heart sounds; carotid, femoral and radial pulses unobtainable without chest compressions.

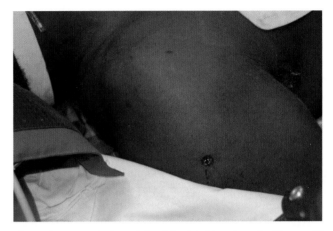

Figure 57.1 Lateral view of the right deltoid region of a 29-year-old male presenting in cardiac arrest.

ABDOMEN: Nondistended.

EXTREMITIES: Wound to lateral aspect of right lower deltoid (Figure 57.1).

NEUROLOGIC: Glasgow Coma Scale (GCS) = 3.

In the ED, the initial rhythm appeared to be pulseless electrical activity (PEA). CPR was continued, and endotracheal intubation was performed. Prior to intubation, emesis mixed with blood was aspirated into the mask during BVM ventilation, as well as suctioned from the oropharynx. As the patient was exposed, a physical exam finding was identified on the right shoulder (Figure 57.1, noted after successful intubation).

What is your diagnosis?

ANSWER

The physical exam finding is a gunshot wound (GSW) to the right shoulder. This arrest requires aggressive management as a traumatic arrest, assuming penetrating trauma to the chest. Following endotracheal intubation of the patient, CPR was continued and a right femoral central venous catheter was placed. Intravenous normal saline was administered rapidly (1-liter bolus) through the line. Needle decompression of the right and left anterior chest walls was performed with 14-gauge angiocatheters without obvious expulsion of air. This was immediately followed by bilateral chest tube thoraco-stomies (Figure 57.2); the right chest tube resulted in signif-icant expulsion of air followed by a large volume of blood. Left chest tube placement resulted in approximately 750 cc of blood. A stat portable chest radiograph was obtained follow-ing bilateral chest tube thoracostomies (Figure 57.3). Despite bilateral chest tube thoracostomies, no palpable pulses or blood pressure was obtainable.

A bedside focused assessment with sonography for trauma (FAST) scan to look for pericardial tamponade from the sub-xyphoid window was attempted but was not of sufficient qual-ity to determine if tamponade was present. At this point, the patient's rhythm deteriorated to asystole. A needle pericar-diocentesis was attempted without return of blood. After ap-proximately 40 minutes, the code was terminated. Upon closer inspection of the body, no other entrance or exit wounds could be found. Neither a chest nor abdominal radiograph performed following cessation of the code resulted in iden-tifying a bullet. A right humerus radiograph demonstrated a humerus fracture near the entrance wound, without any obvi-ous bullet fragments. A subsequent postmortem examination did not identify a bullet fragment or hole in the pericardium.

Penetrating chest trauma, traumatic arrest and ED thoracotomy

Thoracic injuries account for 20–25% of deaths due to trauma.[1] Approximately 16,000 deaths per year may be at-

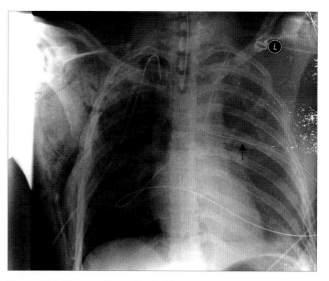

Figure 57.3 Chest radiograph of a 29-year-old male with penetrating traumatic arrest; bilateral chest tube thoracostomies have been per-formed (arrows indicate chest tubes).

tributed to chest trauma. Missiles from GSWs can penetrate all body regions regardless of the point of entry. Any patient with a gunshot entry wound for which a corresponding exit wound cannot be identified should be considered to have a retained projectile, which could embolize to the central or dis-tal vasculature.[1] The patient's clothing should be removed, looking in the axilla, skin folds, and back for occult penetrat-ing injuries. A patient with combined intrathoracic and intra-abdominal wounds has a much greater mortality rate.

Penetrating chest trauma comprises a broad spectrum of injuries and severity (e.g., hemothorax, pneumothorax, dia-phragmatic rupture, pneumomediastinum, cardiac tampo-nade).[2] The clinical consequences depend on mechanism, location, associated injuries and underlying illness. Life-threatening injuries either produce massive hemorrhage, com-promise gas exchange (e.g., hemothorax, pneumothorax), or interfere with cardiac filling (e.g., cardiac tamponade, tension pneumothorax).[3] The emergency physician's initial concern is the airway. Indications for emergency endotracheal intuba-tion include apnea, profound shock and inadequate ventila-tion. Severe bronchial injury or unilateral pulmonary injury may require selective intubation of the opposite mainstem bronchus.[3]

A chest radiograph is not indicated in patients who display clinical signs of a tension pneumothorax (tracheal deviation, unilateral decreased breath sounds, or extreme respiratory or hemodynamic distress). These patients require immediate chest decompression, which may be accomplished by insert-ing a large-bore needle at the second intercostal space, mid-clavicular line, followed by definitive tube thoracostomy.[3] If the needle approach is initially chosen, tube thoracostomy must follow.

The algorithm for management of penetrating chest trauma in the unstable patient involves initial activation of the trauma or surgery team, intubation of patients with apnea, profound shock or inadequate ventilation, followed by

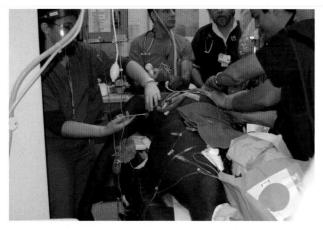

Figure 57.2 Placement of bilateral chest tubes in a 29-year-old male with traumatic arrest following penetrating chest trauma.

recognition of signs of tension pneumothorax with needle or chest tube decompression if present.[3] Any sucking chest wounds should be covered with a "flutter" dressing followed by placement of a chest tube through a separate incision. A chest radiograph should then be obtained, and any significant hemo- or pneumothorax treated with chest tube thoracostomy. Patients with persistent hypotension should be resuscitated to a systolic blood pressure of at least 90 mmHg and the OR should be notified.[3] A bedside transthoracic ultrasound should be performed (if available) to look for signs of pericardial tamponade and cardiac activity; profoundly unstable patients may benefit from ED thoracotomy with ongoing aggressive resuscitation.

The trauma algorithm for unstable patients with transmediastinal GSW involves rapid assessment, endotracheal intubation, placement of two large bore IVs, followed by bilateral chest tube placement and chest radiograph to determine the likely mediastinal trajectory. Patients with continued chest tube drainage, nonevacuated hematoma or suspected cardiac injury should be taken urgently to the operating suite.[3]

ED thoracotomy is a life-saving procedure for an extremely small subset of critically injured patients.[4] Its primary use is in the management of patients in extremis after penetrating chest or abdominal injury and, to a much lesser extent, after blunt injury.[4,5] The therapeutic goals of ED thoracotomy include hemorrhage control, effective cardiac compressions, cross-clamping the pulmonary hilum in the case of air embolism or massive bronchopleural fistula, relief of cardiac tamponade, and cross-clamping the descending aorta for hemorrhage control of the lower torso.[6] Whenever possible, the patient should be stabilized and transported to the operating room where facilities are available for definitive care.

In 2001, practice management guidelines for ED thoracotomy were published by the American College of Surgeons, based upon a detailed literature review of the subject.[7] Several Level II recommendations were set forth in this review:

(1) ED thoracotomy should rarely be performed in patients sustaining cardiopulmonary arrest secondary to blunt trauma because of its very low survival rate and poor neurologic outcomes. ED thoracotomy should be limited to those who arrive with vital signs at the trauma center and experience a witnessed cardiopulmonary arrest.

(2) ED thoracotomy is best performed on patients sustaining penetrating cardiac injuries who arrive at trauma centers after a short scene and transport time with witnessed or objectively measured physiologic parameters (signs of life): pupillary response, spontaneous ventilation, presence of carotid pulse, palpable blood pressure, extremity movement or electrical cardiac activity.

(3) ED thoracotomy should be performed on patients sustaining penetrating noncardiac thoracic injuries, but these patients generally experience a low survival rate. Because it is difficult to ascertain whether the injuries are noncardiac thoracic versus cardiac, ED thoracotomy can be used to establish the diagnosis.

(4) ED thoracotomy should be performed in patients sustaining exsanguinating abdominal vascular injuries, but these patients generally experience a low survival rate. Judicious selection of patients should be exercised. This procedure should be used as an adjunct to definitive repair of the abdominal-vascular injury.

(5) For the pediatric population, guidelines 1–4 are applicable.

In general, patients most likely to respond favorably to ED thoracotomy include victims of penetrating trauma with signs of life upon presentation to the ED or patients who lose signs of life within 10 minutes of arrival.[6] Resuscitative thoracotomy appears to be futile in patients with blunt trauma requiring pre-hospital CPR longer than 5 minutes, and in patients with penetrating trauma with more than 15 minutes of pre-hospital CPR.[8] Pericardiocentesis has no role in patients presenting in traumatic arrest. This procedure often is ineffective in removing clotted blood from the pericardial space, is not a risk-free procedure, potentially delays any surgical procedures, and has negligible diagnostic value with the application of Focused Assessment with Sonography for Trauma (FAST) examination.[6]

KEY TEACHING POINTS

1. It is important to search for occult penetrating injuries (e.g., GSW to axilla, skin folds, or back) in trauma patients.

2. Patients with suspected tension pneumothorax require immediate chest decompression, first by large-bore needle insertion then chest tube thoracostomy.

3. Transthoracic ultrasound (echocardiography) through the subxyphoid approach is a valuable tool to assess for cardiac tamponade in trauma patients (part of the FAST exam).

4. Pericardiocentesis is not recommended for the diagnosis or treatment of traumatic cardiac tamponade.

5. ED thoracotomy is generally indicated for trauma patients who arrest after arrival in the ED, patients with signs of life at the scene but arrest en route to the hospital (who undergo less than 10–15 minutes of CPR), moribund patients who have signs of life present but no (or barely detectable) blood pressure, or in patients who remain unstable despite intubation, tube thoracostomies and adequate volume resuscitation.

REFERENCES

[1] Shahani R. Penetrating chest trauma. eMedicine Website. Available at http://www.emedicine.com/med/topic2916.htm. Accessed June 11, 2008.

[2] Inci I, Ozcelik C, Tacyildiz I, et al. Penetrating chest injuries: unusually high incidence of high-velocity gunshot wounds in civilian practice. *World J Surg* 1998;22:438–42.

[3] Mosesso VN. Penetrating chest trauma. In: Ferrera PC, Colucciello SA, Marx JA, et al. (eds.). Trauma Management, an Emergency Medicine Approach. Philadelphia: Mosby, 2001:259–78.

[4] Mejia JC, Stewart RM, Cohn SM. Emergency department thoracotomy. *Semin Thorac Cardiovasc Surg* 2008;20: 13–8.

[5] Seamon MJ, Pathak AS, Bradley KM, et al. Emergency department thoracotomy: still useful after abdominal exsanguinations? *J Trauma* 2008;64:1–8.

[6] Meredith JW, Hoth JJ. Thoracic trauma: when and how to intervene. *Surg Clin N Am* 2007;87:95–118.

[7] Working Group, Ad Hoc Subcommittee on Outcomes, American College of Surgeons-Committee on Trauma. Practice management guidelines for emergency department thoracotomy. *J Am Coll Surg* 2001;193:303–9.

[8] Powell DW, Moore EE, Cothren CC, et al. Is emergency department resuscitative thoracotomy futile care for the critically injured patient requiring prehospital cardiopulmonary resuscitation? *J Am Coll Surg* 2004;199:211–5.

58

Right lower quadrant abdominal pain in a 36-year-old female

HISTORY OF PRESENT ILLNESS

A 36-year-old female presented to the ED complaining of several days of gradually worsening right lower quadrant abdominal pain. The pain was constant, rated at level of 7 (on a scale of 0 to 10), worse with movement or walking. She denied fevers, nausea, vomiting, diarrhea, constipation, vaginal bleeding or discharge, anorexia or previous abdominal surgeries. Her last normal menstrual period was two weeks earlier; she denied the possibility of pregnancy.

PHYSICAL EXAMINATION

GENERAL APPEARANCE: The patient was a well-nourished, well-hydrated female in no acute discomfort.

VITAL SIGNS

Temperature	98.6°F (37°C)
Pulse	85 beats/minute
Blood pressure	130/85 mmHg
Respirations	18 breaths/minute
Oxygen saturation	100% on room air

HEENT: Unremarkable.

NECK: Supple.

CARDIOVASCULAR: Regular rate and rhythm without rubs, murmurs or gallops.

LUNGS: Clear to auscultation bilaterally.

ABDOMEN: Nondistended, active bowel sounds present, firm and tender to palpation in the right lower quadrant with rebound and guarding, no ecchymosis or obvious masses.

PELVIC: No vaginal bleeding or discharge, os closed, no cervical motion or adnexal tenderness, and no masses appreciated.

RECTAL: Normal tone, soft brown stool, hemoccult negative.

EXTREMITIES: No clubbing, cyanosis or edema.

NEUROLOGIC: Nonfocal.

A peripheral intravenous line was placed, and blood was drawn and sent for laboratory testing. An intravenous normal saline 1-liter bolus was given, as well as morphine sulfate IV for pain. Laboratory tests, including a complete blood count, electrolytes, creatinine, glucose, and liver function tests, were within normal limits. A urinalysis showed no evidence of infection or blood, and a urine pregnancy test returned negative. A CT scan of the abdomen and pelvis with oral and IV contrast was obtained (Figure 58.1).

What is your diagnosis?

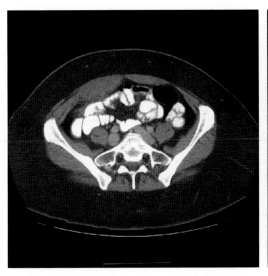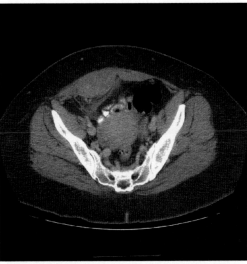

Figure 58.1 CT of the abdomen and pelvis from a 36-year-old female with several days of right lower quadrant abdominal pain.

ANSWER

The diagnosis is rectus sheath hematoma. The CT scan demonstrates enlargement of the right rectus sheath with surrounding stranding, consistent with a rectus sheath hematoma (arrow, Figure 58.2). Upon further questioning, the patient recalled that five days earlier, her 85-lb dog jumped onto her abdomen while she was supine on the ground. Her initial hematocrit was 40%. The patient was observed, and a repeat hematocrit was 36% seven hours after presentation. A third hematocrit two hours later remained stable at 36%. The patient was discharged with close follow up, oral analgesics, instructions to avoid strenuous activity, and to apply ice packs to the area.

Rectus sheath hematoma

Rectus sheath hematoma (RSH) is the result of accumulation of blood in the sheath of the rectus abdominis muscle due to disruption of epigastric vessels or a tear in the muscle itself.[1] Etiologies for RSH include trauma, abdominal operations, trocar site injury after laparoscopic operations, subcutaneous drug injections, anticoagulant therapy, hematological diseases, hypertension, coughing, physical exercise and pregnancy.[1–3] The male to female distribution of RSH is approximately 1:3; it occurs most frequently in the right lower abdomen.[3] It is an uncommon cause of an acute abdomen, and is known to mimic various surgical conditions, including acute cholecystitis, appendicitis, ruptured abdominal aortic aneurysm, sigmoid diverticulitis and abruptio placentae.[2]

RSHs present most commonly with abdominal pain and tenderness, which can be severe and mimic peritonitis.[4] Common presenting signs and symptoms are abdominal pain, abdominal wall mass, decrease in hemoglobin, abdominal wall ecchymosis, nausea, vomiting, tachycardia, peritoneal irritation, fever, abdominal distention and cramping.[1] Fothergill's sign is useful for distinguishing between an intra-abdominal mass and a mass arising in the rectus sheath.[3] It is performed by asking the supine patient to lift their head from the pillow. As the abdominal wall tenses, patients with RSH have increased pain and the mass becomes fixed but is still palpable; an intra-abdominal mass is more difficult to distinguish through the tensed muscle.[3]

Abdominal ultrasound or CT scan can identify RSHs, usually confined to the abdominal wall.[4] Although ultrasonography is one of the first-line investigations with a sensitivity of 80–90%, CT scan remains the gold standard with nearly 100% sensitivity and specificity and the ability to detect other intra-abdominal pathology.[3,5] RSH is usually managed conservatively with rest, analgesics, ice pack application, discontinuation of any anticoagulant therapy and blood (or blood product) transfusion when necessary.[6] Surgical evacuation and hemostasis is necessary if the hematoma fails to resolve. Hemodynamic compromise necessitates operative intervention – clot evacuation and vessel ligation via laparotomy or laparoscopy is usually successful.[7]

KEY TEACHING POINTS

1. Rectus sheath hematoma (RSH) is an accumulation of blood in the sheath of the rectus abdominis muscle due to disruption of epigastric vessels or a tear in the muscle itself.
2. RSH can mimic various surgical conditions, including acute cholecystitis, appendicitis, ruptured abdominal aortic aneurysm, sigmoid diverticulitis and abruptio placentae.
3. RSH most commonly presents with abdominal pain, tenderness, and a palpable abdominal mass often located in the right lower quadrant.
4. Imaging studies used in the diagnosis of RSH include ultrasonography and CT; CT is preferred.
5. Treatment of RSH is conservative in most cases (rest, ice packs, reversal of anticoagulation when needed); surgery is indicated in cases where hemodynamic compromise exists or the hematoma fails to resolve.

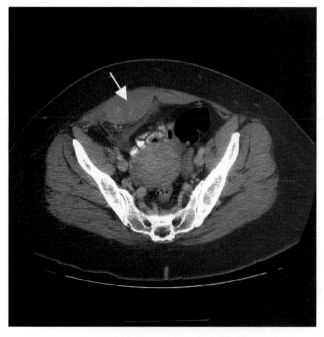

Figure 58.2 CT of the pelvis from a 36-year-old female with large right rectus sheath hematoma (arrow).

REFERENCES

[1] Kapan S, Turhan AN, Alis H, et al. Rectus sheath hematoma: three case reports. *J Med Case Reports* 2008;2:22.
[2] Rajagopal AS, Shinkfield M, Voight S, et al. Massive rectus sheath hematoma. *Am J Surg* 2006;191:126–7.
[3] Luhmann A, Williams EV. Rectus sheath hematoma: a series of unfortunate events. *World J Surg* 2006;30:2050–5.
[4] Raven MC, Hoffman RS. Images in emergency medicine. *Ann Emerg Med* 2005;46:558, 562.
[5] Cherry WB, Mueller PS. Rectus sheath hematoma: review of 126 cases at a single institution. *Medicine* 2006;85:105–10.
[6] James RF. Rectus sheath haematoma. *Lancet* 2005;365:1824.
[7] Costello J, Wright J. Rectus sheath haematoma: 'a diagnostic dilemma?' *Emerg Med J* 2005;22:523–4.

59

Blunt head trauma in a 37-year-old male

HISTORY OF PRESENT ILLNESS

A 37-year-old male was brought to the ED by ambulance after sustaining a head injury in a motor vehicle collision. The patient was a restrained driver of a small truck traveling at moderate speed when another car pulled in front of his vehicle. The patient's truck collided with the passenger side of the other vehicle, causing significant damage to both vehicles. The patient reported a brief loss of consciousness and did not remember the collision. When the paramedics arrived, they found him standing outside his vehicle with a moderate-sized, bleeding laceration to his forehead. He was awake and alert, ambulatory, and denied other injuries. In the ED, the patient reported only a mild headache. He denied neck, chest or abdominal pain, as well as visual changes, focal numbness or weakness, nausea, dizziness, confusion or extreme fatigue.

PHYSICAL EXAMINATION

GENERAL APPEARANCE: The patient was a well-developed male, awake and alert in no acute discomfort.

VITAL SIGNS:

Temperature	98°F (36.6°C)
Pulse	88 beats/minute
Blood pressure	158/90 mmHg
Respirations	18 breaths/minute
Oxygen saturation	98% on room air

HEENT: A 5-cm vertical laceration in the mid-forehead with surrounding edema and ecchymosis without active bleeding, no scalp hematomas noted. PERRL, EOMI, no nystagmus, tympanic membranes clear bilaterally. No Battle's sign or raccoon eyes appreciated.

NECK: Supple, no midline tenderness.

CARDIOVASCULAR: Regular rate and rhythm without rubs, murmurs or gallops.

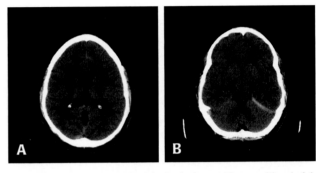

Figure 59.1 Noncontrast CT of the brain from a 37-year-old male following head trauma from a motor vehicle collision.

LUNGS: Clear to auscultation bilaterally.

ABDOMEN: Soft, nontender, nondistended.

EXTREMITIES: No clubbing, cyanosis or edema; no obvious swelling or deformities.

NEUROLOGIC: Alert and oriented to person, place and time; cranial nerves II–XII grossly intact; upper extremity and lower extremity strength 5/5 bilaterally, proximal and distal; sensation grossly intact, no pronator drift, normal gait.

While waiting for CT scan of the brain, the patient's forehead wound was anesthetized with 1% lidocaine with epinephrine, irrigated and closed with simple interrupted nylon sutures using sterile technique. The patient's tetanus status was updated, he was not allowed to have anything to eat or drink, and a noncontrast CT scan of the brain was obtained to evaluate for possible intracranial hemorrhage (Figure 59.1).

What is your diagnosis?

ANSWER

The diagnosis is post-traumatic subarachnoid hemorrhage (SAH). The CT scan in Figure 59.1 demonstrated a small area of increased attenuation along the sulci in the mid-aspect of the left frontal lobe (arrow, panel A, Figure 59.2) consistent with small SAH. Also present on the CT scan is an area of increased attenuation along the left tentorium (panel B, Figure 59.2, arrow) consistent with SAH resulting from a contrecoup injury. No intraparenchymal hemorrhage, midline shift or mass effect was evident. The neurosurgeon on call was consulted and after reviewing the history, physical examination, and CT scan recommended 24-hour observation with frequent neurologic assessments. The patient remained stable and neurologically intact throughout the 24-hour observation period. A repeat CT scan of the brain performed 24 hours later did not reveal an increase in the areas of attenuation noted on the prior CT. The patient was discharged from the hospital and instructed to follow up with his primary care physician in one week, and to return to the ED immediately for any neurologic changes or concerns.

Traumatic brain injury

Traumatic brain injury (TBI) is a nondegenerative, noncongenital insult to the brain from an external mechanical force. It may lead to permanent or temporary impairment of cognitive, physical and psychosocial functions, with diminished or altered states of consciousness.[1] TBI accounts for approximately 40% of all deaths from acute injuries in the United States.[1] Annually, 1.74 million persons sustain mild TBI, requiring a physician visit or temporary disability of at least one day; 200,000 persons sustaining TBI require hospitalization.[1]

Pathologic changes after TBI may be divided into two broad classification schemes: focal versus diffuse and primary versus secondary.[2] Focal injuries involve an injury to a localized area of the brain, whereas diffuse injuries involve a wider region of the brain. Primary injuries occur at the time of impact, whereas secondary injuries occur at some point after the initial blow to the head. Secondary injuries may be avoided or minimized by treatment.[2]

Extra-axial hemorrhages occur frequently after TBI, and include epidural, subdural and SAHs. Epidural hemorrhages (EDH) are frequently caused by laceration of meningeal arteries, often in association with skull fractures.[2,3] The hemorrhage is situated between the skull and the dura, which often limits the extent of bleeding because of the tight adherence of the dura to the skull at the bony sutures.[2] SAHs are located between the pia mater and the arachnoid, predisposing cerebral arteries to vasospasm. This is one reason that worse outcomes occur following TBI with SAH.[2,4] Subdural hemorrhages (SDH) are formed when blood extravasates into the subdural space between the arachnoid and pia mater.[3] SDH surrounds the brain, forming crescent-shaped hyperdense areas on CT that can interdigitate with the gyri of the cortex along the periphery of the hemisphere.[3] Elderly individuals are particularly vulnerable to SDH because bridging veins become more susceptible to shearing forces as the brain naturally atrophies with advancing age.[2]

TBI is commonly categorized using the Glasgow Coma Scale (GCS): severe (GCS ≤ 8), moderate (GCS 9–13) and minor (GCS 14–15).[5,6] Severe and moderate TBI accounts for approximately 10% each of all cases of TBI; the remaining 80% are classified as minor.[5] In the ED, a noncontrast CT scan of the head is the imaging modality of choice for patients with TBI. Research continues to determine which patients with head trauma can safely forego CT. A head CT will determine if an acute traumatic lesion exists, which directs subsequent management. In addition to intracranial and extra-axial lesions, skull fractures – including basilar fractures – can be detected using the bone windows of CT. Plain skull radiographs are generally no longer indicated for patients who have sustained moderate or severe TBI.[5] MRI is better than CT in detecting post-traumatic ischemic infarctions, subacute nonhemorrhagic lesions and contusions, axonal shear injury, and brainstem or posterior fossa lesions.[6]

Traumatic subarachnoid hemorrhage (TSAH) is defined as blood within the CSF and meningeal intima, which likely results from tears of small subarachnoid vessels.[6] TSAH is detected on the first CT scan in up to 33% of patients with severe TBI, with an overall incidence of 44% in all cases of severe head trauma.[5] TSAH is therefore the most common CT scan abnormality seen after head injury. The amount of blood correlates directly with the outcome and inversely with the presenting GCS.[6]

Most low-risk patients who have sustained a minor head injury (with the exception of intoxicated patients and those living alone) can be discharged safely from the ED after a normal examination, although competent observation of at least 4–6 hours is advised.[5] It is helpful to provide a written instruction sheet with a list of symptoms that should prompt a return to the hospital, such as increasing headache, repeated vomiting, weakness, clumsiness, drowsiness, confusion, visual changes, or fluid from the nose or ear that might represent a leak of cerebrospinal fluid.[7] Patients with minor head trauma who are

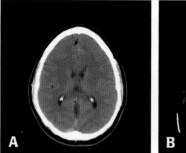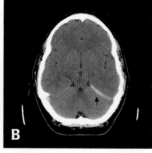

Figure 59.2 Noncontrast CT of the brain from a 37-year-old male demonstrating areas of increased attenuation along the sulci in the mid-aspect of left frontal lobe (arrow, panel A) as well as along the left tentorium (arrow, panel B), consistent with post-traumatic subarachnoid hemorrhage.

discharged from the ED should have early follow up arranged. All patients with moderate TBI should undergo CT scanning and be observed in an ED or hospital setting, even with apparently normal CT scans.[5]

Initial management of patients with severe TBI involves close attention to the airway, breathing and circulation (ABCs), with use of rapid sequence intubation (RSI) to secure the airway in combative, agitated or comatose patients. If hypotension is detected at any time in the emergent management of a head-injured patient, a cause other than the head injury should be sought.[6] If the patient is deteriorating or has signs of increased intracranial pressure (ICP), active interventions must be initiated. These interventions include elevation of the head of the bed, modest hyperventilation to reduce ICP by promoting cerebral vasoconstriction, use of osmotic diuretics such as mannitol, minimizing intravenous fluids, blood pressure and glycemic control, barbiturate therapy to reduce cerebral metabolic demands of the injured brain tissue, and cranial decompression (emergency trephination) when all other attempts at reducing ICP have failed.[6] Seizure prophylaxis with appropriate anticonvulsant agents is recommended in certain patients with severe TBI, particularly in head-injured patients paralyzed during RSI.[6] Neurosurgical consultation should be obtained as soon as possible in all patients with severe TBI to help direct subsequent management.

KEY TEACHING POINTS

1. Traumatic brain injury (TBI) is commonly categorized using the Glasgow Coma Scale as severe (GCS ≤ 8), moderate (GCS 9–13) and minor (GCS 14–15).
2. Extra-axial bleeding occurs frequently after TBI and includes epidural, subdural and subarachnoid hemorrhages.
3. Traumatic SAH is the most common CT scan abnormality seen after TBI.
4. Elderly individuals are particularly vulnerable to SDHs because bridging veins become more susceptible to shearing forces with advancing age.
5. In the ED, a noncontrast CT scan of the head is the imaging modality of choice for patients with TBI; plain skull films have little utility in these patients.
6. Initial management of patients with severe TBI involves close attention to the ABCs, rapid imaging with CT, and prompt neurosurgical consultation.

REFERENCES

[1] Dawodu ST. Traumatic brain injury: definition, epidemiology, pathophysiology. eMedicine Website. Available at http://www.emedicine.com/pmr/topic212.htm. Accessed June 28, 2008.

[2] Flanagan SR, Hibbard MR, Riordan B, et al. Traumatic brain injury in the elderly: diagnostic and treatment challenges. *Clin Geriatr Med* 2006;22:449–68.

[3] Mattiello JA, Munz M. Images in clinical medicine: four types of acute post-traumatic intracranial hemorrhage. *N Engl J Med* 2001;344:580.

[4] Servadi F, Murray GD, Teasdale G, et al. Traumatic subarachnoid hemorrhage: demographic and clinical study of 750 patients from the European brain injury consortium survey of head injuries. *Neurosurgery* 2002;50:261–9.

[5] Heegaard W, Biros M. Traumatic brain injury. *Emerg Med Clin N Am* 2007;25:655–78.

[6] Heegaard WG, Biros MH. Head. In: Marx JA, Hockberger RS, Walls RM, et al. (eds.). *Rosen's Emergency Medicine: Concepts and Clinical Practice*, 6th ed. Philadelphia: Mosby, 2006:349–79.

[7] Ropper AH, Gorson KC. Concussion. *N Engl J Med* 2007;356:166–72.

60

Neck pain after a fall in a 75-year-old female

HISTORY OF PRESENT ILLNESS

A 75-year-old female with a medical history significant for degenerative disc disease and scoliosis of the cervical spine presented to the ED by ambulance after tripping over her dog and falling face first to the ground. The patient struck her forehead but denied loss of consciousness, numbness, tingling or focal weakness to the extremities. She complained of neck pain, which did not feel different from her usual, chronic neck pain. The patient was placed in a cervical spine collar and immobilized on a backboard for transport to the ED by the paramedics.

PHYSICAL EXAMINATION

GENERAL APPEARANCE: The patient was an elderly female lying supine on the backboard in a hard cervical collar, in no acute discomfort.

VITAL SIGNS

Temperature	98.6°F (37°C)
Pulse	88 beats/minute
Blood pressure	140/90 mmHg
Respirations	22 breaths/minute
Oxygen saturation	99% on room air

HEENT: A 2-cm superficial laceration to the forehead, PERRL, EOMI, no Battle's sign or raccoon eyes appreciated. Oropharynx moist, tympanic membranes clear bilaterally without presence of hemotympanum.

NECK: Midline tenderness to palpation of the upper cervical spine.

CARDIOVASCULAR: Regular rate and rhythm without rubs, murmurs or gallops.

LUNGS: Clear to auscultation bilaterally.

ABDOMEN: Soft, nontender, nondistended.

EXTREMITIES: No clubbing, cyanosis or edema; no swelling or deformities.

NEUROLOGIC: Alert and oriented to person, place and time; upper extremity and lower extremity strength 5/5 proximal and distal, bilaterally; sensation grossly intact.

A peripheral intravenous line was placed, blood was drawn and sent for laboratory testing, and a noncontrast CT of the head and cervical spine was obtained while the patient was kept immobilized in the cervical collar. The head CT was normal. The reformatted cervical spine CT is shown in Figure 60.1.

What is your diagnosis?

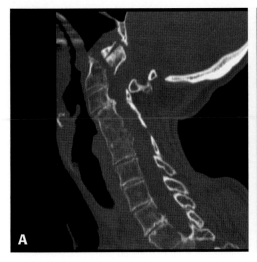 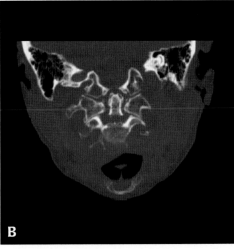

Figure 60.1 Reformatted sagittal (panel A) and coronal (panel B) images from the cervical spine CT of a 75-year-old female with neck pain after a fall.

The diagnosis is a type II fracture through the base of the odontoid process, demonstrated by the CT of the cervical spine (arrows, Figure 60.2). The CT also demonstrates 12-mm dorsal displacement of the C1 ring and odontoid process with respect to C2, as well as posterior displacement of the lateral masses of C1. The patient remained in a hard cervical collar with strict immobilization, and was transferred to the neurosurgical/spine service where she underwent a C1-C2 posterior fusion and facet joint fusion with lateral mass screws at C1 and pedicle screws at C2. A repeat CT of the cervical spine obtained several months after surgery demonstrated healing of the odontoid fracture with no evidence of displacement of the fracture fragments (Figure 60.3).

Odontoid fractures

The overall incidence of odontoid fractures ranges from 7–14% of all cervical fractures. As with most injuries to the upper cervical spine, they are usually the result of falls or motor vehicle collisions.[1] The odontoid, in conjunction with the transverse atlantal ligament, is the prime stabilizer of the atlantoaxial articulation and acts to prevent anterior and posterior dislocation of the atlas and axis. The apophyseal joints of the atlantoaxial complex confer little stability at this level because they lie in a horizontal plane. Thus, with fractures of the odontoid, stability is lost, and anterior and posterior subluxation and dislocation may occur. Despite a large number of autopsy and biomechanical studies, the exact mechanism of injury remains unknown but probably includes a combination of flexion, extension and rotation.[1]

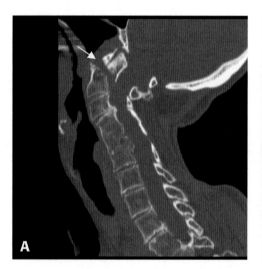
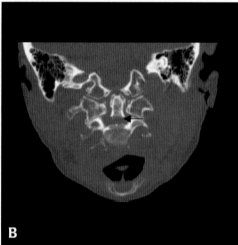

Figure 60.2 Reformatted sagittal (panel A) and coronal (panel B) images from the cervical spine CT of a 75-year-old female with type II odontoid fracture (arrows).

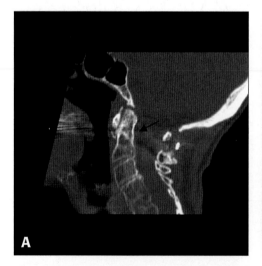
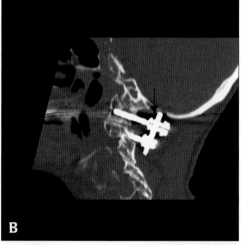

Figure 60.3 Reformatted sagittal images from the cervical spine CT of 75-year-old female several months following C1-C2 posterior fusion and facet joint fusion for type II odontoid fracture demonstrating healed odontoid fracture (arrow, panel A) and lateral mass screws (arrow, panel B).

Anderson and D'Alonzo proposed the most widely accepted classification system for odontoid fractures in the 1970s.[2] Type I fractures were described to be near the tip of the odontoid process, above the transverse ligament. This infrequent fracture is generally thought to occur by avulsion of the apical or alar ligaments. It is considered to be relatively stable.[3] Nonetheless, this fracture type may also herald an inherently unstable occipital-cervical dislocation, particularly if bilateral avulsion of the alar ligaments in type I odontoid fractures or a contralateral occipital condyle fracture is present. Type II fractures occur at the base of the odontoid, between the level of the transverse ligament and the C2 vertebral body. These are the most common types of odontoid fracture and are considered relatively unstable. Type III fractures extend into the vertebral body and are relatively stable unless severely displaced.[2,3]

In the setting of acute spinal trauma, CT scanning has been shown to be more time efficient and significantly more sensitive for fracture detection than plain films.[4] Multidetector CT provides superior evaluation of bony anatomy and pathology. Images may be rapidly acquired and reconstructed at narrow intervals (e.g., 1 minute). Multiplanar and three-dimensional images can subsequently be created. The sensitivity of CT scanning for cervical spine fracture detection has been reported between 90–99%, with specificities ranging from 72–89%.[4] Plain radiography presents limitations in detecting fracture of the cervical spine, particularly at the craniocervical and cervicothoracic junction.[4] In one study, 32 of 88 fractures detected by CT were not seen on limited plain film evaluation, and one-third of those fractures were clinically significant or unstable.[5]

Studies on cervical spine trauma show that elderly patients have different mechanisms and patterns of injury. Older patients are more likely to be injured in falls and have increased likelihood of upper cervical injuries, particularly the odontoid.[6] Degenerative changes of the spine may result in increased risk of spinal fracture, specifically atlantoaxial injury, in older persons. Osteopenia places bones at greater risk from what would otherwise be trivial trauma in younger patients. The presence of senile degenerative disease alters spinal mechanisms, making the upper cervical levels comparatively more mobile and vulnerable to blunt trauma. Cervical spine plain film interpretation in elderly patients is complicated by relative osteopenia, the presence of degenerative changes, and unreliable markers for soft tissue injury.[6] Given the enhanced sensitivity of CT scans and the high incidence of pathology, some physicians have advocated bypassing plain films and going directly to CT in this population. Because elderly patients are more likely to suffer significant head and neck injuries from low-energy mechanisms, particularly falls from standing, and many of these patients have normal neurologic examinations, emergency physicians must take special precautions with elderly patients and have a low threshold for cervical immobilization and imaging.[6–9]

In general, odontoid fractures may be treated with nonoperative immobilization or operatively. Nonoperative treatment generally consists of a collar or halo, whereas operative treatment may be one of several posterior C1-C2 fusion techniques or anterior screw fixation.[3] Although the ideal treatment recommendations for type II odontoid fractures is frequently debated among spine surgeons, surgical intervention is becoming the mainstay of treatment for the majority of patient age groups with this type of fracture.[3]

KEY TEACHING POINTS

1. The emergency physician must have a low threshold for cervical immobilization and imaging in elderly patients with neck pain following low-impact trauma (e.g., a fall from standing).
2. CT scan is superior to plain radiographs for diagnosing cervical spine fractures, especially at the craniocervical junction and in elderly patients with osteopenia and degenerative changes.
3. Elderly patients may have significant cervical spine trauma in the absence of neurologic symptoms.
4. Type II odontoid fractures are generally considered unstable, requiring operative management in most cases.

REFERENCES

[1] Hecht AC, Silcox DH, Whitesides TE. Injuries to the cervicocranium. In: Browner BD, et al. (eds.). *Skeletal Trauma: Basic Science, Management, and Reconstruction*, 3rd ed. Philadelphia: Saunders, 2003:757–90.

[2] Anderson LD, D'Alonzo RT. Fractures of the odontoid process of the axis. *J Bone Joint Surg Am* 1974;56:1663–74.

[3] Maak TG, Grauer JN. The contemporary treatment of odontoid injuries. *Spine* 2006;31:S53–60.

[4] Bagley LJ. Imaging of spinal trauma. *Radiol Clin N Am* 2006;44:1–12.

[5] Nunez DB, Zuluaga A, Fuentes-Bernardo DA, et al. Cervical spine trauma: how much more do we learn routinely by using helical CT? *Radiographics* 1996;16:1307–18.

[6] Kulchycki LK, Edlow JA. Geriatric neurologic emergencies. *Emerg Med Clin N Am* 2006;24:273–98.

[7] Sterling DA, O'Connor JA, Bonadies J. Geriatric falls: injury severity is high and disproportionate to mechanism. *J Trauma* 2001;50:116–9.

[8] Helling TS, Watkins M, Evans LL, et al. Low falls: an underappreciated mechanism of injury. *J Trauma* 2001;46:453–6.

[9] Lomoschitz FM, Blackmore CC, Mirza SK, et al. Cervical spine injuries in patients 65 years old and older: epidemiologic analysis regarding the effects of age and injury mechanism on distribution, type, and stability of injuries. *Am J Roentgenol* 2002;178:573–7.

61

Posterior neck pain in a 77-year-old male

HISTORY OF PRESENT ILLNESS

A 77-year-old male presented to the ED complaining of posterior neck pain for two days after falling out of bed. He hit the back of his head on the floor, and denied loss of consciousness. He reported constant pain on the back of his neck as well as the feeling of neck weakness, as if he needed to support his head with his hands. He described radiation of pain down both shoulders with flexion or extension of his neck. He denied numbness of his upper extremities but reported mild weakness of his left arm.

PHYSICAL EXAMINATION

GENERAL APPEARANCE: The patient was a well-nourished, well-developed male in no acute discomfort, lying supine on the gurney.

VITAL SIGNS

Temperature	98.8°F (37.1°C)
Pulse	72 beats/minute
Blood pressure	141/79 mmHg
Respirations	20 breaths/minute
Oxygen saturation	99% on room air

HEENT: PERRL, EOMI.

NECK: No posterior midline tenderness or deformity noted. Full range of motion with mild pain on flexion and extension.

CARDIOVASCULAR: Regular rate and rhythm without rubs, murmurs or gallops.

LUNGS: Clear to auscultation bilaterally.

ABDOMEN: Soft, nontender, nondistended.

EXTREMITIES: No clubbing, cyanosis or edema.

NEUROLOGIC: Alert and oriented to person, place and time; cranial nerves II–XII grossly intact; upper and lower extremity strength 5/5 proximal and distal bilaterally; sensation grossly intact to light touch throughout.

A cervical spine radiograph series, including anteroposterior, lateral and odontoid views, as well as flexion-extension views (under supervision), was obtained. No fracture was noted on the anteroposterior, lateral or odontoid views, with normal alignment of the vertebral bodies noted. The flexion-extension views are shown (Figure 61.1).

What is your diagnosis?

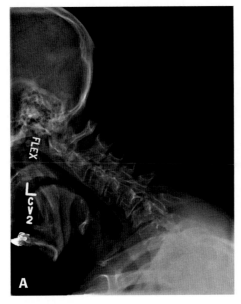 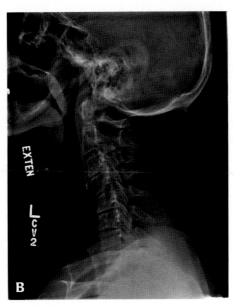

Figure 61.1 Cervical spine flexion (panel A) and extension (panel B) views from a 77-year-old male with posterior neck pain after a fall.

ANSWER

The diagnosis is anterior subluxation of C5 on C6. The lateral flexion radiograph demonstrates a 7-mm anterior subluxation of C5 on C6, with a widened interspinous distance of 20 mm between the C5-C6 spinous processes (8 mm interspinous distance between the other spinous processes; arrows, Figure 61.2). The case was discussed with the spine surgeon. As there was no midline tenderness, no soft tissue swelling anterior to the subluxation, no neurologic findings and the patient was reliable, the decision was made to place the patient in a hard collar and discharge him with oral pain medication and instructions to follow up with the spine surgeon. An MRI of the cervical spine was obtained two days later that demonstrated severe spinal stenosis with compression of the cervical spinal cord by a small posterior central disc protrusion at the C5-C6 level (Figure 61.3). The patient was admitted and underwent successful anterior cervical discectomy and C5-C6 cervical fusion by the spine surgeon.

Cervical spine subluxation

Cervical spine subluxation injury is associated with a flexion mechanism. Pure cervical spinal subluxation occurs when the ligamentous complexes rupture without associated bony injury.[1] This injury begins posteriorly in the nuchal ligament

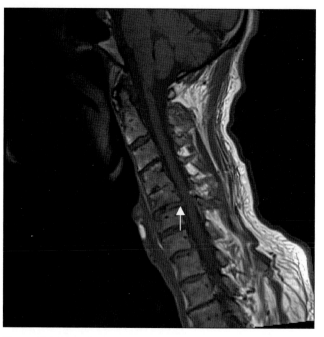

Figure 61.3 MRI (sagittal view) of the C-spine from a 77-year-old male with C5-C6 subluxation, demonstrating an area of severe spinal stenosis with compression of the cervical spinal cord anteriorly by a small, posterior central disc protrusion at the C5-C6 level (arrow).

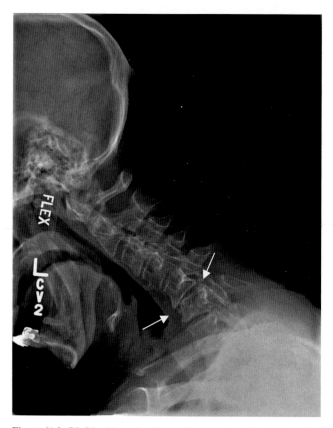

Figure 61.2 C5-C6 subluxation (arrows) demonstrated on flexion view of a 77-year-old male with posterior neck pain after a fall.

and proceeds anteriorly to involve other ligaments. As the anterior longitudinal ligament remains intact, associated bony injury is not seen.[2]

A standard C-spine trauma series is composed of five views: cross-table lateral, swimmer's, oblique, odontoid and anteroposterior. Although the lateral and oblique views may suggest cervical spine subluxation, stability of the cervical spine is best assessed with a functional radiologic examination that includes flexion and extension views during supervision. Flexion and extension radiographs should only be obtained in alert, cooperative patients with normal neurologic function and without radiographic evidence of unstable injuries on AP, lateral or odontoid views.[3] Flexion and extension views may identify true subluxation, as suggested on the lateral view.[1] Radiographically, anterior subluxation is characterized by a localized kyphotic angulation at the level of the injury; anterior rotation or displacement of the subluxed vertebra; anterior narrowing and posterior widening of the disc space; widening of the space between the subluxed vertebral body and the subjacent articular masses; displacement of the inferior articulating facets of the subluxed vertebra with respect to their contiguous subjacent facets; and widening of the interspinous space ("fanning").[4]

The exact role and timing of flexion-extension views are controversial.[1] The National Emergency X-Radiography Utilization Study (NEXUS) enrolled patients with blunt trauma selected for radiographic cervical spine imaging at 21 participating institutions.[5] In the NEXUS cohort, 86 (10.5%) of the 818 patients ultimately found to have cervical spine injury underwent flexion-extension testing.[6] Although two patients had bony injuries and four patients had subluxations demonstrated only on flexion-extension views, all six patients had other cervical spine injuries apparent on routine radiographs. The researchers concluded that flexion-extension imaging added little to the acute evaluation of patients with blunt trauma, and that other approaches, including CT, MRI or delayed flexion-extension imaging, may provide a more reasonable approach to adjunctive imaging.[6]

Anterior subluxation of the cervical spine is rarely associated with neurologic sequelae.[1,2] Nevertheless, most authorities approach this injury as if it were possibly unstable because of the potential for significant displacement with flexion. Although extremely rare, cases of anterior cervical spine subluxation have been associated with neurologic deficit.[2] When anterior subluxation is identified, the patient's cervical spine should be maintained in a hard cervical collar, and an orthopedic spine or neurosurgical consultation should be obtained.

KEY TEACHING POINTS

1. Cervical spine subluxation is associated with a flexion injury and can occur when the ligamentous complexes rupture without associated bony injury.
2. The clinical history of a patient supporting the head with their hands following cervical spine trauma is a clue to the presence of cervical ligamentous injury.
3. Flexion and extension views under supervision may identify true subluxation, as suggested by the lateral and oblique views.
4. The presence of anterior or posterior subluxation greater than 2 mm on one view and not present on the neutral view confirms ligamentous injury.
5. According to NEXUS, routine use of flexion-extension imaging adds little to the acute evaluation of patients with blunt cervical spine trauma.
6. Treatment of anterior cervical subluxation involves stabilizing the cervical spine with a hard collar and urgent consultation with a spine surgeon or neurosurgeon.

REFERENCES

[1] Hockberger RS, Kaji AH, Newton EJ. Spinal injuries. In: Marx JA, Hockberger RS, Walls RM, et al. (eds.). *Rosen's Emergency Medicine: Concepts and Clinical Practice*, 6th ed. Philadelphia: Mosby, 2006:398–439.

[2] Mueller JB, Davenport M, Belaval E, et al. Fractures, cervical spine. eMedicine Website. Available at http://www.emedicine.com/emerg/topic189.htm. Accessed June 29, 2008.

[3] Bagley LJ. Imaging of spinal trauma. *Radiol Clin N Am* 2006;44:1–12.

[4] Green JD, Harle TS, Harris JH. Anterior subluxation of the cervical spine: hyperflexion sprain. *Amer J Neuroradiol* 1981;2:243–50.

[5] Hoffman JR, Mower WR, Wolfson AB, et al. Validity of a set of clinical criteria to rule out injury to the cervical spine in patients with blunt trauma. *N Engl J Med* 2000;343:94–9.

[6] Pollack CV, Hendey GW, Martin DR. Use of flexion-extension radiographs of the cervical spine in blunt trauma. *Ann Emerg Med* 2001;38:8–11.

PART VIII

ORTHOPEDICS

62

Elbow trauma in a 3-year-old male

HISTORY OF PRESENT ILLNESS

A 3-year-old male presented to the ED with his parents after falling on his right elbow while running. The fall was witnessed by his mother, who denied any head trauma, loss of consciousness or other injuries. The child cried immediately and held his right elbow in flexion.

PHYSICAL EXAMINATION

GENERAL APPEARANCE: The patient was a well-nourished and well-developed child holding his right elbow and crying.

VITAL SIGNS

Temperature	98.1°F (36.7°C)
Pulse	120 beats/minute
Blood pressure	not obtained
Respirations	24 breaths/minute
Oxygen saturation	100% on room air

RIGHT UPPER EXTREMITY: Right elbow was swollen and diffusely tender to palpation; a strong radial pulse, brisk capillary refill and normal sensation were present. No tenderness, swelling or deformity to the right shoulder, wrist or hand was noted.

The right arm was placed in a sling for comfort and a radiograph of the elbow was obtained (Figure 61.1).

What is your diagnosis?

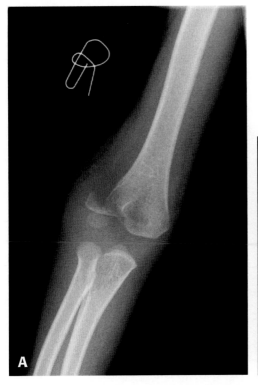
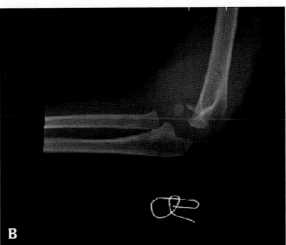

Figure 62.1 Anteroposterior (panel A) and lateral (panel B) views of the right elbow from a 3-year-old male with pain and swelling to the elbow after a fall.

The diagnosis is a Milch type II lateral condyle fracture. The radiographs demonstrate an oblique fracture at the supracondylar portion of distal humerus, with lateral displacement of the distal fracture fragments. Also, the radial shaft is not aligned with the capitellum, indicating subluxation/dislocation of the radius (Figure 62.2, panel B). The orthopedic surgeon was consulted and the patient underwent open reduction and internal fixation (ORIF) of the fracture in the OR. The patient was discharged home the following day.

Supracondylar and lateral condyle fractures in children

Supracondylar humerus fractures are the most common elbow fractures in pediatrics.[1] Classically described as fractures of the distal humerus occurring proximal to the distal humeral condyle through the olecranon fossa, these injuries represent nearly 17% of all childhood fractures and more than 50% of all elbow fractures.[1,2] These fractures occur more frequently in boys and occur typically between the ages of 5–8 years. In most series, the nondominant extremity is more commonly involved.[1] The majority of supracondylar fractures are extension injuries, which are associated with a fall on an outstretched hand, resulting in the proximal ulna transmitting force to the distal humerus.[2]

The child with a supracondylar fracture presents with swelling at the elbow and localized tenderness. With a supra-

condylar extension fracture, a proximal depression is noted over the triceps.[3] The physical examination should focus on the degree of swelling and neurovascular status. Any laceration or skin puncture near the fracture should result in emergent orthopedic consultation and antibiotics. Excessive swelling and ecchymosis at the elbow are concerning signs of extensive soft tissue injury, which is a significant risk factor for compartment syndrome.[3] Neurovascular evaluation includes palpation of the distal pulses and assessment of skin color, temperature and capillary refill, as well as the sensory and motor aspects of the median, radial and ulnar nerves. In the presence of ischemia, emergent reduction of the fracture is required.[3]

Radiographs should be obtained in children who present with a clinical presentation suggesting a supracondylar fracture, an unclear history, or localized tenderness or swelling of the elbow. Both an anteroposterior view in extension and a lateral view at 90° of flexion should be taken.[3] The radiograph should be assessed for the presence of fat pads, the anterior humeral line, and the figure-of-eight at the distal humerus (indicates a true lateral view). Fat pads are a nonspecific marker of hemorrhage and may be an indicator of an occult fracture. A widened anterior fat pad ("sail sign") is indicative of a fracture. The presence of a posterior fat pad is never normal and is indicative of pathology (also indicates a fracture). The anterior humeral line is a line drawn through the anterior cortex of the humerus that intersects the capitellum in its middle third (Figure 62.3). In the presence of a posteriorly displaced supracondylar fracture, the anterior humeral line

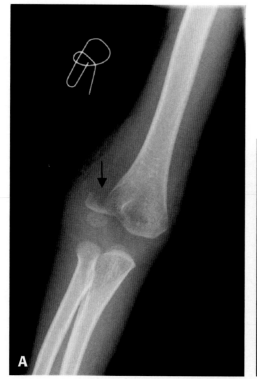
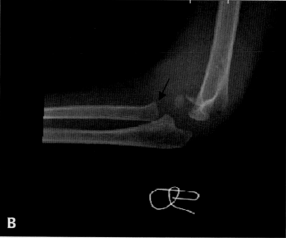

Figure 62.2 Anteroposterior (panel A) and lateral (panel B) views of the right elbow from a 3-year-old male demonstrating oblique fracture at the supracondylar portion of distal humerus, with lateral displacement of the distal fracture fragments (arrow, panel A) and subluxation/dislocation of the radial head (arrow, panel B).

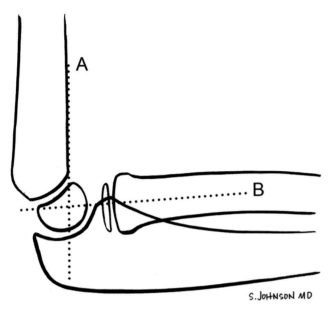

S. JOHNSON MD

Figure 62.3 Illustration of normal anatomic relationships in a pediatric elbow, lateral view (A – anterior humeral line, B – radiocapitellar line).

passes though the anterior third of the capitellum or may entirely miss the capitellum.[3] An assessment of the figure-of-eight requires a true lateral view; disruption of this image indicates a supracondylar fracture.

The Gartland classification system is used for extension-type supracondylar humerus fractures.[4] A type I fracture is essentially a nondisplaced fracture. A type II fracture still has the posterior periosteum intact connecting the distal fragment and the humeral shaft; the anterior humeral line is anterior to the capitellum and does not intersect it. The type III supracondylar fracture has complete displacement of the distal fragment relative to the humeral shaft with fractures of both cortices; there is often significant displacement.[4] Treatment of a type I fracture involves splinting the extremity in a long-arm posterior splint and instructing the patient to return for radiographs in one week; if the fracture remains nondisplaced, the splint is exchanged for a long-arm cast.[4] Type II fractures require pediatric orthopedic evaluation. The choice of therapy for type II fractures, closed reduction versus percutaneous pinning, is based on the degree of deformity as well as the adequacy and stability of the fracture reduction.[3] All type II supracondylar fractures require orthopedic consultation for the evaluation of closed or open reduction with percutaneous pin placement, hospitalization for vigilant neurovascular assessments and close follow up.[3] Treatment of type III fractures is generally surgical.

The two major complications of supracondylar fractures in children include cubitus varus (decreased carrying angle of the upper extremity), which is relatively common, and vascular injury (i.e., from compartment syndrome) leading to Volkmann ischemic contracture, which is less common but has considerable morbidity.[4,5] The potential for significant complications with supracondylar humerus fractures mandates accurate diagnosis and urgent orthopedic consultation.[4] Most children with anything more than the most trivial displacement are admitted for 24–48 hours of observation to frequently reassess their extremity's neurovascular status.

Fractures of the lateral condyle represent 15–17% of pediatric elbow fractures and are the second most common operative elbow fractures in children.[4,6] The lateral condyle functions as the origin of the extensor muscle mass, as well as the lateral collateral ligamentous complex. Most fractures occur in patients 5–7 years of age. The most common mechanism of injury occurs when a varus force is applied to the elbow, causing the extensor muscles and lateral collateral ligaments to avulse the lateral condyle.[4,6] The risk of neurovascular compromise in a lateral condyle fracture is much lower than that of a supracondylar facture.[4]

The Milch classification system is used for describing lateral condyle fractures.[4] A type I fracture extends through the ossification center of the capitellum, entering the joint lateral to the trochlear groove. A type II fracture extends medial to the trochlear groove, making the humeral-ulnar joint less stable. The most important determination is whether or not the fracture is displaced.[4] Only the truly nondisplaced fractures should be treated nonoperatively, with immobilization in a long-arm cast. Plain radiographs of the elbow are obtained two or three times in the first three weeks to assure that reduction is maintained.[6] Any displaced fracture should be treated with open reduction and percutaneous pinning.[4] The most common complications following lateral condyle fractures include nonunion, cubitus varus/valgus, and fishtail deformity of the distal humerus (a rare complication arising from avascular necrosis of the distal fragment).[4]

KEY TEACHING POINTS

1. Supracondylar humerus fractures are the most common elbow fracture in children, accounting for 50–60% of cases.
2. Radiographs of the elbow should be obtained in children who present with a clinical presentation suggesting a supracondylar or lateral condylar fracture, and should include an anteroposterior view in extension and a true lateral view at 90° of flexion.
3. The potential for significant complications with supracondylar humerus fractures mandates accurate diagnosis and urgent orthopedic consultation.
4. The risk of neurovascular compromise in a lateral condyle fracture is much lower than that of a supracondylar facture.
5. The most important determination in assessing lateral condyle fractures is whether or not the fracture is displaced. Only the truly nondisplaced fractures should be treated nonoperatively, with immobilization in a long-arm cast.

REFERENCES

[1] Fayssoux RS, Stankovits L, Domzalski M, et al. Fractures of the distal humeral metaphyseal-diaphyseal junction in children. *J Pediatr Orthop* 2008;28:142–6.

[2]   Shore RM, Grayhack JJ. Elbow trauma, pediatric. eMedicine Website. Available at http://www.emedicine.com/radio/topic 868.htm. Accessed July 6, 2008.

[3]   Carson S, Woolridge DP, Colletti J, et al. Pediatric upper extremity injuries. *Pediatr Clin N Am* 2006;53:41–67.

[4]   Shrader MW. Pediatric supracondylar fractures and pediatric physeal elbow fractures. *Orthop Clin N Am* 2008;39:163–71.

[5]   Rittenberry TJ, Greenfield RH. Injuries of the upper extremities. In: Strange GR, Ahrens WR, Lelyveld S (eds.). *Pediatric Emergency Medicine: A Comprehensive Study Guide*, 2nd ed. New York: McGraw-Hill, 2002:141–3.

[6]   Tamai J, Lou J, Nagda S, et al. Pediatric elbow fractures: pearls and pitfalls. *Univ Penn Orthop J* 2002;15:43–51.

63

Foot trauma in a 12-year-old male

HISTORY OF PRESENT ILLNESS

A 12-year-old male was brought to the ED by ambulance after a car had run over his right foot while crossing a busy street. He reported severe pain to the foot as well as some numbness and tingling, but denied loss of consciousness or other injuries. The right lower extremity was placed in a splint by the paramedics, an IV was placed and 2 mg morphine sulfate had been administered for pain.

PHYSICAL EXAMINATION

GENERAL APPEARANCE: The patient was a well-developed male in moderate discomfort.

VITAL SIGNS

Temperature	98.1°F (36.7°C)
Pulse	110 beats/minute
Blood pressure	120/85 mmHg
Respirations	22 breaths/minute
Oxygen saturation	100% on room air

HEENT: Atraumatic, normocephalic, PERRL, EOMI.

NECK: Supple, no midline tenderness.

CARDIOVASCULAR: Regular rate and rhythm without rubs, murmurs or gallops.

LUNGS: Clear to auscultation bilaterally, no chest wall tenderness.

ABDOMEN: Soft, nontender, nondistended.

RIGHT FOOT: Diffusely swollen, tense and tender to touch, ecchymotic and slightly dusky at the medial/dorsal aspect. Sensation to light touch was grossly intact. The patient was unable to move his toes secondary to pain and swelling. Severe pain was elicited on passive dorsiflexion of the toes. A dorsalis pedis pulse could not be palpated on the right foot, nor could it be elicited by Doppler stethoscope. There was no obvious deformity to the ankle or the remainder of the right lower extremity.

NEUROLOGIC: Nonfocal.

An additional dose of morphine sulfate IV was administered; blood was drawn and sent for laboratory testing, whereas the foot remained splinted and elevated with ice packs applied. Radiographs of the foot were obtained (Figure 63.1). The patient was not allowed anything by mouth.

What is your diagnosis?

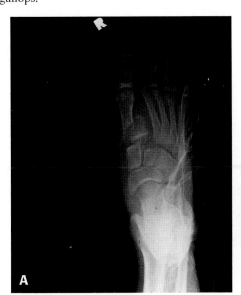
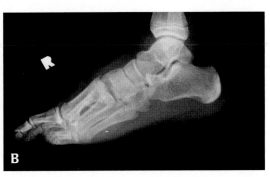

Figure 63.1 Anteroposterior (panel A) and lateral (panel B) radiographs of the right foot from a 12-year-old male with right foot trauma.

ANSWER

Radiographs of the right foot demonstrate a comminuted, displaced fracture at the base of the first metatarsal, as well as distal fractures of the second through fourth metatarsals with substantial displacement. These injuries are consistent with a Lisfranc fracture-dislocation. The podiatry service was urgently consulted and the patient was taken to the OR. Compartment pressures of the right foot were measured and found to be 58–62 mmHg (normal compartment pressures of foot 5.0 ± 2.5 mmHg),[1] consistent with right foot compartment syndrome. The patient underwent compartment fasciotomies, as well as an open reduction and internal fixation of the right foot fractures and dislocation. The final postoperative diagnosis was right foot compartment syndrome, right foot Lisfranc fracture-dislocation, and fractures of the right second, third and fourth metatarsal heads (postoperative radiograph, Figure 63.2).

Lisfranc injuries

Although fractures of the proximal first through fourth metatarsals are less common than other metatarsal fractures, they warrant special consideration because they are often associated with injury to the Lisfranc ligament complex (Figure 63.3).[2, 9] These crucial ligaments hold the metatarsal bases rigidly in place, maintaining the arch of the foot and anchoring the metatarsals to the rest of the body. Injuries to this ligament complex, even if subtle, can cause long-term disability and are important to detect.[2]

Complex forces, usually high-energy, may result in injury to the metatarsal-tarsal (Lisfranc) joint.[3,4] Direct crushing blows can displace the metatarsals in the direction of the force. More commonly, indirect or rotational mechanisms can result in injury to the Lisfranc joint. Examples include falls from a height, striking a fixed plantar-flexed foot on the floorboard in a motor vehicle collision, or even a misstep onto an uneven surface with axial force transmitted up the metatarsals displacing them dorsally relative to the tarsals.[4] The patient with Lisfranc injury is unable to bear weight on the affected foot. The dorsum of the midfoot shows swelling, ecchymosis, deformity and tenderness.[5] Pedal pulses may be difficult to palpate because of the swelling, but assessment of perfusion of the foot distal to the injury should be made based on warmth, color, and hand-held Doppler.[5]

Standard anteroposterior and lateral radiographs of the foot are usually sufficient to demonstrate the fracture.[5] Fractures of the second metatarsal, cuboid or navicular should increase suspicion of disruption to the Lisfranc joint. The most consistent radiographic finding is loss of the usual alignment between the medial borders of the second metatarsal and second cuneiform.[4] After assessing distal neurovascular status, immobilize patients with suspected Lisfranc joint injuries but normal radiographic findings with a posterior splint, prohibit weight-bearing, and consult orthopedics or podiatry for urgent follow up.

Consult orthopedic surgery for displaced fractures requiring reduction, casting or operative fixation. Open reduction and fixation is necessary if adequate reduction cannot be achieved or maintained.

Compartment syndrome of the foot

Compartment syndrome can occur in the foot as in other parts of the body. The mechanism of injury is usually severe

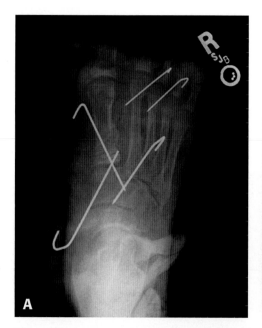
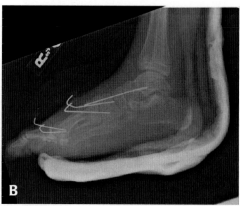

Figure 63.2 Anteroposterior (panel A) and lateral (panel B) radiographs of the right foot from a 12-year-old male following compartment fasciotomies, open reduction and internal fixation of a Lisfranc fracture-dislocation.

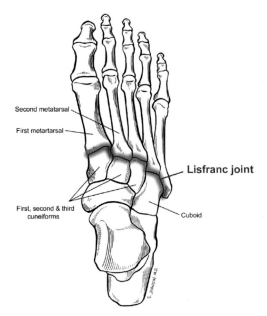

Figure 63.3 Lisfranc joint.

local trauma and associated skeletal injury. Classic symptoms and signs are progressive pain, numbness in the toes and decreased motion.[6] However, these are the same symptoms that one expects to find with concomitant foot fractures and severe injury. Tense tissue bulging may be the most reliable symptom.[6] Compartment pressures are elevated.

The nine compartments of the foot can be placed into four groups: the intrinsic compartment, which comprises the four intrinsic muscles between the first and fifth metatarsals; the medial compartment, which comprises the abductor hallucis and flexor hallucis brevis; the central calcaneal compartment, which comprises the flexor digitorum brevis, the quadratus plantae and the adductor hallucis; and the lateral compartment, which comprises the flexor digiti minimi brevis and the abductor digiti minimi.[6]

In examining a patient with potential compartment syndrome of the foot, pain alone is not sufficient for the diagnosis.[6] Patients with a burning quality of pain, delayed onset or increasing severity of pain, or pain on passive stretch of the compartment merit evaluation for compartment syndrome.[7] Increased pain on passive dorsiflexion of metatarsophalangeal joints is a key finding, indicating myoneural ischemia in the intrinsic muscles.[6] The soft tissues are often visibly swollen, and the compartment will usually have a tense ("woody") feeling on palpation.[7] Poor capillary refill and absent pulses are late findings. In the presence of massive swelling of the foot, which usually accompanies these injuries, pulses may not be palpable. Currently, the most reliable means of diagnosing compartment syndrome is to directly measure pressure in the compartment using an automated device such as a Stryker manometer.[7] Appropriate treatment for a suspected compartment syndrome of the foot is urgent and complete fasciotomy.

Silas et al. reviewed the cases of seven children and teenagers identified as having compartment syndrome of the foot during a five-year period.[8] The average age at the time of diagnosis was 10 years (range 4–16 years). The cause of the compartment syndrome was a crush injury in six patients and a motor vehicle collision in one. All patients had swelling and pain with passive motion but none had neurovascular deficits. Only the two oldest children had an osseous injury that necessitated open reduction and internal fixation, but all had elevated compartment pressures ranging from 38–55 mmHg. All seven patients had fasciotomies of the nine compartments of the foot, and the skin was closed primarily within five days following the operation. No patients had complications or required skin grafting. All patients had a good or excellent result after an average duration of follow up of 41 months (range 23–53 months).

KEY TEACHING POINTS

1. Lisfranc fracture-dislocations of the foot generally result from high-energy forces, such as crushing trauma to the foot (often in flexion or rotation).
2. Patients with Lisfranc fracture-dislocations commonly present with midfoot pain, swelling and decreased ability to bear weight.
3. The most consistent radiographic finding in Lisfranc joint dislocations is loss of the usual alignment between the medial borders of the second metatarsal and second cuneiform.
4. Patients with Lisfranc injuries require urgent consultation with an orthopedic or podiatric specialist.
5. In compartment syndrome of the foot, findings on examination include increased pain on passive dorsiflexion of the metatarsophalangeal joints, poor capillary refill and absent pulses (late findings).
6. Appropriate treatment for suspected compartment syndrome of the foot is urgent and complete fasciotomy.

REFERENCES

[1] Dayton P, Goldman FD, Barton E. Compartment pressure in the foot. Analysis of normal values and measurement technique. *J Am Podiatr Med Assoc* 1990;80:521–5.
[2] Hatch RL, Alsobrook JA, Clugston JR. Diagnosis and management of metatarsal fractures. *Am Fam Physician* 2007;76:817–26.
[3] Hays EP. Ankle and foot injuries. In: Ferrera PC, Colucciello SA, Marx JA, et al. (eds.). *Trauma Management, an Emergency Medicine Approach*. Philadelphia: Mosby, 2001:460–2.
[4] Simon RR, Koenigsknecht SJ. Fractures and dislocations of the foot. In: Simon RR, Koenigsknecht SJ (eds.). *Emergency Orthopedics of the Extremities*, 4th ed. New York: McGraw-Hill, 2001:549–51.
[5] Newton EJ, Love J. Emergency department management of selected orthopedic injuries. *Emerg Med Clin N Am* 2007;25:763–93.

[6] Compartment syndrome of the foot. In *Wheeless' Textbook of Orthopedics*. Available online at http://www.wheelessonline.com/ortho/compartment_syndrome_of_the_foot. Accessed June 23, 2008.

[7] Newton EJ. Acute complications of extremity trauma. *Emerg Med Clin N Am* 2007;25:751–61.

[8] Silas SI, Herzenberg JE, Myerson MS, et al. Compartment syndrome of the foot in children. *J Bone and Joint Surg* 1995;77:356–61.

[9] Schofer JM, O'Brien S. Images in emergency medicine: Lisfranc fracture-dislocation. *West JEM* 2008;9:56–7.

64

Forearm pain and swelling in a 14-year-old male

HISTORY OF PRESENT ILLNESS

A 14-year-old left-hand dominant male presented to the ED after falling backward on his outstretched left hand during a martial arts match. The patient experienced the sudden onset of severe pain with significant deformity to the left forearm. Upon presentation to the ED, the patient complained of severe pain to his distal left forearm but denied numbness, tingling or weakness.

PHYSICAL EXAMINATION

GENERAL APPEARANCE: The patient was a well-developed male in moderate discomfort.

VITAL SIGNS

Temperature	98.5°F (36.9°C)
Pulse	110 beats/minute
Blood pressure	120/85 mmHg
Respirations	20 breaths/minute

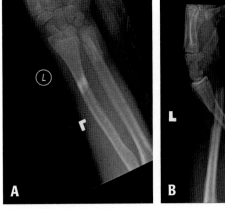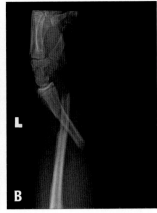

Figure 64.2 Anteroposterior (panel A) and lateral (panel B) radiographs of the left wrist and forearm from a 14-year-old male after a fall on the outstretched hand.

RIGHT UPPER EXTREMITY: Significant dorsal displacement of the distal forearm ("dinner fork deformity"), with a small puncture wound noted on the volar aspect of the forearm just proximal to the deformity (arrow, Figure 64.1). The radial and ulnar pulses were easily palpable, and sensation and motor function distal to the deformity were intact. The right shoulder, elbow, wrist and hand were without deformity or tenderness.

Anteroposterior and lateral radiographs of the wrist and forearm were obtained (Figure 64.2).

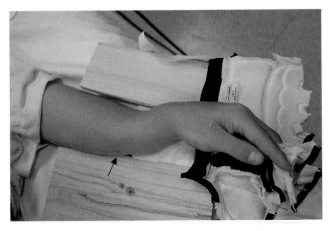

Figure 64.1 Left forearm of a 14-year-old male after falling backward on his outstretched hand (arrow indicates puncture wound).

What is your diagnosis?

ANSWER

The diagnosis is open distal radial and ulnar fracture (both bone forearm fracture) with significant shortening, dorsal displacement and volar angulation of the distal fracture fragments. Treatment is urgent closed reduction followed by definitive open reduction and internal fixation (ORIF). The patient received cefazolin intravenously prior to closed reduction, as well as multiple doses of morphine sulfate for pain control. Urgent closed reduction was performed in the ED using intravenous fentanyl and midazolam for procedural sedation (post-reduction radiographs, Figure 64.3). The patient was admitted to the orthopedic service for definitive ORIF of the fractures that same evening.

Open forearm fractures

Fractures of the shaft of the radius or ulna have been reported to account for 10–45% of pediatric fractures; 75–84% of pediatric forearm fractures occur distally.[1,2] These injuries vary greatly; they may involve one or both bones, and may be complete or greenstick fractures (fracture through only one cortex or incomplete, seen in pediatric cases) in as high as 50%. Pediatric forearm fractures are usually successfully treated with closed reduction because the substantial remodeling potential of pediatric bone allows for excellent healing. Forearm fractures are usually the result of a fall on an outstretched hand, but direct trauma of significant force can cause forearm fractures as well.[1]

Forearm fractures are classified according to location, degree of displacement, and degree of angulation.[2] Patients

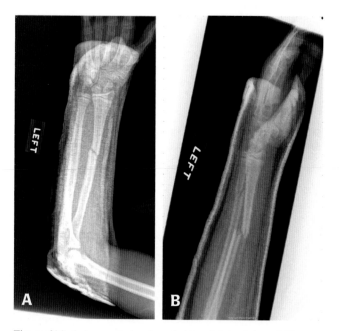

Figure 64.3 Anteroposterior (panel A) and lateral (panel B) post-reduction radiographs of a left both bone forearm fracture from a 14-year-old boy following a fall on the outstretched hand.

TABLE 64.1 Gustilo classification of open fractures[5]	
Type I	Puncture wound of 1 cm or less, with minimal contamination or muscle crushing.
Type II	Laceration more than 1 cm long with moderate soft tissue damage and crushing. Bone coverage is adequate and comminution is minimal.
Type IIIA	Extensive soft tissue damage, often caused by a high-energy injury with a severe crushing component. Massively contaminated wounds and severely comminuted or segmental fractures are included in this subtype. Bone coverage is adequate.
Type IIIB	Extensive soft tissue damage with periosteal stripping and bone exposure, usually with severe contamination and bone comminution. Flap coverage is required.
Type IIIC	Arterial injury requiring repair.

with fractures of the distal one-third (the most common) present with the classic "dinner fork" deformity. The skin requires careful examination for any in-to-out puncture because such an injury requires immediate orthopedic consultation and operative treatment.[1,2] It is essential that at least two radiographic views be obtained to determine an accurate measurement of displacement and angulation. If only one forearm bone is fractured, radiographs of the wrist and elbow should be obtained to exclude a Galeazzi (fracture of the radial shaft with dislocation of the radioulnar joint) or Monteggia (fracture of the ulna with dislocation of the radial head) fracture-dislocation.[1] Surgical indications for forearm fractures include open fractures, failed or unstable reductions, and vascular injuries, as well as fractures in skeletally-mature individuals (older children where remodeling is not likely).[2,3]

An open fracture is characterized by soft tissue disruption that results in communication of the fracture site with the outside environment.[4] Open fractures are severe injuries with a potential for serious complications, such as infection or nonunion. The main principles of open fracture management include careful evaluation of the injury, prevention of infection, wound management with soft tissue coverage, fracture stabilization, and promotion of healing by early bone grafting or other supplemental procedures.[4] A classification system for open fractures has been devised by Gustilo and colleagues (Table 64.1).[5]

Intravenous antibiotic administration should start as soon as possible, tetanus status should be updated and surgical management should begin as soon as the patient has been adequately evaluated and resuscitated. Approximately 65% of patients with open fractures have wound contamination with microorganisms; therefore, antibiotics are not used for prophylaxis but rather for treatment of wound contamination. Delayed surgical management in children and adults has not been associated with an increased infection rate in patients who receive early antibiotic therapy.[4] Aggressive intraoperative irrigation is of critical importance.

KEY TEACHING POINTS

1. Fractures of the shaft of the radius or ulna may account for 10–45% of pediatric fractures; 75–84% of pediatric forearm fractures occur distally.

2. Forearm fractures are usually the result of a fall on an outstretched hand, but direct trauma of significant force can also cause forearm fractures.

3. Pediatric forearm fractures are usually treated successfully with closed reduction because of the substantial remodeling potential of pediatric bone.

4. Open fractures are injuries with a potential for serious complications, including infection and nonunion, and require prompt antibiotic administration and surgical management.

5. Neurovascular status should be evaluated for all extremity injuries (including fractures); if vascular compromise is present, immediate reduction is necessary before radiographic evaluation.

REFERENCES

[1] Carson S, Woolridge DP, Colletti J, Kilgore K. Pediatric upper extremity injuries. *Pediatr Clin N Am* 2006;53:41–67.

[2] Benjamin HJ, Hang BT. Common acute upper extremity injuries in sports. *Clin Ped Emerg Med* 2007;8:15–30.

[3] Canale ST. Fractures and dislocations in children; forearm fractures. In: Canale ST (ed.). *Campbell's Operative Orthopedics*, 10th ed. Philadelphia: Mosby, 2003:1405–7.

[4] Zalavras CG, Patzakis MJ, Holtom PD, Sherman R. Management of open fractures. *Infect Dis Clin N Am* 2005;19: 915–29.

[5] Gustilo RB, Mendoza RM, Williams DN. Problems in the management of type III (severe) open fractures: a new classification of type III open fractures. *J Trauma* 1984;24:742–6.

65

Foot pain while playing soccer in a 22-year-old male

HISTORY OF PRESENT ILLNESS

A 22-year-old male presented to the ED complaining of left foot pain after an inversion injury to the foot while playing soccer. He reported the sudden onset of severe pain followed by swelling and inability to bear weight on his right foot immediately following the injury. He denied numbness or tingling to the foot.

PHYSICAL EXAMINATION

GENERAL APPEARANCE: The patient was a well-developed male lying supine on the gurney with his right foot raised, in no acute discomfort.

VITAL SIGNS

Temperature	98.6°C (37°C)
Pulse	74 beats/minute
Blood pressure	130/85 mmHg
Respirations	20 breaths/minute
Oxygen saturation	100% on room air

LEFT FOOT AND ANKLE: Swelling of the dorsal-lateral and plantar aspects of the left foot, with tenderness to palpation at the base of the fifth metatarsal on the plantar aspect. No tenderness or swelling of the ankle; the patient was unable to bear weight on the left foot. The right foot was neurovascularly intact.

Radiographs of the left foot were obtained (Figure 65.1).

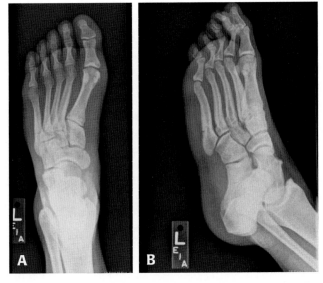

Figure 65.1 Anteroposterior (panel A) and oblique (panel B) radiographs of a 22-year-old male after inversion injury to the left foot playing soccer.

What is your diagnosis?

ANSWER

The diagnosis is a Jones fracture (fracture of the base of the fifth metatarsal). The radiographs demonstrate a transverse fracture of the proximal fifth metatarsal at the junction of the diaphysis and metaphysis (arrows, Figure 65.2). The patient's foot was elevated with ice packs applied, and subsequently placed in a short-leg splint. The patient was given crutches and pain medication and instructed to continue non-weight-bearing and elevation of the foot at rest. Follow up was arranged with the orthopedist, at which time a short-leg cast was placed. The fracture was treated nonsurgically, with immobilization and non-weight-bearing for six weeks.

Jones fracture

In 1902, Sir Robert Jones was the first to describe a fracture of the proximal fifth metatarsal.[1] A true Jones fracture is defined as a transverse fracture of the proximal fifth metatarsal at the junction of the diaphysis and metaphysic, without extension distal to the intermetatarsal articulation of the fourth and fifth metatarsals. Fractures generally begin laterally in the more distal portion of the tuberosity and extend transversely or obliquely into the area of the medial cortex, where the fifth metatarsal articulates with the fourth metatarsal.[1] The injury is believed to occur when a large adduction force is applied to the forefoot with the ankle plantar flexed (e.g., pivoting or cutting with most of the body weight on the metatarsal heads). When high load on the plantar aspect of the fifth metatarsal head creates a large bending motion, the bone fractures at the junction of the proximal diaphysis and the metaphysis.[1]

A Jones fracture is located within 1.5 cm distal to the tuberosity of the fifth metatarsal, and should not be confused with the more common avulsion fracture of the fifth

metatarsal styloid process.[2] It is not due to peroneus brevis tendon avulsion but rather a twisting inversion injury of the foot. More proximal injuries are frequently misinterpreted as Jones fractures but really are avulsion fractures caused by the peroneus brevis tendon. These fractures heal quickly, whereas more distal fractures may undergo fibrous union only.[2] Radiographically, acute fractures should show sharp fracture margins and no intramedullary sclerosis. Delayed union will show a persistent fracture line in both cortices, periosteal callus and intramedullary sclerosis. A stress fracture is revealed by a widened fracture line and varying degrees of medullary sclerosis.[2]

Emergency treatment of Jones fractures involves ice, elevation, splinting of the injured foot and pain control.[3] The definitive treatment of Jones fractures may be nonoperative or operative. Nonoperative treatment varies from functional bracing to casting, but typically involves the application of a non-weight-bearing short-leg cast for six weeks for best results.[1,4] The time needed to achieve union is a minimum of two months, with delayed union or nonunion reported in up to 50% of cases. Operative treatment involves intramedullary screw fixation or bone grafting. These allow earlier weight-bearing and generally result in union in less than three months. As many as 50% of patients with this fracture develop persistent nonunions, requiring bone grafting and internal fixation.[3]

KEY TEACHING POINTS

1. A Jones fracture is a transverse fracture of the proximal fifth metatarsal at the junction of the diaphysis and metaphysis without extension distal to the intermetatarsal articulation of the fourth and fifth metatarsals.
2. The mechanism of injury in a Jones fracture involves a large adduction force applied to the forefoot with the ankle plantar flexed, causing the fifth metatarsal to fracture.
3. Emergent treatment of Jones fractures involves ice, elevation, splinting of the injured foot and pain control.
4. The definitive treatment of Jones fractures may be nonoperative (bracing or casting and non-weight-bearing for six weeks) or operative (intramedullary screw fixation or bone grafting).

REFERENCES

[1] Fetzer GB, Wright RW. Metatarsal fractures and fractures of the proximal fifth metatarsal. *Clin Sports Med* 2006;25:139–50.
[2] Jones fracture. In *Radiographic Pathology Index X-Ray* 2000. Available online at http://www.e-radiography.net/radpath/j/jones_fracture.htm. Accessed June 30, 2008.
[3] Silbergleit R. Fractures, foot. eMedicine Website. Available at http://www.emedicine.com/emerg/topic195.htm. Accessed June 30, 2008.
[4] Ortiguera CJ, Fischer DA. A review of the current treatment for fracture of the proximal fifth metatarsal first described by Jones. *Ortho Tech Rev* 2000;2:1–2.

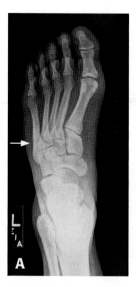
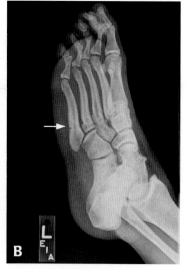

Figure 65.2 Anteroposterior (panel A) and oblique (panel B) radiographs of a 22-year-old male with a Jones fracture (arrows).

66

Elbow trauma in a 29-year-old male

HISTORY OF PRESENT ILLNESS

A 29-year-old right-handed male presented to the ED one day after falling on his right elbow while skating. The patient reported pain and swelling to the elbow, as well as limited ability to flex and extend his elbow secondary to pain. He denied weakness or numbness of his right upper extremity or other injuries.

PHYSICAL EXAMINATION

GENERAL APPEARANCE: The patient was a well-developed male holding his right elbow in a flexed position, in no acute discomfort.

VITAL SIGNS

Temperature	98.6°F (37°C)
Pulse	75 beats/minute
Blood pressure	125/85 mmHg
Respirations	20 breaths/minute
Oxygen saturation	100% on room air

RIGHT UPPER EXTREMITY: Swelling to the elbow and tenderness over the radial head, as well as pain and limited range of motion with attempted supination or pronation of the right forearm. Mild ecchymosis to the elbow, no wound present. The right shoulder, forearm, wrist and hand were nontender, without swelling or deformity. The forearm, wrist and hand were neurovascularly intact.

An ice pack was applied to the elbow, and an elbow radiograph was obtained (Figure 66.1).

What is your diagnosis?

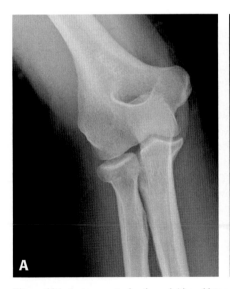
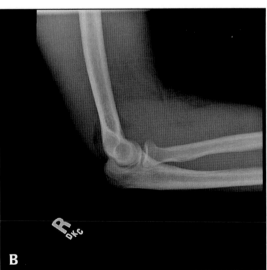

Figure 66.1 Anteroposterior (panel A) and lateral (panel B) radiographs of the right elbow from a 29-year-old male after a fall.

ANSWER

The diagnosis is a radial head fracture. The lateral radiograph demonstrates both a posterior and anterior ("sail sign") fat pad (arrows, Figure 66.2) resulting from intra-articular hemorrhage. This is indicative of intra-articular pathology, most commonly caused by a radial head fracture in adults. The subtle radial head fracture can be appreciated on the anteroposterior view of the elbow (arrow, Figure 66.3). The patient was placed in a sling and referred to the orthopedic clinic, where recommendations were made to continue using the sling as needed with frequent range of motion exercises.

The fat pad sign and radial head fractures

Normally, on a lateral radiograph of the elbow held in 90° of flexion, a lucency that represents fat is present along the anterior surface of the distal humerus; on a normal radiograph, no lucency is visualized along its posterior surface.[1] An elevated anterior lucency or a visible posterior lucency on a true lateral radiograph of an elbow flexed at 90° is described as a positive fat pad sign.[1] Fat pad signs provide radiological evidence of a joint effusion in the elbow joint, appearing as translucent areas on the lateral radiograph of the elbow flexed to a right angle.[2]

In obtaining radiographs of the elbow, the lateral view is probably the most useful. In this view, the anterior humeral line should bisect the middle third of the capitellum.[3] In minimally displaced supracondylar fractures, the distal humerus is displaced posteriorly so that the anterior humeral line bisects the anterior third of the capitellum (or misses it completely), therefore alerting the physician to the presence of

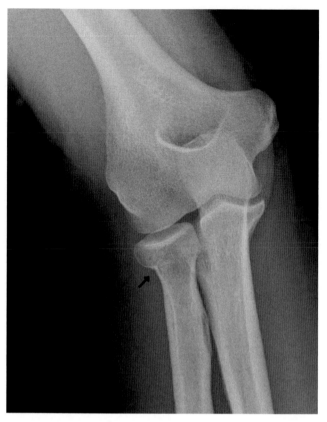

Figure 66.3 Anteroposterior view of the right elbow demonstrating a radial head fracture (arrow).

this fracture.[3] The lateral radiograph may show an anterior fat pad protruding from the coronoid fossa at the distal humerus. This finding is normal unless the pad is bulging or in the shape of a ship's sail.[4] This sail sign may indicate fluid in the joint, although alone it may not be a reliable predictor of a fracture. However, the posterior fat pad sits snugly within the olecranon fossa, and is never seen without a fracture around the elbow.[4] In this case, blood pushes the fat pad laterally, making it visible on lateral radiograph of the elbow. Therefore, visualization of a posterior fat pad on a true lateral radiograph of the elbow suggests the presence of an occult fracture around the elbow and, if the fracture is not seen, warrants oblique views of the elbow, splinting and close follow up.[4]

The presence of a fat pad sign following elbow trauma in adults is most commonly associated with the presence of a radial head fracture (86% of fractures associated with a fat pad sign were radial head fractures in one study).[5] The fat pad sign has been shown to be sensitive in detecting radial head fractures but is not specific to these fractures.[2] Fat pad signs can also be seen in cases of inflammation, infection or neoplasm associated with the elbow joint.[1,2] The absence of a fat pad sign on the lateral elbow radiograph is a reliable indicator that a fracture around the elbow is not present.[2]

In the acute setting, occult radial head fractures can be treated with a sling for comfort.[3] For nondisplaced radial head fractures, results are generally good with a short period of immobilization followed by early range of motion.[6] Conversely,

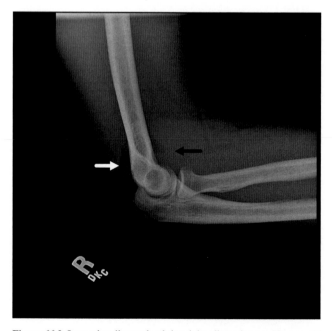

Figure 66.2 Lateral radiograph of the right elbow from a 29-year-old male demonstrating anterior (dark arrow) and posterior (white arrow) fat pads from a radial head fracture.

any significantly displaced fracture merits orthopedic consultation and referral.

KEY TEACHING POINTS

1. An elevated anterior lucency or visible posterior lucency on a true lateral radiograph of an elbow flexed at 90° is described as a positive fat pad sign; the presence of a fat pad sign following elbow trauma in adults is most commonly associated with a radial head fracture.
2. The absence of a positive fat pad sign on the lateral elbow radiograph is reliable evidence for the absence of a fracture around the elbow.
3. In the acute setting, occult radial head fractures can be treated with a sling for comfort and a short period of immobilization, followed by early range of motion.

REFERENCES

[1] Goswami GK. The fat pad sign. *Radiology* 2002;222:419–20.
[2] Irshad F, Shaw NJ, Gregory RJH. Reliability of fat-pad sign in radial head/neck fractures of the elbow. *Injury* 1997; 28:433–5.
[3] Benjamin HJ, Hang BT. Common acute upper extremity injuries in sports. *Clin Ped Emerg Med* 2007;8:15–30.
[4] McQuillen KK. Musculoskeletal disorders. In: Marx JA, Hockberger RS, Walls RM, et al. (eds.). *Rosen's Emergency Medicine: Concepts and Clinical Practice*, 6th ed. Philadelphia: Mosby, 2006:2694–5.
[5] O'Dwyer H, O'Sullivan P, Fitzgerald D, et al. The fat pad sign following elbow trauma in adults: its usefulness and reliability in suspecting occult fracture. *J Comput Assist Tomogr* 2004;28:562–5.
[6] Rizzo M, Nunley JA. Fractures of the elbow's lateral column radial head and capitellum. *Hand Clin* 2002;18:21–42.

67

Forearm trauma in a 32-year-old male

HISTORY OF PRESENT ILLNESS

A 32-year-old right-hand dominant male arrived by ambulance to the ED after colliding his motorcycle with another vehicle. The patient was helmeted, awake and alert and complained of left forearm and elbow pain. He denied numbness to his left forearm, wrist or hand. He did not lose consciousness, and denied other injuries.

PHYSICAL EXAMINATION

GENERAL APPEARANCE: The patient was a well-developed male holding his left forearm in moderate discomfort.

VITAL SIGNS

Temperature	98.2°F (36.8°C)
Pulse	95 beats/minute
Blood pressure	140/95 mmHg
Respirations	22 breath/minute
Oxygen saturation	100% on room air

HEENT: Atraumatic, normocephalic, PERRL, EOMI.

NECK: Supple, no midline tenderness.

CARDIOVASCULAR: Regular rate and rhythm without rubs, murmurs or gallops.

CHEST: No chest wall tenderness, lungs clear to auscultation bilaterally.

ABDOMEN: Soft, nontender, nondistended.

LEFT FOREARM: Swelling and deformity to the mid-portion of the left forearm with tenderness to palpation. A small wound was noted over the deformity (Figure 67.1), as well as tenderness to the elbow over the radial head. The forearm, wrist and hand were neurovascularly intact.

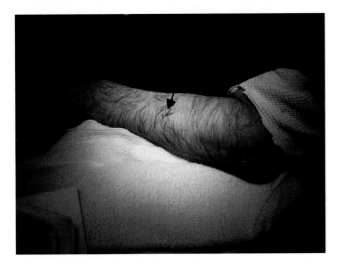

Figure 67.1 Left forearm of a 32-year-old man after motorcycle collision (arrow indicates wound).

A peripheral intravenous line was placed, morphine sulfate was administered for pain control, and radiographs of the forearm, elbow and wrist were obtained (Figure 67.2).

What is your diagnosis?

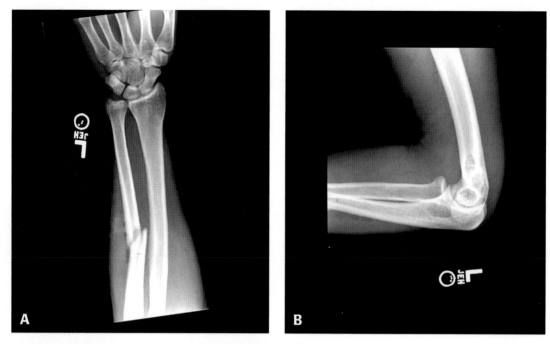

Figure 67.2 Anteroposterior (panel A) and lateral (panel B) radiographs of the left forearm and wrist from a 32-year-old-male with left forearm pain following a motorcycle collision.

The diagnosis is an open, oblique, comminuted mid-shaft ulnar fracture with subluxation of the radial head with respect to the proximal humerus (Monteggia fracture-dislocation, type I). The patient received intravenous cefazolin and a tetanus booster following temporary splinting of the forearm. He was taken to the operating room by the orthopedic surgeon, where open reduction and internal fixation of the fracture-dislocation was performed (postoperative radiograph, Figure 67.3).

Monteggia fracture-dislocations

Monteggia fracture-dislocation (first described by Giovanni Battista Monteggia in 1814) refers to a fracture of the proximal third of the ulnar shaft combined with a radial head dislocation.[1] These injuries are relatively uncommon, accounting for less than 5% of all forearm fractures.[2] The ulna fracture is usually clinically and radiographically apparent. The key to successful diagnosis of a Monteggia fracture-dislocation is clinical suspicion. Diagnosis is made with radiographs of the entire forearm and elbow.[3]

The Bado classification of Monteggia fracture-dislocations is:

- Type I: Fracture of the proximal or middle third of the ulna with anterior dislocation of the radial head.
- Type II: Fracture of the proximal or middle third of the ulna with posterior dislocation of the radial head.
- Type III: Fracture of the ulnar metaphysis with lateral dislocation of the radial head.
- Type IV: Fracture of the proximal or middle third of the ulna and radius with anterior dislocation of the radial head.[1–4]

Of the Monteggia fracture-dislocations, Bado type I is the most common (59%), followed by type III (26%), type II (5%) and type IV (1%).[2,3] Monteggia fracture-dislocations are one-third as common as the more familiar Galeazzi fracture-dislocations (fracture of distal radius and concomitant dislocation of the distal radioulnar joint). The radial head dislocation in Monteggia fracture-dislocations may not be

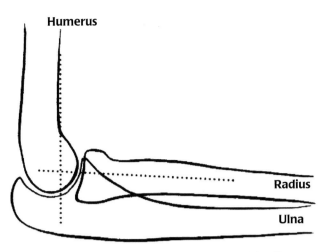

Figure 67.4 Normal interarticular relationships of the elbow.

apparent, and may be missed if radiographs of the elbow are not included. Separate radiographs (including a true lateral) should be taken of the elbow. In a normal elbow, the radial head points toward the capitellum on the lateral radiograph (Figure 67.4).

Monteggia fracture-dislocations are primarily associated with falls on an outstretched hand with forced pronation.[1–4] High-energy trauma (e.g., motor vehicle collisions) and low-energy trauma (e.g., falls from standing) can result in these injuries; thus, a high index of suspicion should be maintained with any ulna fracture.

In pediatric patients, many Monteggia fracture-dislocation patterns can be managed conservatively with closed reduction and long-arm casting.[4] However, most adult Monteggia fracture-dislocations require open reduction and internal fixation techniques. The radial head dislocation should be reduced by closed reduction under sedation within 6–8 hours of the injury. This is usually achieved with supination of the forearm, but may require traction and direct pressure on the radial head.[3]

If closed reduction is unsuccessful, the patient should be taken to the operating room within the same timeframe (6–8 hours) for open reduction. Delay in reduction of the radius may lead to permanent articular damage, further nerve injury or both. An open fracture requires emergent operative intervention, intravenous antibiotic administration and tetanus immunization (if necessary). In closed injuries, once the radial head is reduced the forearm is splinted and operative fixation of the ulna fracture may be carried out in a semi-elective fashion.

KEY TEACHING POINTS

1. Monteggia fracture-dislocations are primarily associated with falls on an outstretched hand with forced pronation; high- and low-energy trauma can result in these types of injuries.

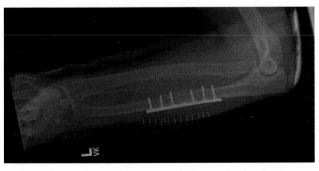

Figure 67.3 Lateral radiograph of the left forearm following open reduction and internal fixation of a Monteggia fracture-dislocation.

2. The radial head dislocation may not be clinically apparent, and may be missed if the elbow is not included in the radiograph. The keys to successful diagnosis of a Monteggia fracture-dislocation include a high clinical suspicion and radiographs of the entire forearm and elbow.

3. With Monteggia fracture-dislocations, most pediatric fracture patterns can be managed conservatively with closed reduction and long-arm casting. However, most adult fractures require open reduction and internal fixation.

4. Consider any wound overlying a fracture site as a potential open fracture, requiring antibiotic administration, updating tetanus status and operative repair.

REFERENCES

[1] Simon R, Koenigsknecht SJ. Fractures of the radius and ulna. *Emergency Orthopedics, the Extremities*, 4th ed. New York: McGraw-Hill, 2001:217–8.

[2] Jupiter JB, Kellam JF. Diaphyseal fractures of the forearm. *Skeletal Trauma: Basic Science, Management, and Reconstruction*, 3rd ed. Philadelphia: Saunders, 2003:1383–8.

[3] Putigna F. Monteggia fracture. eMedicine Website. Available at http://www.emedicine.com/orthopedic/topic201.htm. Accessed July 6, 2008.

[4] Smith WR, Agudelo JF, Parekh A, et al. Musculoskeletal trauma surgery. In: Skinner, HB (ed.). *Current Concepts and Treatment in Orthopedics*, 4th ed. New York: McGraw-Hill, 2006:111–2.

68

Left knee pain following trauma in a 68-year-old male

HISTORY OF PRESENT ILLNESS

A 68-year-old male presented to the ED by ambulance after being struck by a slow-moving vehicle while crossing the street. The patient fell to the ground, landing on his knees. He reported significant left knee and left lower leg pain, and was unable to bear weight at the scene. He denied head trauma, loss of consciousness, neck, chest, abdominal or hip pain, shortness of breath, and other injuries. The patient's tetanus status was unknown.

PHYSICAL EXAMINATION

GENERAL APPEARANCE: The patient was an elderly male sitting on the gurney, in mild discomfort.

VITAL SIGNS

Temperature	97.5°F (36.4°C)
Pulse	86 beats/minute
Blood pressure	153/82 mmHg
Respirations	18 breaths/minute
Oxygen saturation	99% on room air

HEENT: Atraumatic, PERRL, EOMI.

NECK: Supple, no midline tenderness.

CARDIOVASCULAR: Regular rate and rhythm without rubs, murmurs or gallops.

LUNGS: Clear to auscultation bilaterally.

ABDOMEN: Soft, nontender, nondistended.

HIPS: Stable, nontender, full range of motion.

KNEES: Abrasions to both knees. Minimal tenderness to palpation of the right knee, with full active range of motion without pain. Tenderness to palpation of left knee anteriorly and

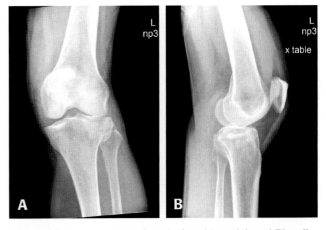

Figure 68.1 Anteroposterior (panel A) and lateral (panel B) radiographs of the left knee from a 68-year-old male with left knee pain following trauma.

medially; patient unable to actively range left knee secondary to pain; small effusion of the left knee.

EXTREMITIES: No clubbing, cyanosis or edema; strong peripheral pulses present.

NEUROLOGIC: Nonfocal.

A peripheral intravenous line was placed, morphine sulfate IV was administered for pain and tetanus immunization was given. Radiographs of the right and left knees were obtained; radiographs of the right knee were normal. Radiographs of the left knee are shown (Figure 68.1).

What is your diagnosis?

ANSWER

The diagnosis is a depressed left lateral tibial plateau fracture. A comminuted, intra-articular fracture at the lateral tibial plateau with depression of fracture fragments is evident on the anteroposterior radiograph of the left knee (arrow, panel A, Figure 68.2). Orthopedics was consulted, and a non-contrast CT scan of the left knee was obtained for preoperative planning (Figure 68.3). The CT demonstrated a comminuted, depressed fracture of the lateral tibial plateau with displacement and distraction of the fracture fragments, as well as a large amount of fluid in the joint seen with a fat-fluid level (consistent with lipohemarthrosis). This lipohemarthrosis can be identified on the lateral view radiograph when the film is viewed in its anatomic position (arrows, panel B, Figure 68.2). The patient underwent open reduction and internal fixation

(ORIF) of the fracture, with plate and screw fixation (Figure 68.4).

Tibial plateau fractures

The tibial plateau is composed of the medial and lateral tibial condyles, which form the inferior articular surfaces of the knee. Fractures of the plateau are relatively common in elderly persons (comprising almost 8% of all fractures in older persons) as a result of osteoporosis, and can occur with minor trauma.[1,2] Fractures in younger persons are usually the result of high-energy motor vehicle trauma, falls or contact-sports injuries; associated injuries are often present. Lateral plateau fractures are more common than medial plateau fractures, resulting from valgus stress and abduction forces.[3] Medial plateau fractures are the result of varus stress and adduction forces. Both plateaus are fractured in 11–31% of cases.[1]

The Segond fracture is a type of tibial plateau fracture that results from forced internal rotation of the tibia with varus stress. It is associated with an anterior cruciate ligament tear in 75–100% of cases.[1] The resultant tension on the lateral knee capsule avulses a small vertical fragment from the margin of the lateral tibial condyle, and is a reliable sign of anterior cruciate ligament tear. A "reverse Segond" fracture has also been described. This is a bony avulsion from the medial condyle, which has a strong association with a posterior cruciate ligament tear.[1]

Several methods have been developed to classify tibial plateau fractures. The Schatzker system is the best known (Table 68.1).[2] In this system, tibial plateau fractures are classified by the presence or absence of a sagittal split, a depressed articular segment, the presence or absence of a medial condylar fragment, and attachment to the tibial shaft.[4] Clinically, patients with tibial plateau fractures present with pain, knee effusion and the inability to bear weight.[1] Neurovascular

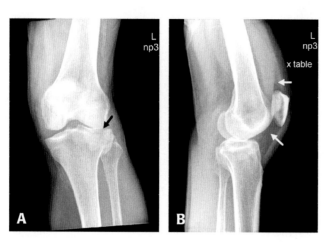

Figure 68.2 Anteroposterior (panel A) and lateral (panel B) radiographs of the left knee from a 68-year-old male demonstrating a depressed, comminuted lateral tibial plateau fracture (arrow, panel A) and joint effusion (arrows, panel B).

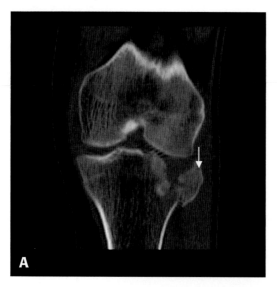
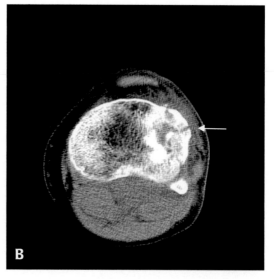

Figure 68.3 Coronal (panel A) and transverse (panel B) images from a noncontrast CT of the left tibial plateau fracture from a 68-year-old male (arrows indicate fracture).

TABLE 68.1 Schatzker classification system for tibial plateau fractures[2]

Type I	Split fractures of the lateral tibial plateau, usually in younger patients. No depression is seen at the articular surface.
Type II	Split fractures with depression of the lateral articular surface, typically seen in older patients with osteoporosis.
Type III	Fractures characterized by depression of the lateral tibial plateau, without splitting through the articular surface.
Type IV	Fractures involving the medial tibial plateau, and may be split fractures with or without depression.
Type V	Fractures characterized by split fractures through both the medial and lateral tibial plateaus.
Type VI	Fractures as the result of severe stress and resulting dissociation of the tibial plateau region from the underlying diaphysis.

injury is uncommon but compartment syndrome can occur. Physical examination reveals a joint effusion from hemarthrosis, decreased range of motion, and knee laxity and instability if an associated ligamentous injury is present.[1,3] Most tibial plateau fractures are diagnosed by conventional radiography (anteroposterior and lateral views, with oblique views added for the diagnosis of minimally or nondisplaced fractures not readily apparent on anteroposterior or lateral views).[2] CT is often used in more complex fractures to confirm the anatomic relationship of fracture fragments, especially at the articular surface of the tibia where precise three-dimensional anatomy is critical to the success of surgical repair. Less comminuted and depressed fractures may not require CT imaging. MRI is also useful to detect associated ligamentous injury and to more accurately delineate the extent of the fracture.[1]

Initial emergency management of tibial plateau fractures includes immobilization of the knee with splinting in full extension, ice to reduce swelling and parenteral pain medication. The patient should be kept NPO in anticipation of possible surgical repair. Indications for nonoperative treatment of tibial plateau fractures include incomplete or nondisplaced fractures (usually after a low-energy injury), a displaced lateral plateau fracture without articular instability, and some unstable lateral plateau fractures in osteoporotic patients.[5] Absolute indications for surgery include an open tibial plateau fracture and a tibial plateau fracture combined with either acute compartment syndrome or acute vascular injury. Relative indications for surgery include most displaced bicondylar fractures, displaced medial condylar fractures, lateral plateau fractures that result in joint instability, and plateau fractures in the context of patients with multiple injuries.[5]

KEY TEACHING POINTS

1. Fractures of the tibial plateau are relatively common, comprising almost 8% of all fractures in older persons, and can occur with minor trauma in this age group.
2. Clinically, patients with tibial plateau fractures present with knee effusion, inability to bear weight, decreased range of motion, and knee laxity and instability if ligamentous injury is present.
3. Most tibial plateau fractures are diagnosed by conventional radiography. CT can confirm the anatomic relationship of fracture fragments with more complex fractures; MRI is useful to detect associated ligamentous injury.
4. Initial emergent management of tibial plateau fractures includes immobilization of the knee, ice to reduce swelling and parenteral pain medication.
5. Indications for surgery include an open fracture, a fracture combined with an acute compartment syndrome or vascular injury, most displaced bicondylar fractures, displaced medial condylar fractures, lateral plateau fractures resulting in joint instability, and plateau fractures in multiply injured patients.

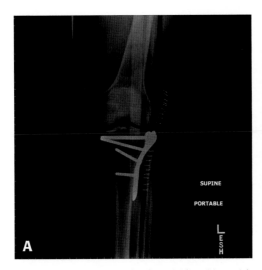 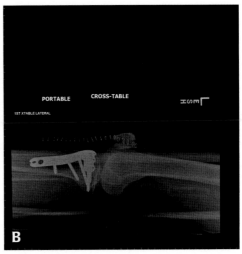

Figure 68.4 Anteroposterior (panel A) and lateral (panel B) radiographs of the left knee following ORIF for a depressed lateral tibial plateau fracture.

REFERENCES

[1] Newton EJ, Love J. Emergency department management of selected orthopedic injuries. *Emerg Med Clin N Am* 2007; 25:763–93.

[2] Sorenson SM, Gentili A, Masih S. Tibial plateau fractures. eMedicine Website. Available at http://www.emedicine.com/radio/topic698.htm. Accessed June 30, 2008.

[3] Pimentel L. Orthopedic trauma: office management of major joint injury. *Med Clin N Am* 2006;90:355–82.

[4] Zura RD, Browne JA, Black MD, et al. Current management of high-energy tibial plateau fractures. *Curr Orthop* 2007;21:229–35.

[5] Watson JT, Schatzker J. Tibial plateau fractures. In: Browner BD, Jupiter JB, Levine AM, et al. (eds.). *Skeletal Trauma: Basic Science, Management, and Reconstruction*, 3rd ed. Philadelphia: Elsevier, 2003:2074.

69

Left hip pain in a 70-year-old male

HISTORY OF PRESENT ILLNESS

A 70-year-old male with a medical history significant for diabetes, hypertension, hyperlipidemia and obesity presented to the ED complaining of six weeks of left hip pain that had acutely worsened over the past several days. The patient rated his pain at a level of 7 (on a scale of 0 to 10). His pain was worse with movement, and he was unable to ambulate secondary to pain. He denied redness or swelling over the hip, as well as any recent trauma. He denied fevers or chills, but reported that his left hip felt warm at times.

PHYSICAL EXAMINATION

GENERAL APPEARANCE: The patient appeared well hydrated, alert and in moderate discomfort.

VITAL SIGNS

Temperature	98.9°F (37.2°C)
Pulse	105 beats/minute
Blood pressure	171/79 mmHg
Respirations	22 breaths/minute
Oxygen saturation	97% on room air

HEENT: Unremarkable.

NECK: Supple, no jugular venous distension.

CARDIOVASCULAR: Tachycardic rate, regular rhythm without rubs, murmurs or gallops.

LUNGS: Clear to auscultation bilaterally.

ABDOMEN: Soft, nontender, nondistended.

LEFT HIP: Tender to palpation, slight warmth, no redness or swelling, pain elicited on passive range of motion. Normal position of hip at rest, without abnormal rotation; no length discrepancy of the lower extremities.

EXTREMITIES: No clubbing, cyanosis or edema; strong radial and dorsalis pedis pulses bilaterally.

NEUROLOGIC: Nonfocal.

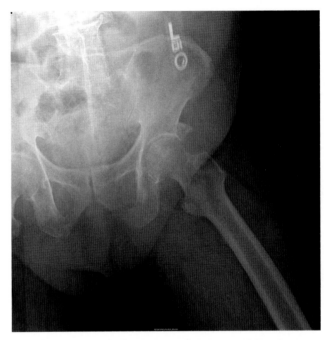

Figure 69.1 Left hip radiograph from a 70-year-old male with left hip pain.

A peripheral intravenous line was placed, blood was drawn and sent for laboratory testing, and radiographs of the left hip were obtained (Figure 69.1). Morphine sulfate IV was administered for pain. Laboratory evaluation revealed a leukocyte count of 8.9 K/μL (normal 3.5–12.5 K/μL) with 68% neutrophils (normal 50–70%), hematocrit of 35% (normal 39–51%), erythrocyte sedimentation rate (ESR) of 95 mm/Hr (normal 0–20 mm/Hr) and C-reactive protein (CRP) of 8.2 mg/dL (normal less than 0.9 mg/dL). A random blood glucose was 199 mg/dL (normal 61–159 mg/dL); the remainder of the chemistry panel, BUN and creatinine were within normal limits.

What is your diagnosis?

ANSWER

The diagnosis is septic arthritis of the left hip. The left hip radiograph did not reveal any fracture or acute abnormality. MRI of the left hip was obtained (Figure 69.2), which demonstrated a moderate amount of fluid in the left hip joint as well as increased signal (hyperdensity) in the joint and adjoining periarticular soft tissue of the left hip on T2-weighted images. The patient received vancomycin IV empirically and underwent fine needle aspiration of joint fluid from the left hip under fluoroscopy. Joint fluid revealed 12,250 leukocytes/μL, with 91% neutrophils; the Gram stain demonstrated many white blood cells without the presence of bacteria. A culture of the joint fluid subsequently grew out group B beta-hemolytic streptococcus (*Streptococcus agalactiae*) on hospital day #3; antibiotics were changed to penicillin and ceftriaxone IV according to sensitivities. The patient was taken to the OR by an orthopedic surgeon and underwent incision and drainage of the left hip joint with washout of the affected joint and placement of drains. The patient was discharged to a skilled nursing facility on hospital day #5 to continue IV antibiotics for four weeks.

Septic arthritis

Bacterial (septic) arthritis is the most rapidly destructive joint disease. The yearly incidence of bacterial arthritis varies from 2–10 per 100,000 in the general population to 30–70 per 100,000 in patients with rheumatoid arthritis or a joint prosthesis.[1] Septic arthritis is most commonly the result of hema-

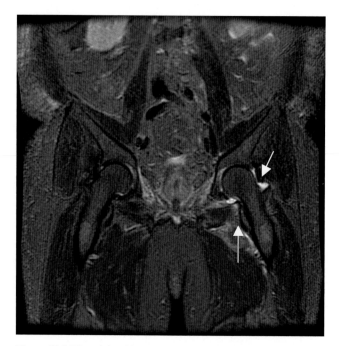

Figure 69.2 T2-weighted images of MRI of the hips in a 70-year-old male with left hip pain, demonstrating increased signal in the left hip joint and adjoining periarticular soft tissue (arrows).

togenous seeding of joints from bacteremia; less frequently, it is the result of joint surgery, direct inoculation by steroid injection, joint aspiration, animal or human bite, or direct extension from contiguous osteomyelitis.[2] Irreversible loss of joint function develops in 25–50% of patients. Despite better antimicrobial agents and improved hospital care, the case fatality rate for bacterial arthritis has not changed substantially in the past 25 years, ranging from 5–15%.[1]

A high index of suspicion for septic arthritis should be considered in patients with other rheumatic diseases, such as rheumatoid arthritis, osteoarthritis, gout, pseudogout and systemic lupus erythematosus.[3] Of these, rheumatoid arthritis is the most common, probably because of the combination of joint damage and immunosuppressive medications. Polyarticular disease is common, functional outcomes are worse and mortality is high in rheumatoid arthritis patients with septic joints.[3] Diagnosis is often delayed because physicians (and patients) confuse septic arthritis for an acute flare of rheumatoid arthritis.

The two major classes of bacterial arthritis are gonococcal and nongonococcal. Overall, although *Neisseria gonorrhoeae* remains the most frequent pathogen among younger sexually active individuals (75% of cases), *Staphylococcus aureus* is the most common cause of the vast majority of cases of acute bacterial arthritis in adults and children older than 2 years.[4] *S. aureus* is the pathogen in 80% of infected joints affected by rheumatoid arthritis. Streptococcal species, such as *Streptococcus viridans*, *Streptococcus pneumoniae* and group B streptococci, account for 20% of cases; aerobic Gram-negative rods are involved in 20–25% of cases.[4]

A patient with septic arthritis may complain of the acute onset of fever and chills. A prodromal phase of several days duration with malaise, arthralgia and low-grade fever can be encountered.[5] Pain, tenderness, redness, warmth and soft tissue swelling about the involved joint are common. The knee is the site of infection in 50% of cases but any joint may be involved.[1] In hip infections, the hip is often held in a flexed and externally rotated position, and there is extreme pain on motion. It is often difficult to detect an effusion of the hip, although the joint is frequently warm and very tender.[3] Ten percent to 20% of infections are polyarticular, usually affecting two or three joints.[1] Polyarticular septic arthritis most likely occurs in patients with rheumatoid arthritis, systemic connective-tissue disease or overwhelming sepsis.[1]

The key to the diagnosis of bacterial arthritis is the identification of bacteria in the synovial fluid by Gram stain or culture. At the clinical suspicion of joint infection, synovial fluid aspiration should be performed.[3] The synovial fluid of septic arthritis is usually purulent, with an average leukocyte count of 50,000–150,000 cells/mm³ (most of which are neutrophils). Gram stain smears are positive only 60–80% of the time.[3] The glucose level in synovial fluid is often depressed; lactic acid and lactate dehydrogenase levels are raised in septic arthritis (although values may also be elevated in inflammatory joint disease). Synovial fluid cultures are positive 90% of the time with nongonococcal infection, only 50% of the time with gonococcal infection.[2] Blood cultures should be obtained in any patient with suspected bacterial arthritis, and are positive in about half of the patients with nongonococcal septic arthritis.[3] Other laboratory findings, such as an increased white blood cell count and an elevated ESR are common but nonspecific. An ESR or CRP is useful to follow response to therapy, as well as to detect an acute process in chronically infected joints.[4]

Radiographic abnormalities parallel the pathologic changes. Initially, radiographs can be completely normal.[5] The first detectable abnormalities are soft tissue swelling that accompany local hyperemia, edema and joint distension secondary to effusion.[5] These abnormalities are followed by joint space narrowing (frequently diffuse) that reflects damage to the chondral surface and osseous erosions at the margins of the joint, related to the effects of diseased synovium on bone. Advanced and severe cases of infection are associated with subluxation or dislocation and massive bone destruction.

Early manifestations of septic arthritis seen on CT scan include joint effusions, synovial thickening and soft tissue swelling.[5] Once the infectious process has caused destruction of the articular cartilage, irregularity and narrowing of the joint, articular erosion and subchondral bone destruction are also noted. Ultrasound is an extremely sensitive modality for demonstrating joint effusions and has been successfully used by emergency physicians for bedside, ultrasound-guided hip arthrocentesis.[6] Septic effusions may be completely anechoic or associated with septations and debris. However, neither the size nor the relative echogenicity of the fluid can be used to distinguish an infected inflammatory effusion from one that is not infected.[5]

With MRI, effusions appear as regions of decreased signal intensity in T1-weighted images, and increased signal intensity in fluid-sensitive T2-weighted images.[5] The effusion tends to be homogeneous, although loculation and inhomogeneity may be seen in more chronic septic processes. Radionuclide scans are used to nonspecifically localize areas of inflammation; they cannot be used to distinguish infectious from sterile processes. However, they may be of use in diagnosing septic arthritis in relatively sequestered areas, such as the hip and sacroiliac joints.[4]

Septic arthritis is considered a medical emergency requiring early and aggressive intervention. Optimal therapy includes systemic antibiotics and surgical drainage.[1–5] A young, healthy, sexually active individual should be treated with penicillin or a high-generation cephalosporin (e.g., ceftriaxone, ceftizoxime or cefotaxime) for suspected disseminated gonococcal infection. Elderly patients with suspected nongonococcal infections should be treated more broadly for the most common causes of infection, namely *S. aureus,* streptococcal species and Gram-negative pathogens.[2] Empiric treatment generally includes a beta-lactam in combination with either an aminoglycoside or quinolone. Special consideration should be given to the treatment of joint infections in patients with prostheses. In addition to antibiotics, therapy usually requires open drainage and prosthesis removal because of the difficulty eradicating infection because bacteria attach to the prosthetic material.[2]

KEY TEACHING POINTS

1. Septic arthritis is a medical emergency requiring aggressive management, including systemic antibiotics, surgical drainage and hospitalization.
2. Pain, tenderness, redness, warmth and soft tissue swelling about the involved joint are common in septic arthritis but may not be specific.
3. The diagnostic test of choice in the evaluation of a septic joint is synovial fluid aspiration, with Gram stain and culture of the fluid.
4. CT, MRI and ultrasound are more sensitive in identifying early manifestations of septic arthritis compared with plain radiography.
5. Young, healthy, sexually active patients with septic arthritis should be treated for possible gonococcal infection; elderly patients should be treated for nongonococcal infections with broad-spectrum antibiotics pending culture results.

REFERENCES

[1] Goldenberg DL. Septic arthritis. *Lancet* 1998;351:197–202.
[2] Harrington L, Schneider JI. Atraumatic joint and limb pain in the elderly. *Emerg Med Clin N Am* 2006;24:389–412.
[3] Garcia-De La Torre I. Advances in the management of septic arthritis. *Infect Dis Clin N Am* 2006;20:773–88.
[4] Brusch JL. Septic arthritis. eMedicine Website. Available at http://www.emedicine.com/med/topic3394.htm. Accessed June 20, 2008.
[5] Mohana-Borges AVR, Chung CB, Resnick D. Monoarticular arthritis. *Radiol Clin N Am* 2004;42:135–49.
[6] Freeman K, Dewitz A, Baker WE. Ultrasound-guided hip arthrocentesis in the ED. *Am J Emerg Med* 2007;25:80–6.

70

Thigh trauma in an 81-year-old female

HISTORY OF PRESENT ILLNESS

An 81-year-old female with a medical history significant for osteoporosis presented to the ED by ambulance after falling to the ground, twisting her right thigh. She reported sudden, sharp pain to her right thigh with significant swelling. She was unable to bear weight. She rated her pain at a level of 7 (on a scale of 0 to 10). She denied loss of consciousness, head or neck trauma, or other injuries.

PHYSICAL EXAMINATION

GENERAL APPEARANCE: The patient was lying supine on the gurney in moderate discomfort.

VITAL SIGNS

Temperature	98.6°F (37°C)
Pulse	90 beats/minute
Blood pressure	150/90 mmHg
Respirations	20 breaths/minute
Oxygen saturation	100% on room air

HEENT: Unremarkable.

NECK: Supple, no midline tenderness.

CARDIOVASCULAR: Regular rate and rhythm without rubs, murmurs or gallops.

LUNGS: Clear to auscultation bilaterally.

ABDOMEN: Soft, nontender, nondistended.

RIGHT LOWER EXTREMITY: Obvious deformity to the right thigh with swelling and tenderness (Figure 70.1); the right thigh compartments were soft without wounds. No tenderness or deformity to the right hip or knee; patient unable to move right lower extremity at the hip or knee secondary to severe pain in the thigh, although she could move her ankle and foot. The right lower extremity was neurovascularly intact.

EXTREMITIES: No clubbing, cyanosis or edema; no other musculoskeletal injuries noted.

NEUROLOGIC: Nonfocal.

An intravenous line was placed, blood was drawn and sent for laboratory tests, and morphine sulfate was administered for pain control. Ice packs were applied to the right thigh, and the patient was not allowed to eat or drink. Radiographs of the right femur were obtained (Figure 70.2).

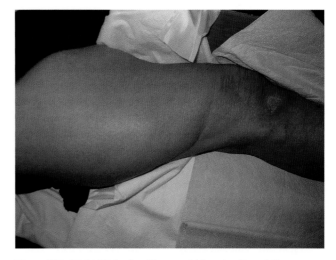

Figure 70.1 Right thigh of an 81-year-old female after a fall.

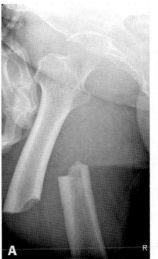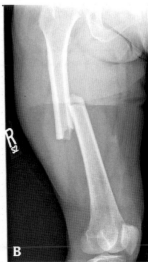

Figure 70.2 Anteroposterior (panel A) and lateral (panel B) radiographs of the right femur from an 81-year-old female after a fall onto her right side.

What is your diagnosis?

ANSWER

The diagnosis is a right femur fracture. The radiographs demonstrated a completely displaced, overriding fracture at the mid-shaft of the right femur. The proximal femoral head and neck were intact, and the hip joint was not dislocated. The affected limb was placed in a Sager traction splint, and the orthopedic surgeon was urgently consulted. The patient was taken to the OR and the fracture was repaired using a closed intramedullary nailing procedure (Figure 70.3).

Femoral shaft fractures

The femoral shaft extends from an area 5 cm distal to the lesser trochanter to a point 6 cm proximal to the adductor tubercle.[1] It is a strong bone with an excellent blood supply and therefore good healing potential.[2] Femoral shaft fractures are more common in children and adolescents. The extensive musculature surrounding the femoral shaft is often the source of displacement. Mid-shaft fractures undergo a varus deformity because of the pull by the medial adductors, which is resisted by the lateral thigh muscles and fascia lata.

Femoral shaft fractures are classified into three types: type I, spiral or transverse shaft fractures (most common); type II, comminuted femoral shaft fractures; and type III, open femoral shaft fractures.[3] Femoral shaft fractures are usually secondary to severe forces, such as a direct blow or an indirect

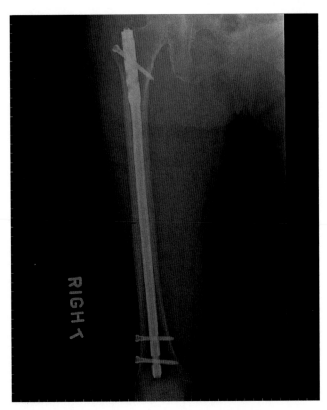

Figure 70.3 Anteroposterior radiograph of the right femur following closed intramedullary nailing.

force transmitted through the flexed knee. Pathologic fractures may occur with relatively little force, as a result of bone weakness from osteoporosis or lytic lesions.[3]

On examination, the patient will present with severe pain in the involved extremity and usually visible deformities. The extremity may be shortened, and there may be crepitation with movement.[1] The thigh may be swollen and tense secondary to hemorrhage and hematoma formation. The skin should be examined for open wounds and to check the soft tissues. It is important to establish whether the injury had a crushing component, as prolonged crushing may cause myonecrosis necessitating muscle resection or amputation.[4] Extensive bleeding into the muscle may also occur, and can be exacerbated by anticoagulant medications. Although rare, thigh compartment syndrome can occur.[4] A thorough neurovascular examination of the affected limb must occur; femoral nerve damage is unusual after femoral shaft fractures, but sciatic nerve injury can occur.[4] Because of extensive blood supply to the musculature surrounding the femur, femoral shaft fractures may be associated with significant blood loss (i.e., one liter or more), resulting in tachycardia and hypotension.[3]

Routine anteroposterior and lateral radiographic views are usually adequate in demonstrating the fracture. Hip and knee views should be included, as there is significant incidence of associated injury. Initial management of femoral shaft fractures includes reducing fractures to near-anatomic alignment with in-line traction (reduces pain and helps prevent hematoma formation).[3] Traction devices (e.g., Hare, Thomas, Buck or Sager) can be used to hold reduction of the affected leg. Pain medication (parenteral opiate analgesics) should be administered, and ice packs applied to the fracture site. Antibiotics should be promptly administered for open fractures, as well as tetanus toxoid (if not current).

The definitive treatment for type I fractures is closed intramedullary nailing.[1,2] Immediate nailing of the femoral shaft allows for early patient mobilization and reduces the incidence of complications, including fat embolism and acute respiratory distress syndrome (ARDS). Open fractures require emergent operative debridement with delayed intramedullary nailing. Complications of femoral shaft fractures include nonunion or infection (less than 1% of patients), malunion or delayed union, malrotation of the extremity leading to permanent deformity, knee stiffness, breakage of nails and plates, arterial injury with delayed thrombosis or aneurysm, peroneal nerve contusion, refracture of the initial site, and development of thigh compartment syndrome.[1–4] Patients over age 60 with closed shaft fractures have a mortality rate of 16–20% and a complication rate near 50%.[1]

KEY TEACHING POINTS

1. Femoral shaft fractures are classified into three types: type I, spiral or transverse shaft fractures (most common); type II, comminuted femoral shaft fractures; and type III, open femoral shaft fractures.

2. Patients with femoral shaft fractures generally present with severe pain and visible deformity of the involved extremity; the extremity may be shortened with a tense and swollen thigh secondary to hemorrhage and hematoma formation.

3. Routine anteroposterior and lateral radiographic views of the femur (including the hip and knee) are generally adequate in demonstrating the fracture.

4. Initial management of femoral shaft fractures includes application of an in-line traction device, ice packs to the affected limb and pain control with opiate analgesics.

5. The definitive treatment for type I fractures is closed intramedullary nailing.

REFERENCES

[1] Simon RR, Koenigsknecht SJ. Fractures of the femoral shaft. In: Simon RR, Koenigsknecht SJ. *Emergency Orthopedics, the Extremities*, 4th ed. New York: McGraw-Hill, 2001:391–4.

[2] Aukerman DF, Deitch JR, Ertl JP. Femur injuries and fractures. eMedicine Website. Available at http://www.emedicine.com/sports/topic38.htm. Accessed June 30, 2008.

[3] Keany JE. Fractures, femur. eMedicine Website. Available at http://www.emedicine.com/emerg/topic193.htm. Accessed June 30, 2008.

[4] Court-Brown CM, Robinson CM, Tornetta P. Femoral diaphyseal fractures. In: Browner BD, Jupiter JB, Levine AM (eds.). *Skeletal Trauma: Basic Science, Management, and Reconstruction*, 3rd ed. Philadelphia: Saunders, 2003:1893.

PART IX

HAND

71

Right thumb pain and swelling in a 20-year-old female

HISTORY OF PRESENT ILLNESS

A 20-year-old right-hand dominant female presented to the ED complaining of three days of worsening right thumb redness, swelling and pain. The patient denied recent trauma or puncture wounds to the thumb, fevers, chills, or drainage from the thumb or thumbnail. On the day of presentation, she noticed a red streak spreading up her right forearm. She worked as a hairdresser, and had not experienced similar symptoms in the past. The patient's last tetanus prophylaxis booster was unknown.

PHYSICAL EXAMINATION

GENERAL APPEARANCE: The patient appeared uncomfortable, holding her right hand with her left hand.

VITAL SIGNS

Temperature	98.1°F (36.7°C)
Pulse	88 beats/minute
Blood pressure	130/80 mmHg
Respirations	22 breaths/minute
Oxygen saturation	99% on room air

RIGHT FOREARM/WRIST/HAND: Significant redness and swelling of the distal phalanx, extending proximal to the distal interphalangeal joint (DIP) of the right thumb (panel A, Figure 71.1). The thumb was held in extension for comfort. The volar pad was tense, warm and tender to palpation. Neither drainage nor a paronychia was noted. Artificial nails of the digits were present. The patient had limited range of motion at the DIP joint. Neither tenderness, redness nor swelling to the volar surface of the thumb proximal to the DIP joint was present. Examination of the right forearm revealed a faint, erythematous line extending from the volar wrist to the antecubital fossa (panel B, Figure 71.1).

An intravenous line was placed, blood was drawn and sent for laboratory testing, and cefazolin 1 gm was administered intravenously. All laboratory tests, including a complete blood count, erythrocyte sedimentation rate (ESR) and C-reactive protein (CRP), returned within normal limits. Radiographs of the right thumb were obtained (Figure 71.2).

What is your diagnosis?

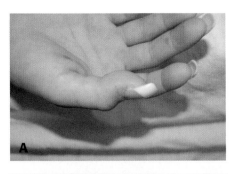
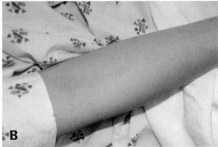

Figure 71.1 Right thumb (panel A) and forearm (panel B) of a 20-year-old female with right thumb pain and swelling.

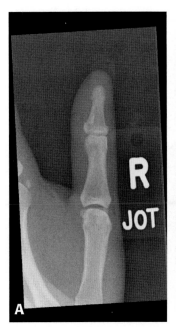
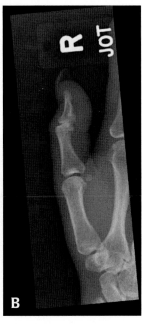

Figure 71.2 Anteroposterior (panel A) and lateral (panel B) radiographs of the right thumb from a 20-year-old female with right thumb pain and swelling.

ANSWER

The diagnosis is subungual abscess of the right thumb. The right thumb radiographs were normal except for soft tissue swelling of the distal phalanx. In the ED, a digital block of the right thumb was performed using 0.5% bupivacaine (panel A, Figure 71.3), and incision and drainage of the thumb using sterile technique was performed with a vertical incision into the volar pad of the distal phalanx (panel B, Figure 71.3). Pus was not expressed from the incision site.

The right thumb was cleaned and sterile dressing applied. The right hand and wrist were placed in a thumb spica splint, and the patient was discharged home to continue oral antibiotics (Augmentin® 875 mg orally twice per day) with instructions to soak the right thumb in warm water and Epsom salts two to three times per day. The patient was seen the following day by a hand surgeon; no improvement of the swelling and erythema of the thumb was appreciated despite antibiotics.

There was still no improvement in the swelling and erythema on a second visit to the hand surgeon three days following the initial incision and drainage. The patient still complained of considerable pain. The patient was therefore admitted to the hospital for intravenous antibiotics. After two doses of IV antibiotics, splinting, elevation and warm soaks, there was still no improvement. At this time, the nail and overlying artificial nail were removed, despite no evidence of erythema or swelling at or around the nail bed. Upon removal of the nails, frank pus was expressed from the nail bed. The eponychial fold was stented with sterile foil from a suture package. Dramatic improvement in the patient's symptoms were noted the following morning. The thumb and nail bed were dressed with xeroform and sterile gauze, and the patient was discharged to continue 10 days of oral moxifloxacin.

Subungual abscesses

Subungual abscesses are generally the result of an acute paronychia that has extended underneath the nail plate.[1] Paronychiae and subungual abscesses are most commonly caused by *Staphylococcus aureus* or *Streptococcus* species.[1] Patients with a subungual abscess generally present with severe, throbbing pain of the affected distal phalanx.[2] The presence of a subungual abscess requires nail plate removal, with the degree of subsequent debridement commensurate with the degree of nail bed infection. Trephination of the nail plate with a cautery device may also be performed to relieve pressure underneath the nail bed by expressing pus from the abscess.[2] Although nail plate removal or trephination are the treatments of choice to achieve adequate drainage of the subungual abscess, antibiotics (e.g., cephalexin) are indicated in cases where associated cellulitis is present. If left untreated, a subungual abscess can progress to a felon of the affected digit.[1] Paronychial infections and subungual abscesses have been reported in patients with sculptured nails (e.g., placement of artificial nails), which may be a risk factor for the development of both of these infections.[3]

KEY TEACHING POINTS

1. A subungual abscess generally results from an acute paronychia that has extended underneath the nail plate.
2. Patients with subungual abscesses present with severe, throbbing pain of the distal portion of the affected digit.
3. Treatment of a subungual abscess involves nail plate removal or trephination to achieve adequate and drainage.
4. Antibiotics (e.g., cephalexin) are indicated in cases of subungual abscesses with an associated cellulitis.

REFERENCES

[1] Murphy-Lavoie H. Paronychia. eMedicine Website. Available at http://www.emedicine.com/emerg/topic357.htm. Accessed June 23, 2008.
[2] Fleming TE, Brodell RT. Subungual abscess: a bacterial infection of the nail bed. *J Am Acad Derm* 1997;37:486–7.
[3] Roberge RJ, Weinstein D, Thimons MM. Perionychial infections associated with sculptured nails. *Am J Emerg Med* 1999;17:581–2.

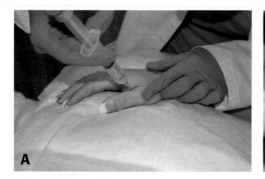 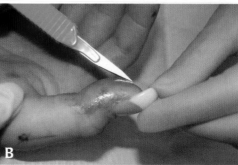

Figure 71.3 Digital block (panel A) and incision and drainage (panel B) of suspected felon of the right thumb in a 20-year-old female.

72

Paint gun injury to the hand in a 22-year-old male

HISTORY OF PRESENT ILLNESS

A 22-year-old right-hand dominant male presented to the ED complaining of left hand pain and swelling following injury to his left hand from a paint gun hose. The patient was attempting to cover up a hole in the hose of a pressurized paint sprayer (containing water-based paint) with his left hand, when he noted the sudden onset of pain in and swelling of his left hand. He denied numbness or weakness of the hand. His tetanus immunization was current.

PHYSICAL EXAMINATION

GENERAL APPEARANCE: The patient was a well-developed male holding his left hand in his right hand, in moderate discomfort.

VITAL SIGNS

Temperature	98.6°F (37°)
Pulse	88 beats/minute
Blood pressure	135/85 mmHg
Respirations	18 breaths/minute
Oxygen saturation	100% on room air

LEFT HAND: A small puncture wound was noted over the web space between the index and middle finger. Moderate swelling of the hand near the puncture site both dorsally and ventrally was noted, as well as swelling to the proximal phalanges of the index and ring finger. White paint was oozing from the wound.

A peripheral intravenous line was placed, morphine sulfate IV was administered for pain, and a radiograph of the left hand was obtained (Figure 72.1).

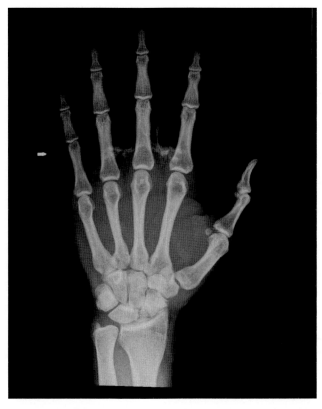

Figure 72.1 Left hand radiograph from a 22-year-old male following injury with a paint gun hose.

What is your diagnosis?

ANSWER

The diagnosis is high-pressure injection injury to the hand (left second web space). The radiograph demonstrated a moderate degree of soft tissue swelling along the dorsal aspect of the left hand, with the presence of a patchy radio-opaque density consistent with paint between the web spaces of the index and middle, and middle and ring fingers. The patient received intravenous antibiotics (piperacillin/tazobactam 3.375 gm IV) and a hand surgeon was consulted. The patient was taken to the OR where exploration, debridement and irrigation of the wound occurred using incisions over the volar aspects of the index and middle digits extending into the second web space. Upon exploration, a significant amount of paint was noted in the second web space, traversing in the ulnar direction. The paint was debrided and the wound copiously irrigated. No tendon injury was noted. The incisions were closed intraoperatively and the hand splinted. The patient was discharged on hospital day #2 to continue cephalexin orally, with follow up arranged with the hand surgeon in 10 days. Cultures taken from the wound were positive for moderate growth *Pseudomonas aeruginosa*.

High-pressure injection injuries to the hand

High-pressure injection injuries to the hand hide the true extent of tissue damage behind an apparently harmless puncture of the finger or hand.[1] However, these injuries are potentially devastating and frequently lead to permanent functional loss or amputation.[2] Many types of hydraulic paint-spraying guns and greasing apparatuses with high working pressures have been produced, and have led to injuries after breaching the skin from the considerable dissipation of energy. This often distributes toxic material throughout the tissues. A pressure of about 7 bar (100 psi or 700 kN/m^2) can breach the skin; most grease guns operate around this pressure.[1] Airless spray guns work at service pressures around 200 bar (3000 psi).[1,3] The pinpoint nozzle ending the gun shrinks the output from 0.18–1.00 mm, causing fluid to leave at a velocity of 183 m/sec.[1,3]

Upon initial evaluation, most high-pressure injection injuries present as innocuous wounds with very few symptoms. Patients are typically young men, usually manual workers, with the most common site of injection the terminal segment of the nondominant index finger.[4] Pain is often mild or absent, which can lead to delays in seeking medical attention.[2] The affected body part swells, both from the presence of injected material and from the inflammatory response that many injected materials provoke.[2] The increased tissue pressure, combined with the irritant nature of many of the injected materials, compromises blood flow to the digit, leading to vasospasm and thrombosis.

High-pressure injections into the fingers are nearly three times more likely to require amputation than the same injuries to the palm or thumb.[2] The anatomic characteristics of the hand and fingers offer explanations for the increased

morbidity of digital injection. Digital injection injuries do worse than palmar injuries because of the limited space available for expansion caused by inflammation and swelling.[5] The nature of the injected material is also important in determining the extent of injury. Paint and paint thinners cause an especially intense inflammatory reaction.[6] When delivered under high pressure, such substances may spread widely through fascial planes and along tendon and nerve sheaths to produce vascular compression and subsequent necrosis.[6] There is also a distinction in the extent of tissue damage produced based on the type of paint injected. Spirit-based paints cause damage by disintegrating cell membranes, whereas oil-based paints cause an intense inflammatory response.[5] Water-based latex paints are the least noxious. Injuries with water, air or low-volume vaccines (e.g., chicken vaccine) may be amenable to nonoperative treatment.[5]

ED management of high-pressure injection injuries to the hand should include careful examination and documentation of the injury (including mechanism, material injected and time of injury), the patient's hand dominance and occupation, and the neurovascular status of the affected digit or limb. Any constricting jewelry on the fingers or wrist should be removed. Tetanus prophylaxis should be updated if necessary. Prophylactic intravenous broad-spectrum antibiotics should be administered, and plain radiographs of the affected digit and hand should be obtained. These radiographs will assist in delineating the extent of injury and spread of foreign body, as radiography reveals varying distributions of radio-opaque densities associated with paint or grease injections, and air density (subcutaneous emphysema) after air or water injection.[1] The use of immediate high-dose systemic corticosteroids followed by high-dose oral steroids in tapered doses has been suggested to decrease the chemical inflammation and deleterious tissue responses to the injected material.[7] However, the relative rarity and wide variation of severity of this injury precludes a proper controlled trial of the effect of steroids, and a theoretical risk of sepsis due to immunosuppression exists. Therefore, routine steroid administration is not considered the current standard of care.[4] Finally, a hand surgeon should be contacted immediately in preparation for prompt surgical exploration.

Wide surgical debridement, the recommended treatment for high-pressure injection injuries to the hand and fingers, relieves the external pressure created by the injected material, attenuates the local inflammatory response and reduces bacterial counts.[2] This not only improves circulation but also diminishes the risk of infection. Intuitively, the greatest benefit is achieved from immediate removal of the offending material. In a review of 435 cases of high-pressure injection injury to the upper extremity, the amputation rate after injection of benign material was independent of time to surgical debridement.[2] These injuries resulted in less tissue damage, tended toward greater delays in clinical presentation due to milder symptoms, and carried a relatively lower amputation risk compared to patients injected with organic solvents. In contrast, time to debridement had a significant impact upon survival of the body part in patients who had sustained injections with the most toxic substances (paint, diesel, oil, paint thinner, gasoline, automotive undercoating). In this study, surgery within six hours of injury resulted in amputation 40% of the time, compared with 57% of the time if surgery was delayed greater than six hours.[2] If debridement was delayed greater than one week, the amputation rate rose to 88%.

KEY TEACHING POINTS

1. High-pressure injection injuries to the fingers and hand are potentially devastating injuries that frequently lead to permanent functional loss or amputation.
2. Key points to history and physical examination include hand dominance, occupation, tetanus status, mechanism and time of injury, substance involved, and neurovascular status of the affected limb.
3. High-pressure injections into the fingers are almost three times more likely to require amputation than injuries to the palm or thumb.
4. The nature of the injected material is important in determining the extent of injury, with paint and paint thinners causing an especially intense inflammatory reaction.
5. Emergency care of high-pressure injection injuries includes removal of constricting jewelry, elevation of the affected extremity, radiographs of the affected limb, administration of prophylactic antibiotics and pain medications, and prompt consultation with the hand surgeon.
6. Aggressive, prompt debridement is the key to success in treating high-pressure injection injuries of the hand.

REFERENCES

[1] Vasilevski D, Noorbergen M, Depierreux M. High-pressure injection injuries to the hand. *Am J Emerg Med* 2000;18: 820–4.
[2] Hogan CJ, Ruland RT. High-pressure injection injuries to the upper extremity: a review of the literature. *J Orthop Trauma* 2006;20:503–11.
[3] Neal NC, Burke FD. High-pressure injection injuries. *Injury* 1991;22:467–70.
[4] Lewis HG, Clarke P, Kneafsey B, et al. A 10-year review of high-pressure injection injuries to the hand. *J Hand Surg* 1998;23B:479–81.
[5] Christodoulou L, Melikyan EY, Woodbridge S, et al. Functional outcome of high-pressure injection injuries of the hand. *J Trauma* 2001;50:717–20.
[6] O'Sullivan ST, Beausang JM, O'Donoghue JM, et al. The importance of open wound management in high-pressure injection injuries of the upper limb. *J Hand Surg* 1997;22B: 542–3.
[7] Wong TC, Ip FK, Wu WC. High-pressure injection injuries of the hand in a Chinese population. *J Hand Surg* 2005;30B: 588–92.

73

Finger pain and swelling in a 34-year-old male

HISTORY OF PRESENT ILLNESS

A 34-year-old right-hand dominant male presented to the ED complaining of four days of pain and swelling to the distal portion of his left middle finger. The patient initially noted mild redness, swelling and slight drainage around his nail four days prior to presentation. The volar pad of his finger had become increasingly red, painful and swollen. He denied fevers, redness spreading from the fingertip, trauma to the finger or similar episodes in the past. The patient worked as a musician playing guitar, and his tetanus status was unknown.

PHYSICAL EXAMINATION

GENERAL APPEARANCE: The patient was a well-developed male in no acute discomfort.

VITAL SIGNS

Temperature	98.6°F (37°C)
Pulse	77 beats/minute
Blood pressure	125/85 mmHg
Respirations	20 breaths/minute
Oxygen saturation	100% on room air

LEFT MIDDLE FINGER: The distal volar pad of the affected digit was tense, swollen and erythematous, with marked tenderness to palpation (Figure 73.1). No erythema was noted below the distal interphalangeal (DIP) joint. The patient maintained full active motion at the proximal interphalangeal (PIP) joint, with limited range of motion at the DIP joint secondary to pain and swelling. Swelling and exudate were noted adjacent to the nail's insertion on the radial aspect of the distal phalanx.

What is your diagnosis?

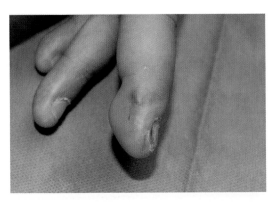 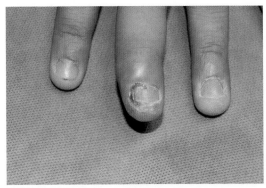

Figure 73.1 Left middle finger from a 34-year-old male with pain and swelling for four days.

ANSWER

The diagnosis is a felon of the distal phalanx. A digital block of the affected digit was performed with 0.5% bupivacaine, a tourniquet was placed proximal to the PIP joint, and an incision and drainage (I&D) of the distal phalanx using a medial approach on the radial aspect of the volar pad was performed with a #11 scalpel and sterile technique (Figure 73.2). Kelly clamps were used to open the incision; no pus was expressed from the incision site. The digit was soaked in warm water and Betadine solution, dressed with bacitracin and xeroform dressing, and splinted in extension. The patient's tetanus status was updated; he was discharged on amoxicillin/clavulanate 875 mg orally two times per day and instructed to continue warm water and Epsom salt soaks three times per day.

The patient was seen two days later in the hand surgery clinic with improvement of his swelling and symptoms. A second I&D using an anterior approach was performed following a digital block; again, no pus was expressed. The patient continued soaking the digit, with resolution of the felon noted on a return visit to the hand surgeon one week later.

Felon

A felon is an infection of the distal finger or thumb pulp. It differs from other types of subcutaneous abscesses because of the presence of multiple vertical septae that divide the pulp into small fascial compartments.[1] The thumb and index finger are the most commonly affected digits.[2] Penetrating trauma with secondary bacterial invasion is the usual cause. A felon may also arise when an untreated paronychia spreads into the pad of the fingertip.[2] The most common pathogen is *Staphylococcus aureus*, although Gram-negative organisms have also been identified.[1] Felons are characterized by throbbing pain, tenseness and edema of the fingertip pad.[3] The swelling does not extend proximally to the DIP joint.[2] Occasionally, the high pressure in the fingertip pad will cause a felon to spontaneously drain, resulting in a visible sinus.

If diagnosed during the early stages of cellulitis, a felon may be amenable to treatment with elevation, oral antibiotics, and warm water or saline soaks.[2] Tetanus prophylaxis should be administered when necessary. Proper treatment of a mature

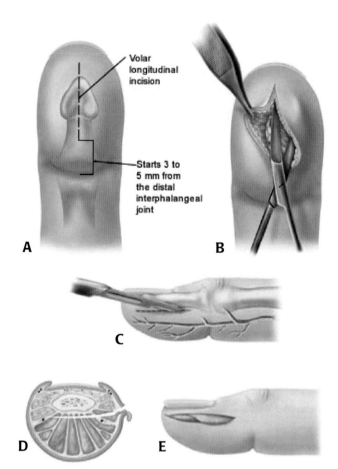

Figure 73.3 Felon drainage (from Clark DC, *Am Fam Phys* 2003;68: 2167–76).

felon consists of early and complete incision and drainage.[4] The preferred initial approach is a simple longitudinal incision over the area of greatest fluctuance, either laterally or along the volar surface.[4] A potential drawback to an incision in the middle of the fat pad is the production of a scar in a very sensitive and commonly traumatized area. The incision must not extend to the DIP crease because of the danger of injuring the flexor tendon mechanism. The subcutaneous tissue is bluntly dissected using a hemostat to provide adequate drainage (Figure 73.3). A gauze pack may be placed in the wound for

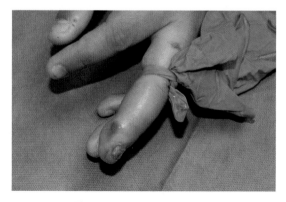
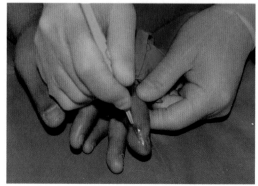

Figure 73.2 Incision and drainage of a felon on the left middle finger of a 34-year-old male.

24–48 hours to ensure continued drainage.[4] A snug dressing and splint should be placed, and opioid analgesia provided. The patient should be rechecked in two to three days.

KEY TEACHING POINTS

1. A felon is an infection involving the pulp of the distal volar pad of the digits (fingers or thumb).
2. Felons are characterized by throbbing pain, tenseness and edema of the fingertip pulp; the swelling does not extend proximally to the DIP joint.
3. If diagnosed early, felons may be treated by elevation, oral antibiotics and warm water soaks.
4. If fluctuance is present, incision and drainage of the felon at the point of maximal fluctuance is appropriate.

REFERENCES

[1] Lyn E, Antosia RE. Hand. In: Marx JA, Hockberger RS, Walls RM, et al. (eds.). *Rosen's Emergency Medicine: Concepts and Clinical Practice*, 6th ed. Philadelphia: Mosby, 2006:576–619.

[2] Clark DC. Common acute hand infections. *Am Fam Phys* 2003;68:2167–76.

[3] Vaughn G. Felon. eMedicine Website. Available at http://www.emedicine.com/emerg/topic178.htm. Accessed July 8, 2008.

[4] Butler KH. Incision and drainage. In: Roberts JR, Hedges JR, Chanmugan AS, et al. (eds.). *Roberts: Clinical Procedures in Emergency Medicine*, 4th ed. Philadelphia: Saunders, 2004:741–4.

74

Finger laceration in a 50-year-old female

HISTORY OF PRESENT ILLNESS

A 50-year-old right-hand dominant female employed as an OR nurse presented to the ED with a laceration to her right index finger, sustained with a sterile scalpel while assisting in the OR. She reported significant bleeding from the wound, which was now controlled with pressure. The patient reported numbness around the wound and the inability to extend her index finger at the proximal joint. Her tetanus status was current.

PHYSICAL EXAMINATION

GENERAL APPEARANCE: The patient was a well-appearing female in no acute discomfort.

VITAL SIGNS

Temperature	98.2°F (36.8°C)
Pulse	85 beats/minute
Blood pressure	130/80 mmHg
Respirations	20 breaths/minute
Oxygen saturation	100% on room air

RIGHT INDEX FINGER: A 1.5-cm oblique laceration was noted over the radial portion of the proximal interphalangeal (PIP) joint (Figure 74.1), with minimal bleeding from the wound. The patient was unable to extend her finger at this joint but was able to extend the metacarpophalangeal (MCP) joint. There was no obvious deformity to the finger or PIP joint, and the wound edges were clean without erythema. Brisk capillary refill of the distal phalanx was present. Numbness around the laceration was noted, although sensation to light touch and pinprick was present over the distal phalanx, volar pad and the remainder of the digit.

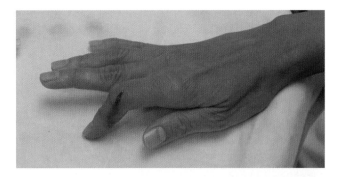

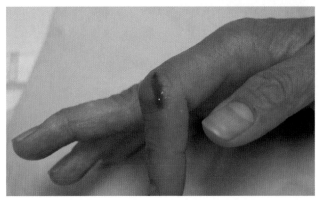

Figure 74.1 Laceration to the right index finger of a 50-year-old female attempting to extend the injured finger.

What is your diagnosis?

The diagnosis is extensor tendon laceration of the right index finger (zone 3). A digital block of the finger was performed following the initial physical examination, and the wound was copiously irrigated with normal saline. Upon careful exploration of the wound, near complete laceration of the extensor hood at the level of the PIP joint was noted. The wound was loosely approximated with two simple interrupted 5.0 nylon sutures. The finger was splinted in extension and the patient was started on amoxicillin/clavulanate 875 mg orally twice per day, pending definitive tendon repair. Two days later, the tendon laceration was repaired in the OR using seven 4.0 monocryl sutures. The patient was placed in a volar hand splint for four weeks with close follow up in the hand clinic, and referred for subsequent physical therapy.

Extensor tendon laceration of the fingers

The extensor tendons course over the dorsal side of the forearm, wrist and hand. Nine extensor tendons pass under the extensor retinaculum and separate into six compartments.[1] In the dorsum of the hand, the extensors digitorum communis are connected by junctura. Because of this, a complete tendon laceration proximal to the junctura may still result in normal extensor function.[1] In the finger, the extensor expansion divides into a central slip that attaches to the middle phalanx, and into two lateral bands that join with the tendons of the lumbricals and interosseous muscles that attach to the base of the distal phalanx.

The most common site of tendon injury is the extensors over the dorsum of the hand.[1,2] These extensors are predisposed to laceration because of their superficial location and the minimal amount of subcutaneous tissue between these tendons and overlying skin.[2] Because the extensor tendons are not constrained in tight fibro-osseous canals (except in the wrist), they are generally easily located and repaired. Closed injuries to extensor tendons of the hand and digits may appear innocuous at first but may result in tendon injuries that lead to severe deformities or dysfunction if undetected.[3] Closed injuries are also commonly associated with fractures. A hand radiograph is recommended in closed hand injuries when a fracture is suspected, or in open hand injuries where fracture or a foreign body is suspected.[3]

Injuries to the extensor tendons have been grouped into anatomic zones to improve classification and communication.[1–5] In the Verdan system, there are eight zones: zone I at the distal interphalangeal (DIP) joint level to zone VIII at the distal forearm level.[2] Zone III is the area of the PIP joint. The central tendon is the most commonly injured structure in this zone, and represents the second most common closed tendon injury in athletes.[2] The mechanisms for closed rupture of the central tendon include forced flexion of an actively extended finger, a direct blow to the dorsum of the PIP joint, or hyperextension with volar dislocation of the PIP joint.[2]

Disruption of the central tendon of the digit causes an imbalance in the extensor mechanism. The flexor digitorum superficialis (FDS) becomes unopposed and flexes the PIP joint. The lateral bands displace volarly to the axis of the PIP joint and become joint flexors. In addition, the extensor hood retracts proximally, causing extension of the MCP and DIP joints. The resulting tendon imbalance leads to a buttonhole (or *boutonnière*) deformity, with flexion of the PIP joint and hyperextension of the DIP and MCP joints.[2] Although open injuries of the central tendon may cause an acute *boutonnière* deformity, this is usually delayed several weeks after a closed athletic injury.

Although emergency physicians may repair many extensor tendon injuries immediately, some injuries are best managed with delayed repair.[3] In cases of extensor tendon lacerations, a hand surgeon should be consulted to determine the best course of management.[4] A hand specialist may recommend primary closure of the skin after wound irrigation, splinting the digit in extension and use of prophylactic antibiotics until definitive repair of the tendon is undertaken (usually within 24–48 hours). It is imperative the wounds occurring in zone III be carefully explored in the ED to rule out penetration of the joint capsule.[3] Patients with wounds that are suspected of penetrating the joint or joint capsule are generally taken to the OR for surgical exploration, irrigation and treatment with IV antibiotics, although protocols vary.[3]

Zone III tendon lacerations can result in long-term deformity if not carefully repaired, and patients with such injuries are commonly referred to a hand surgeon.[3] Tendons in zone III are free without ligamentous attachment, and are covered only by paratenon (tissue between a tendon sheath and its tendon) and fascia.[4] These tendons are generally sutured individually with a mattress suture of monofilament or other suture material that does not require removal as there is much less reaction to foreign materials in this area.[4] Lacerations over the PIP joint are best repaired with the PIP joint fixed in full extension. For contaminated wounds, repair is best delayed.[5] The extensor tendons should be splinted even longer than the flexor tendons to prevent damage to the repair resulting from the more powerful action of the flexor tendons.[5]

KEY TEACHING POINTS

1. Important components in the evaluation of patients presenting with hand injuries include obtaining a history of hand dominance, occupation, mechanism of injury and tetanus status.

2. The most common site of tendon injury is the extensors over the dorsum of the hand, which are predisposed to laceration because of their superficial location and the minimal amount of subcutaneous tissue between the overlying skin and tendon.

3. Disruption of the central extensor tendon may result in a *boutonnière* deformity of the finger.

4. In cases of extensor tendon lacerations, consultation with a hand or plastic surgeon should be considered; all flexor tendon injuries of the hand require specialty consultation.

5. In cases of extensor tendon laceration where repair of the tendon is not done in the ED, primary closure of the skin after irrigating the wound, splinting the digit in extension and prophylactic antibiotics until definitive repair are appropriate.

REFERENCES

[1] Muelleman RL, Wadman MC. Injuries to the hand and digits. In: Tintinalli JE, Kelen GD, Stapczynski JS (eds.). *Emergency Medicine: A Comprehensive Study Guide*, 6th ed. New York: McGraw-Hill, 2004;1665–73.

[2] Lyn E, Antosia RE. Hand. In: Marx JA, Hockberger RS, Walls RM (eds.). *Rosen's Emergency Medicine: Concepts and Clinical Practice*, 6th ed. Philadelphia: Mosby, 2006;576–619.

[3] Sokolove PE. Extensor and flexor tendon injuries of the hand, wrist, and foot. In: Roberts JR, Hedges JR, Chanmugam AS (eds.). *Roberts: Clinical Procedures in Emergency Medicine*, 4th ed. Philadelphia: Elsevier, 2004;928–30.

[4] Wright PE. Flexor and extensor tendon injuries. In: Canale TE, et al. (eds.). *Campbell's Operative Orthopedics*, 10th ed. Philadelphia: Mosby, 2003:3469.

[5] Bolitho DG. Hand, tendon lacerations: extensors. eMedicine Website. Available at http://www.emedicine.com/plastic/topic324.htm. Accessed June 23, 2008.

75

Cat bite to the finger of a 52-year-old male

HISTORY OF PRESENT ILLNESS

A 52-year-old right-hand dominant male presented to the ED three days after being bitten by his cat on his right index finger. One day following the cat bite, the patient presented to an urgent care clinic complaining of pain and a small area of redness around the bite. The patient was prescribed amoxicillin/clavulanate orally twice per day. Despite six doses, the patient continued to have pain, increased swelling and redness to the finger, which had spread to the back of his hand. He denied fevers or chills. His last tetanus immunization was unknown.

PHYSICAL EXAMINATION

GENERAL APPEARANCE: The patient was a well-developed, well-nourished male in no acute discomfort.

VITAL SIGNS

Temperature	99°F (37.2°C)
Pulse	95 beats/minute
Blood pressure	140/90 mmHg
Respirations	22 breaths/minute
Oxygen saturation	100% on room air

RIGHT HAND: A healing puncture wound on the dorsal surface of the right index finger was noted, as well as significant erythema and swelling to the finger and dorsum of the hand (Figure 75.1). The area was warm and tender to touch. The patient could flex his index finger and was able to make a fist, but experienced significant discomfort.

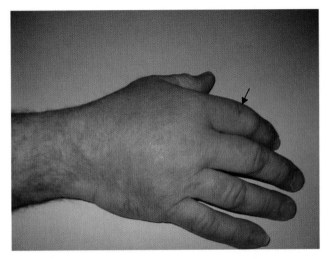

Figure 75.1 Right hand of a 52-year-old male three days after a cat bite to his right index finger (arrow indicates site of bite).

What is your diagnosis?

ANSWER

The diagnosis is cellulitis and lymphangitis of the hand from a cat bite. The patient received intravenous piperacillin/tazobactam and his tetanus status was updated. A radiograph of the right hand did not show subcutaneous air, osteomyelitis or a foreign body (e.g., cat tooth) (Figure 75.2). A complete blood count was normal. The right hand was splinted in neutral position and the patient was admitted to the plastic surgery service for additional intravenous antibiotics and hand elevation.

Mammalian bites of the hand

Mammalian bites of the hand generally have a high risk for infection because of the relatively poor blood supply of many structures and anatomic considerations that make adequate cleansing of the wound difficult. In general, the better the vascular supply and the easier the wound is to clean (i.e., laceration versus puncture), the lower the risk of infection.[1] Infections from mammalian bites can be caused by nearly any group of pathogens (bacteria, viruses, rickettsia, spirochetes or fungi). Common bacteria involved in cat bite wound infections include *Pasteurella, Actinomyces, Propionibacterium, Bacteroides, Fusobacterium, Clostridium, Wolinella, Peptostreptococcus, Staphylococcus* and *Streptococcus*.[1]

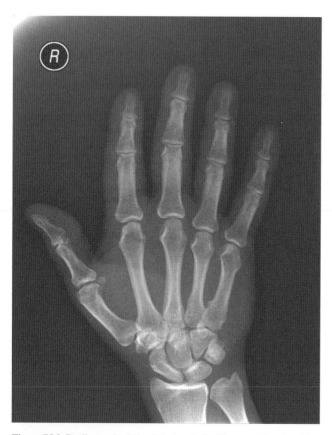

Figure 75.2 Radiograph of the right hand of a 52-year-old male with a cat bite to his right index finger.

Of an estimated 3–6 million animal bites in the United States, approximately 5–15% are from cats.[2] Approximately 6% of cat bite wounds require hospitalization. Women are more frequently bitten by cats, whereas men are more often bitten by dogs. Nearly half of all victims of cat bites are older than 20 years, and up to two-thirds of cat bite injuries occur on the upper extremity, typically the hand.[2] *Pasteurella multocida* infection, the most common pathogen contracted from cat bites, may be complicated by sepsis in rare cases. Meningitis, osteomyelitis and septic arthritis are additional concerns in bite wounds.

In taking a history for mammalian bites, note the type of animal and its immunization status (e.g., rabies vaccination), health and behavior. Note the time and location of the event, circumstances surrounding the bite (i.e., provoked or defensive bite versus unprovoked), current whereabouts of the animal (i.e., quarantined) and what pre-hospital treatment for the bite has been rendered. The victim's comorbidities (e.g., diabetes, peripheral vascular disease), immune status, tetanus status and allergies to medications should be carefully noted. In examination of the bite, consider distal neurovascular status, tendon and tendon sheath involvement, bone injury (particularly of the skull in infants and young children), joint space violation, visceral injury and foreign bodies.

A clenched fist injury that occurs when one person strikes another person's mouth is referred to as a "fight bite." This is a serious injury, where a tooth typically penetrates the dorsum of the hand over the third or fourth metacarpophalangeal (MCP) joint.[3] Although initial findings may reveal a small, seemingly innocuous puncture or laceration, the penetration often injures the soft tissue, extensor tendon and sheath, and may disrupt the MCP joint. If deep structures have been penetrated, a hand surgeon should be consulted immediately because of the high risk of spreading infection.[3]

Fresh wounds are not generally cultured, whereas infected wounds should be cultured. Other laboratory tests are generally not indicated in simple wound infections.[1] Radiographs are indicated if any concerns exist that deep structures are at risk (hand wounds, deep punctures, crush injuries), especially over joints. Radiographs may reveal occult fractures or osteomyelitis, as well as foreign bodies.

Bite wounds should be cleaned initially with soap and water; subsequently, all wounds should be copiously irrigated with normal saline or lactated Ringer's solution under high pressure with an 18- or 19-gauge catheter tip and large syringe. Devitalized tissue should be debrided.[1,4] Infected wounds and those first seen more than 24 hours after the bite should be left open. Some physicians recommend consideration of wound closure after irrigation and debridement in patients presenting less than eight hours after the injury if there is no visible evidence of infection.[4] For bite wounds in anatomic regions where there are significant cosmetic concerns (such as the face), a primary closure approach is often undertaken to prevent significant scarring. However, wounds with high risk of complication or infection, such as hand wounds, are generally left open even in patients who present early. Other important elements of treatment include elevation and immobilization

TABLE 75.1 Guide to tetanus prophylaxis in routine wound management among adults aged 19–64 years[7]

Characteristic History of absorbed	Clean, minor wound		All other wounds[a]	
Tetanus toxoid	Tdap or Td[b]	TIG	Tdap or Td[b]	TIG
Unknown or < 3	Yes	No	Yes	Yes
≥ 3	No[c]	No	No[d]	No

[a] Such as, but not limited to, wounds contaminated with dirt, feces, soil and saliva; puncture wounds; avulsions; and wounds resulting from missiles, crushing, burns and frostbite.

[b] Tdap is preferred to Td for adults who have never received Tdap. Td is preferred to TT for adults who received Tdap previously, or when Tdap is not available. If TT and TIG are both used, tetanus toxoid absorbed rather than tetanus toxoid for booster use only (fluid vaccine) should be used.

[c] Yes, if more than 10 years since last tetanus toxoid-containing vaccine dose.

[d] Yes, if more than 5 years since the last tetanus toxoid-containing vaccine dose.

of the wound, early removal of jewelry such as rings (which may cause constriction after edema occurs), and close follow up after discharge.

Whether antibiotics prevent infection after mammalian bites remains controversial. Although early studies reported rates of infection as high as 45% after dog or cat bites, the incidence was closer to 2–3% among patients who were not selected on the basis of risk factors for infection in subsequent studies.[5] Currently, antibiotic prophylaxis is indicated in all human bites and in selected cat and dog bite wounds (e.g., bites on the hand from a cat or dog).[5,6] If an antibiotic is prescribed, in most cases a β-lactam antibiotic such as amoxicillin combined with a β-lactamase inhibitor (e.g., amoxicillin/clavulanate) would be the appropriate choice.[2,5] Doxycycline may be considered in patients who are allergic to penicillin, although the anaerobic coverage may be less than ideal.[4]

In the case of infected bites, physicians must distinguish the normal inflammatory response from the erythema and swelling of infection. If a wound is obviously infected, some or all of the sutures should be removed (if present) and fluctuant collections of pus should be drained. Intravenous antibiotics should be administered in the majority of cases. Given the risk of tetanus after bites of all kinds, tetanus immune globulin (TIG) and tetanus toxoid (Td) should be administered to patients with two or fewer primary immunizations. Tetanus, diphtheria and pertussis toxoid (Tdap) is preferred to Td for adults 19–64 years of aged vaccinated more than five years ago who require a tetanus toxoid-containing vaccine as part of wound management, and who have not previously received Tdap (Table 75.1).[7] For adults previously vaccinated with Tdap, Td should be used if a tetanus toxoid-containing vaccine is indicated for wound care.

KEY TEACHING POINTS

1. Mammalian bites of the hand generally have a high risk of infection because of the relatively poor blood supply of many structures and anatomic considerations that make adequate cleansing of the wound difficult.

2. Evaluation of patients with mammalian bites should include noting patient comorbidities, tetanus status, medication allergies and hand dominance (in cases of hand or upper extremity bites).

3. In examination of the bite, consider distal neurovascular status, tendon and tendon sheath involvement, bone injury, joint space violation, visceral injury and foreign bodies (e.g., teeth or debris) in the wound.

4. Currently, antibiotics are recommended for all human bites and for high-risk wounds, such as deep punctures (particularly if inflicted by cats), those requiring surgical repair, and those involving the hand.

5. Wounds with high risk of complications or infection (such as hand wounds) are generally left open, even in patients who present early.

REFERENCES

[1] Stump JL. Bites, animal. eMedicine Website. Available at http://www.emedicine.com/emerg/topic60.htm. Accessed July 3, 2008.

[2] Talan DA, Citron DM, Abrahamian FM, et al. Bacteriologic analysis of infected dog and cat bites. *N Engl J Med* 1999;340:85–92.

[3] Daniels JM, Zook EG, Lynch JM. Hand and wrist injuries: Part II. Emergent evaluation. *Am Fam Physician* 2004;69:1949–56.

[4] Tapiltz RA. Managing bite wounds: currently recommended antibiotics for treatment and prophylaxis. *Postgrad Med* 2004;116:49–59.

[5] Fleisher GR. Editorial: the management of bite wounds. *N Engl J Med* 1999;340:138–40.

[6] Turner TWS. Do mammalian bites require antibiotic prophylaxis? *Ann Emerg Med* 2004;44:274–6.

[7] Kretsinger K, Broder KR, Cortese MM. Preventing tetanus, diphtheria, and pertussis among adults: use of tetanus toxoid, reduced diphtheria toxoid and acellular pertussis vaccine. Recommendations of the Advisory Committee on Immunization and Practices (ACIP) and recommendation of ACIP, supported by the Healthcare Infection Control Practices Advisory Committee (HICPAC), for use of Tdap among health-care personnel. *MMWR Recomm Rep* 2006; 55(RR-17):1–37.

PART X

PEDIATRICS

76

Rapid heart rate in an 8-week-old male

HISTORY OF PRESENT ILLNESS

An 8-week-old male with a medical history significant for fetal supraventricular tachycardia and Wolff-Parkinson-White syndrome (diagnosed in utero) was brought to the ED by his mother when she noted a rapid heart rate while holding her baby and feeling his chest. According to the mother, the child did not appear short of breath, and was not sweating during the episode. He had been feeding well prior to the onset of the rapid heart rate. The patient's only medication was sotalol 6 mg orally every eight hours; he had not missed any doses.

PHYSICAL EXAMINATION

GENERAL APPEARANCE: The patient appeared well nourished and well hydrated, was nontoxic and in no acute discomfort.

VITAL SIGNS

Temperature	98.0°F (36.6°C) rectal
Pulse	240 beats/minute
Blood pressure	not obtained
Respirations	30 breaths/minute
Oxygen saturation	99% on room air
Weight	11 lbs (5 kg)

HEENT: PERRL, EOMI, oropharynx moist.

NECK: Supple.

CARDIOVASCULAR: Tachycardic rate, regular rhythm, unable to assess for rubs, murmurs or gallops. Palpable and rapid brachial and femoral pulses.

LUNGS: Clear to auscultation bilaterally.

ABDOMEN: Soft, nontender, nondistended.

EXTREMITIES: No cyanosis or edema, capillary refill less than 2 sec.

SKIN: Pink, warm, well perfused, no rashes.

NEUROLOGIC: Nonfocal, age-appropriate exam.

The patient was placed on the cardiac monitor and a 12-lead ECG was obtained (Figure 76.1).

What is your diagnosis?

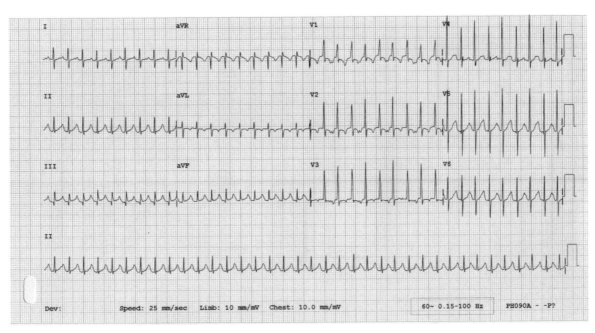

Figure 76.1 12-lead ECG from an 8-week-old male with a rapid heart rate.

ANSWER

The diagnosis is paroxysmal supraventricular tachycardia (PSVT). The 12-lead ECG demonstrated supraventricular tachycardia with a ventricular rate of 223 beats per minute. An ice bag was firmly placed over the child's face, which successfully converted the rhythm back to normal sinus rhythm (Figure 76.2). The patient's pediatric cardiologist was consulted, and a decision was made to maintain the current dosage of sotalol. The child was discharged home after a brief, uneventful observation period. Several hours later, the mother returned with her child stating that he had experienced another episode of PSVT, which had resolved by the time the patient arrived at the ED. The child was admitted to the pediatric intensive care unit overnight for observation and monitoring. The sotalol dose was increased from 6 mg orally three times per day to 7 mg orally three times per day. The child did not experience further episodes of PSVT, and was discharged the following morning.

Supraventricular Tachycardia

Supraventricular tachycardia (SVT) is the most common symptomatic dysrhythmia in infants and children, with a frequency of 1 in 250–1000 patients.[1,2] The peak incidence of SVT occurs during the first two months of life.[2] In newborns and infants who have SVT, the heart rate is usually greater than 220 beats/minute.[1] In older children, SVT is defined as a heart rate of more than 180 beats/minute. The ECG shows a narrow complex tachycardia, either without discernable P waves or with retrograde P waves with an abnormal axis. The

QRS duration is normal but may occasionally be increased with aberrant conduction. SVT is further characterized by little or no variation in the heart rate.[1]

In infants, the most common cause of SVT is idiopathic (approximately 50%), likely secondary to a concealed accessory atrioventricular pathway.[3] Approximately 25% have associated conditions such as infection, fever or drug exposure, 23% have previously diagnosed congenital heart disease, and 22% have Wolff-Parkinson-White syndrome (WPWS). Typical ECG findings of WPWS are a short PR interval, a wide QRS, and a positive deflection in the upstroke of the QRS complex. These findings are only evident after the SVT is converted to a sinus rhythm.[1] In older children and adolescents, atrioventricular node re-entry tachycardia (AVNRT) becomes more prevalent as a cause of SVT.[3]

Infants with SVT typically present with nonspecific complaints, such as fussiness, poor feeding, pallor or lethargy.[2] Older children may complain of chest pain, pounding in their chest, dizziness, shortness of breath or may demonstrate an altered level of consciousness. The diagnosis often begins in triage, with the nurse reporting that the "heart rate is too fast to count."[2] If congestive heart failure (CHF) is present, caretakers may describe pallor, cough and respiratory distress. Although many infants can tolerate SVT for 24 hours, 50% of infants with SVT will develop heart failure within 48 hours and may rapidly decompensate.[1]

The management of pediatric SVT begins with ensuring that the patient is maintaining airway, breathing and cardiovascular status. In a child presenting with unstable SVT with severe heart failure and poor perfusion, synchronized cardioversion is initiated at 0.5 J/kg, which can be increased up to

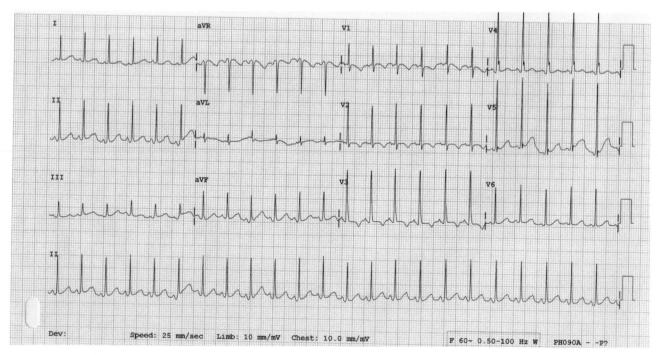

Figure 76.2 12-lead ECG from an 8-week-old male with a rapid heart rate after applying an ice bag over his face.

1 J/kg.[1] Adenosine may be administered before cardioversion if intravenous access has already been established. In unstable patients, cardioversion should not be delayed by attempts at IV access or sedation.[1] If the patient is stable, vagal maneuvers may be attempted. Vagal stimulatory maneuvers such as carotid massage, gagging, pressure on an eyeball, headstand or Valsalva may be effective in older children; these maneuvers are rarely effective in infants.[4,5] In infants, the only practical way to perform a vagal maneuver is by inducing the diving reflex with an ice bag over the face.[3] Reported complications of this maneuver include profound vagal response, retinal detachment if pressure is placed on the eye, and fat necrosis from cold injury to the face.[3]

Although intravenous calcium-channel blockers may be used as therapy for SVT in adults, they are contraindicated in children, especially those under 1 year of age. Hemodynamic compromise and sudden death have been reported in infants who were given verapamil.[5] Adenosine, an endogenous nucleoside, has negative chronotropic, dromotropic and inotropic actions of very short duration (half-life less than 1.5 sec), with minimal hemodynamic consequences.[4] It transiently blocks AV conduction and sinus node pacemaking activity. Adenosine is therefore the drug of choice in the treatment of SVT, terminating almost all SVT in which the AV node forms part of the reentry circuit. Adenosine is given as a rapid intravenous bolus followed by a saline flush, starting at 0.1 mg/kg (maximum dose 6 mg).[3] If the initial dose is unsuccessful, an increased dose of 0.2 mg/kg (maximum dose 12 mg) can be tried. An effective response results in a brief period of asystole on ECG, followed by the immediate return of a normal sinus rhythm.[1] Failure to terminate the dysrhythmia after the second dose of adenosine in a stable pediatric patient should prompt consultation with a pediatric cardiologist.

Alternative medications for pediatric SVT include procainamide (15 mg/kg IV over 30–60 min or 20–80 μg/kg/min) or amiodarone (5 mg/kg over 20–60 min, with a maximum single dose of 150 mg and a maximum daily dose of 15 mg/kg).[1] Amiodarone should not be used in newborns during the first month of life because it contains the preservative benzyl alcohol, which has been associated with a gasping syndrome characterized by metabolic acidosis, gasping respirations, hypotension, bradycardia and cardiovascular collapse.[1] Beta-blockers such as propranolol or esmolol should be used with caution because they may induce hypotension. Digoxin is not recommended in patients with WPWS because it can precipitate ventricular fibrillation.[3] Because WPWS cannot be diagnosed during the tachydysrhythmia, digoxin is discouraged in patients presenting with SVT for the first time.

Any infant found to have an initial episode of SVT should be thoroughly evaluated by a pediatric cardiologist to rule out SVT-induced CHF, anatomic anomalies (i.e., Ebstein's anomaly), or a re-entrant/aberrant pathway such as WPWS.[6] The prognosis for infants with SVT is excellent, with 60–90% of patients experiencing complete remission of symptoms by 6–12 months of age.[6] The long-term management of SVT may include beta-blockers, procainamide, sotalol, amiodarone or flecainide.[1] When pharmacologic treatment fails, radiofrequency catheter ablation has an 85–95% success rate of preventing recurrent SVT.[1]

KEY TEACHING POINTS

1. Supraventricular tachycardia (SVT) is the most common symptomatic dysrhythmia in infants and children, with a frequency of 1 in 250–1000 patients.
2. The ECG in SVT shows a narrow complex tachycardia either without discernable P waves or with retrograde P waves with an abnormal axis, a normal QRS duration (except when aberrancy is present), and little or no variation in the heart rate.
3. Infants with SVT typically present with nonspecific complaints, such as fussiness, poor feeding, pallor, or lethargy; older children may complain of chest pain, pounding in their chest, dizziness, shortness of breath or an altered level of consciousness.
4. In a child presenting with unstable SVT and severe heart failure or poor perfusion, synchronized cardioversion should be performed immediately at 0.5 J/kg, and can be increased up to 1 J/kg.
5. In stable patients with SVT, vagal maneuvers may be attempted, followed by intravenous adenosine if necessary.

REFERENCES

[1] Doniger SJ, Sharieff GQ. Pediatric dysrhythmias. *Pediatr Clin N Am* 2006;53:85–105.
[2] Sharieff GQ, Rao SO. The pediatric ECG. *Emerg Med Clin N Am* 2006;24:195–208.
[3] Brown K. The infant with undiagnosed cardiac disease in the Emergency Department. *Clin Ped Emerg Med* 2005;6:200–6.
[4] Park MK, Troxler RG. Cardiac arrythmias. In: Zorab R, Fletcher J (eds.). *Pediatric Cardiology for Practitioners*, 4th ed. Philadelphia: Mosby, 2002;338–41.
[5] Kaltman J, Shah M. Evaluation of the child with an arrhythmia. *Pediatr Clin N Am* 2004;51:1537–51.
[6] Woods WA, McCulloch MA. Cardiovascular emergencies in the pediatric patient. *Emerg Med Clin N Am* 2005;23:1233–49.

77

Cough, fever and poor feeding in a 4-month-old male

HISTORY OF PRESENT ILLNESS

A 4-month-old male was brought to the ED by his parents for four days of cough, fever, breathing difficulty and poor feeding. The patient would breastfeed for only a short time before becoming agitated with rapid breathing and sweating, and had produced only two wet diapers over the past 24 hours. The family denied any sick contacts or recent travel, and the infant's immunizations and routine medical appointments were current.

PHYSICAL EXAMINATION

GENERAL APPEARANCE: The patient appeared lethargic and dusky, with a rapid respiratory rate, visible grunting, nasal flaring and sternal retractions.

VITAL SIGNS

Temperature	95.4°F (35.2°C) rectal
Pulse	180 beats/minute
Blood pressure	not obtained
Respiratory rate	60 breaths/minute
Oxygen saturation	91% on room air

HEENT: PERRL, oropharynx moist, nasal flaring, no perioral cyanosis appreciated.

CARDIOVASCULAR: Tachycardic, regular rate, unable to appreciate rubs, murmurs or gallops. Weak femoral pulses noted.

LUNGS: Coarse breath sounds present bilaterally, with markedly diminished breath sounds on the left.

ABDOMEN: Soft, nontender, nondistended, no masses.

EXTREMITIES: Cool, delayed capillary refill (more than 3 sec).

SKIN: Dusky and clammy, no rashes.

NEUROLOGIC: Awake, crying, moving all extremities.

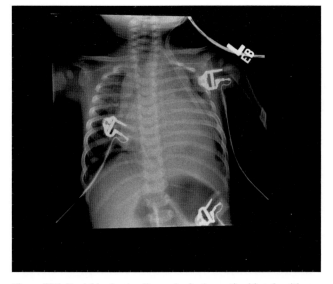

Figure 77.1 Portable chest radiograph of a 4-month-old male with respiratory distress.

The patient was placed on the cardiac monitor, a peripheral intravenous line was placed and blood was sent for laboratory testing. He initially received nebulized bronchodilator treatments (albuterol) and oral corticosteroids (prednisolone), and a portable chest radiograph was obtained (Figure 77.1).

What is your diagnosis?

ANSWER

The diagnosis is dilated cardiomyopathy. The initial chest radiograph demonstrated marked cardiomegaly. As the patient's respiratory status continued to deteriorate, the patient was emergently intubated (post-intubation radiograph, Figure 77.2). Two 20 mL/kg boluses of intravenous normal saline were administered with improvement of his hemodynamic status. Laboratory tests revealed a leukocyte count of 14.1 K/µL (normal 6.0–17.0 K/µL), hematocrit of 32.4% (normal 28–42%), and a post-intubation arterial blood gas on 100% inspired oxygen with pH of 7.14 (normal 7.32–7.43), pCO_2 of 37 mmHg, pO_2 of 207 mmHg and bicarbonate of 12.6 mmol/L with a base excess of −16.0 mmol/L, consistent with a metabolic acidosis. The troponin I returned elevated at 0.72 ng/mL (normal 0.00–0.09 ng/mL). The patient was admitted to the Pediatric Intensive Care Unit (PICU).

A transthoracic echocardiogram showed a left ventricular end-diastolic dimension of 46 mm (mean for age 23 mm), with a calculated ejection fraction of 33% consistent with severe dilated cardiomyopathy (Figure 77.3). The patient was started on a dobutamine drip (10 mcg/kg/min IV) in the PICU, as well as a regimen of digoxin, furosemide, spironolactone, captopril, levocarnitine and aspirin per pediatric cardiology recommendations. The patient remained intubated until hospital day #10, after which he was weaned to nasal cannula and finally room air. The patient was discharged home on hospital day #18.

Pediatric dilated cardiomyopathy

Dilated cardiomyopathy (DCM) is a myocardial disorder characterized by a dilated left ventricular chamber and systolic dysfunction. It commonly results in congestive heart failure

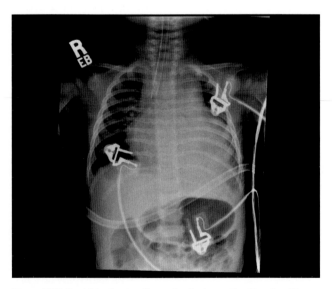

Figure 77.2 Portable chest radiograph of a 4-month-old male with respiratory distress post-intubation.

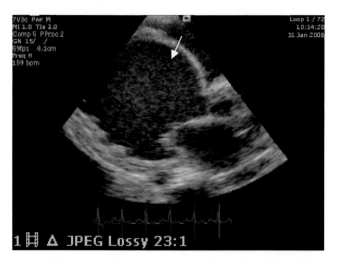

Figure 77.3 Transthoracic echocardiogram from a 4-month-old male showing a dilated left ventricle (arrow).

(CHF), and is the most common form of cardiomyopathy and reason for cardiac transplantation in adults and children.[1,2] The incidence of DCM in children in North America has been estimated to be 0.56 cases per 100,000 per year, ten-fold lower than in adults.[1] The cause in the vast majority of pediatric cases is still unknown (idiopathic dilated cardiomyopathy) but may have a genetic basis. A remote history of viral illness in many patients suggests that the disease may be a sequela of a previous episode of myocarditis.[3] In as many as 20% of cases, the disease is recognized as familial, having autosomal dominant, autosomal recessive, X-linked and mitochondrial inheritance patterns.[3] Nearly 40% of children with symptomatic cardiomyopathy receive a transplant or die within 2 years. Outcomes have not improved substantially, despite advances in medical care and technology.[4,5]

Dilated cardiomyopathy is a common etiology of CHF in children.[6] CHF exists when the heart is unable to provide an output sufficient to meet the metabolic demands of the body. Although CHF is often a chronic condition, acute decompensation may occur when compensatory mechanisms are overwhelmed.[6] Clinical symptoms of CHF vary depending on age and underlying cardiac pathophysiology. Neonates and infants may have failure to thrive, feeding difficulties, diaphoresis and tachypnea. Viral upper respiratory tract infections and fevers or dehydration may be poorly tolerated. Older children with failure of the left ventricle may have dyspnea on exertion, exercise intolerance or syncope. Common signs of left-sided decompensated heart failure include rales on lung auscultation and tachycardia. In advanced cases, patients may have evidence of cardiogenic shock (poor perfusion, hypotension), severe pulmonary edema and other end-organ insufficiency.[6]

The electrocardiogram in DCM shows a combination of atrial enlargement, varying degrees of left or right ventricular hypertrophy, and nonspecific T-wave abnormalities.[3] The chest radiograph confirms cardiomegaly. Pulmonary congestion and pleural effusions may be present. Echocardiography shows dilatation of the left atrium and ventricle, and poor contractility. Doppler studies show decreased flow velocity through the aortic valve and mitral regurgitation.[3]

Treatment of acute decompensated CHF of infants and children in the emergency department includes supplemental oxygen to keep saturations about 95%.[7] Over-oxygenating the patient may lead to pulmonary vascular dilation and worsened failure. The infant should be kept in a semi-reclining position if possible, although older children will generally find their own best position. Fluid and sodium restriction are necessary, and furosemide should be given at 0.5–2.0 mg/kg intravenously as diuretic therapy.[6] Patients may require sedation, but careful attention must be paid to maintaining airway, breathing and circulation. Preparations should be made for endotracheal intubation and ventilatory support in the event they are needed. If the patient is in shock, fluids must be used judiciously (boluses of only 5 mL/kg, if at all), and inotropic support with dopamine (3–10 µg/kg/min) or dobutamine (starting dose of 5 µg/kg/min) may be more appropriate.[6,7] Complete blood count, chemistry panel, calcium level, rapid bedside glucose test and arterial blood gas should be assessed. Vital signs, including blood pressure, cardiac rhythm and oxygen saturation, should be monitored continuously. It is important to involve the pediatric intensivist as well as a pediatric cardiologist early in the evaluation of any child in acute decompensated CHF.

KEY TEACHING POINTS

1. The cause of pediatric dilated cardiomyopathy (DCM) in the vast majority of cases is unknown but may have a genetic basis; a remote history of viral illness suggests that the disease may be a sequela of a previous episode of myocarditis.
2. The onset of DCM is usually insidious but symptoms of heart failure may occur suddenly. Irritability, anorexia, abdominal pain, cough from pulmonary congestion and dyspnea with exertion (such as during feeding) are common.
3. The electrocardiogram in DCM shows a combination of atrial enlargement, varying degrees of left or right ventricular hypertrophy, and nonspecific T-wave abnormalities, whereas the chest radiograph confirms cardiomegaly.
4. Emergency treatment of decompensated CHF includes supplemental oxygen, proper positioning, fluid and sodium restriction, and diuretic administration. Early involvement of a pediatric cardiologist or intensivist is essential.
5. In patients with shock, fluids must be used judiciously; inotropic support with dopamine or dobutamine may be necessary.

REFERENCES

[1] Towbin JA, Lowe AM, Colan SD, et al. Incidence, causes, and outcomes of dilated cardiomyopathy in children. *JAMA* 2006;296:1867–76.
[2] Tsirka AE, Trinkaus K, Chen S-C, et al. Improved outcomes of pediatric dilated cardiomyopathy with utilization of heart transplantation. *J Am Coll Cardiol* 2004;44:391–7.
[3] Bernstein D. Diseases of the myocardium. In: Behrman RE, Kliegman RM, Jensen HB (eds.). *Nelson Textbook of Pediatrics*, 17th ed. Philadelphia: Elsevier, 2004; 1572–5.
[4] Cox GF, Sleeper LA, Lowe AM, et al. Factors associated with establishing a causal diagnosis for children with cardiomyopathy. *Pediatrics* 2006;118:1519–31.
[5] Lipshultz SE, Sleeper LA, Towbin JA, et al. The incidence of pediatric cardiomyopathy in two regions of the United States. *N Engl J Med* 2003;348:1647–55.
[6] Costello JM, Almodovar MC. Emergency care for infants and children with acute cardiac disease. *Clin Ped Emerg Med* 2007;8:145–55.
[7] Young KD. Congenital heart disease. In: Strange GR, Ahrens WR, Lelyveld S, Schafermeyer RW (eds.). *Pediatric Emergency Medicine, A Comprehensive Study Guide*, 2nd ed. New York: McGraw-Hill, 2002;241–2.

78

Head trauma in a 5-month-old male

HISTORY OF PRESENT ILLNESS

A 5-month-old male was brought to the ED by his parents after falling out of his car safety seat, which had been on the kitchen counter. The patient fell approximately 4 feet onto the floor, striking the back of his head. The child was noted to cry immediately, and had not experienced any episodes of vomiting following the injury. The parents reported a bump on his scalp but denied other associated injuries.

PHYSICAL EXAMINATION

GENERAL APPEARANCE: The patient was awake and alert, playful, smiling and interactive with the examiner.

VITAL SIGNS

Temperature	98.3°F (36.8°C) rectal
Pulse	115 beats/minute
Blood pressure	not obtained
Respirations	26 breaths/minute
Oxygen saturation	100% on room air

HEENT: 4 cm × 4 cm hematoma over the left occipital region without lacerations or crepitance. PERRL, conjugate gaze, oropharynx moist.

NECK: Supple.

CARDIOVASCULAR: Regular rate and rhythm without rub, murmur or gallop.

LUNGS: Clear to auscultation bilaterally.

ABDOMEN: Soft, nontender, nondistended, active bowel sounds present, no bruising or masses.

EXTREMITIES: No cyanosis or edema, brisk capillary refill, no deformities or swelling.

NEUROLOGIC: Alert, moving all four extremities, age appropriate.

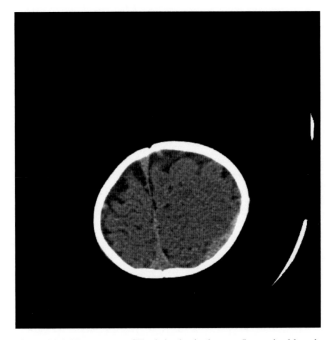

Figure 78.1 Noncontrast CT of the brain from a 5-month-old male after a fall from 4 feet.

The parents were instructed not to give the child anything by mouth, and a noncontrast CT of the brain was obtained (Figure 78.1).

What is your diagnosis?

ANSWER

The diagnosis is subdural hematoma (SDH). The noncontrast CT demonstrated a hyperdense region in the left occipital area just underneath the occipital hematoma, consistent with a subdural hematoma (Figure 78.2). The patient was transferred to the pediatric neurosurgery service, and was observed for 24 hours in the pediatric intensive care unit. The patient's neurologic status remained stable, and a repeat CT scan obtained the following day demonstrated dramatic improvement in the SDH (Figure 78.3). The patient was discharged home on hospital day #2, with close follow up in the pediatric neurosurgery clinic.

Pediatric head injury

Pediatric head injury comprises a large portion of pediatric trauma cases seen in EDs. Among children up to 14 years of age, traumatic brain injury (TBI) results in over 400,000 ED visits each year.[1] Injury rates are highest among children up to 4 years of age. A total of 1–2% of all pediatric patients seen in the ED present with minor head trauma; only 3–5% of those patients have intracranial injury, and less than 1% of these patients require neurosurgical intervention.[1] Nonetheless, TBI accounts for the single largest source of childhood mortality, with an additional 29,000 children suffering permanent neurologic disability.[2]

Child abuse is a common etiology of head injury in young children, and must be considered when evaluating a child with a head injury. In one study, 24% of head injuries in infants resulted from inflicted trauma; among infants with severe injuries, the proportion was even higher.[3] In cases of acciden-

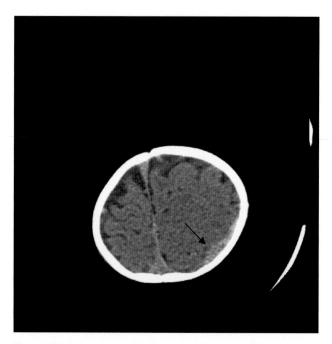

Figure 78.2 Noncontrast CT of the brain from a 5-month-old male with a left occipital subdural hematoma (arrow).

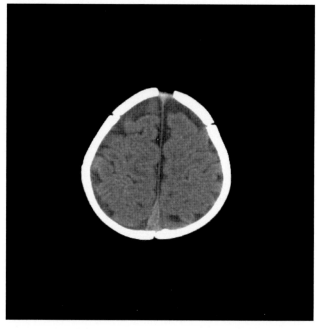

Figure 78.3 Repeat noncontrast CT of the brain from a 5-month-old male following head trauma the following day.

tal head injury, falls account for the most common mechanism of injury, particularly in children less than 2 years old.[1] One study of head-injured infants demonstrated a relationship between mechanism of injury and likelihood of intracranial injury (ICI), with direct falls from heights greater than or equal to 3 feet and falls on stairs being more likely to result in ICI than falls less than 3 feet.[4]

Children who sustain head trauma often have more pronounced physical signs and symptoms than adults. Despite apparent "trivial" trauma, children may appear pale, lethargic, have frequent emesis, and complain of headaches and dizziness.[2] Conversely, the clinical presentation of post-traumatic intracranial lesions in infants can be extremely subtle, especially in those younger than 6 months.[2] Clinical signs and symptoms are poor indicators of ICI in infants, and occult ICIs are more common among younger infants.[1] In asymptomatic infants, the presence of a scalp hematoma on physical examination has been shown to be a clinical indicator of a potential underlying skull fracture, and warrants further investigation.[4]

A noncontrast CT should be strongly considered in pediatric patients with minor head trauma who have history of vomiting, abnormal mental status or lethargy, clinical signs of skull fracture, obvious scalp hematomas in children 2 years old or younger, and increasing headache.[2] The use of skull radiography to screen infants for skull fractures is still controversial because skull radiographs do not detect underlying brain injury.[1] If a fracture is detected on radiographs, a head CT is required to evaluate for underlying intracranial pathology.

In an effort to derive a decision rule for identifying children at low risk for traumatic brain injuries, Palchak et al. enrolled 2043 children with blunt head trauma in an observational cohort study.[5] Of the children who underwent CT (62%),

98 (7.7%) had traumatic brain injuries on CT scan. Of the 2043 patients, 105 had traumatic brain injuries requiring acute intervention (29 of those patients did not have a traumatic brain injury identified on the initial CT scan). Abnormal mental status, clinical signs of skull fracture, history of vomiting, scalp hematoma (in children younger than 2 years) or headache identified 97/98 of those children with traumatic brain injuries on CT scan and 105/105 of those with traumatic brain injuries requiring acute intervention. The authors concluded that the absence of all of these findings were important factors for identifying children at low risk for traumatic brain injuries after blunt head trauma.

KEY TEACHING POINTS

1. Although less than 1% of pediatric patients with head injury require neurosurgical intervention, TBI accounts for the single largest source of childhood mortality, with 29,000 children suffering permanent neurologic disability each year.

2. Child abuse is a common etiology of head injury in young children, and must be considered when evaluating any child with a head injury.

3. The clinical presentation of post-traumatic intracranial lesions in infants can be extremely subtle, especially in those younger than 6 months.

4. In asymptomatic infants, presence of scalp hematomas on physical examination has been shown to be a clinical indicator of a potential underlying skull fracture, and warrants further investigation.

5. Abnormal mental status, clinical signs of skull fracture, history of vomiting, scalp hematoma (in children younger than 2 years) or headache following minor head injury may indicate significant intracranial pathology in these patients.

REFERENCES

[1] Thiessen ML, Woolridge DP. Pediatric minor closed head injury. *Pediatr Clin N Am* 2006;53:1–26.

[2] Heegaard WG, Biros MH. Head. In: Marx, JA, Hockberger, RS, Walls, RM, et al. (eds.). *Rosen's Emergency Medicine: Concepts and Clinical Practice*, 6th ed. Philadelphia: Mosby, 2006;349–82.

[3] Duhaime AC, Christian CW, Rorke LB, et al. Nonaccidental head injury in infants – the "shaken-baby syndrome." *N Engl J Med* 1998;338:1822–9.

[4] Greenes DS, Schutzman SA. Clinical indicators of intracranial injury in head-injured infants. *Pediatrics* 1999;104: 861–7.

[5] Palchak MJ, Holmes JF, Vance CW, et al. A decision rule for identifying children at low risk for brain injuries after blunt head trauma. *Ann Emerg Med* 2003;42:492–506.

79

PEG tube complication in a 7-month-old female

HISTORY OF PRESENT ILLNESS

A 7-month-old female with a medical history significant for Treacher Collins syndrome presented to the ED one day following percutaneous endoscopic gastrostomy (PEG) tube replacement in the gastroenterology clinic. The PEG tube had been in place since 3 months of age for enteral feedings. Her mother noted significant leakage of formula around the PEG tube site on the day of presentation, as well as several episodes of nonbloody, watery diarrhea.

PHYSICAL EXAMINATION

GENERAL APPEARANCE: The child appeared well nourished, well hydrated and in no acute discomfort.

VITAL SIGNS

Temperature	98.4°F (36.9°C)
Pulse	110 beats/minute
Blood pressure	not obtained
Respirations	26 breaths/minute
Oxygen saturation	100% on room air
Weight	26.4 lbs (12 kg)

HEENT: Downward slanting eyes, a small lower jaw and malformed ears consistent with Treacher Collins syndrome. PERRL, EOMI, oropharynx moist.

NECK: Supple.

CARDIOVASCULAR: Regular rate and rhythm without rubs, murmurs or gallops.

LUNGS: Clear to auscultation bilaterally.

ABDOMEN: Soft, nontender, nondistended. PEG tube site clean and intact, no erythema, slight leakage of formula at the PEG tube insertion site was noted.

EXTREMITIES: No cyanosis or edema, brisk capillary refill (less than 2 sec).

NEUROLOGIC: Nonfocal.

An abdominal radiograph was obtained (Figure 79.1), followed by observing flow of contrast through the PEG tube under fluoroscopy (Figure 79.2).

What is your diagnosis?

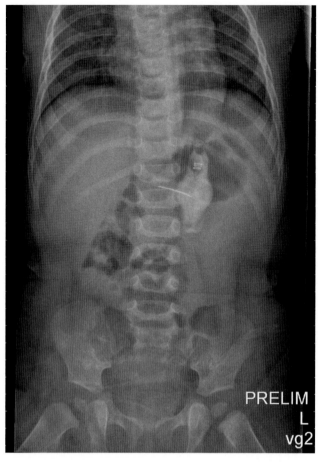

Figure 79.1 Abdominal radiograph from a 7-month-old female with leakage around the PEG tube site.

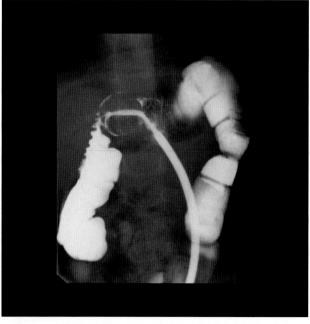

Figure 79.2 KUB radiograph under fluoroscopy following instillation of contrast into the PEG tube in a 7-month-old female with recent PEG tube replacement.

ANSWER

The diagnosis is translocation of the PEG tube into the transverse colon during recent replacement. The contrast fluoroscopy demonstrates opacification of the colon, with neither uptake of contrast into the stomach nor leakage of contrast into the peritoneum. Placement of the tip of the tube was at the level of the hepatic flexure (Figure 79.2). The patient received prophylactic intravenous antibiotics and was taken to the OR by the pediatric surgeon where an exploratory laparotomy was performed. Upon surgical exploration, the gastrostomy tube button was in the colon; it appeared that the initial gastrostomy tube had been placed such that it perforated through the transverse colon into the stomach. In fact, it had functioned normally for several months in this position until the tube was replaced in the clinic one day prior to presentation. No leakage of formula or stool was noted into the peritoneum. The section of transverse colon that the tube had transversed was resected with the colon re-anastamosed; the gastrostomy tube was replaced intraoperatively in the correct position in the stomach.

Colocutaneous fistula as a PEG tube complication

Colocutaneous fistula is a rare PEG tube-related complication.[1] In some reported cases of colocutaneous fistula, the tip of the gastrostomy tubes were in the stomach at the time of insertion and functioned normally until they migrated to the colon.[1] After this migration, the patients exhibited symptoms including diarrhea, malnutrition, formula in their stools due to the direct passage of feedings into the colon, and fecal material in the gastrostomy tube. The fistula is thought to form during insertion of the original PEG tube, when the colon becomes interposed between the stomach and the abdominal wall.[2,3] The fistula initially functions normally, and the patient can remain asymptomatic for several months. The transverse colon is tightly compressed but not completely obstructed, enabling feces and flatus to pass. Such colocutaneous fistulae often remain asymptomatic until the tube is exchanged.[2]

Appreciation of a colocutaneous fistula is important for clinicians who insert PEG tubes. The occurrence of such a complication should be taken into consideration whenever this procedure is performed for the initial placement or subsequent replacement of the cannulae.[4] Early accidental dislodgement of a PEG tube in a patient with a colocutaneous fistula, in whom the tract is not yet mature, may lead to fecal peritonitis and death. At the time of changing a PEG tube, the correct position of the new tube must be confirmed before feeding commences. The development of feculent emesis, severe diarrhea, formula in the stool or fecal material in the gastrostomy tube after replacement of a PEG tube should alert clinicians to the possibility of this rare complication.[4]

KEY TEACHING POINTS

1. Colocutaneous fistula is a rare but significant complication of PEG tube placement.
2. The presence of a colocutaneous fistula is generally not recognized until the tube dislodges into the colon or upon replacement of the tube.
3. Signs and symptoms of colocutaneous fistula following PEG tube placement include diarrhea, malnutrition, appearance of formula in the stool, and fecal material in the gastrostomy tube.
4. Passage of contrast through the PEG tube visualized under fluoroscopy is the test of choice for diagnosing a colocutaneous fistula.
5. The gastroenterology and surgical services should be consulted upon diagnosis of a colocutaneous fistula after PEG tube placement.

REFERENCES

[1] Siddique I, Krishnamurthy M, Choubey S, et al. Colocutaneous fistula: a rare and silent complication of percutaneous endoscopic gastrostomy. *Dig Dis Sci* 1996;41:301–4.
[2] Sakai H, Inamori M, Sato T, et al. Colocutaneous fistula after percutaneous endoscopic gastrostomy (Letter to the Editor). *Digestion* 2007;75:103.
[3] Karhadkar AS, Schwartz HJ, Dutta SK. Jejunocutaneous fistula manifesting as chronic diarrhea after PEG tube replacement. *J Clin Gastroenterol* 2006;40:560–1.
[4] Smyth GP, McGreal GT, McDermott EWN. Delayed presentation of gastric colocutaneous fistula after percutaneous endoscopic gastrostomy. *Nutrition* 2003;19:905–6.

80

Cough and fever in a 10-month-old female

HISTORY OF PRESENT ILLNESS

A 10-month-old female born at 31 weeks gestation presented to the ED with three days of cough, runny nose, rapid breathing and fevers to 102°F (38.9°C). The mother reported her infant was acting normal for her age, feeding and urinating well. Neither vomiting nor diarrhea had occurred. Her last dose of acetaminophen was 12 hours earlier. The patient's mother denied any recent travel or sick contacts, and her immunizations were current.

PHYSICAL EXAMINATION

GENERAL APPEARANCE: The child appeared well nourished, well hydrated, active and nontoxic, although she was breathing rapidly.

VITAL SIGNS

Temperature	102°F (38.9°C) rectal
Pulse	173 beats/minute
Blood pressure	not obtained
Respirations	70 breaths/minute
Oxygen saturation	92% on room air
Weight	23 lbs (10.5 kg)

HEENT: PERRL, nasal flaring, oropharynx pink and moist.

NECK: Supple, no meningeal signs.

CARDIOVASCULAR: Tachycardic rate, regular rhythm without rubs, murmurs or gallops.

LUNGS: Intercostal retractions, mild expiratory wheezing and crackles present bilaterally, with good air movement.

ABDOMEN: Soft, nontender, nondistended.

EXTREMITIES: No clubbing, cyanosis or edema; brisk capillary refill (less than 2 sec).

SKIN: Pink, warm and dry.

NEUROLOGIC: Age-appropriate.

The patient was placed on the cardiac monitor with continuous pulse oximetry, and supplemental oxygen was administered by face mask. Acetaminophen 160 mg rectal suppository was administered, albuterol nebulized treatments were begun and a chest radiograph was obtained (Figure 80.1).

What is your diagnosis?

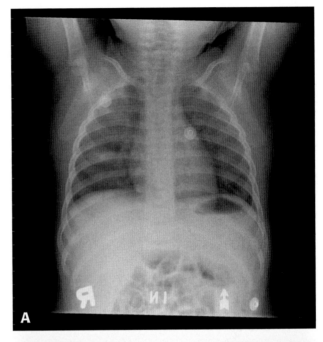
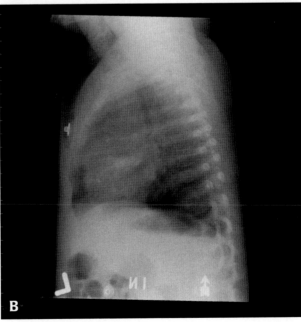

Figure 80.1 Anteroposterior (panel A) and lateral (panel B) views of the chest radiograph from a 10-month-old female with three days of cough, fevers and rapid breathing.

ANSWER

The diagnosis is respiratory syncytial virus (RSV) bronchiolitis with concomitant bacterial pneumonia. The chest radiograph demonstrates mild hyperinflation of the lungs with peribronchial infiltrates in a central, symmetric pattern consistent with a viral-type pattern of pneumonitis. There is also a focal infiltrate in the medial segment of the right middle lobe consistent with pneumonia (arrow, Figure 80.2). The patient received amoxicillin suspension orally (500 mg) and was admitted to the pediatric service. A nasopharyngeal swab obtained in the ED returned positive for RSV by reverse transcriptase-polymerase chain reaction (RT-PCR). The patient's respiratory status improved, and she was discharged home on hospital day #3 to complete a ten-day course of oral amoxicillin.

Pediatric pneumonia

Community-acquired pneumonia (CAP) is one of the most common serious infections in children, with an annual incidence of 34–40 cases per 1000 children in North America.[1-3] Group B streptococcus and Gram-negative enteric bacteria are the most common pathogens in neonates (i.e., birth to 20 days), and are transmitted from the mother during birth.[3] Anaerobic organisms may be acquired from chorioamnionitis (inflammation of the fetal membranes). Pneumonia in infants three weeks to three months of age is most often bacterial; *Streptococcus pneumonia* is the most common pathogen.[2] From three months of age to the preschool years, viruses are the predominant causative organisms, with RSV the most common viral cause.[2,3] The etiology of bacterial pneumonia during this age range is still predominantly *S. pneumoniae*. Other potential bacterial causes of pediatric pneumonia include *Mycoplasma pneumoniae, Haemophilus influenza* type B and non-typeable strains, *Staphylococcus aureus*, and *Moraxella catarrhalis*.[1,2]

Pneumonia can be defined clinically as the presence of lower respiratory tract dysfunction in association with radiographic opacity.[4] Bacterial pneumonia generally has an abrupt onset with fever and chills, productive cough, and chest pain.[2] However, infants may have poor feeding, disturbed sleep or symptoms less typical than older children. Regarding clinical findings indicative of pneumonia, tachypnea has good clinical reproducibility compared with observation of retractions or auscultatory findings such as crackles or wheezes.[4] However, no finding in itself can be used to diagnose or rule out pneumonia. The absence of the symptom cluster of respiratory distress, tachypnea, crackles and decreased breath sounds accurately excludes the presence of pneumonia.[4] Assessment of oxygenation gives a good indication of disease severity. Although the respiratory rate is neither sensitive nor specific for identifying hypoxia, the children's general well-being and ability to be consoled typically indicate normal oxygenation. Oximetry should be used in the assessment of a child with suspected pneumonia in the outpatient or hospital setting because these results correlate well with clinical outcome and length of hospital stay.[4]

In an immunocompetent patient with an uncomplicated lower respiratory tract infection who is otherwise stable, laboratory testing is not necessary.[2] The complete blood count (CBC) with differential does not differentiate bacterial from viral infection, and should not be measured routinely.[3] Rapid antigen tests are available for RSV, parainfluenza 1, 2 and 3, influenza A and B, and adenovirus. These assays, performed on specimens collected from the nasopharynx, can help determine the etiology of viral pneumonia.[3] A confirmatory chest radiograph is necessary to diagnose pneumonia. Both bronchiolitis and asthma may cause hyperinflation and atelectasis, and must therefore be distinguished from pneumonia.[4] Two main patterns of pneumonia are recognized: interstitial and alveolar. However, these patterns cannot be used to identify the etiology. Peribronchial thickening, diffuse interstitial infiltrates and hyperventilation tend to be seen with viral infections.[4] Lobar infiltrates, particularly with pneumatoceles and pulmonary abscesses, strongly suggest bacterial pneumonia.

In the majority of mild to moderate cases of pediatric bacterial pneumonia, oral antimicrobial therapy is adequate. Antibiotics should be initiated based on the presumptive causative organism. For infants less than 28 days old, empiric ampicillin 50 mg/kg every six hours and a third-generation cephalosporin such as cefotaxime at 50 mg/kg every six hours should be considered.[2] For patients older than three months who are stable, amoxicillin may be prescribed as an outpatient at 100–120 mg/kg/day divided in three doses.[2] In children older than three years, oral azithromycin at a dose of 10 mg/kg the first day followed by 5 mg/kg/day for the next four days is appropriate therapy to cover atypical pneumonias.

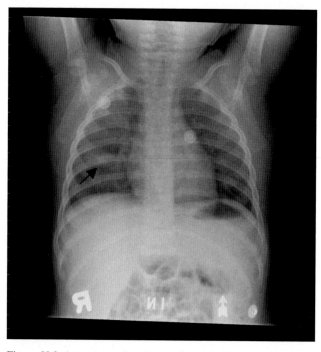

Figure 80.2 Anteroposterior chest radiograph from a 10-month-old female with RSV bronchiolitis and coexisting bacterial pneumonia (arrow indicates focal infiltrate within the medial segment of the right middle lobe).

Intravenous antibiotics are usually reserved for neonates and patients with severe pneumonia who warrant hospitalization. The ultimate decision to admit a patient must be based on the overall clinical picture and the reliability of parents. Given the rise in incidence of organisms resistant to antibiotics, prescribing antibiotics for nonbacterial (i.e., viral) infections should be actively discouraged.

Bronchiolitis

Bronchiolitis is a common, usually self-limited, lower respiratory tract infection caused by RSV observed in all geographic areas, usually between October and April.[5] The underlying pathophysiology of viral bronchiolitis is inflammation of the small airways (bronchioles). Infection of the bronchiolar and ciliated epithelial cells produces increased mucous secretion, cell death and sloughing, followed by a peribronchial lymphocytic infiltrate and submucosal edema.[6] This combination of debris and edema results in distal airway obstruction, which in turn results in increased work of breathing due to increased end expiratory lung volume and decreased lung compliance. Although bronchiolitis may occur in all age groups, the larger airways in older children better accommodate mucosal edema; thus, severe symptoms are usually seen in children less than two years of age.[2]

The incubation period of RSV varies from two to eight days and, after a prodrome of several days, results in an acute illness characterized by rhinorrhea, cough and low-grade fever.[5] Young children may be restless or lethargic and drink less than normal. The physical examination is marked by tachypnea, accessory muscle use, wheezes or crackles.[5] Hypoxemia may be seen secondary to ventilation-perfusion mismatch. Respiratory distress in these children manifests as tachypnea, with respiratory rates as high as 80–100 breaths/minute, nasal flaring, intercostal and supraclavicular retractions, apnea, grunting and cyanosis.[2] The natural course of this illness is about 7–10 days but can last several weeks to a month.[2]

The chest radiograph in patients with bronchiolitis typically shows lung hyperinflation with flattening of the diaphragm.[2] Diagnosis of RSV can be confirmed by nasopharyngeal aspirates. Because the diagnosis of bronchiolitis is a clinical one, routine RSV antigen testing has little value in outpatient management. Respiratory viral antigen testing may be helpful for infection control in patients admitted to inpatient units.[5] Some centers are using rapid nasopharyngeal swabs to test for RSV to gain confidence that the etiology of presentation is not due to an alternate source, such as the urine or CNS; however, this strategy has not gained full acceptance.

Treatment of patients with bronchiolitis is largely supportive, paying attention to hydration and maintaining satisfactory oxygenation.[2,6] Because most children with bronchiolitis will have some degree of hypoxia, oximetry monitoring and provision of oxygen are important.[7] Many of these children will have difficulty drinking secondary to their increased work of breathing. Intravenous hydration should be considered if the child is not able to take adequate oral fluids.[7] A chest radiograph will often reveal areas of opacity suggestive of pneumonia. Deciding whether to use antibiotics in these patients is often difficult; no significant benefit has been demonstrated from routine antibiotic use. In the severely-ill patient, a broad-spectrum antibiotic (i.e., cefuroxime) may be warranted to cover the possibility of bacterial superinfection until ruled out by appropriate cultures.[7]

No study to date has convincingly documented the benefit of steroid use in bronchiolitis.[7] Steroids are therefore not recommended for routine use by most authors. Inhaled steroids in children with bronchiolitis have also been studied, and have not demonstrated any benefit. The use of bronchodilators (i.e., albuterol, nebulized epinephrine) in bronchiolitis is also controversial. Most authors recommend that patients with bronchiolitis, especially those with a history of wheezing, should be given at least a trial of adrenergic bronchodilators. If there is no response to the trial dose, then therapy should be discontinued.[7]

The antiviral drug ribavirin, delivered by small-particle aerosol for three to five days, probably has a modest beneficial effect on the course of RSV pneumonia.[8] However, neither shortened hospital stay nor reduced mortality have been demonstrated, and trials in intubated infants have not shown efficacy. Therefore, its use is rarely indicated except in selected cases of severe immunodeficiency, in which unrestricted viral replication is clearly important in the pathogenesis of severe disease.[8] Intravenous immunoglobulin (RSV-IGIV) as well as humanized monoclonal antibody (palivizumab) have been used to treat severely immunodeficient patients with pneumonia and RSV infection. Although there is no clear evidence of efficacy, these treatments reduce virus titers in the respiratory tract and may offer a rational therapeutic approach in situations with otherwise poor prognoses.[8]

KEY TEACHING POINTS

1. Pneumonia can be defined clinically as the presence of infection and lower respiratory tract dysfunction in association with radiographic opacity.

2. Bacterial pneumonia in older children generally has an abrupt onset with fever and chills, productive cough and chest pain, whereas infants may present with signs and symptoms less typical than older children, such as poor feeding, disturbed sleep, irritability or tachypnea.

3. In the majority of mild-to-moderate cases of pediatric bacterial pneumonia, oral antimicrobial therapy is appropriate; intravenous antibiotics are usually reserved for neonates and patients with severe pneumonia who warrant hospitalization.

4. Bronchiolitis is a common, self-limited, lower respiratory tract infection in infants caused by RSV, usually occurring between October and April in all geographic areas.

5. Because the diagnosis of bronchiolitis is clinical, routine RSV antigen testing has little utility in the outpatient setting but may be helpful for infection control in patients admitted to inpatient units.

6. Treatment of patients with bronchiolitis is largely supportive; attention to and addressing both hydration and oxygenation status are of particular importance.

REFERENCES

[1] McIntosh K. Current concepts: community-acquired pneumonia in children. *N Engl J Med* 2002;346:429–37.

[2] Shah S, Sharieff GQ. Pediatric respiratory infections. *Emerg Med Clin N Am* 2007;25:961–79.

[3] Ostapchuk M, Roberts DM, Haddy R. Community-acquired pneumonia in infants and children. *Amer Fam Phys* 2004;70:899–908.

[4] Jadavji T, Law B, Lebel MH, et al. A practical guide for the diagnosis and treatment of pediatric pneumonia. *Can Med Assoc J* 1997;156:S703–11.

[5] Rafei K, Lichenstein R. Airway infectious disease emergencies. *Pediatr Clin N Am* 2006;53:215–42.

[6] Meates-Dennis M. Best practice: bronchiolitis. *Arch Dis Child Educ Pract Ed* 2005;90:81–6.

[7] Brown K. Bronchiolitis. In: Strange GR, Ahrens WR, Lelyveld S, et al. (eds.). *Pediatric Emergency Medicine, a Comprehensive Study Guide*. New York: McGraw-Hill, 2002;215–8.

[8] McIntosh K. Respiratory syncytial virus. In: Behrman RE, Kliegman RM, Jensen HB, (eds.). *Nelson Textbook of Pediatrics*, 17th ed. Philadelphia: Saunders, 2004;1076–9.

81

Vomiting in a 21-month-old male

HISTORY OF PRESENT ILLNESS

A 21-month-old male presented to the ED following several episodes of vomiting that began in the middle of the night. The patient had been having intermittent bouts of vomiting beginning two weeks earlier. He had been seen on three separate occasions, diagnosed with acute gastroenteritis. The parents reported that between the bouts of vomiting, their son maintained a very poor appetite and had experienced some weight loss. On this visit, the parents reported the first episode of emesis beginning 10 hours prior to arrival, followed by three more episodes. The patient had refused to take fluids during this period. The family denied recent travel or sick contacts, and the child had not experienced fevers, cough, congestion or diarrhea.

His medical history was significant for a similar episode occurring three months earlier and lasting approximately one week. The patient had no other medical problems and had been prescribed Phenergan® suppositories and Zantac® for his symptoms; no Phenergan® was given prior to this visit.

PHYSICAL EXAMINATION

GENERAL APPEARANCE: The patient was awake, making good eye contact, but appeared listless and very fatigued.

VITAL SIGNS

Temperature	98.9°F (37.2°C)
Pulse	64 beats/minute
Blood pressure	110/60 mmHg
Respirations	24 breaths/minute
Oxygen saturation	100% on room air

HEENT: Atraumatic, normocephalic, PERRL, EOMI, oropharynx moist.

NECK: Supple, no meningeal signs.

CARDIOVASCULAR: Bradycardic, regular rate and rhythm without rubs, murmurs or gallops.

LUNGS: Clear to auscultation bilaterally.

ABDOMEN: Soft, nontender, nondistended, active bowel sounds present.

EXTREMITIES: No clubbing, cyanosis or edema, capillary refill less than 2 sec.

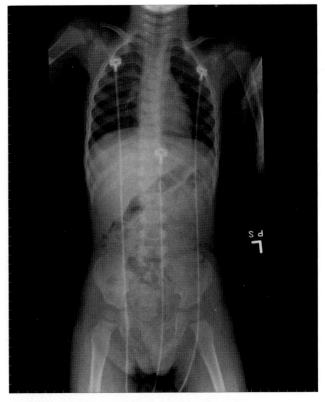

Figure 81.1 Portable chest and abdominal radiograph of a 21-month-old male with persistent vomiting.

NEUROLOGIC: Awake, following commands, moving all extremities.

An ECG, chest and abdominal radiograph were obtained. The ECG demonstrated sinus bradycardia, otherwise normal for age. The combined chest and abdominal radiograph is shown in Figure 81.1. A peripheral intravenous line was placed, and blood was drawn and sent for laboratory testing. A 20 mL/kg bolus of normal saline IV was administered. Laboratory tests, including a complete blood count, electrolytes, glucose, creatinine and urinalysis, were all within normal limits.

What is your diagnosis?

ANSWER

The diagnosis is obstructive hydrocephalus from a posterior fossa brain tumor (ependymoma), determined following admission to the pediatric service. The chest and abdominal radiograph was normal. The pediatrics service was consulted, and the patient was admitted for observation. Approximately nine hours after admission, the patient had a witnessed tonic-clonic seizure that resolved with intravenous lorazepam. After resolution of the seizure, the patient underwent a CT scan of the brain with and without contrast, which demonstrated obstructive hydrocephalus with a posterior fossa mass, most likely tumor (Figure 81.2). The patient was transferred to the pediatric neurosurgical service, where he had an apneic episode and was intubated for airway protection. He continued to have brief seizures, which were treated with lorazepam and fosphenytoin. An MRI of the brain was obtained (Figure 81.3), which demonstrated a posterior fossa tumor. The

patient was taken to the OR and underwent resection of the tumor; pathology results confirmed the tumor to be an ependymoma.

Posterior fossa brain tumors and ependymomas in children

Primary brain tumors are the most common solid neoplasms of childhood, comprising 15–20% of all malignancies occurring in childhood and adolescence.[1,2] The best current estimates of primary brain tumors place the incidence between 2.76–4.28 per 100,000 children per year.[1] Compared with brain tumors in adults, a much higher percentage of pediatric brain tumors arise in the posterior fossa. The most frequent types of posterior fossa tumors diagnosed in children are medulloblastoma, ependymoma, cerebellar astrocytoma and brainstem glioma.[1] Most symptomatic children require several visits to a physician before the correct diagnosis is made. One retrospective study demonstrated that the mean time interval between

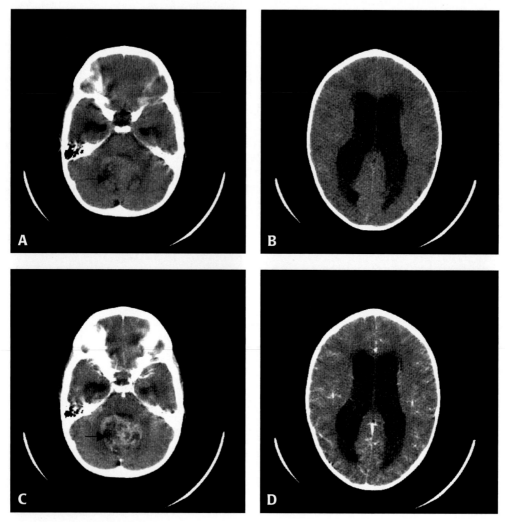

Figure 81.2 Noncontrast (panels A, B) and contrast (panels C, D) CT of the brain from a 21-month-old male demonstrating posterior fossa brain tumor (arrows, panels A, C) and obstructive hydrocephalus (panels B, D).

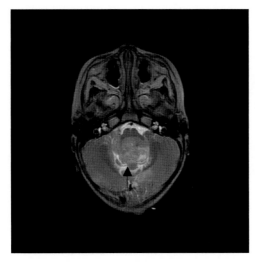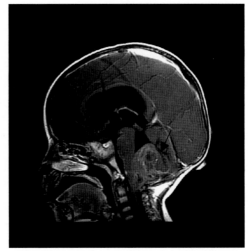

Figure 81.3 MRI of the brain from a 21-month-old male with vomiting and bradycardia, demonstrating posterior fossa brain tumor (arrows).

first chart-documented symptoms from posterior fossa tumors and radiographic diagnosis was 142 days.[3]

Regardless of histology, posterior fossa tumors in children characteristically present with symptoms of increased intracranial pressure (ICP) caused by hydrocephalus. At least 90% of patients with medulloblastoma or cerebellar astrocytomas and 65% of patients with ependymomas present with symptoms of hydrocephalus.[1] Generally, these symptoms include headache and recurrent vomiting, although irritability, lethargy and feeding intolerance may also be noted, especially in infancy.[1–3] Symptoms are typically worse in the morning because recumbency and a relatively elevated $PaCO_2$ increases ICP.[1] Cerebellar symptoms, particularly ataxia, are a frequent complaint of patients with posterior fossa tumors that invade or exert mass effect on the cerebellum or cerebral peduncles. Bradycardia is particularly ominous because it signifies that ventilatory arrest is imminent.[4]

CT is often the first imaging technique obtained for children with suspected intracranial pathology. If properly done, CT will detect 95% or more of brain tumors.[2] However, because of the superior image contrast of MRI it is essential in the diagnosis of brain tumors, and its multiplanar capabilities offer far superior localization. In selected cases, PET scanning may provide additional information but is most useful in supplying baseline diagnostic information as a means to follow the tumor over time.[2]

Ependymomas comprise 5–10% of all childhood brain tumors.[2,5] Most (70–80%) arise in the posterior fossa. Because of a relative predilection for the cerebellopontine angle and lateral portion of the lower brainstem, these often cause multiple cranial nerve deficits, including sixth and seventh nerve palsies, hearing loss, and swallowing difficulties.[2] Ependymomas arising in the fourth ventricle, brainstem or lateral ventricles can present with headaches or other symptoms of hydrocephalus (especially nausea and vomiting), ataxia, and increased head circumference.[5] Because ependymomas may

be present for as long as three to six months before they come to clinical attention, symptoms may sometimes be labeled as "chronic."[5]

Surgery is the primary treatment for ependymoma, with the extent of surgical resection a major prognostic factor.[6] Two other major prognostic factors are age, with younger children having poorer outcomes, and tumor location, with localization in the posterior fossa often seen in young children associated with poorer outcomes.[6] After surgery, radiotherapy is the mainstay of treatment for patients with residual tumor.[5] Some advocate watchful waiting after surgery, administering radiotherapy only when there is evidence of tumor recurrence or growth, especially if a gross, total resection of tumor has been achieved and confirmed with MRI.[5] Ependymoma is sensitive to a spectrum of chemotherapeutic agents; however, the role of chemotherapy in multimodal therapy (surgery, radiation therapy) remains unclear.[6]

KEY TEACHING POINTS

1. Posterior fossa tumors in children characteristically present with symptoms of increased intracranial pressure (ICP) caused by hydrocephalus, including (but not limited to) headache, vomiting, irritability, feeding intolerance and cerebellar symptoms (e.g., ataxia).

2. Symptoms of posterior fossa tumors in children are often subtle, and are commonly missed initially by physicians.

3. Bradycardia in patients with posterior fossa tumors is a particularly ominous sign, indicating imminent brainstem herniation and respiratory arrest.

4. Treatment of patients diagnosed with posterior fossa tumors includes airway management, seizure prophylaxis, measures to reduce ICP in cases of impending herniation (e.g., mannitol), and urgent neurosurgical consultation and evaluation.

5. Treatment of ependymoma involves surgery followed by radiotherapy in most cases; the role of chemotherapy remains unclear.

REFERENCES

[1] Maher CO, Raffel C. Neurosurgical treatment of brain tumors in children. *Pediatr Clin N Am* 2004;51:327–57.

[2] Packer RJ, MacDonald T, Vezina G. Central nervous system tumors. *Pediatr Clin N Am* 2008;55:121–45.

[3] Dorner L, Fritsch MJ, Stark AM, et al. Posterior fossa tumors in children: how long does it take to establish the diagnosis? *Childs Nerv Syst* 2007;23:887–90.

[4] Piatt JH. Recognizing neurosurgical conditions in the pediatrician's office. *Pediatr Clin N Am* 2004;51:237–70.

[5] Janus TJ, Yung WKA. Primary neurological tumors. In: Goetz CG (ed.). *Textbook of Clinical Neurology*, 3rd ed. Philadelphia: Saunders, 2007:1604–5.

[6] Kuttesch JF, Ater JL. Brain tumors in children. In: Bherman RE, Kliegman RM, Jenson HB (eds.). *Nelson Textbook of Pediatrics*, 17th ed. Philadelphia: Saunders, 2004:1705–6.

82

Choking episode in a 21-month-old male

HISTORY OF PRESENT ILLNESS

A 21-month-old male was noted by his mother to be choking at home. He was found sitting next to some loose change, which was left on the coffee table. The mother patted the child on the back and the choking slowly resolved. The patient was brought to the ED by his mother for evaluation. According to her, he did not appear short of breath, nor had he been drooling, stridorous or have any change to his cry. He was tolerating sips of liquids.

PHYSICAL EXAMINATION

GENERAL APPEARANCE: The child appeared well nourished, well hydrated, was smiling and playful during the examination, and was tolerating his secretions.

VITAL SIGNS

Temperature	98.6°F (37°C)
Pulse	120 beats/minute
Blood pressure	90/50 mmHg
Respirations	24 breaths/minute
Oxygen saturation	100% on room air

HEENT: The oropharynx was moist, pink and clear without uvular or tonsillar swelling; no pooling of secretions was noted.

NECK: Supple, nontender without anterior swelling. No stridor noted upon auscultation of the anterior neck.

LUNGS: Clear to auscultation bilaterally without the presence of rales, rhonchi or wheezes.

CARDIOVASCULAR: Regular rate and rhythm without rubs, murmurs or gallops.

ABDOMEN: Soft, nontender, nondistended with active bowel sounds present.

EXTREMITIES: No cyanosis or edema; capillary refill less than 2 sec.

A radiograph of the neck, chest and abdomen was obtained (Figure 82.1).

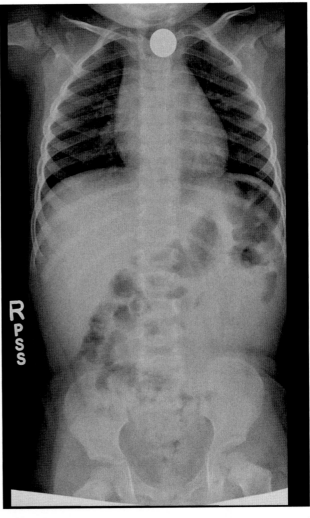

Figure 82.1 Anteroposterior radiograph of the neck, chest and abdomen from a 21-month-old male following a choking episode.

What is your diagnosis?

ANSWER

The diagnosis is esophageal foreign body. The radiograph demonstrates a small coin most likely in the esophagus. The pediatric gastroenterologist was consulted. Because the patient was tolerating liquids, the patient was kept in the ED overnight for observation and kept NPO. A repeat radiograph was performed the following morning to determine if the coin had passed into the stomach. The radiograph showed the coin in the same location as the previous evening. The patient was taken to the OR by the pediatric gastroenterologist, where an upper endoscopy was performed to retrieve the foreign body under general endotracheal anesthesia. The scope was passed through the mouth into the upper esophagus without difficulty, where a dime was located in the esophagus 12 cm from the incisors (panel A, Figure 82.2). The dime was carefully grasped with toothed forceps and removed (panel B, Figure 82.2). No major lesions, erosions, rings or strictures were noted throughout the esophagus (panels C and D, Figure 82.2). The patient was discharged from the pediatrics ward later that day.

Esophageal coins in children

Coins are the most common foreign body ingested by pediatric patients according to Poison Control, with more than 3000 pediatric cases annually.[1] Because the condition is under-reported, the actual number of cases is most likely much higher. Not surprisingly, coins are also the most common foreign body lodged in the esophagus.[1] As many as 35% of the children who have esophageal coins will be asymptomatic.[2] Because lodged coins can result in life-threatening complications, determining the location of ingested coins is important. Anteroposterior and lateral chest radiographs can confirm the diagnosis of a coin in the esophagus. Esophageal coins generally align so as to appear as a circular disc (en face) on the anteroposterior view, and as a thick line (on edge) on the lateral view. Coins in the trachea generally align to appear on edge on the anteroposterior view and en face on the lateral view. A mnemonic has been proposed to remember the presentation on the anteroposterior view: "Is it SAFE?" – Side Airway, Face Esophagus.[2]

The main anatomic locations of esophageal coin retention are the level of the cricopharyngeus muscle, the thoracic inlet, the aortic arch and the lower esophageal sphincter.[3] Radiographically, these anatomic areas correlate with the proximal third (cricopharyngeus and aortic thoracic inlet), middle third (aortic arch) and distal third (lower esophageal sphincter) of the esophagus. Esophageal coins lodge at relatively equal frequencies at these locations.[3] Patients with airway symptoms (cough, stridor, respiratory distress) generally have the coins retained in the proximal esophagus. Pain, drooling and dysphagia are generally seen in patients with coins in the middle or distal third of the esophagus.[3] Children less than 2 years

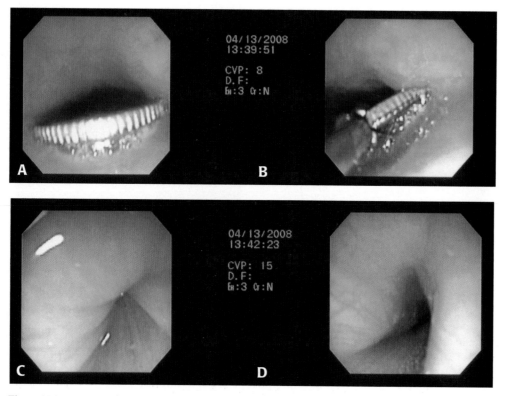

Figure 82.2 Images during upper endoscopy of the upper esophagus with foreign body (dime) and removal of the foreign body with toothed forceps (panels A and B); images of the normal lower esophagus following removal of the foreign body (panels C and D).

of age with wheezing, rhonchi, stridor or retractions must be considered to have a retained foreign body, even if there is no witness to or history of foreign body ingestion.

Severe complications are possible from esophageal foreign bodies. These include esophageal stricture, mediastinitis, lung abscess, esophagoaortic fistula, respiratory distress and death.[4,5] Perforation of the esophagus due to swallowed foreign bodies is rare, representing only 12–25% of all cases.[4] It is important to try to determine how long a foreign body has been present, because those lodged for greater than 24 hours represent a greater risk of erosion or other damage.[4] This will affect the choice and timing of procedure for removing the foreign body. One study found the risk of perforation to be highest in children who had swallowed coins more than 36 hours prior to presentation.[4]

There are several strategies available for the management of esophageal coins in children. The most common modalities are endoscopic coin retrieval, a brief period of observation to monitor spontaneous passage of the coin into the stomach, fluoroscopically guided removal with a balloon catheter, and immediate esophageal bougienage.[1] Endoscopy has been the mainstay of management of esophageal foreign bodies in children.[3] Although spontaneous passage of esophageal coins occurred in 30% of children in one study (range of 8–16 hours), greater than two-thirds of patients managed by expectant observation will require endoscopic coin removal.[1,5] Spontaneous passage is more likely to occur in older, male patients, and when the coin is lodged in the distal third of the esophagus.[5]

One special circumstance of ingested foreign bodies in children involves the ingestion of button batteries. These may appear as coins on the radiograph but, if suspected, must be removed immediately. Button batteries generally contain a heavy metal like mercury, silver or lithium and a strong hydroxide of sodium or potassium.[6] Although they are sealed, occasional leakage of these corrosive substances is not uncommon, leading to mucosal damage by ulceration, stricture formation or perforation.

KEY TEACHING POINTS

1. Coins are the most common foreign body ingestion by children reported to Poison Control, and are also the most common foreign body lodged in the esophagus.
2. On chest radiographs, esophageal coins generally align so as to appear as a circular disc (en face) on the anteroposterior view and as a thick line (on edge) on the lateral view; coins in the trachea generally align to appear on edge on the anteroposterior view and en face on the lateral view.
3. Symptoms indicating a possible esophageal foreign body include throat, neck or chest pain, drooling, dysphagia, cough, stridor and respiratory distress.
4. Severe complications may result from esophageal foreign bodies, such as esophageal stricture, mediastinitis, lung abscess, esophagoaortic fistula, respiratory distress and death.
5. Endoscopy by a skilled pediatric endoscopist under general anesthesia is the preferred management of an esophageal coin in most pediatric patients.

REFERENCES

[1] Arms JL, Mackenberg-Mohn MD, Bowen MV, et al. Safety and efficacy of a protocol using bougienage or endoscopy for the management of coins acutely lodged in the esophagus: a large case series. *Ann Emerg Med* 2008;51:367–72.

[2] Raney LH, Losek JD. Child with esophageal coin and atypical radiograph. *J Emerg Med* 2008;34:63–6.

[3] Waltzman ML. Management of esophageal coins. *Curr Opin Pediatr* 2006;18:571–4.

[4] Balci AE, Eren S, Eren MN. Esophageal foreign bodies under cricopharyngeal level in children: an analysis of 1116 cases. *Interact CardioVasc Thorac Surg* 2004;3:14–8.

[5] Waltzman ML, Baskin M, Wypij D, et al. A randomized trial of the management of esophageal coins in children. *Pediatrics* 2005;116:614–9.

[6] Banerjee R, Rao GV, Sriram PVJ, et al. Button battery ingestion. *Indian J Pediatr* 2005;72:173–4.

83

Abdominal pain and vomiting in a 23-month-old male

HISTORY OF PRESENT ILLNESS

A 23-month-old male presented to the ED with intermittent abdominal pain and vomiting for two days. The patient first presented to his pediatrician's office one day earlier, where the mother reported several episodes of crying followed by three episodes of nonbilious, nonbloody emesis. The mother denied fevers or diarrhea, and between the episodes the patient tolerated sips of fluids. On examination by the pediatrician, the patient was afebrile and nontoxic-appearing, with the abdomen reported to be soft, nontender and nondistended. A diagnosis of viral gastroenteritis was made, and the mother was instructed to encourage fluid intake. The following day the patient returned to his pediatrician where the mother again reported several episodes of intermittent abdominal pain, as well as decreased stool output with small, hard stools without blood. The patient was afebrile, and examination again revealed a well-appearing infant with a soft, nontender abdomen. The patient was diagnosed with constipation versus viral syndrome, and was discharged home. That evening, the child was brought to the ED where the mother reported intermittent episodes of abdominal pain, each lasting 15–20 minutes, during which the child seemed to be clutching his abdomen in pain. Each episode was followed by nonbilious, nonbloody emesis.

PHYSICAL EXAMINATION

GENERAL APPEARANCE: The child was nontoxic in appearance, well hydrated, and in no acute discomfort.

VITAL SIGNS

Temperature	98°F (36.6°C) rectal
Pulse	100 beats/minute
Blood pressure	not obtained
Respirations	26 breaths/minute
Oxygen saturation	100% on room air

HEENT: PERRL, conjugate gaze, oropharynx pink and moist.

NECK: Supple, no meningeal signs.

CARDIOVASCULAR: Regular rate and rhythm without rubs, murmurs or gallops; capillary refill less than 2 sec.

LUNGS: Clear to auscultation bilaterally.

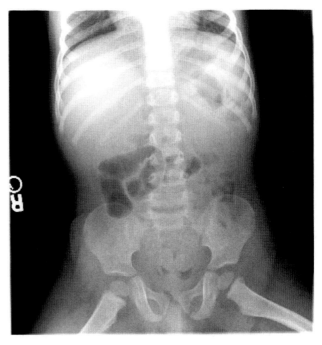

Figure 83.1 Plain radiograph of the abdomen from a 23-month-old male with intermittent abdominal pain.

ABDOMEN: Slightly distended, hypoactive bowel sounds, tenderness in the right upper quadrant.

GENITOURINARY: Normal genitalia, circumcised, testes descended bilaterally, no hernias.

RECTAL: Brown stool, hemoccult negative.

EXTREMITIES: No clubbing, cyanosis or edema.

NEUROLOGIC: Nonfocal.

An intravenous line was placed, blood was drawn and sent for laboratory testing, and an IV fluid bolus of normal saline was administered (20 mL/kg). Laboratory tests, including a complete blood count, chemistry panel and urinalysis, were within normal limits. A plain radiograph of the abdomen was obtained (Figure 83.1).

What is your diagnosis?

ANSWER

The diagnosis is intestinal (ileocolic) intussusception. The plain radiograph in Figure 83.1 demonstrates a dilated loop of bowel in the right upper quadrant, with paucity of gas in the right lower quadrant. The patient underwent a contrast enema study under fluoroscopy after notification of the pediatric surgeon, which demonstrated an intussusception in the right, mid-ascending colon (panel A, Figure 83.2). The intussusception was successfully reduced by the contrast enema (panel B, Figure 83.2), with a post-procedural KUB radiograph demonstrating opacification of the terminal ileum (panel C, Figure 83.2). The patient was admitted to the hospital for observation; he was discharged home 24 hours later doing well and tolerating feedings.

Intussusception

Intussusception is the most common etiology for bowel obstruction in children less than 2 years of age.[1] It is the prolapse of one part of the intestine into the lumen of an immediately distal adjoining part. The most common type of intussusception is ileocolic invagination.[2] During the invagination, the mesentery is dragged along into the distal lumen, obstructing venous return. This leads to bowel wall edema, bleeding of the intestinal mucosa, increased pressure in the area and eventually obstruction to arterial flow.[2] Gangrene and perforation may result.

Intussusception is estimated to occur in about 1 in 2000 infants and children.[1] The typical age distribution is between 3 months and 6 years of age, with the peak incidence between 5 months and 1 year of age. There is a 3:2 male to female distribution.[1] Approximately 90% of intussusceptions are ileocolic and do not have a pathologic lead point. Common lead points include an appendix, lipoma, intestinal polyp, Meckel's diverticulum, enlarged Peyer's patch and Henoch-Schönlein purpura (HSP)-associated submucosal hematoma.[1] The second most common type, representing 4% of intussus-

ceptions, is ileoileocolic. Approximately 40% of ileoileocolic intussusceptions will have a pathologic lead point.[1]

The "classic" symptoms and signs of intussusception (vomiting, abdominal pain, red currant jelly stool and a palpable abdominal mass) are frequently not all present in children with intussusception.[3] Reliance on "classic" symptoms alone might therefore lead to a delay in diagnosis. Vomiting is frequently the first symptom of intussusception, particularly in infants under 4 months of age.[4] Initially, the emesis consists of gastric contents; if the diagnosis is delayed and intestinal obstruction occurs, it may become bile-stained or even feculent. The "classic" abdominal pain associated with intussusception is described as severe, intermittent, and cramping.[4] Episodes may persist for 4–5 minutes, with a period of 10–20 minutes of relief. During episodes of pain, infants may pull their knees up toward the abdomen, and may become pale, sweaty and lethargic.[4] Episodes of intermittent lethargy have been named a "cardinal symptom" of intussusception.[5] These episodes are typically associated with episodes of pallor. Presentation with hypovolemic shock has been associated with prolonged duration of symptoms and high mortality.[4] In fact, intussusception should be part of the differential diagnosis in infants presenting with altered mental status.

On physical examination, the abdomen may be distended and tender, but usually the pain appears to be out of proportion to the physical findings.[2] There may be an elongated mass in the right upper or lower quadrants. Any type of blood in the stool may be caused by intussusception. Rectal examination may reveal either occult blood or bloody, foul-smelling stool, classically described as "currant jelly."[2] However, frank rectal bleeding is a late and unreliable sign; its absence should not deter physicians from pursuing this diagnosis. A period of observation for the recurrence of a painful episode may prove helpful in equivocal cases.[2]

No laboratory test reliably rules in or rules out the diagnosis of intussusception. If the bowel has become ischemic or necrotic, acidosis may be present. Initial radiographic studies for patients with suspected intussusception might include plain

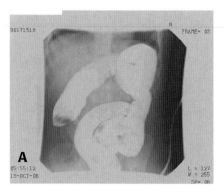
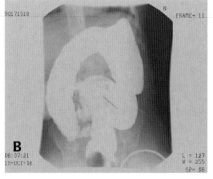
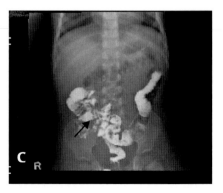

Figure 83.2 Contrast enema in a 23-month-old male demonstrating ileocolic intussusception (panel A) and reduction of intussusception (panel B); plain radiograph demonstrates opacification of the terminal ileum following procedure (arrow, panel C).

radiographs of the abdomen, although their use remains controversial.[1] Nevertheless, certain radiographic findings have become almost pathognomonic for intussusception. These include a soft-tissue mass in the right upper quadrant, the meniscus sign (a crescent of gas within the colonic lumen outlining the apex of the intussusception), and the target sign (a soft-tissue mass outlined by a lucency of peritoneal fat).[1] These findings are not common and, more importantly, an infant with intussusception may have a normal radiograph.

The use of ultrasonography to diagnose intussusception is noninvasive, avoids radiation exposure and is accurate in experienced hands; unfortunately, interpretation and study quality are operator-dependent.[6] Findings on ultrasound are distinct; on cross-section, a 3-cm to 5-cm diameter mass is seen in the shape of a target or doughnut.[1] Sonography has also been shown effective in diagnosing pathologic lead points and determining other causes of abdominal pain in children, such as appendicitis, hernias, ovarian torsion and small bowel volvulus.[1]

Barium contrast enema can be both diagnostic and therapeutic and, until recently, has traditionally been the study of choice.[7] More recently, air or saline hydrostatic reductions have become preferred. Infants with ileocolic intussusception can be successfully managed by nonoperative reduction in the vast majority of cases (85–90%).[6] Enema reduction with either hydrostatic barium contrast technique or pneumatic reduction with air under fluoroscopic or ultrasonographic guidance should be attempted only in clinically stable, well-hydrated patients without evidence of peritonitis.[6] The pediatric surgery team should be available to intervene if the attempted reduction fails or perforation occurs; therefore, it is important to notify them once the diagnosis is entertained, in advance of any contrast or hydrostatic study. The recurrence rate of intussusception after successful reduction is approximately 10%, with two-thirds occurring within the first few days.[6]

KEY TEACHING POINTS

1. Intussusception is the most common etiology for bowel obstruction in children less than 2 years of age, with the peak incidence occurring between 5 months and 1 year of age.
2. The "classic" symptoms and signs of intussusception (vomiting, abdominal pain, red currant jelly stool and a palpable, sausage-shaped abdominal mass) are frequently not all present in children with intussusception.
3. Signs and symptoms of intussusception include intermittent episodes of crampy, severe abdominal pain, vomiting, intermittent lethargy and bloody stools.
4. Ultrasonography is noninvasive, avoids radiation exposure and can be highly accurate in diagnosing intussusception.
5. Barium contrast or air enema is both diagnostic and therapeutic in cases of intussusception.

REFERENCES

[1] Louie JP. Essential diagnosis of abdominal emergencies in the first year of life. *Emerg Med Clin N Am* 2007;25:1009–40.
[2] McCollough M, Sharieff GQ. Abdominal pain in children. *Pediatr Clin N Am* 2006;53:107–37.
[3] Blanch AJM, Perel SB, Acworth JP. Paediatric intussusception: epidemiology and outcome. *Emerg Med Austral* 2007;19:45–50.
[4] Bines JE, Ivanoff B, Justice F, et al. Clinical case definition for the diagnosis of acute intussusception. *J Pediatr Gastroenterol Nutr* 2004;39:511–8.
[5] Knudson M. Intussusception. A case that suggests a new cardinal symptom – lethargy. *Postgrad Med* 1988;83:201–2.
[6] Grosfeld JL. Intussusception then and now: a historical vignette. *J Am Coll Surg* 2005;201:830–3.
[7] Herman M, Le A. The crying infant. *Emerg Med Clin N Am* 2007;25:1137–59.

84

Vomiting, diarrhea and seizure in a 3-year-old male

HISTORY OF PRESENT ILLNESS

A 3-year-old male came to the ED by ambulance after having a generalized seizure lasting 30 seconds. The father woke to a noise in his child's room, and upon entering found the child with his neck arched, eyes rolled back and both arms shaking. The seizure lasted approximately 30 seconds, after which the child was slow to arouse. Three days earlier, the child developed a low-grade fever, crampy abdominal pain, diarrhea and vomiting. He was seen one day previously by his pediatrician, diagnosed with acute gastroenteritis and prescribed Phenergan® suppositories for the vomiting. The parents denied recent travel or sick contacts. The patient's immunizations were current, and he was otherwise healthy. He had neither a history of seizures nor any family history of the same.

PHYSICAL EXAMINATION

GENERAL APPEARANCE: The patient appeared dehydrated and lethargic but arousable.

VITAL SIGNS

Temperature	97°F (36.1°C)
Pulse	117 beats/minute
Blood pressure	115/60 mmHg
Respirations	26 breaths/minute
Oxygen saturation	97% on room air

HEENT: Atraumatic, normocephalic, PERRL, EOMI, oropharynx dry.

NECK: Supple, no meningeal signs.

CARDIOVASCULAR: Regular rate and rhythm without rubs, murmurs or gallops.

LUNGS: Clear to auscultation bilaterally.

ABDOMEN: Soft, nontender, nondistended, hyperactive bowel sounds.

EXTREMITIES: No clubbing, cyanosis or edema, capillary refill approximately 3 sec.

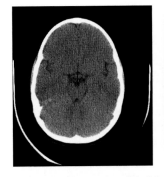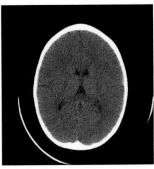

Figure 84.1 Noncontrast CT of the brain from a 3-year-old male with vomiting, diarrhea and seizure.

SKIN: Warm, good skin turgor.

NEUROLOGIC: Lethargic, arousable but minimally able to follow commands, moving all extremities.

A bedside blood glucose was 112 mg/dL. A peripheral intravenous line was placed, and blood was drawn and sent for laboratory testing. Lorazepam 0.05 mg/kg IV and ceftriaxone 50 mg/kg IV, followed by a 20 mL/kg normal saline IV bolus were administered. A chest radiograph was normal, and noncontrast CT of the brain was obtained (Figure 84.1). The patient's laboratory tests revealed a leukocyte count of 21.8 K/μL (normal 5.0–15.5 K/μL), hematocrit of 26% (normal 34–40%) with presence of schistocytes and platelet count of 98 K/μL (normal 140–400 K/μL). The creatinine was 6.6 mg/dL (normal 0.30–0.70 mg/dL), BUN 119 mg/dL (normal 9–20 mg/dL), potassium 5 mEq/L (normal 3.5–5.3 mEq/L), sodium 131 mEq/L (normal 137–145 mEq/L), bicarbonate 15 mEq/L (normal 22–30 mEq/L) and an anion gap 21 mEq/L (normal 5–16 mEq/L).

What is your diagnosis?

ANSWER

The diagnosis is hemolytic uremic syndrome (HUS). The CT of the brain was normal. The patient was started on dilantin IV (loading dose 18 mg/kg) for seizures, continued on intravenous fluids and admitted to the Pediatric Intensive Care Unit (PICU) for close monitoring of fluid and electrolyte status. Rectal swabs for stool culture were obtained in the ED, and returned one day later positive for *E. coli* O157:H7. Hemodialysis was initiated in the PICU. The patient began to produce urine two weeks following admission, at which time hemodialysis was discontinued and he was discharged home. His creatinine had nearly normalized (1.0 mg/dL) one week following discharge.

Hemolytic uremic syndrome

Hemolytic uremic syndrome (HUS) is a disease primarily of infancy and early childhood, generally occurring in children 1–10 years of age.[1,2] It is caused primarily by Shiga toxin-producing *Escherichia coli* O157:H7, and is characterized by the triad of microangiopathic hemolytic anemia, thrombocytopenia and acute renal failure.[1,2] HUS occurs in 9–30% of infected children about one week after an episode of bloody diarrhea caused by *E. coli* O157:H7.[3] The incubation period for *E. coli* O157:H7 is usually three to four days; however, the incubation also can range from just one day to eight days.[2] Infections with other *E. coli* serotypes, *Shigella dysenteriae* and (occasionally) other microbes may cause HUS in children and adults. HUS occurs with an average annual incidence of 1–3 cases per 100,000 children, and a survival rate of nearly 95%.[2] The use of antimotility drugs may increase the risk of developing HUS, as the gut is exposed to a greater number of toxins for a longer period due to slowed intestinal motility.[1,2]

HUS and thrombotic thrombocytopenic purpura (TTP) represent different ends of what is probably the same disease continuum.[1] In TTP, systemic microvascular aggregation of platelets causes ischemia in the brain and other organs. In the HUS, platelet-fibrin thrombi predominantly occlude the renal circulation.[3] However, nonrenal complications of HUS should be anticipated; neurologic complications are the most ominous and are important determinants of morbidity and mortality.[4] Irritability, lethargy and confusion could be caused by fatigue, cerebral microvascular thrombi, cerebral hypoxia, or the direct neuronal effects of Shiga toxin; stroke (thrombotic or hemorrhagic), seizures and coma occur in about 10% of patients.[4] Cranial imaging should be used to assess neurologic complications.

Typically, *E. coli* O157:H7 infections cause one to three days of nonbloody diarrhea, after which the diarrhea becomes bloody.[4] Bloody diarrhea, which occurs in about 90% of cases, is generally the sign that prompts patients or their families to seek medical attention. Most patients with *E. coli* O157:H7 are afebrile when investigated in a medical setting, even though about half of all infected patients report fever before assessment.[4] Leukocytes are found in only half of examined

fecal samples, and are rarely described as abundant if present. Normal testing for stool cultures does not reveal *E. coli* O157:H7; the physician must specifically request this analysis.[1] Abdominal pain is greater than is generally seen in other forms of bacterial gastroenteritis (physicians commonly note abdominal tenderness during their examination), and defecation tends to be painful.[4] About half of the patients will have nausea and vomiting.[5] Infection with *E. coli* O157:H7 must be immediately reported to local public health officials.[2,4]

HUS cannot be diagnosed without evidence of hemolytic anemia.[1,2] Hematologic findings include destruction and fragmentation of erythrocytes that result in microangiopathic hemolytic anemia. A mean hemoglobin concentration of 6 g/dL is common, and often requires red blood cell transfusion.[2] Ninety-two percent of patients with HUS develop thrombocytopenia, which results from entrapment of platelets in organs.[1,2] Acute renal failure results when microthrombi are deposited in kidney parenchyma. This manifests in the form of hypertension associated with oliguria and anuria, which are early signs of acute renal failure. Prothrombin time (PT), activated partial thromboplastin time (aPTT), fibrinogen and a disseminated intravascular coagulation (DIC) panel are generally within the reference ranges.[1]

HUS is typically a self-limiting disease with spontaneous recovery, although close monitoring and treatment of symptoms are essential.[2] Because HUS has a wide spectrum of presentation, supportive therapy and close monitoring of fluid and electrolyte status are crucial for a good outcome. Strict fluid monitoring is important in detecting early renal failure; if it develops, it should be handled aggressively with peritoneal or hemodialysis. Hypertension is treated with antihypertensives. Antibiotics are ineffective except for certain cases caused by *Shigella dysenteriae*.[1] In fact, antibiotic therapy may increase the risk of developing HUS in children with *E. coli* O157:H7 colitis. Platelet transfusion is not recommended because it could exacerbate the thrombotic process; however, risks and benefits should be considered when platelet transfusion is necessary (e.g., invasive vascular procedures, active bleeding).[2]

Plasma infusion or exchange has been tried as treatment for HUS with equivocal results.[3] Other modalities, such as antithrombotic agents, steroids and Shiga toxin-binding agents have proved ineffective and remain controversial.[2] Infection-induced HUS presenting with a diarrheal prodrome has a good prognosis; the average length of hospitalization in children is 11 days, with a range of 1 to 388 days.[6] Predictors of the severity of HUS include elevated peripheral leukocyte count, a severe gastrointestinal prodrome, anuria early in the course of the illness and an age under 2 years.[5] Currently, the mortality rate for all patients with HUS is less than 10%.[2]

KEY TEACHING POINTS

1. Hemolytic uremic syndrome (HUS), a disease primarily of infancy and early childhood, is characterized by the triad

of microangiopathic hemolytic anemia, thrombocytopenia and acute renal failure.

2. The most common cause of HUS is a toxin produced by *Escherichia coli* serotype O157:H7, transmitted by contaminated food, such as undercooked ground beef and other cattle products and unpasteurized dairy products.

3. HUS is primarily a clinical diagnosis coupled with consistent laboratory findings, including a microangiopathic hemolytic anemia (hemoglobin typically less than 8 g/dL and presence of schistocytes on peripheral smear), thrombocytopenia that is mild to moderate in severity, and marked elevations in BUN and creatinine.

4. Emergency care should focus on supportive management, treatment of blood pressure elevation, blood transfusions and admission to the hospital with arrangement for prompt dialysis.

5. Antibiotics should be avoided in children with bloody diarrhea if suspicion for infection with *E. coli* O157:H7 exists, as they may increase the risk of developing HUS.

6. Infection with *E. coli* O157:H7 (and HUS) must be immediately reported to local public health officials.

REFERENCES

[1] Shapiro W. Hemolytic uremic syndrome. eMedicine Website. Available at http://www.emedicine.com/emerg/topic238.htm. Accessed June 21, 2008.

[2] Razzaq S. Hemolytic uremic syndrome: an emerging health risk. *Am Fam Physician* 2006;74:991–6, 998.

[3] Moake, JL. Mechanisms of disease: thrombotic microangiopathies. *N Engl J Med* 2002;347:589–600.

[4] Tarr PI, Gordon CA, Chandler WL. Shiga-toxin-producing Eschericia coli and hemolytic uraemic syndrome. *Lancet* 2005;365:1073–86.

[5] Boyce TG, Swerdlow DL, Griffin PM. Current concepts: Eschericia coli O157:H7 and the hemolytic-uremic syndrome. *N Engl J Med* 1995;333:364–8.

[6] Banatvala N, Griffin PM, Greene KD, et al. The United States Prospective Hemolytic Uremic Syndrome Study: microbiologic, serologic, clinical, and epidemiologic findings. *J Infect Dis* 2001;183:1063–70.

85

Left arm and leg weakness in a 6-year-old female

HISTORY OF PRESENT ILLNESS

A 6-year-old female with no significant medical history presented to the ED with one day of weakness and inability to move her left arm. She denied trauma to the arm, pain or numbness. On examination, her left arm was completely flaccid (strength 0/5) with intact sensation and a normal radial pulse. Radiographs of the left arm and a noncontrast CT of the brain were obtained. Both tests were normal, and the patient was admitted to the pediatric service. On hospital day #2 an MRI of the neck was obtained, which was normal. By this time, the patient had regained most of the strength in her left arm, and was discharged home with the diagnosis of left brachial plexitis.

Eight days following discharge, the patient again presented to the ED, now with the chief complaint of left leg weakness, as well as worsening weakness in her left arm. She was having difficulty walking secondary to the leg weakness. She denied pain or numbness to the arm, and her parents denied recent trauma, fevers, illnesses, travel or sick contacts.

PHYSICAL EXAMINATION

GENERAL APPEARANCE: The patient appeared well nourished, well hydrated, nontoxic and in no acute discomfort.

VITAL SIGNS

Temperature	98.2°F (36.8°C)
Pulse	95 beats/minute
Blood pressure	100/60 mmHg
Respirations	20 breaths/minute
Oxygen saturation	100% on room air

HEENT: PERRL, EOMI, oropharynx pink and moist.

NECK: Supple, no midline tenderness, no meningeal signs.

CARDIOVASCULAR: Regular rate and rhythm without rubs, murmurs or gallops.

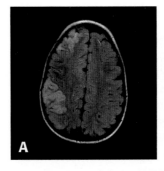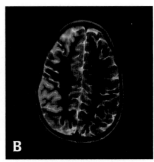

Figure 85.1 Coronal views of MRI of the brain (FLAIR image, panel A; T2-weighted image, panel B) from a 6-year-old female with left arm and leg weakness.

LUNGS: Clear to auscultation bilaterally.

ABDOMEN: Soft, nontender, nondistended.

EXTREMITIES: No clubbing, cyanosis or edema; strong and equal peripheral pulses, upper and lower extremities.

NEUROLOGIC: Alert and oriented to person, place and time; cranial nerves II–XII grossly intact. Right upper and lower extremity strength 5/5 proximal and distal, left upper extremity strength 3/5, left lower extremity strength 2/5. Bilateral knee, ankle and biceps reflexes 2+. Patient could ambulate but with a slow, wide-based gait.

A peripheral intravenous line was placed, blood was drawn and sent for laboratory testing, and MRI of the brain was obtained (Figure 85.1). Laboratory tests, including a complete blood count, electrolytes, creatinine, glucose and INR, were within normal limits.

What is your diagnosis?

ANSWER

The diagnosis is Moyamoya disease (MMD). The MRI images (Figure 85.1) demonstrate extensive hypoxic/ischemic insult involving the right frontal, parietal and occipital cerebral cortices (bright signal intensities). The patient underwent magnetic resonance angiogram (MRA) of the brain (Figure 85.2), which demonstrated occlusion of the supraclinoid portion of the right internal carotid artery with Moyamoya-associated collaterals. The patient was transferred to the pediatric neurosurgical service, where she underwent a nuclear single photon emission computed tomography (SPECT) perfusion study (Figure 85.3). This demonstrated moderate to severe reversible ischemia and decreased cerebrovascular reserve involving the majority of her right cerebral hemisphere. The patient's weakness improved during hospitalization. A cerebral angiogram was performed that confirmed extensive Moyamoya-like changes in the right anterior circulation with occlusion of the supraclinoid internal carotid artery (Figure 85.4). She underwent an encephaloduroarteriosynangiosis (EDAS) for external revascularization of the right cerebral circulation, with a complete and uneventful recovery.

Moyamoya disease

Moyamoya disease is a cerebrovascular disorder that features a narrowing or stenosis of the cerebral circulation, starting at the distal internal carotid artery and involving proximal portions of the anterior and middle cerebral arteries.[1] The term *moyamoya* means a "wavering puff of smoke," and is used to describe the abnormal collateral vasculature present at the base of the brain in patients with this disease. MMD is characterized by progressive intracranial vascular obliterations of the circle of Willis, resulting in successive ischemic or hemorrhagic events.[2] It is an extremely rare disorder in most parts of the world (except Japan and Korea), and tends to affect children as well as adults in their third or fourth decades.

The etiology of MMD is unknown, although a number of factors have been postulated to play a role (e.g., fibroblast growth factor, transforming growth factor beta-1, prostaglandins, Epstein-Barr virus infection, hypercoagulable states).[1] A

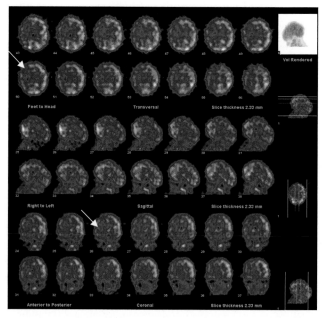

Figure 85.3 Nuclear SPECT perfusion study from a 6-year-old female with Moyamoya disease, demonstrating moderate to severe reversible ischemia and decreased cerebrovascular reserve involving the majority of the right cerebral hemisphere (white arrows).

genetic predisposition exists in endemic areas, with a familial predilection in about 10% of cases.[3] There are two age peaks for disease presentation: between 6–15 years of age and around the fourth decade, with a higher incidence among

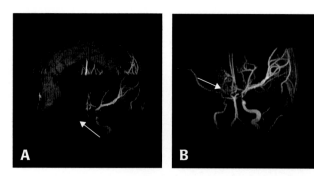

Figure 85.2 MRA of the brain demonstrating occlusion of the supraclinoid portion of the right internal carotid artery (arrow, panel A) and Moyamoya-associated collaterals (arrow, panel B).

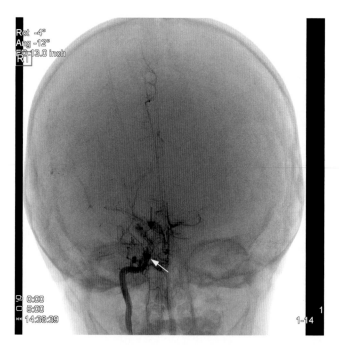

Figure 85.4 Cerebral angiogram of the right internal carotid artery demonstrating occlusion of the supraclinoid internal carotid artery (white arrow) and Moyamoya-associated collateral vessels (dark arrow).

females in all age groups affected.[3] Progressive vascular stenosis causes cerebral hypoperfusion and a reduced hemodynamic reserve. Children usually present with cerebral ischemic events, causing transient (or less often, permanent) motor, sensory, cognitive-behavioral deficits, endocrine dysfunction, incontinence, migraine-like symptoms and seizures.[3,4] In adults, ischemic events usually manifest as an infarction rather than a transient ischemic attack (TIA). Hemorrhagic stroke related to MMD is more frequent in adults than in children.[4]

Traditionally, cerebral angiography has been used to diagnose MMD. MRA is being used more frequently to confirm the diagnosis because of its excellent accuracy and noninvasive nature, especially in children.[1] Moyamoya vessels are visualized as multiple small, round or tortuous low-intensity areas extending from the suprasellar cisterns to the basal ganglia. Occlusive changes in the distal internal carotid, anterior cerebral and middle cerebral arteries, as well as ischemic cerebral lesions and collateral vessels, can also be visualized using MRI.[1]

Surgical options exist for the treatment of MMD and are generally recommended in symptomatic patients.[1] The treatment goal is to improve blood flow to hypoperfused cerebral regions by neurosurgery. EDAS, also known as pial synangiosis, has shown excellent postoperative results in the surgical treatment of MMD.[5] This procedure involves sewing the superficial temporal artery to the inside edge of the dura such that it remains in contact with the exposed cortex. Over time, angiogenesis results in the formation of small arteries to the brain.[5] Several studies have demonstrated 100% revascularization of the brain using this technique in pediatric patients, with excellent neurologic short-term outcomes.[5-8]

KEY TEACHING POINTS

1. Moyamoya disease (MMD) is characterized by progressive intracranial vascular obliterations of the circle of Willis, resulting in recurrent and progressive ischemic or hemorrhagic events.

2. Children with MMD usually present with cerebral ischemic events, causing transient (or less often, permanent) motor, sensory, cognitive-behavioral deficits, endocrine dysfunction, incontinence, migraine-like symptoms and seizures.

3. MRA is the imaging test of choice for diagnosing MMD, as it can visualize occlusive changes in the distal internal carotid, anterior and middle cerebral arteries, as well as ischemic cerebral lesions and collateral vessels.

4. Surgical treatment of MMD (e.g., EDAS) is generally recommended in symptomatic patients, and has shown excellent revascularization and improved neurologic outcomes, particularly in pediatric populations.

REFERENCES

[1] Gosalakkal JA. Moyamoya disease: a review. *Neurol India* 2002;50:6–10.

[2] Marcinkevicius E, Liutkus D, Gvazdaitis A. Experience of treatment of moyamoya disease at the clinic of neurosurgery of Kaunas University of Medicine. *Medicina (Kaunas)* 2006;42:130–6.

[3] Nissim O, Bakon M, Ben Zeev B, et al. Moyamoya disease – diagnosis and treatment: indirect cerebral revascularization at the Sheba Medical Center. *IMAJ* 2005;7:661–6.

[4] Kornblihtt LI, Cocorullo S, Miranda C, et al. Moyamoya syndrome in an adolescent with essential thrombocythemia. *Stroke* 2005;36:e71–3.

[5] Tripathi P, Tripathi V, Naik RJ, et al. Moya moya cases treated with encephaloduroarteriosynangiosis. *Indian Pediatr* 2007;44:123–7.

[6] Fung LW, Thompson D, Ganesan V. Revascularisation surgery for pediatric moyamoya: a review of the literature. *Child Nerv Syst* 2005;21:358–64.

[7] Matsushima Y, Inaha Y. Moya moya disease in children and its surgical treatment: the introduction of a new surgical procedure and its follow up angiograms. *Child Brain* 1984;11:155–70.

[8] Houkin K, Nakayama N, Kuroda S, et al. How does angiogenesis develop in pediatric moyamoya disease after surgery. A prospective study with MR angiography. *Child Nerv Syst* 2004;20:734–41.

86

Chest pain in a 9-year-old female

HISTORY OF PRESENT ILLNESS

A 9-year-old female with a medical history significant for congenital, progressive sensorineural hearing loss presented to the ED complaining of chest pain that woke her from sleep. She denied shortness of breath but reported nausea and a mild headache related to her chest pain. Her chest pain was located on the left lower chest, was not pleuritic and (according to the mother) was reproducible by pressing on the left chest. The patient was recently diagnosed with a left knee sprain after twisting her knee; she was seen four days previously in the ED with normal knee radiographs and given crutches. She returned to the ED two days later after noting significant swelling to her knee and left leg. The patient was diagnosed with nonspecific leg swelling, instructed to continue conservative management of her injury, and was referred to the orthopedics clinic. The patient had recently visited relatives in Pennsylvania, where a cousin had been diagnosed with Lyme disease. The patient denied any rashes.

PHYSICAL EXAMINATION

GENERAL APPEARANCE: The patient appeared awake and alert, and in no acute discomfort.

VITAL SIGNS

Temperature	98°F (36.6°C)
Pulse	46 beats/minute
Blood pressure	110/60 mmHg
Respirations	20 breaths/minute
Oxygen saturation	99% on room air

HEENT: Unremarkable.

NECK: Supple, no jugular venous distension.

CARDIOVASCULAR: Bradycardic rate, regular rhythm without rubs, murmurs or gallops.

LUNGS: Clear to auscultation bilaterally.

ABDOMEN: Soft, nontender, nondistended.

LEFT KNEE: Moderate swelling anteriorly, no warmth or erythema; tenderness to medial aspect of knee with full range of motion; patient was weight-bearing on left knee.

EXTREMITIES: No clubbing, cyanosis or edema.

NEUROLOGIC: Nonfocal.

SKIN: No rashes.

The patient was placed on the cardiac monitor, a peripheral intravenous line was placed, and blood was drawn and sent for laboratory testing. A rhythm strip (Figure 86.1) and a 12-lead ECG (Figure 86.2) were obtained. Laboratory tests, including a complete blood count, electrolytes, creatinine, glucose, troponin-I and D-dimer, were all within normal limits. A chest radiograph was normal.

What is your diagnosis?

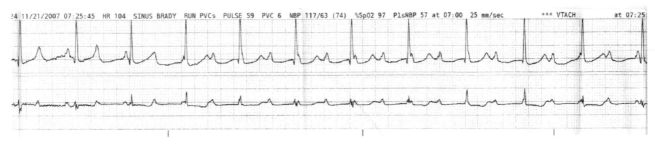

Figure 86.1 Rhythm strip from a 9-year-old female with chest pain.

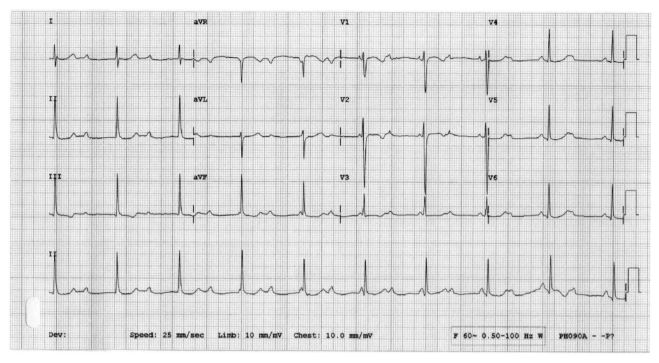

Figure 86.2 12-lead ECG from a 9-year-old female with chest pain.

The diagnosis is third-degree atrioventricular (AV) block (complete heart block) secondary to Lyme carditis. The initial rhythm strip and 12-lead ECG demonstrate a third-degree AV block. A repeat ECG was obtained four hours after the initial ECG (Figure 86.3) that demonstrated sinus bradycardia with first-degree AV block and the presence of blocked premature atrial contractions (partially buried in the T waves). Pediatric cardiology was consulted and recommended to set the patient up for an outpatient Holter monitor as well as close follow up with her pediatrician and pediatric cardiology. At the time of discharge (approximately eight hours after presentation), a third ECG (Figure 86.4) demonstrated only first-degree AV block.

The patient was referred to the pediatric infectious disease specialist by her pediatrician. During that clinic visit (approximately six days following her initial ED visit), she was found to be in third-degree AV block (Figure 86.5) without symptoms. The presumptive diagnosis of Lyme carditis was made based on her travel history (she spent the summer in Pennsylvania with a relative diagnosed with Lyme disease), her recent history of arthralgias and the intermittent high-grade AV blocks. The patient was admitted to the Pediatric Intensive Care Unit (PICU) for monitoring and PICC line placement to begin daily intravenous ceftriaxone administration (1 gm IV daily for 28 days). The patient was seen by the pediatric cardiologist at this time, who agreed with the diagnosis of Lyme carditis. An initial Lyme screen by enzyme-linked

immunosorbent assay (ELISA) returned positive, which was confirmed by western blot technique.

Third-degree heart block and Lyme carditis

Complete heart block (also referred to as third-degree heart block) may be an isolated anomaly. It may be congenital, associated with structural lesions such as in L-transposition of the great arteries or maternal connective tissue disorders.[1] Acquired heart block may result from cardiac surgery, especially when there is suturing in the atrium. This effect can be either transient, generally resolving within eight days postoperatively, or permanent. Other causes include myocarditis, Lyme disease, rheumatic fever, diphtheria or inflammatory disorders such as Kawasaki disease and systemic lupus erythematosus.[1] Complete heart block has also been associated with myocardial infarction, cardiac tumors, muscular dystrophies, hypocalcemia and drug overdoses.

Lyme disease is the most commonly reported vector-born disease in the United States.[2] Lyme borreliosis is a multiorgan infection caused by the spirochete *Borrelia burgdorferi*, which is transmitted by ticks of the species *Ixodes*.[3] Although Lyme disease has been reported in 49 states and the District of Columbia, 92% of cases have been reported to occur in only 10 states (Massachusetts, Rhode Island, Connecticut, Delaware, Pennsylvania, Maryland, New York, New Jersey, Wisconsin and Minnesota).[2] Late extracutaneous manifestations of Lyme borreliosis are characterized by carditis, neuroborreliosis and arthritis. Carditis due to *B. burgdorferi*

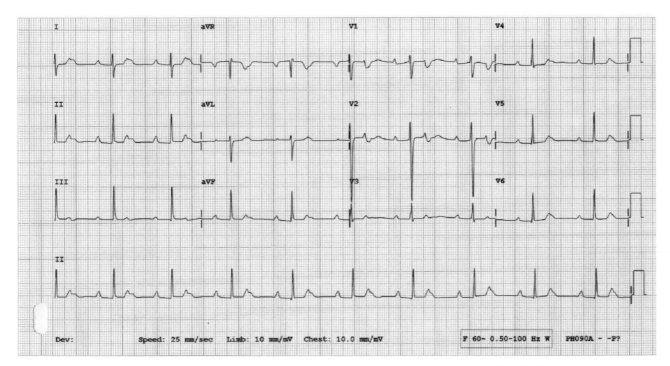

Figure 86.3 Second ECG obtained four hours after ED presentation of a 9-year-old female with chest pain demonstrating sinus bradycardia with first-degree AV block and the presence of blocked premature atrial contractions.

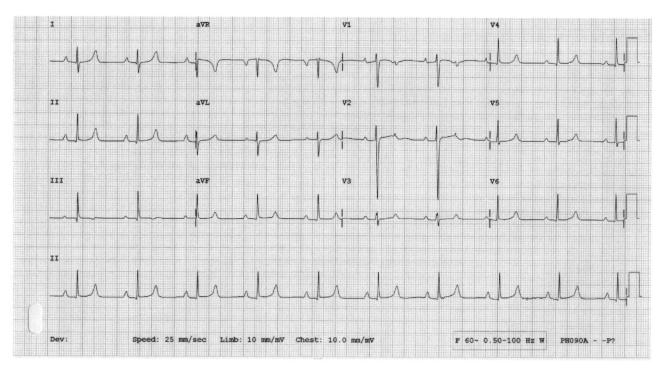

Figure 86.4 Third ECG obtained eight hours after initial presentation of a 9-year-old female with chest pain demonstrating first-degree AV block.

typically occurs weeks to months after infection (commonly between June and December), and is usually manifested by atrioventricular block.[2,3] The patient may not recall either the rash or the tick bite. Complete heart block has been reported as the sole manifestation of Lyme carditis.[2]

Autopsy and biopsy specimens demonstrate that cardiac Lyme disease can affect all layers of the heart. The histology of Lyme carditis shows a transmural, inflammatory infiltrate.[2] In hyperacute disease, small inflammatory nodules composed primarily of neutrophils and macrophages have been seen.

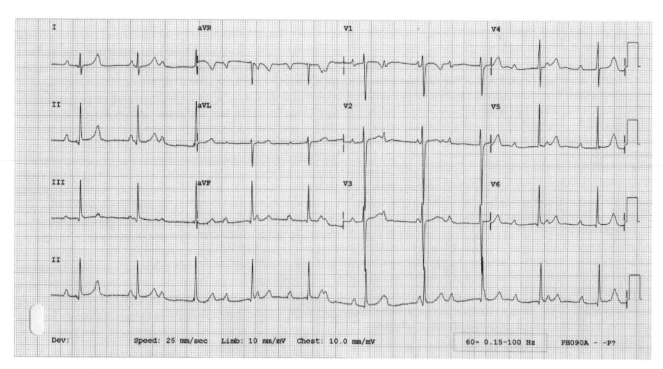

Figure 86.5 12-lead ECG obtained on return visit to pediatric infectious disease specialist six days following initial ED visit demonstrating third-degree AV block.

Later, lymphoid cells infiltrate the endocardium, creating a characteristic band- or plaque-like pattern. Isolated myocyte necrosis and evolution to endocardial fibrosis can be seen.[2]

Patients with Lyme carditis most commonly present with fluctuating degrees of AV block, but occasionally present with acute myopericarditis or mild left ventricular dysfunction. Rarely, cardiomegaly or fatal pancarditis occurs.[4] Common complaints are lightheadedness, syncope, dyspnea and palpitations.[2] The level of AV block varies and fluctuates; the symptoms may be intermittent. As the block rarely lasts longer than a week, a temporary pacemaker is rarely required.[5]

In the United States, the diagnosis of Lyme disease is usually based on the recognition of characteristic clinical findings, a history of exposure in an endemic area and, except in patients with erythema migrans, an antibody response to *B. burgdorferi* by ELISA and western blotting.[4] The most common test is an ELISA assay to detect serum antibodies (IgM and IgG) to *B. burgdorferi*. IgM and IgG antibodies to outer-surface protein A, B or C can also be measured by western blot immunoblot assays, which are generally more sensitive and specific than ELISA assays. However, only one-third of patients with a single erythema migrans lesion have detectable antibodies to *B. burgdorferi* during the first six to eight weeks after transmission of the spirochete. Moreover, if the disease is treated appropriately, antibodies develop in only a few patients.[6] By the time carditis, arthritis and neuroborreliosis develop, most patients have positive serologic tests. More specific tests can be performed on tissue samples from affected organs. In cases of Lyme disease with cardiac involvement, biopsy and autopsy specimens of the myocardium show changes that are characteristic of myocarditis.[6] In addition, *B. burgdorferi* organisms have been isolated from endomyocardial biopsy samples of patients with chronic dilated cardiomyopathy.[3]

Common antibiotic regimens for the treatment of Lyme carditis include amoxicillin (500 mg orally three or four times daily for 30 days), doxycycline (100 mg orally twice daily for 30 days), and ceftriaxone (2 g intravenously daily for two to four weeks).[2] Patients with minor cardiac involvement (i.e., first-degree AV block with P-R interval less than or equal to 0.3 seconds) and no other symptoms should receive antibiotic therapy with doxycycline, tetracycline or amoxicillin as for early disease. Patients with more severe conduction system disease (such as P-R interval greater than 0.3 seconds, second- or third-degree AV block, or clinical evidence of congestive heart failure) should be hospitalized because of the increased risk of complete heart block or asystole.[2] These

patients should be given intravenous ceftriaxone or high-dose penicillin G. Temporary pacing may be necessary for patients with high-grade or symptomatic heart block; the indications for pacing are the same as in other causes of heart block. Complete heart block generally resolves within one week; lesser conduction disturbances typically resolve within six weeks.[2] The overall prognosis of Lyme carditis is very good, although recovery may be delayed and late complications such as dilated cardiomyopathy may occur.[7]

KEY TEACHING POINTS

1. Causes of third-degree heart block in children include congenital anomalies, cardiac surgery, infectious etiologies (such as Lyme carditis), inflammatory disorders, myocardial infarction, cardiac tumors, muscular dystrophies, hypocalcemia and drug overdoses.
2. Lyme carditis typically develops weeks to months following infection with *B. burgdorferi*, and usually manifests with various degrees of AV block.
3. By the time carditis, arthritis and neuroborreliosis develop, most patients have positive serologic tests for antibodies to *B. burgdorferi*.
4. Treatment for patients with Lyme carditis presenting with second- or third-degree AV block or P-R interval greater than 0.3 seconds is intravenous antibiotics (ceftriaxone or penicillin G) and telemetry monitoring.
5. Complete heart block in patients with Lyme carditis generally resolves within one week.

REFERENCES

[1] Doniger SJ, Sharieff GQ. Pediatric dysrhythmias. *Pediatr Clin N Am* 2006;53:85–105.
[2] Pinto DS. Cardiac manifestations of Lyme disease. *Med Clin N Am* 2002;86:285–96.
[3] Hengge UR, Tannapfel A, Tyring SK, et al. Lyme borreliosis. *Lancet Infect Dis* 2003;3:489–500.
[4] Steere AC. Lyme disease. *N Engl J Med* 2001;345:115–25.
[5] Meyerhoff J. Lyme disease. eMedicine Website. Available at http://www.emedicine.com/med/topic1346.htm. Accessed June 26, 2008.
[6] Harris NL, McNeely WF, Shepard JO. Case records of the Massachusetts General Hospital: case 17-2002. *N Engl J Med* 2002;346:1732–8.
[7] Rosenfeld ME, Beckerman B, Ward MF, Sama A. Lyme carditis: complete AV dissociation with episodic asystole presenting as syncope in the emergency department. *J Emerg Med* 1999;17:661–4.

87

Headache and vomiting in a 12-year-old female

HISTORY OF PRESENT ILLNESS

A 12-year-old female with no significant medical history was brought to the ED by her parents after experiencing the sudden onset of a severe headache that began earlier that day at school. The patient described the pain as a throbbing, severe pain rated at a level of 10 (on a scale of 0 to 10), localized to the forehead. She had experienced several episodes of vomiting, as well as dizziness and difficulty walking. She also reported sensitivity to light and neck stiffness, but denied focal weakness or numbness, visual or hearing changes.

PHYSICAL EXAMINATION

GENERAL APPEARANCE: The patient appeared well developed, well nourished and in moderate discomfort.

VITAL SIGNS

Temperature	98.6°F (37°C)
Pulse	95 beats/minute
Blood pressure	130/90 mmHg
Respirations	22 breaths/minute
Oxygen saturation	99% on room air

HEENT: PERRL, EOMI, no nystagmus, mild photophobia present.

NECK: Supple, no meningeal signs.

CARDIOVASCULAR: Regular rate and rhythm without rubs, murmurs or gallops.

LUNGS: Clear to auscultation bilaterally.

ABDOMEN: Soft, nontender, nondistended.

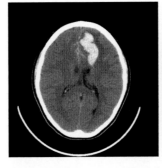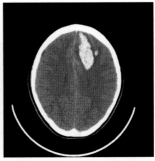

Figure 87.1 Noncontrast CT of the brain from a 12-year-old female with the sudden onset of a frontal headache, vomiting, dizziness and difficulty walking.

EXTREMITIES: No clubbing, cyanosis or edema.

NEUROLOGIC: Alert and oriented to person, place and time; cranial nerves II–XII grossly intact; left upper and lower extremity strength 5/5, right upper and lower extremity strength 4/5, pronator drift present in the right upper extremity; sensation grossly intact.

A peripheral intravenous line was placed, and blood was drawn and sent for laboratory testing. Morphine sulfate as well as Phenergan® IV were administered for pain and nausea, respectively. Laboratory tests, including a complete blood count, electrolytes, BUN, creatinine and glucose, were within normal limits. A noncontrast CT of the brain was obtained (Figure 87.1).

What is your diagnosis?

ANSWER

The diagnosis is intracerebral hemorrhage (ICH) secondary to an arteriovenous malformation of the brain. The noncontrast cranial CT (Figure 87.1) demonstrates a left frontal ICH with diffuse calcifications, edema and mass effect, with displacement of the anterior falx toward the right by 7 mm. Careful assessment of the patients ABCs was undertaken (patient was awake, breathing and protecting her airway). Her head was kept elevated at 45°, and she was given mannitol to decrease intracranial pressure (ICP) in consultation with the pediatric neurosurgeon, as well as phenytoin for seizure prophylaxis. Intravenous fluids were held to a minimum, and

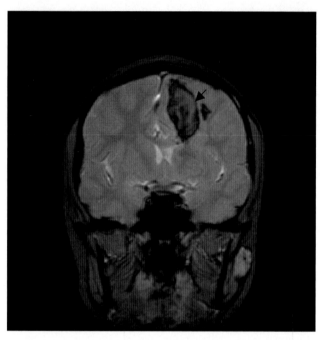

Figure 87.2 MRI of the brain from a 12-year-old female with the sudden onset of a headache, vomiting, dizziness and difficulty walking, demonstrating intracerebral hematoma in the left frontal lobe (arrow).

the blood pressure was carefully monitored. The patient was transferred to the pediatric neurosurgical service for further evaluation and treatment. She subsequently underwent an MRI/MRA of the brain (Figure 87.2), which demonstrated the ICH in the left frontal lobe with the presence of mild heterogeneous enhancement of multiple tubular structures within the parenchymal hematoma, consistent with an arteriovenous malformation (AVM).

Cerebral angiography was performed, which demonstrated a complex AVM in the left frontal lobe (Figure 87.3). The patient's clinical condition improved, and a repeat CT scan performed several days later demonstrated minimal resolution in the edema and hematoma. The patient was discharged home with precautions given to the parents to seek immediate medical attention if symptoms recurred, as well as instructions to avoid strenuous activity. A repeat CT scan was performed as an outpatient four weeks later, which demonstrated near complete resolution of the hematoma. Seven months following the initial presentation for her ICH, the patient underwent gamma knife radiation resection of her AVM.

Pediatric hemorrhagic stroke

Intracerebral hemorrhage (ICH) may occur in the subarachnoid space, or may be primarily located in the parenchyma of the brain.[1] Subarachnoid bleeding is generally characterized by severe headache, nuchal rigidity and progressive loss of consciousness. Intracerebral bleeding is more often characterized by focal neurologic signs and seizures. ICH is more common in premature infants than older children.[1]

Pediatric stroke is caused by heterogeneous diseases; no specific cause can be determined in approximately one-third to one-half of the children affected.[2] The predominant risk factors for stroke in children are congenital heart disease, prothrombic and metabolic disorders, vascular abnormalities, and infections.[2] Hemorrhagic stroke accounts for approximately half of strokes in childhood.[3] Intraparenchymal hemorrhage is the most common type of hemorrhagic stroke. Retrospective

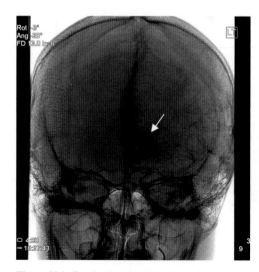
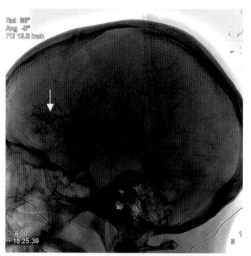

Figure 87.3 Cerebral angiogram from a 12-year-old female with a left frontal intraparenchymal hemorrhage, demonstrating a left frontal AVM (arrows).

studies suggest that intraparenchymal hemorrhage in childhood is most often the result of AVM, hypertension, hematologic abnormality or brain tumor.[3,4] Other etiologies include cavernous hemangioma, vasculopathy, vasculitis, cerebral and systemic infections, and (rarely) illicit drug use.[3] In children, AVMs are 10 times more frequent than saccular aneurysms.[5] The overall mortality from hemorrhagic stroke is approximately 25% in children; significant disability is present in 42% of those who survive.[3]

AVMs result from failure of normal capillary bed development between arteries and veins during embryogenesis.[1] AVMs produce abnormal shunting of blood, which causes an expansion of vessels resulting in space-occupying effect or rupture of a vein and intracerebral bleeding. AVMs are typically located in the cerebral hemispheres, but may be situated in the cerebellum, brainstem or spinal cord.[1] Although the AVM may remain asymptomatic throughout life, rupture and bleeding can occur at any age. Children with AVMs frequently have a history of seizures and migraine-like headaches. Typical migraine headache pain alternates from one side of the head to the other, whereas headaches associated with an AVM classically occur on the same side.[1] A contrast CT scan, or MRI with gadolinium followed by an MRA, are useful for identifying large AVMs; however, four-vessel cerebral angiography is the study of choice for investigating most AVMs and cerebral aneurysms.[1]

Unenhanced CT is considered the initial imaging study of choice in children with suspected ICH because it is rapid, widely available and clearly distinguishes hemorrhagic from ischemic stroke.[3] MRI sequences such as susceptibility-weighted images clearly identify hemorrhage, but are not universally available and require experience and training to correctly identify the hemorrhage.[3] Once an ICH is identified, the pediatric neurosurgical service should be consulted and cerebral angiography performed to identify the source of bleeding (e.g., AVM, cerebral aneurysm).

Medical management guidelines do not currently exist for pediatric patients with spontaneous intraparenchymal hemorrhage, but most guidelines for adults from the American Heart Association are applicable to children.[6] Fluid management to maintain euvolemia and maintenance of body temperature at normal levels with acetaminophen and cooling blankets are recommended.[3,6] Careful monitoring for and treatment of hydrocephalus is essential. Perihematomal edema is typical with intraparenchymal hemorrhage, and osmotherapy (e.g., mannitol) is recommended to treat elevated intracranial pressure. Corticosteroids are not recommended because randomized trials in adults with intraparenchymal hemorrhage have failed to demonstrate efficacy.[3] Additionally, hyperglycemia in this setting has been demonstrated to be detrimental.[3]

Treatment of children with intraparenchymal hemorrhage has primarily been guided by extrapolation from the adult literature.[3] Treatment of brain AVMs depend on their size, venous drainage pattern and location. In general, small, superficial AVMs are microsurgically resected. Embolization may facilitate microsurgery or radiosurgery of larger AVMs in critical areas by reducing the size of the AVM; rarely, it may obliterate the AVM entirely.[3] Radiosurgery typically results in involution of an AVM over three to five years to achieve angiographic obliteration. A particular form of radiotherapy known as gamma knife surgery has recently been shown effective for the treatment of intracranial AVMs in children, yielding high obliteration and low complication rates.[7]

KEY TEACHING POINTS

1. Intraparenchymal hemorrhage is the most common type of hemorrhagic stroke in children, most often the result of an arteriovenous malformation (AVM).

2. Intracerebral bleeding is generally characterized by headache, nausea and vomiting, focal neurologic signs and seizures.

3. Unenhanced CT is considered to be the initial imaging study of choice in children with suspected ICH.

4. Immediate treatment of children with ICH includes assessment and stabilization of the airway, breathing and circulation, maintenance of euvolemia, use of osmotic agents to control elevated ICP, seizure prophylaxis, and tight temperature and glycemic control.

5. Children diagnosed with a spontaneous ICH should undergo urgent neurosurgical consultation and cerebral angiography to identify the source of bleeding.

REFERENCES

[1] Johnston MV. Acute stroke syndromes. In: Behrman RE, Kliegman RM, Jenson HB (eds.). *Nelson Textbook of Pediatrics*, 17th ed. Philadelphia: Elsevier, 2004:2036–7.

[2] Simma B, Martin G, Muller T, et al. Risk factors for pediatric stroke: consequences for therapy and quality of life. *Pediatr Neurol* 2007;37:121–6.

[3] Jordan LC, Hillis AE. Hemorrhagic stroke in children. *Pediatr Neurol* 2007;36:73–80.

[4] Awada A, Daif A, Obeid T, et al. Nontraumatic cerebral hemorrhage in the young: a study of 107 cases. *J Stroke Cerebrovasc Dis* 1998;7:200–4.

[5] Meyer-Heim AD, Boltshauser E. Spontaneous intracranial hemorrhage in children: aetiology, presentation and outcome. *Brain Dev* 2003;25:416–21.

[6] Broderick JP, Adams HP Jr, Barsan W, et al. Guidelines for the management of spontaneous intracerebral hemorrhage: a statement for healthcare professionals from a special writing group of the Stroke Council, American Heart Association. *Stroke* 1999;30:905–15.

[7] Kiran NA, Kale SS, Vaishya S, et al. Gamma knife surgery for intracranial arteriovenous malformations in children: a retrospective study of 103 patients. *J Neurosurg* 2007;107 (6 Suppl):479–84.

PART XI

INFECTIOUS DISEASE

88

Back pain and fever in a 24-year-old male

HISTORY OF PRESENT ILLNESS

A 24-year-old male with no significant medical history presented to the ED by ambulance complaining of several days of mid-lower back pain. The patient reported that the pain started gradually and had worsened over the past several days, to the point were he could not bear weight. He denied leg weakness or numbness, problems with bowel or bladder function, abdominal pain, dysuria or hematuria. He similarly denied any recent trauma, heavy lifting or previous back injuries. He had developed tactile fevers and chills over the past 24 hours. The patient denied intravenous drug use, alcohol, a history of diabetes and had no HIV risk factors.

PHYSICAL EXAMINATION

GENERAL APPEARANCE: The patient was an obese male lying supine on the gurney in moderate discomfort.

VITAL SIGNS

Temperature	101.6°F (38.7°C)
Pulse	100 beats/minute
Blood pressure	135/85 mmHg
Respirations	20 breaths/minute
Oxygen saturation	99% on room air

HEENT: Unremarkable.

NECK: Supple, no meningeal signs, no midline tenderness.

CARDIOVASCULAR: Tachycardic rate, regular rhythm without rubs, murmurs or gallops.

LUNGS: Clear to auscultation bilaterally.

ABDOMEN: Soft, nontender, nondistended.

RECTAL: Normal tone, no perianal anesthesia; brown stool, hemoccult negative.

BACK: Left paraspinous tenderness in the lumbar region with the presence of midline tenderness over the lumbar spinous processes. No thoracic spine tenderness. Lower back pain exacerbated by movement.

EXTREMITIES: No clubbing, cyanosis or edema.

NEUROLOGIC: Alert and oriented to person, place and time; cranial nerves II–XII grossly intact; upper and lower extremity strength 5/5 bilaterally, proximal and distal; sensation grossly intact. Patellar reflexes were brisk bilaterally. The patient was unable to ambulate secondary to low back pain.

A peripheral intravenous line was placed, blood was drawn and sent for laboratory testing and cultures, and Dilaudid® was administered for pain as well as acetaminophen for fever. Laboratory results were significant for a leukocyte count of 12.5 K/µL (normal 3.5–12.5 K/µL) with 94% neutrophils (normal 50–70%) and C-reactive protein (CRP) of 3.5 mg/L (normal less than 0.9 mg/L); the erythrocyte sedimentation rate (ESR), electrolytes, BUN, creatinine and liver function tests were all within normal limits. A urinalysis was negative for blood or infection.

The patient continued to experience significant pain despite multiple repeat doses of intravenous Dilaudid®, and his temperature rose to 102.5°F (39.2°C). A noncontrast CT of the abdomen and pelvis did not reveal evidence of renal or ureteral calculi, hydronephrosis, or abnormal fluid collections in the abdomen or retroperitoneum. The patient was given empiric antibiotics intravenously (vancomycin and piperacillin/tazobactam), and the medicine service was consulted for admission and further evaluation.

What is your diagnosis?

The diagnosis is vertebral osteomyelitis. MRI of the lumbo-sacral spine was obtained, which demonstrated mild increase in T2-weighted signal and enhancement of the L4 and L5 vertebral bodies, without significant disc enhancement (Figure 88.1). The patient's blood cultures subsequently grew out *Serratia marcescens*, and the patient's antibiotics were changed to ciprofloxacin and meropenem upon recommendation of the infectious disease specialist. The patient's symptoms continued to improve during hospitalization, and he was discharged home on hospital day #10, at which time he remained afebrile and was able to ambulate with minimal pain. A PICC line was placed prior to discharge, and the patient continued a three-week course of intravenous ertapenem and oral ciprofloxacin as an outpatient.

Vertebral osteomyelitis

Vertebral osteomyelitis is defined as the inflammation of a vertebral body due to a pyogenic organism.[1] Bacterial osteomyelitis is the most common type of spinal vertebral infection.[2] It is notoriously difficult to diagnose early because of its insidious nature and lack of localizing symptoms and signs. Frequently, the infection spreads to the adjacent disc space, resulting in spondylodiscitis.[1] The vertebral body is the most common site of bacterial seeding, with the posterior elements (such as lamina or facet joints) rarely involved.[2] The lumbar spine is involved most frequently, followed by the thoracic and cervical spinal regions.

Hematogenous bacterial dissemination is the most common mechanism for vertebral osteomyelitis.[2] Staphylococcal species are the major infectious organisms, although mycobacterial organisms are also common in some populations.[3] Compared with younger hosts, elderly patients are more likely to be infected with Gram-negative organisms (particularly urinary tract organisms) and to have had recent surgery.[3] Some well-known predisposing factors of vertebral osteomyelitis are male gender, diabetes mellitus, immunocompromised state, sickle cell anemia, hemodialysis, spinal instrumentation and intravenous drug use.[2]

Most patients who have vertebral osteomyelitis present with back pain, which typically develops in an indolent fashion over a period of weeks to months.[1] Nocturnal pain, symptoms of malaise, generalized fatigue and depressed appetite are commonly seen with fever.[2] Neurologic symptoms are not seen until later stages, when infection extends directly into the epidural space and an epidural abscess begins to compress adjacent neural tissue. Physical examination usually reveals tenderness to percussion of the spinous process of the involved vertebral body. Nearly all patients report localized pain and tenderness of the involved bone segments.[4] Fever and peripheral leukocytosis are present in approximately half of patients, and ESR is usually elevated. Following the ESR provides a prognostic guide during treatment.[4] The CRP level is also usu-

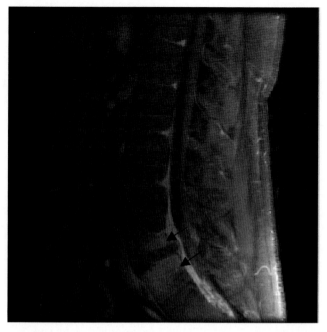

Figure 88.1 MRI of the lumbar spine from a 24-year-old male demonstrating enhancement of L4 and L5 vertebral bodies on T2-weighted images (arrows), consistent with vertebral osteomyelitis.

ally elevated in cases of vertebral osteomyelitis; it may be more useful than the ESR because it generally shows elevation earlier than the ESR.[5] Because the most frequent mode of infection is hematogenous spread, blood cultures should be obtained in every patient. Depending on the study, blood cultures are positive in up to 70% of patients, and should guide antibiotic therapy.[1]

Plain radiographs should be obtained in all patients suspected of having a spinal infection.[6] These may reveal the degree of bony destruction, and may identify any corresponding coronal or sagittal deformity due to the disease process. Radionuclide studies are more sensitive than radiographs in detecting early disease. Three-phase ^{99m}Tc bone scans are sensitive (about 90%) but nonspecific (about 78%) for spinal infections, particularly in older patients with some degree of spondylosis and degenerative disc disease present.[6] CT provides excellent detail of bony anatomy, and can also identify and delineate the presence of adjacent soft tissue masses or abscesses. However, CT is inferior to MRI in evaluating disc spaces and the neural elements. MRI is the gold standard for evaluating spinal infections, and is especially useful in the early stages of infection when other modalities are still normal (radiography) or nonspecific (nuclear medicine). Early in the disease process, MRI demonstrates signs of edema and inflammation.[1] Additional advantages of MRI include its ability to identify the extent of disease and spinal cord involvement.

Once the diagnosis of vertebral osteomyelitis is made, treatment with broad-spectrum antibiotics should be initiated and a spine surgeon should be consulted.[3] Antibiotics should be given for 6–12 weeks, and should be modified based on culture results. Nonoperative management with antibiotics and analgesia is appropriate in patients who have a stable spine and minor or no neurologic deficit; this strategy is effective in 60–95% of such patients.[3] In pyogenic vertebral osteomyelitis, surgical intervention is reserved for the management of complications (e.g., presence of fluid collection, impending cord compression) or for the failure of medical therapy.[7] However, in spinal epidural abscess, decompressive laminectomy with antibiotics is the treatment of choice.

KEY TEACHING POINTS

1. Predisposing factors for vertebral osteomyelitis include male gender, diabetes mellitus, immunocompromised state, sickle cell anemia, hemodialysis, spinal instrumentation and intravenous drug use.

2. Signs and symptoms of vertebral osteomyelitis include indolent back pain (over a period of weeks to months), nocturnal back pain, malaise, generalized fatigue, depressed appetite and fever.

3. ESR, CRP and leukocyte count are useful but nonspecific laboratory tests in the diagnosis of vertebral osteomyelitis.

4. MRI is the gold standard for diagnosing vertebral osteomyelitis and related spinal infections.

5. Treatment of vertebral osteomyelitis is primarily with a prolonged course of broad-spectrum antibiotics; surgery is reserved for the management of complications or when medical management fails.

REFERENCES

[1] Winters ME Kluetz P, Zilberstein J. Back pain emergencies. *Med Clin N Am* 2006;90:505–23.

[2] Meleger AL, Krivickas LS. Neck and back pain: musculo-skeletal disorders. *Neurol Clin* 2007;25:419–38.

[3] Broder J, Snarski JT. Back pain in the elderly. *Clin Geriatr Med* 2007;23:271–89.

[4] Calhoun JH, Manring MM. Adult osteomyelitis. *Infect Dis Clin N Am* 2005;19:765–86.

[5] King RW. Osteomyelitis. eMedicine Website. Available at http://www.emedicine.com/emerg/topic349.htm. Accessed July 10, 2008.

[6] An HS, Seldomridge JA. Spinal infections: diagnostic tests and imaging studies. *Clin Orthop Relat Res* 2006;444:27–33.

[7] Lew DP, Waldovegel FA. Current concepts: osteomyelitis. *N Engl J Med* 1997;336:999–1007.

89

Intermittent fevers, chills and headache in a 26-year-old male

HISTORY OF PRESENT ILLNESS

A 26-year-old male visiting the United States from India presented to the ED complaining of several days of intermittent fevers, shaking chills and headaches. He denied shortness of breath or cough, neck stiffness, abdominal pain or dysuria. He reported mild nausea, diarrhea and anorexia, as well as a sore throat and decreased oral intake during this time. He was seen two days previously in an outside clinic, diagnosed with streptococcal pharyngitis and started on oral amoxicillin-clavulanate. His symptoms had not improved. The patient arrived from India five days prior to presentation in the ED. He denied chronic medical problems and took no medications. He denied tobacco, alcohol or illicit drugs, and was traveling on business. According to the patient, his immunizations were up to date.

PHYSICAL EXAMINATION

GENERAL APPEARANCE: The patient was awake and alert, although he appeared ill and dehydrated.

VITAL SIGNS

Temperature	104.4°F (40.2°C)
Pulse	123 beats/minute
Blood pressure	115/64 mmHg
Respirations	22 breaths/minute
Oxygen saturation	99% on room air

HEENT: PERRL, EOMI, sclera anicteric, oropharynx dry, without oral lesions or exudates.

NECK: Supple, no meningeal signs, no cervical lymphadenopathy.

CARDIOVASCULAR: Tachycardic rate, regular rhythm without rubs, murmurs or gallops.

LUNGS: Clear to auscultation bilaterally.

ABDOMEN: Soft, nontender, nondistended, without hepato- or splenomegaly.

EXTREMITIES: No clubbing, cyanosis or edema.

SKIN: Warm and moist, no rashes.

NEUROLOGIC: Nonfocal.

A peripheral intravenous line was placed, and blood was drawn and sent for cultures and laboratory testing. Intravenous fluids were administered (2 liters of normal saline) along with acetaminophen orally for the fever and morphine sulfate IV for the headache. A 12-lead ECG demonstrated sinus tachycardia, rate 120, without acute ST-T wave changes.

Laboratory tests revealed a leukocyte count of 4.5 K/μL (normal 3.5–12.5 K/μL) with 12% bands (presence of bands abnormal), 53% neutrophils, 16% lymphocytes, 19% monocytes, and hematocrit of 41% (normal 39–51%) with 77 K/μL platelets (normal 140–400 K/μL). The serum glucose was slightly elevated at 170 mg/dL (normal 60–159 mg/dL), whereas the serum sodium was slightly decreased at 131 mEq/L (normal 137–145 mEq/L). The remainder of the electrolytes were within normal limits. Liver function tests revealed an AST of 72 U/L (normal 17–59 U/L), ALT of 81 U/L (normal 11–66 U/L) and total bilirubin of 1.7 mg/dL (normal 0.2–1.3 mg/dL). A chest radiograph and noncontrast CT of the brain were performed (Figures 89.1 and 89.2, respectively).

A lumbar puncture to evaluate for possible meningitis was performed. Examination of the cerebrospinal fluid (CSF) revealed 1 white blood cell (WBC) and 1 red blood cell (RBC) per μL, slight elevation in CSF glucose at 86 mg/dL (normal 40–73 mg/dL) and normal CSF protein. Gram stain of the CSF revealed neither organisms nor white blood cells.

What is your diagnosis?

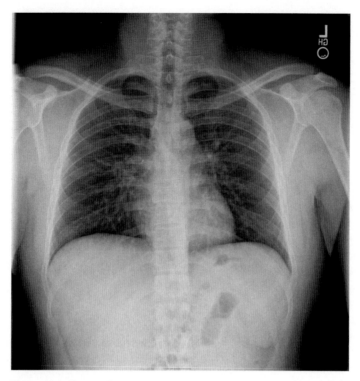

Figure 89.1 Chest radiograph of a 26-year-old male with fevers, chills and headache.

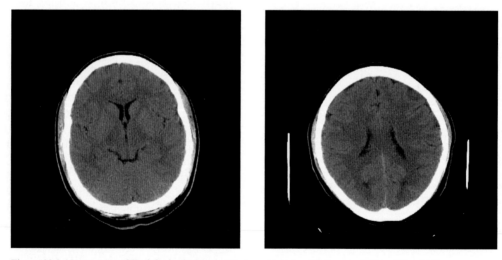

Figure 89.2 Noncontrast CT of the brain from a 26-year-old male with fevers, chills and headache.

ANSWER

The diagnosis is malaria caused by *Plasmodium vivax*. The head CT and chest radiograph were normal. Thin and thick blood smears were performed, which were positive for malaria. The patient received one oral dose of Malarone® (atovaquone and proguanil chloride) in the ED, and was admitted to the medicine service to continue intravenous hydration, hemodynamic monitoring and daily oral doses of Malarone®. Two days after admission to the hospital, blood cultures returned positive for *Plasmodium vivax*. By hospital day #4, the patient's condition had improved considerably; he was tolerating food and was afebrile. The patient was seen in the infectious disease clinic two weeks after discharge, at which time he was asymptomatic with normal liver function tests. The patient was prescribed primaquine 30 mg orally daily for two weeks as terminal prophylaxis.

Malaria

Malaria is an infection caused by the coccidian protozoan parasite of the genus *Plasmodium*, carried by female *Anopheles* species mosquitoes.[1] The clinical disease in humans may vary widely according to the species of parasite – *Plasmodium falciparum, vivax, ovale* or *malariae* – as well as the genetics, immune status, and age of the host. These variables have a major influence on all aspects of the disease, including epidemiology, pathogenesis, clinical features and management.[1] The annual global clinical caseload of malarial infections is estimated at nearly 500 million, with 1–3 million deaths (mainly among young children in Africa).[2] Malaria occurs annually in about 25,000 cases of travelers; about half of these are reported and about 150 (less than 1%) are fatal.[2] About 1000 cases of malaria occur in the United States annually, whereas the United Kingdom has over 2000 cases each year, with 10–20 deaths.[2]

The female *Anopheles* mosquito is the arthropod vector that can transmit malaria after ingesting gametocytes from infected persons.[3] After sexual reproduction in the gut of the mosquito, sporozoites are released from the salivary glands of the arthropod into the human host during a blood meal. The sporozoites rapidly penetrate the liver parenchymal cells. The protozoans, now termed cryptozoites or exoerythrocytic schizonts, rapidly multiply. Eventual lysis of the hepatic cells results in the release of merozoites into the bloodstream, where they invade erythrocytes. In *P. vivax* and *P. ovale* infections, a dormant hypnozoite can reside in hepatocytes, allowing for recrudescent infection many months to years later.[3]

After invading red blood cells (RBC), the merozoites transform into trophozoites, which feed on the cell's hemoglobin. These trophozoites mature into schizonts, which may divide asexually into additional merozoites. The RBCs undergo lysis, releasing many merozoites into the blood. Although some merozoites are destroyed by the body's immune apparatus, many enter new erythrocytes. After several repetitions of this erythrocytic cycle, the cyclic process changes, and male mi-crogametocytes or female macrogametocytes may develop instead of merozoites.[3] These gametes subsequently complete the reproductive cycle by fusion within the gut of a new female *Anopheles* mosquito after she has taken a blood meal from an infected host (Figure 89.3).[3]

Plasmodium falciparum causes most malaria deaths and can be rapidly fatal.[4] Although malaria is found throughout the tropics, various countries are endemic to specific species. *P. falciparum* is the predominant species in Africa, causing the development of symptoms within one month. In contrast, *P. vivax* is rare in Africa because Africans generally lack the Duffy antigen on the surface of the red blood cell necessary for the parasite to penetrate.[4] *P. vivax* predominates in Asia and Latin America; here, symptoms develop within one month only 50% of the time.[5]

Travelers with malaria are usually male and female adults, who may be elderly.[2] Most patients become symptomatic 10 days to four weeks after infection, although patients may present many months later.[4] The clinical presentation of malaria is nonspecific, with fever, cough, sore throat and flu-like illness. Headaches, myalgias, fatigue and rigors occur, as may nausea, vomiting and diarrhea. Although a history of fever is typically present, 10–40% of persons with malaria may be afebrile when first examined.[5] Patterns of fever are rarely diagnostic, but fevers at regular 48–72 hour intervals are virtually pathognomonic of *P. vivax*, *P. ovale*, and *P. malariae* infections.[5] In severe cases, malaria may present with shock, renal failure, hypoglycemia, pulmonary edema, acidosis, seizures, abnormal bleeding and disseminated intravascular coagulation (DIC).[4]

The definitive diagnosis of malaria is made by microscopic examination of thick and thin blood films.[1–5] There is no need to wait for the fever to peak before carrying out a blood film, as parasites are often present throughout the red cell cycle (Figure 89.4). Malarial chemoprophylaxis should be withheld during investigation for malaria, as antimalarials can suppress peripheral parasitemia.[1] The most common abnormality on full blood count is thrombocytopenia, especially in the nonimmune host. This is due largely to splenic pooling of platelets and platelet activation.[1] The total WBC count is usually in the normal range, but lymphopenia may be present due to lymphocytic redistribution. More recently, apoptosis of lymphocytes has been identified in *P. falciparum* malaria.[1]

Chloroquine remains the treatment of choice for *P. falciparum* acquired in areas without chloroquine-resistant strains.[6] In areas with chloroquine resistance, a combination of atovaquone and proguanil (Malarone®) or quinine plus either tetracycline, doxycycline or clindamycin are the best treatment options. Chloroquine remains the treatment of choice for all other malarial species, with the exception of *P. vivax* acquired in Indonesia or Papua New Guinea. In these areas, atovaquone-proguanil is best, with either mefloquine alone or a combination of quinine plus tetracycline or doxycycline as alternatives. Quinidine is currently the recommended treatment for severe cases of malaria in the United States.[6]

Infections with *P. vivax* and *P. ovale* should be treated with primaquine to prevent potential relapses.[6,7] To achieve

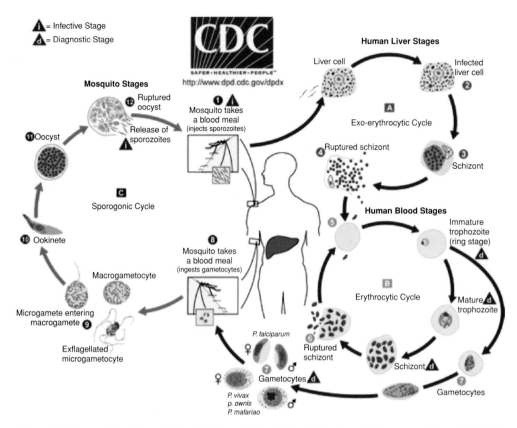

Figure 89.3 Plasmodium life-cycle (from CDC, available at http://dpd.cdc.gov/dpdx, accessed June 23, 2008).

more reliable eradication of hypnozoites, the CDC currently recommends a regimen of 0.5 mg/kg to a maximum of 30 mg of primaquine base daily for 14 days.[6] The most common severe adverse effect associated with primaquine is intravascular hemolysis in persons with glucose-6-phosphate dehydrogenase (G6PD) deficiency, a contraindication to using this drug. Patients must be screened for G6PD deficiency prior to use of primaquine. If possible, primaquine treatment should overlap with the blood schizonticidal treatment.[6]

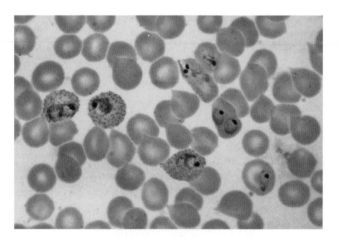

Figure 89.4 Photomicrograph of red blood cells infected with *P. vivax* (available at http://health.howstuffworks.com/malaria1.htm, accessed June 23, 2008).

For travelers, malarial chemoprophylaxis should start one week before entering an endemic area (to ensure adequate blood levels and to identify any potential side effects), and continue while within an endemic area and for four weeks after return. Malarone can be commenced on the day before entry, and continued for one week after leaving.[3] Chloroquine, two tablets (300 mg base) once a week, together with proguanil, two tablets (200 mg) daily, is one of the safest and most inexpensive regimens, but has diminishing efficacy. These drugs have only minor side effects, the most common being difficulty in visual accommodation (chloroquine) and mouth ulcers (proguanil).[3] There is increasing use of mefloquine one tablet (250 mg) weekly, or doxycycline one tablet (100 mg) daily, or Malarone® one tablet daily, by travelers to sub-Saharan Africa, Papua New Guinea and the Solomon Islands because of chloroquine resistance. The main side effects of mefloquine are neuropsychiatric and are of varying severity; doxycycline can lead to light sensitization and Malarone® can cause gastrointestinal upset.[3] Because of constantly changing malarial resistance patterns, it is necessary to consult an updated resource or consultant for current treatment recommendations.

KEY TEACHING POINTS

1. Malaria is a parasitic infection whose vector is carried by female *Anopheles* species mosquitoes. It is caused by one

of four species of parasite – *Plasmodium falciparum*, *vivax*, *ovale* or *malariae*.

2. *P. falciparum*, the predominant species of parasite responsible for malaria in Africa, causes most malaria deaths and can be rapidly fatal.

3. The nonspecific clinical presentation of malaria includes fever, cough, sore throat and flu-like illness.

4. The definitive diagnosis of malaria is made by prompt microscopic examination of thick and thin blood films.

5. Chloroquine remains the treatment of choice for *P. falciparum* acquired in areas without chloroquine-resistant strains.

6. It is important to identify areas with chloroquine resistance, and to consult appropriate malarial sites or infectious disease specialists regarding the most updated treatment and chemoprophylactic regimens.

REFERENCES

[1] Pasvol G. Malaria. In: Cohen J, Powderly WG, et al. (eds.). *Cohen and Powderly: Infectious Diseases*, 2nd ed. Philadelphia: Mosby, 2004:1579–91.

[2] Pasvol G. Management of severe malaria: interventions and controversies. *Infect Dis Clin N Am* 2005;19:211–40.

[3] Becker BM, Cahill JD. Parasites. In: Marx JA, Hockberger RS, Walls RM, et al. (eds.). *Rosen's Emergency Medicine: Concepts and Clinical Practice*, 6th ed. Philadelphia: Mosby, 2006:2096–104.

[4] Lowenstein R. Deadly viral syndrome mimics. *Emerg Med Clin N Am* 2004;22:1051–65.

[5] Ryan ET, Wilson ME, Kain KC. Current concepts: illness after international travel. *N Engl J Med* 2002;347:505–16.

[6] Griffith KS, Lewis LS, Mali S, et al. Treatment of malaria in the United States. *JAMA* 2007;297:2264–77.

[7] Baird JK. Effectiveness of antimalarial drugs. *N Engl J Med* 2005;352:1565–77.

90

Fever and rash in a 39-year-old male

HISTORY OF PRESENT ILLNESS

A 39-year-old male with a medical history significant for hypertension presented to the ED complaining of one day of fevers, chills, malaise, headache, nausea, vomiting, and a purple rash on his face and extremities. He had recently been traveling in rural China for two weeks. His symptoms began prior to boarding his return flight to the United States one day prior to presentation. Upon return to the United States, his symptoms became progressively worse. He was brought to the ED by a friend. He denied chest pain, cough, shortness of breath or abdominal pain. He denied alcohol, tobacco, intravenous or illicit drug use. He denied recent ill contacts or sexual activity, and traveled alone while in China.

PHYSICAL EXAMINATION

GENERAL APPEARANCE: The patient was a well-developed, ill-appearing male breathing rapidly yet able to speak in full sentences.

VITAL SIGNS

Temperature	101.8°F (38.8°C) rectal
Heart rate	118 beats/minute
Blood pressure	118/79 mmHg
Respiratory rate	30 breaths/minute
Oxygen saturation	91% on room air

HEENT: PERRL, EOMI, oropharynx dry.

NECK: Supple, no meningeal signs.

CARDIOVASCULAR: Tachycardic rate, regular rhythm without rubs, murmurs or gallops.

TABLE 90.1 Laboratory results from a patient with fever and rash

WBC 6.6 K/μL	Fibrin split products > 20	Lactic acid >12 mmol/L
RBC 5.2 M/μL	Fibrinogen 118 mg/dL (L)	Glucose 40 mg/dL
Hemoglobin 16.3 g/dL	PT 31.1 sec	Potassium 3.9 mEq/L
Hematocrit 48.1%	INR 3.1	Sodium 135 mEq/L
Platelets 19 K/μL		Chloride 88 mEq/L
Neutrophils 82%	Alkaline phos 78 U/L	CO_2 9 mEq/L
Lymphocytes 17%	Amylase 93 U/L	BUN 27 mg/dL
Monocytes 1%	Bilirubin 1.9 mg/dL	Creatinine 5.4 mg/dL
Metamyelocytes 13%	AST 2752 U/L	Anion gap 38 mEq/L
Bands 41%	ALT 1075 U/L	
	LDH 10,562 U/L	

CHEST: Clear to auscultation bilaterally.

ABDOMEN: Soft, nontender, nondistended, active bowel sounds present.

EXTREMITIES: Weak peripheral pulses, extremities cool and cyanotic, with markedly delayed capillary refill.

SKIN: Mottled with evidence of large, coalesced areas of purpura on the face and extremities (Figure 90.1).

NEUROLOGIC: Nonfocal.

Two peripheral intravenous lines were placed, blood was drawn and sent for laboratory testing and culture, and intravenous fluid boluses (2 liters of normal saline) were given. A portable chest radiograph was obtained (Figure 90.2). Laboratory test results returned as shown in Table 90.1 (abnormal test results in red).

What is your diagnosis?

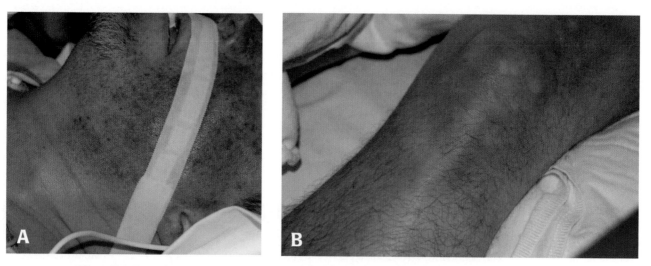

Figure 90.1 Purpuric rash on the face (panel A) and leg (panel B) of a 39-year-old male with fevers, chills and vomiting for one day.

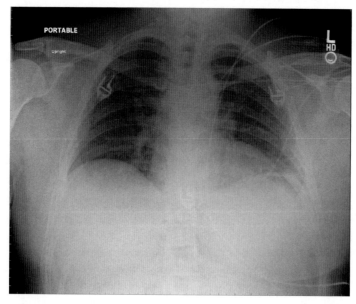

Figure 90.2 Portable chest radiograph from a 39-year-old male with fevers, chills, rash and vomiting for one day.

ANSWER

The diagnosis is purpura fulminans and multi-organ failure due to pneumococcal sepsis (*Streptococcus pneumoniae*). Following initial examination, intravenous antibiotics (ceftriaxone and vancomycin) were given along with IV steroids (Decadron®) due to concern for meningococcemia. Strict isolation precautions were instituted, and the medical intensivist and infectious disease specialists were consulted. Early during the ED encounter, the patient began wheezing and developed respiratory distress. An arterial blood gas performed while his oxygen saturation was 88% on a 100% non-rebreather mask demonstrated a pH of 6.99 (normal 7.35–7.45), pCO_2 of 19 mmHg (normal 35–45 mmHg), pO_2 of 82 mmHg (normal 80–95 mmHg), bicarbonate of 4.5 mmol/L (normal 23–28 mmol/L) with a base excess of −27 (normal −2.4 to +2.3). The patient was orotracheally intubated using rapid sequence induction. Pressors (dopamine and norepinephrine) were started along with continuation of intravenous fluids, and the patient was transferred to the ICU. A portable chest radiograph performed four hours after the initial radiograph (following intubation) demonstrated the development of acute respiratory distress syndrome (ARDS) (Figure 90.3). Repeat laboratory tests performed five hours following the initial tests demonstrated an AST of 1,000,000 U/L. The patient expired approximately seven hours after presentation, despite aggressive antibiotics and resuscitative efforts. Blood cultures returned positive for Gram-positive cocci in pairs and chains, identified as *Streptococcus pneumoniae*.

Sepsis-induced purpura fulminans

Purpura fulminans (PF) is an acute illness commonly associated with meningococcemia or invasive streptococcal dis-

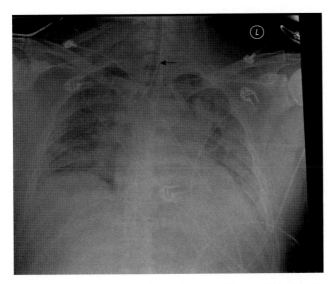

Figure 90.3 Portable chest radiograph from a 39-year-old male with purpura fulminans and *Streptococcus pneumoniae* sepsis, performed four hours after initial chest radiograph (arrow indicates endotracheal tube).

ease. It is typically characterized by disseminated intravascular coagulation (DIC) and purpuric lesions.[1] More specifically, PF can be identified in three clinical conditions: patients with pre-existing inherited or acquired abnormality of the protein C or S anticoagulant pathway; patients with acute severe infection, predominantly Gram-negative bacterial infections, called acute infectious purpura fulminans; and patients without known infections, termed idiopathic purpura fulminans.[2] The last subtype occurs primarily in children, usually after benign infections.[2] In sepsis-induced PF, there are four primary features: large purpuric skin lesions, fever, hypotension and DIC.[1]

Most cases of PF have been reported in children, although it can occur at all ages. PF sometimes represents a fatal disorder.[3] Most cases develop in childhood during an acute infection, particularly meningococcal sepsis.[4] PF occurs only rarely in the course of infection with other organisms, for example group A and B *Streptococcus*, varicella, rubella and *Streptococcus pneumoniae*.[4] Skin and soft tissue infections due to *Streptococcus pneumoniae* are reported mainly in patients with immunosuppression or other underlying conditions.[4]

Regardless of the precipitating condition, PF initially presents with erythematous macules and petechiae, which rapidly evolve into painful, indurated and well-demarcated purpuric plaques.[3] Late findings include hemorrhagic bullae, skin necrosis and eschars. Necrosis may extend to subcutaneous tissue, muscles and bones. A characteristic histologic feature is dermal vessel thrombosis.[3] Vascular changes may be widespread and involve multiple organ systems, rendering PF a life-threatening disorder.

DIC is present in more than 90% of cases of sepsis-induced PF, supporting the notion that PF is a cutaneous marker of DIC.[2] DIC is the clinical manifestation of inappropriate thrombin activation.[5] The development of DIC is mediated by several simultaneously occurring mechanisms, initiated by the proinflammatory cytokines TNF-α, IL-1 and IL-6.[2] The mechanisms include ongoing generation of thrombin, the inhibition of natural anticoagulant mechanisms, and the impairment of fibrinolysis caused by plasminogen activator inhibitor-1.[2]

PF is a syndrome, not a specific disease; therefore, treatment must be aimed at the underlying infection, along with supportive management.[2] Early administration of antibiotics as soon as the diagnosis of PF is entertained provides a significant therapeutic advantage. Patients presenting with PF should receive antibiotic therapy active not only against *Neisseria meningitides* and streptococci but also against methicillin-resistant *Staphylococcus aureus* (MRSA).[1] Some authors also recommend considering early administration of activated protein C (i.e., drotrecogin-alpha) in an attempt to minimize purpuric skin injury and down-regulate the inflammatory cascade before irreparable tissue injury occurs.[1] Despite early antibiotic intervention and intensive care treatment, the mortality rate for PF remains high, averaging 40% (range 20–70%).[2]

All patients with sepsis-induced PF should be treated in an intensive care setting for optimal supportive management.

Hemodynamic monitoring of blood pressure and arterial blood gases is necessary. Aggressive fluid resuscitation to restore intravascular volume, inotropic and ventilatory support, and continuous renal replacement therapy (when required) are major therapeutic interventions.[2] If patients survive the acute phase of PF, attention is turned to the treatment of cutaneous manifestations. Most authors agree that debridement and subsequent coverage with skin grafts are the mainstays of managing necrotic lesions resulting from PF.[4]

KEY TEACHING POINTS

1. Sepsis-induced purpura fulminans (PF) is characterized by large purpuric skin lesions, fever, hypotension and disseminated intravascular coagulation (DIC).
2. DIC is present in more than 90% of cases of sepsis-induced PF, supporting the notion that PF is a cutaneous marker of DIC.
3. PF presents initially with erythematous macules and petechiae, which rapidly evolve into painful, indurated and well-demarcated purpuric plaques.
4. Treatment of sepsis-induced PF includes early administration of antibiotics, aggressive fluid, inotropic and ventilatory support in an ICU setting, and consideration of activated protein C administration.
5. Despite early antibiotic intervention and intensive care treatment, the mortality rate for PF remains high.

REFERENCES

[1] Kravitz GR, Dries DJ, Peterson ML, Schlievert PM. Purpura fulminans due to *Staphylococcus aureus*. *Clin Infect Dis* 2005;40:941–7.
[2] Betrosian AP, Berlet T, Agarwal B. Purpura fulminans in sepsis. *Amer J Med Sci* 2006;332:339–45.
[3] Galimberti R, Pietropaolo N, Galimberti G, et al. Adult purpura fulminans associated with staphylococcal infection and administration of colony-stimulating factors. *Euro J Derm* 2003;13:95–7.
[4] Meiners PM, Leon-Villapalos J, Dziewulski P. Pneumococcal septicemia with purpura fulminans in an 11-month-old child (case report). *J Plast Recon Aesthet Surg* 2006;59:1377–80.
[5] Davis MDP, Dy KM, Nelson S. Presentation and outcome of purpura fulminans associated with peripheral gangrene in 12 patients at Mayo Clinic. *J Am Acad Dermatol* 2007;57:944–56.

91

Fever, abdominal pain and diarrhea in a 51-year-old male

HISTORY OF PRESENT ILLNESS

A 51-year-old male with a medical history significant for hypertension presented to the ED complaining of several days of crampy abdominal pain, nausea and loose stools. He reported that two weeks earlier, he began developing fevers with shaking chills and mild right upper quadrant abdominal pain. The patient was seen two days previously by his primary care provider and diagnosed with gastroenteritis. He continued to experience abdominal pain, nausea and mild diarrhea, as well as fevers to 104°F (40°C), chills and anorexia. His only medication was atenolol, which he had not taken for several days. He had no known allergies, did not smoke or drink, and had no history of abdominal surgeries. He was originally from India, and his last travel to that country was one year ago. The patient denied cough, chest pain, headache, neck stiffness, sore throat or urinary symptoms.

PHYSICAL EXAMINATION

GENERAL APPEARANCE: The patient appeared pale and acutely ill. He was awake and alert and responded appropriately to questioning.

VITAL SIGNS

Temperature	103°F (39.4°C)
Pulse	130 beats/minute
Blood pressure	70/40 mmHg
Respirations	26 breaths/minute
Oxygen saturation	97% on room air

HEENT: PERRL, EOMI, slight scleral icterus, oropharynx dry.

NECK: Supple, no nuchal rigidity.

CARDIOVASCULAR: Tachycardic, regular heart sounds without rubs, murmurs or gallops.

LUNGS: Clear to auscultation bilaterally.

ABDOMEN: Soft, nondistended, hypoactive bowel sounds; epigastric and right upper quadrant tenderness, no Murphy's sign or pulsatile masses.

EXTREMITIES: Cool, delayed capillary refill, weak pulses.

SKIN: Pale and dry, no rashes.

NEUROLOGIC: Nonfocal.

The patient was placed on the cardiac monitor, a peripheral intravenous line was placed, and blood as well as blood cultures were drawn and sent for laboratory testing. A 1-liter normal saline IV bolus was infused. An initial 12-lead ECG demonstrated sinus tachycardia, rate 130, with nonspecific ST-T wave changes. A portable chest radiograph revealed no focal consolidation. Initial laboratory tests were significant for a leukocyte count of 2.0 K/μL (normal 3.5–12.5 K/μL) with 27% immature bands (presence of bands abnormal), hematocrit of 29% (normal 39–51%), platelets of 81 K/μL (normal 140–400 K/μL), creatinine of 1.6 mg/dL (normal 0.8–1.5 mg/dL), total bilirubin of 2.9 mg/dL (normal 0.2–1.3 mg/dL), AST of 84 U/L (normal 17–59 U/L), ALT of 93 U/L (normal 11–66 U/L), alkaline phosphatase of 205 U/L (normal 38–126 U/L) and troponin I of 0.18 ng/dL (normal 0.00–0.09 ng/dL).

What is your diagnosis?

ANSWER

The diagnosis is septic shock secondary to a hepatic abscess. Additional laboratory tests revealed a lactate level of 4.6 mmol/L (normal 0.7–2.1 mmol/L), INR of 1.3, fibrinogen of 516 mg/dL (normal 189–434 mg/dL) and an arterial blood gas demonstrating a pH of 7.46 (normal 7.35–7.45), pCO_2 of 22 (normal 35–45), pO_2 of 79 (normal 80–95), bicarbonate of 18 mmol/L (normal 23–28 mmol/L) and base excess of −8.1 (normal −2.4 to +2.3). The patient received a total of 5 liters normal saline IV; a norepinephrine IV drip was started after minimal improvement in the patient's blood pressure following IV fluids. A central venous catheter and $ScVO_2$ monitor were placed, and empiric broad-spectrum antibiotics were given.

The patient was admitted to the ICU, and a noncontrast CT of the abdomen showed ill-defined, fluid-filled areas of low attenuation in the left lobe of the liver. CT of the abdomen with IV contrast demonstrated a 4-cm multiloculated left hepatic abscess (Figure 91.1). The liver abscess was drained under CT guidance by an interventional radiologist. Cloudy, brownish fluid was aspirated and sent for culture. A Jackson-Pratt drain was left in place at the drainage site. Blood and abscess fluid cultures both grew out *Streptococcus constellatus* (viridans group). The patient's antibiotic regimen was switched to metronidazole and cefotaxime IV based on abscess fluid cultures and sensitivities, and a PICC line was placed for long-term antibiotic treatment. On hospital day #8, the patient's vital signs had normalized and he was discharged home to complete his course of IV antibiotics.

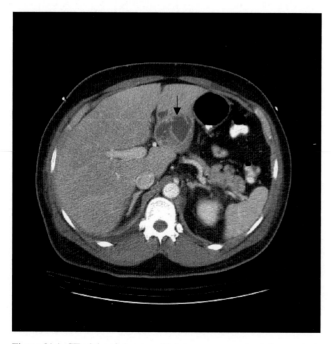

Figure 91.1 CT of the abdomen with intravenous contrast demonstrating a 4-cm multiloculated left hepatic abscess (arrow).

Sepsis and hepatic abscesses

Sepsis has been defined as a suspected or proven infection plus the systemic inflammatory response syndrome (SIRS): fever, tachycardia, tachypnea and leukocytosis.[1,2] Severe sepsis may be defined as sepsis with organ dysfunction (hypotension, hypoxemia, oliguria, metabolic acidosis, thrombocytopenia or obtundation). Septic shock is generally defined as severe sepsis with hypotension, despite adequate fluid resuscitation. The mortality rates associated with severe sepsis and septic shock are 25–30% and 40–70%, respectively.[1]

The cornerstone of emergency management of sepsis is early, goal-directed therapy (EGDT), plus lung-protective ventilation, broad-spectrum antibiotics and possibly activated protein C.[1] Rivers and colleagues conducted a randomized controlled trial in which patients with severe sepsis and septic shock received either early, goal-directed, protocol-guided therapy during the first six hours after enrollment or "standard" therapy.[3] Crystalloids were administered to maintain central venous pressure at 8–12 mmHg. Vasopressors were added if the mean arterial pressure (MAP) was less than 65 mmHg; if central venous oxygen saturation was less than 70%, erythrocytes were transfused to maintain a hematocrit of greater than 30%. Dobutamine was added if the central venous pressure (CVP), MAP and hematocrit were optimized yet venous oxygen saturation remained below 70%. EGDT in that study decreased mortality at 28 and 60 days, as well as the duration of hospitalization.[3] The mechanisms of the benefit of EGDT are unclear, but may include reversal of tissue hypoxia and a decrease in inflammation and coagulation defects.[1]

The use of lactate as a biomarker for tissue oxygenation and perfusion has enhanced the early identification of patients with severe sepsis.[2] Lactate greater than or equal to 4 mmol/L, independent of blood pressure, was used as a major criteria for the EGDT study.[2,3] Nguyen et al. found that for each 10% decrease in serum lactate, mortality decreased by 11%.[2,4] Additionally, 29% of infected patients with elevated lactates were normotensive – yet if the lactate was not cleared within six hours, their mortality was 55%. These results underscore two major points: a normal blood pressure does not equate to effective end-organ perfusion, and when serum lactate is elevated, the patient is in a critical but potentially reversible situation in which oxygen delivery is not meeting demand.[2]

Once EGDT has been initiated, lung-protective ventilation should be considered.[1] Lung-protective mechanical ventilation, with the use of a tidal volume of only 6 cc/kg (compared with 12 cc/kg of ideal body weight) has been shown to decrease the mortality rate from 40% to 31%, to reduce organ dysfunction, and to lower levels of cytokines.[1,5] Therapy with activated protein C (24 μg/kg/hour for 96 hours) has been reported to decrease mortality and to ameliorate organ dysfunction in patients with severe sepsis (APACHE II score greater than 25 or dysfunction of two or more organs). Patients with severe sepsis had the greatest benefit from this therapy – an absolute decrease in the mortality rate of 13%.[6]

However, a subsequent trial of activated protein C in patients having a low risk of death was halted after an interim analysis demonstrated its lack of effectiveness.[7] This outcome strongly suggests that activated protein C is not beneficial in low-risk patients.

The use of corticosteroids in septic patients remains controversial. Because adrenal insufficiency is being reconsidered as part of septic shock, there has been renewed interest in therapy including corticosteroids, with focus on timing, dose and duration.[1] A patient may be tested for adrenal insufficiency using cosyntropin stimulation testing. Because this testing may not be feasible in the ED, the emergency physician may empirically treat patients for adrenal insufficiency by administering an initial bolus of dexamethasone (5–10 mg IV), as this exogenous cortisol analog will not interfere with cosyntropin stimulation testing done after ICU admission. Alternative steroid therapies, such as methylprednisolone or prednisone, should not be used as they mimic endogenous serum cortisol and will falsely elevate serum cortisol assays.[2] In a recent multicenter, randomized, double-blind, placebo-controlled trial, hydrocortisone did not improve survival or reversal of shock in patients with septic shock, either overall or in patients who did not have a response to corticotropin, although hydrocortisone hastened reversal of shock in patients in whom shock was reversed.[8]

Bacterial (pyogenic) abscesses of the liver are relatively rare; mortality rates are currently 5–30%.[9] When not diagnosed early and treated promptly, pyogenic liver abscess can be fatal, with reported mortality rates as high as 80–100%.[10] There are three forms of liver abscesses: pyogenic, most often polymicrobial, accounts for 80% of hepatic abscesses in the United States; amebic abscesses, due to *Entamoeba histolytica*, account for 10% of cases; fungal abscesses, most often due to Candida species, account for less than 10% of cases.[9] The most frequent symptoms of hepatic abscess include fever, chills, right upper quadrant pain, anorexia and malaise. Cough or hiccups and referred pain to the right shoulder may be present. Fever of unknown origin can frequently be an initial diagnosis in indolent cases.

Physical sequelae of hepatic abscesses most commonly include fever and tender hepatomegaly. Mid-epigastric tenderness, with or without a mass, is suggestive of left lobe involvement. Decreased breath sounds in the right lung base with signs of atelectasis and effusion on examination or chest radiograph may be present. Jaundice may be present in as many as 25% of cases. A complete blood count may show anemia of chronic disease and neutrophilic leukocytosis. Hypoalbuminemia and elevated alkaline phosphatase are the most common liver function test abnormalities, whereas elevated transaminases and bilirubin levels are variable. Blood cultures are positive in roughly 50% of cases of hepatic abscess.[9] Cultures of abscess fluid should be the goal in establishing a microbiologic diagnosis.

CT evaluation with contrast and ultrasonography remain the radiologic modalities of choice as screening procedures.

Both can also be used as techniques for guided percutaneous aspiration and drainage.[9–11] CT scan is 95–100% sensitive, whereas ultrasound is 80–90% sensitive in identifying hepatic abscesses.[8] Percutaneous catheter drainage with antimicrobial therapy is the standard of care for treating hepatic abscesses, although open surgical treatment is occasionally required.[9,10] Empiric antimicrobial therapy (before culture identification) must be comprehensive and should cover all likely pathogens in the context of the clinical setting. Meropenem appears to be a good first choice for hepatic abscesses, as it is a broad-spectrum bactericidal agent effective against most Gram-positive and Gram-negative bacteria. Metronidazole or clindamycin should be added to cover *Bacteroides fragilis* if other antibiotics do not offer anaerobic coverage.

KEY TEACHING POINTS

1. Sepsis is defined as suspected or proven infection plus a systemic inflammatory response syndrome (SIRS).

2. The mortality rates associated with severe sepsis and septic shock are 25–30% and 40–70%, respectively, although EGDT has decreased these rates.

3. The cornerstone of emergency management of sepsis involves EGDT, lung-protective ventilation, broad-spectrum antibiotics, and the use of activated protein C in selected patients with severe sepsis.

4. The most frequent symptoms of hepatic abscess include fever, chills, right upper quadrant abdominal pain, anorexia and malaise.

5. CT and ultrasonography remain the radiologic modalities of choice to screen for hepatic abscesses, whereas CT-guided percutaneous catheter drainage with broad-spectrum antimicrobial therapy remain the standard of care for this condition.

REFERENCES

[1] Russell JA. Drug therapy: management of sepsis. *N Engl J Med* 2006;355:1699–713.

[2] Heavey J, Osborn TM. Acute management of severe sepsis and septic shock. EmedHome Website. Available at http://www.EmedHome.com. Accessed February 10, 2007.

[3] Rivers E, Nguyen B, Havstad S, et al. Early goal-directed therapy in the treatment of severe sepsis and septic shock. *N Engl J Med* 2001;345:1368–77.

[4] Nguyen HB, Rivers EP, Knoblich BP, et al. Early lactate clearance is associated with improved outcome in severe sepsis and septic shock. *Crit Care Med* 2004;32:1637–42.

[5] Ranieri VM, Suter PM, Tortorella C, et al. Effect of mechanical ventilation on inflammatory mediators in patients with acute respiratory distress syndrome: a randomized control trial. *JAMA* 1999;282:54–61.

[6] Ely EW, Laterre PF, Angus DC, et al. Drotrecogin alfa (activated) administration across clinically important subgroups of patients with severe sepsis. *Crit Care Med* 2003;31: 12–9.

[7] Abraham E, Laterre PF, Garg R, et al. Drotrecogin alfa (activated) for adults with severe sepsis and low risk of death. *N Engl J Med* 2005;353:1332–41.

[8] Sprung CL, Annane D, Keh D, et al. Hydrocortisone therapy for patients with septic shock. *N Engl J Med* 2008;358:111–24.

[9] Peralta R, Lisgaris MV. Liver abscess. eMedicine Website. Available at http://www.emedicine.com/med/topic1316.htm. Accessed January 8, 2009.

[10] Ng SS, Lee JF, Lai PB. Role and outcome of conventional surgery in the treatment of pyogenic liver abscess in the modern era of minimally invasive therapy. *World J Gastroenterol* 2008;14:747–51.

[11] Wang CL, Guo XJ, Qiu SB, et al. Diagnosis of bacterial hepatic abscess by CT. *Hepatobiliary Pancreat Dis Int* 2007;6:271–5.

92

Right groin pain and swelling in a 56-year-old female

HISTORY OF PRESENT ILLNESS

A 56-year-old female with a history of diabetes, hypertension, asthma and hypothyroidism presented to the ED complaining of one month of intermittent fevers and chills, right lower quadrant pain and nausea. The patient had noted increased pain and swelling in her right lower abdomen and right groin area. She denied vomiting, diarrhea or constipation, as well as dysuria or abnormal vaginal bleeding. She also denied any back pain or focal weakness. She did not drink alcohol, smoke or use intravenous drugs.

PHYSICAL EXAMINATION

GENERAL APPEARANCE: The patient appeared well developed, well hydrated and in moderate discomfort.

VITAL SIGNS

Temperature	98.2°F (36.8°C)
Pulse	92 beats/minute
Blood pressure	130/90 mmHg
Respirations	22 breaths/minute
Oxygen saturation	98% on room air

HEENT: Unremarkable

NECK: Supple, no jugular venous distension.

CARDIOVASCULAR: Regular rate and rhythm without rubs, murmurs or gallops.

LUNGS: Clear to auscultation bilaterally.

ABDOMEN: Moderate swelling in right lower quadrant and right groin without erythema; tenderness to palpation in this area, without rebound or guarding. No hernias noted, no pulsatile masses.

RECTAL: Normal tone, normal perianal sensation, brown stool, hemoccult negative.

EXTREMITIES: No clubbing, cyanosis or edema.

BACK: Mild tenderness to palpation over spinous processes and paraspinous area in lower thoracic/upper lumbar area.

NEUROLOGIC: Alert and oriented to person, place and time; upper and lower extremity strength 5/5 proximal and distal, bilaterally; sensation grossly intact throughout; abnormal gait with patient favoring her right side secondary to pain.

A peripheral intravenous line was placed, and blood was drawn and sent for laboratory testing. Laboratory tests, including a complete blood count, chemistry panel with BUN, creatinine, glucose and urinalysis, were all within normal limits. A C-reactive protein (CRP) was mildly elevated at 1.4 mg/dL (normal less than 0.9 mg/dL), as was an erythrocyte sedimentation rate (ESR) at 35 mm/Hr (normal 0–30 mm/Hr). A CT of the abdomen and pelvis with oral and intravenous contrast was obtained (Figure 92.1).

What is your diagnosis?

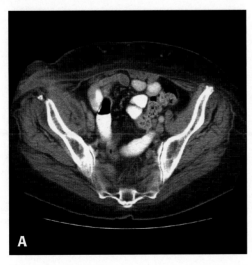
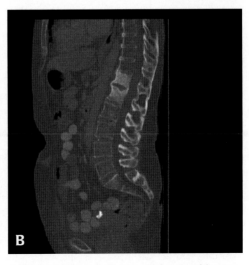

Figure 92.1 CT of the abdomen and pelvis with oral and IV contrast from a 56-year-old female with a one-month history of right lower quadrant abdominal and groin pain (transverse view, panel A; sagittal view, panel B).

The diagnosis is psoas muscle abscess with discitis and osteomyelitis at the T12-L1 spine. The CT demonstrates a right psoas abscess extending into the soft tissue of the pelvic brim, as well as sclerosis of the T12 and L1 vertebral bodies with widening of the disc space, concerning for discitis (arrows, Figure 92.2). An MRI of the lumbosacral spine was obtained (Figure 92.3), which demonstrated definite discitis at the T12-L1 level with some mild, early vertebral osteomyelitis involving the T12 and L1 vertebral bodies. There was no evidence of an associated epidural abscess. The patient was given intravenous empiric antibiotics (piperacillin/tazobactam and vancomycin), and the abscess was drained under CT guidance by interventional radiology. Cultures from the abscess fluid grew *Staphylococcus aureus*. The patient continued to improve and was discharged on hospital day #7 to continue IV antibiotics for six weeks through a PICC line.

Psoas muscle abscess

Because the psoas muscle lies in close relationship with all the major abdominal and pelvic structures, any infectious process in these regions can spread to the psoas muscle, resulting in psoas abscess formation.[1] Primary psoas muscle abscess usually arises in young persons, generally without a definable etiology. Eighty-three percent of cases occur under the age of 30 years, with males more often affected than females.[1] Intravenous drug use and HIV-positive individuals are at increased risk to develop a psoas abscess.[2] Hematogenous spread is the presumed cause, and *Staphylococcus aureus* is identified in 88% of positive blood cultures in patients with primary psoas abscesses.[1]

Secondary psoas abscess results from the spread of infection from adjacent gastrointestinal (e.g., Crohn's disease, appendicitis, diverticulitis, typhlitis, neoplasms), urological (e.g., perinephric abscess, pyelonephritis) or skeletal (e.g., osteomyelitis, discitis, Pott's disease) regions.[2] Microorganisms normally in the bowel flora (*Escherichia coli*, bacteroides and enterococcus) are frequently isolated from these secondary psoas muscle abscesses.[1] Secondary infections occur in older and more debilitated people with pre-existing diseases, particularly diabetic patients.[1,3]

The classic triad of psoas muscle abscess includes lower back pain, anterior thigh or groin pain, and persistent fever with daily spikes.[1,2] The abscess may present as back pain, fever of unknown origin, groin pain, hip pain, increased frequency of urination, or abdominal pain.[4] Onset is usually subacute, and symptoms are generally present for a few weeks. Patients usually present with flexion of the hip and lumbar lordosis.[1,4] Distal extension of a psoas abscess may present as a mass in the inguinal region. Proximity to the hip capsule can precipitate symptoms that mimic a septic hip. Clinically, it may be possible to distinguish a septic hip from a psoas abscess, as hip flexion does not generally cause pain in cases of psoas abscess, but hip flexion or extension is very painful in cases of septic arthritis.[4]

Chern et al. reported their one-year experience in which 10 ED patients were diagnosed with psoas abscesses; in seven cases, diagnoses were established in the ED.[5] Patients' mean age was 64.6 years. Pain was the most frequently encountered symptom (80%), with five patients (50%) complaining of flank pain. The triad of fever, flank pain and limitation of hip movement, which is specific for psoas abscess, was present in only three patients (30%). The mean duration of symptoms was 10.6 days (range 1 to 30 days). The diagnosis of psoas abscess

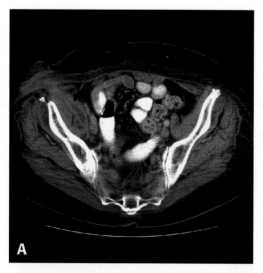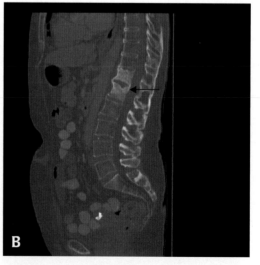

Figure 92.2 CT of the abdomen and pelvis from a 56-year-old female demonstrating right psoas abscess extending into the soft tissue of the pelvic brim (arrow, panel A), as well as sclerosis of the T12 and L1 vertebral bodies with widening of the disc space (arrow, panel B).

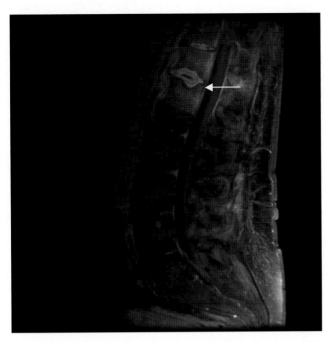

Figure 92.3 MRI of the lumbosacral spine (sagittal view) from a 56-year-old female demonstrating discitis and early osteomyelitis at the T12 and L1 vertebrae (arrow).

was established by ultrasound in six patients, CT in three patients and during surgery in one patient. Only three patients presented to the ED with an initial diagnosis of psoas abscess; the remaining seven had the following initial ED diagnoses: fever of unknown origin (2), septic shock (2), shock (1), sepsis (1) and peritonitis (1). All but one patient had manifestations of sepsis. Two patients died of septic shock; these two patients were not drained.

Psoas abscesses should be initially treated with antibiotics and CT- or ultrasound-guided percutaneous drainage; smaller abscesses may be treated with antibiotics alone.[6] In the past, open drainage of the abscess through an iliac crest incision was the treatment of choice. Surgical drainage should be reserved only for complicated recurrences.[6]

KEY TEACHING POINTS

1. Psoas abscess may present as back pain, fever of unknown origin, groin pain, hip pain, increased frequency of urination or abdominal pain; in other words, a broad constellation of presenting complaints.
2. Risk factors for development of a psoas abscess include infective spondylitis, infections of sacroiliac joint, renal infections, vertebral osteomyelitis, IV drug use, HIV infection and diabetes.
3. The triad of fever, flank pain and limitation of hip movement, which is specific for psoas abscess, may be present in only 30% of patients.
4. Ultrasound and CT are useful in establishing the diagnosis of psoas abscess.
5. CT- or ultrasound-guided drainage and appropriate antibiotic therapy are the mainstays of treatment in cases of suppurative psoas muscle abscess.

REFERENCES

[1] Gezer A, Erkan S, Saygi Erzik B, et al. Primary psoas muscle abscess diagnosed and treated during pregnancy: case report and literature review. *Infect Dis Obstet Gynecol* 2004;12: 147–9.
[2] Roberge RJ, Park AJ. Flank and groin pain in a pregnant intravenous drug user: iliopsoas abscess. *J Emerg Med* 2006;31:225–6.
[3] Gupta S, Koirala J, Khardori R, et al. Infections in diabetes mellitus and hyperglycemia. *Infect Dis Clin N Am* 2007;21:617–38.
[4] Todkar M. Case report: psoas abscess – unusual etiology of groin pain. Medscape General Medicine 2005;7. Available at http://www.medscape.com/viewarticle/507610. Accessed June 23, 2008.
[5] Chern CH, Hu SC, Kao WF, et al. Psoas abscess: making an early diagnosis in the ED. *Am J Emerg Med* 1997;15:83–8.
[6] Yacoub WN, Sohn HJ, Chan S, et al. Psoas abscess rarely requires surgical intervention. *Am J Surg* 2008 (in press).

93

Fatigue, weight loss, intermittent fevers and sweats in a 74-year-old male

HISTORY OF PRESENT ILLNESS

A 74-year-old male with a medical history significant for hypertension, hyperlipidemia, diabetes and gout presented to the ED complaining of several months of fatigue, intermittent tactile fevers, sweats and an unintentional 15-pound weight loss over two months. He had traveled to the Philippines four months prior to presentation for three weeks. The patient denied chest pain, cough or shortness of breath, as well as abdominal pain, nausea or vomiting. He reported decreased appetite and poor oral intake over the same time period. The patient did not drink alcohol or smoke cigarettes. His medications included Lipitor®, atenolol, aspirin and allopurinol.

PHYSICAL EXAMINATION

GENERAL APPEARANCE: The patient was a slightly cachectic, elderly male in no acute discomfort.

VITAL SIGNS

Temperature	100.1°F (37.8°C)
Pulse	81 beats/minute
Blood pressure	132/72 mmHg
Respirations	18 breaths/minute
Oxygen saturation	97% on room air

HEENT: PERRL, EOMI, sclera anicteric, oropharynx moist.

NECK: Supple, no jugular venous distension.

CARDIOVASCULAR: Regular rate and rhythm without rubs, murmurs or gallops.

LUNGS: Clear to auscultation bilaterally without presence of rales, rhonchi or wheezes.

ABDOMEN: Soft, nontender, nondistended.

EXTREMITIES: No clubbing, cyanosis or edema.

NEUROLOGIC: Nonfocal.

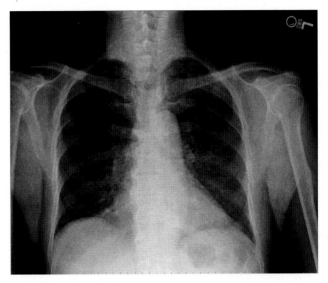

Figure 93.1 Chest radiograph from a 74-year-old male with several months of fatigue, unintentional weight loss, fevers and sweats.

A peripheral intravenous line was placed, and blood was drawn and sent for laboratory testing. A 12-lead ECG showed a normal sinus rhythm, rate 81 without presence of any acute ST-T wave changes. Laboratory tests revealed a leukocyte count of 9.8 K/μL (normal 3.5–12.5 K/μL) with 74% neutrophils, 9% lymphocytes, 14% monocytes, 3% eosinophils, hematocrit of 30% (decreased from 37% one month previously; normal 39–51%) and alkaline phosphatase at 234 U/L (normal 38–126 U/L); amylase, AST, ALT, lipase and total bilirubin were within normal limits. A urinalysis was normal. A chest radiograph was obtained (Figure 93.1).

What is your diagnosis?

ANSWER

The diagnosis is miliary tuberculosis (TB) from *Mycobacterium tuberculosis*. The chest radiograph demonstrated diffuse reticular nodular interstitial disease and innumerable tiny interstitial nodules throughout both lungs, consistent with an infectious etiology such as miliary TB. The patient was admitted to the hospital and placed in a negative pressure room. A sputum sample and sputum culture demonstrated rare acid-fast bacilli, positive for *Mycobacterium tuberculosis* by RNA amplification method. The public health department was immediately notified, and he was started on a four-drug regimen for tuberculosis (isoniazid, rifampin, ethambutol and pyrazinamide). He had several repeat sputum cultures during hospitalization, which were all negative for *M. tuberculosis*. He continued to have intermittent, low-grade fevers to 101°F. On hospital day #17, he was pan-cultured and underwent a noncontrast CT of the chest to rule out possible lung abscess or effusion (Figure 93.2). The CT did not show evidence of lung abscesses or effusions but demonstrated diffuse, fine alveolar densities within the upper lung zones consistent with the clinical history of miliary TB. By hospital day #18, the fevers had subsided, three subsequent sputum cultures had returned negative for TB, and the patient was discharged home to continue his four-drug regimen as an outpatient. Close follow up was arranged with the infectious disease specialist, to which the patient agreed prior to hospital discharge.

Miliary tuberculosis

Tuberculosis is a global infection. The World Health Organization estimates that approximately 1.7 billion persons are infected with *Mycobacterium tuberculosis* (approximately one-third of the world's population).[1] A total of 16,377 cases (5.8 cases per 100,000 population) were reported to the CDC in the United States in 2000, a 45% decrease from the peak rate in 1992.[2] This decline was largely attributable to a comprehensive strengthening of control activities and the resulting decrease in the transmission of *M. tuberculosis* from persons with active disease. As the rates of tuberculosis have declined in the United States, the distribution of cases has been limited to identifiable populations, such as in urban and immigrant communities.[2]

Virtually all *M. tuberculosis* is transmitted by airborne particles that are 1–5 μm in diameter.[2] Transmission is greatly influenced by characteristics of the source case (such as the number of bacteria excreted) and the nature of the encounter (such as the duration and closeness of exposure). Regardless of these factors, it is thought that infection results when as few as one to five bacteria are deposited in a terminal alveolus.[2] Primary TB, a self-limited, mild pneumonic illness that generally goes undiagnosed, may develop in a subgroup of infected persons. During this illness, bacillemia and seeding of other organs may occur, setting the stage for subsequent reactivation in extrapulmonary sites.

Miliary TB is the widespread dissemination of *M. tuberculosis* from hematogenous spread.[3] Classic miliary TB is defined as millet-like (mean size 2 mm) seeding of TB bacilli in the lung, as can be seen on chest radiograph. This pattern is seen in 1–3% of all TB cases.[1,3] Miliary TB may occur in an individual organ (less than 5%), in several organs or throughout the entire body, including the brain.[3] Up to 25% of patients with miliary TB have meningeal involvement.

Patients diagnosed with miliary TB usually do not have a prior history of TB. The onset of this disease is often subtle.[4] Generalized symptoms of fever, anorexia, weakness and weight loss are nonspecific. When present, headache may indicate meningitis, abdominal pain may be due to peritonitis, and pleural pain may result from pleuritis. Clinical manifestations depend on the organs involved. Fulminant disease (septic shock, acute respiratory distress syndrome and multi-organ failure) has been described.[5]

Physical findings are usually nonspecific but a careful search for cutaneous eruptions, sinus tracts, scrotal masses

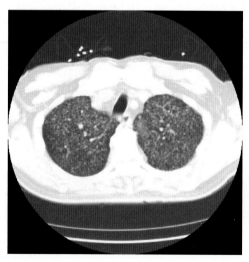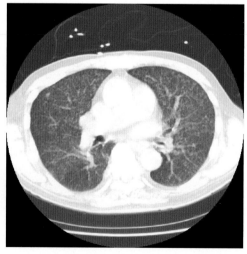

Figure 93.2 Noncontrast chest CT from a 74-year-old male with miliary TB, demonstrating diffuse, fine alveolar densities within the upper lung zones.

or lymphadenopathy may yield a prompt biopsy diagnosis.[4] A "miliary" infiltrate on chest radiograph is the most helpful finding, and is typically the reason miliary TB is suspected. High-resolution CT scans have improved the antemortem diagnosis of miliary tuberculosis, revealing the classic miliary pattern even when the chest radiograph appears normal.[6]

Common laboratory abnormalities include normochromic anemia, leukopenia or leukocytosis, elevated sedimentation rate and hyponatremia.[5] Examination of the sputum, bronchoalveolar lavage, gastric washings, CSF, blood culture, or biopsies of liver and bone marrow may be necessary to make the diagnosis. Sputum induction has low sensitivity, as findings are smear- and culture-negative in 80% of patients with miliary TB because of hematogenous spread.[3] Fiberoptic bronchoscopy is the most effective procedure for obtaining cultures through bronchoalveolar lavage, whereas the culture yield for transbronchial biopsies is 90%.[3] A tuberculin skin test is not a useful diagnostic test in patients with miliary TB, as the result is positive in less than 50% of patients.[5,6]

Miliary TB is uniformly fatal if not treated.[6] Antituberculosis treatment is the cornerstone of management. Directly observed therapy is strongly recommended to encourage medication compliance.[5] Because treatment differs for persons infected with drug-resistant strains, every effort should be made to obtain adequate specimens for culture and susceptibility testing before treatment is initiated.[2] In the absence of associated meningeal involvement, the American Thoracic Society (ATS), the Centers for Disease Control and Prevention (CDC), the Infectious Disease Society of America (IDSA) and the British Thoracic Society (BTS) guidelines state that six months of treatment (two-month intensive phase with isoniazid, rifampin, pyrazinamide and ethambutol or streptomycin, followed by a four-month continuation phase with isoniazid and rifampin) is adequate in miliary tuberculosis.[6] The American Academy of Pediatrics (AAP) advocates nine months of treatment for children with miliary TB.[7] In the presence of associated tuberculosis meningitis, treatment needs to be given for at least 12 months in all patients.[6]

Patients diagnosed with miliary TB should be admitted to the hospital and placed in a negative pressure room with strict respiratory precautions for initiation and direct observation of therapy. All states require that cases of tuberculosis be reported to public health authorities.[2] Such reports set in motion a range of activities designed not only to treat the individual patient but also to protect the health of others in the community. The treatment of patients with tuberculosis should be monitored by public health officials to ensure compliance, prevent the emergence of drug-resistant organisms, coordinate the evaluation of contacts, monitor patterns of drug resistance in the community, provide patient education and identify possible outbreaks.[2] Patients who discontinue their medications may be remanded to custody and ordered to continue therapy if judged to be a public health risk.[3]

In persons with positive sputum cultures, conversion to negative cultures provides the only objective measure of successful treatment. Cultures should be obtained monthly until conversion is documented.[2] Once the patient receives several weeks of effective therapy, experiences significant clinical improvement and has three consecutive negative acid-fast bacillus sputum smears, restrictions are minimal.[3] More than 85% of patients who receive both isoniazid and rifampin have negative sputum cultures within two months after the initiation of treatment.[2] If cultures remain positive for more than three months, nonadherence, malabsorption of drugs, drug resistance or some combination of these factors should be suspected.[2]

KEY TEACHING POINTS

1. Miliary tuberculosis (TB) is a potentially lethal form of TB resulting from massive lymphohematogenous dissemination of *Mycobacterium tuberculosis* bacilli.
2. Presenting symptoms include fever, chills, night sweats, weight loss and anorexia; fulminant disease including septic shock, acute respiratory distress syndrome and multi-organ failure has been described.
3. A chest radiograph or CT scan reveals numerous 2- to 3-mm nodules (millet-seed in appearance) scattered throughout the lung in more than 85% of patients.
4. Patients diagnosed with miliary TB should be placed in negative pressure isolation rooms and hospitalized with respiratory precautions.
5. Examination of sputum, bronchoalveolar lavage, gastric washings, CSF, blood culture, or biopsies of liver and bone marrow may be necessary for diagnosis.
6. Treatment of miliary TB initiated under direct observation should include current four drug regimen according to local and individual sensitivities.

REFERENCES

[1] Tanoue LT, Mark EJ. Case 1-2003: a 43-year-old man with fever and night sweats. *N Engl J Med* 2003;348:151–61.

[2] Small PM, Fujiwara PI. Medical progress: management of tuberculosis in the United States. *N Engl J Med* 2001;345: 189–200.

[3] Lessnau KD. Miliary Tuberculosis. eMedicine Website. Available at http://www.emedicine.com/med/topic1476.htm. Accessed June 23, 2008.

[4] Fitgerald D, Haas DW. Mycobacterium tuberculosis. In: Mandell GL, Bennett JE, Dolin R (eds.). *Principles and Practice of Infectious Disease*, 6th ed. New York: Churchill Livingston, 2005;2582–883.

[5] Golden MP, Vikram HR. Extrapulmonary tuberculosis: an overview. *Amer Fam Physician* 2005;72:1761–8.

[6] Sharma SK, Mohan A, Sharma A, et al. Miliary tuberculosis: new insights into an old disease. *Lancet Infect Dis* 2005;5:415–30.

[7] American Academy of Pediatrics Committee on Infectious Diseases: Chemotherapy for tuberculosis in infants and children. *Pediatrics* 1992;89:161–5.

PART XII

TOXICOLOGY/ENVIRONMENTAL

94

Acute agitation and confusion in a 13-year-old male

HISTORY OF PRESENT ILLNESS

A 13-year-old male was brought to the ED by paramedics after being found acutely agitated and confused by his parents. He had been outside playing with friends most of the day and returned home very agitated, confused and complaining of visual hallucinations. The patient had no significant medical problems, took no medications, and denied drug or alcohol use. The parents did not report finding illicit drugs or medications at home.

PHYSICAL EXAMINATION

GENERAL APPEARANCE: The patient appeared alert, agitated and unable to keep still.

VITAL SIGNS

Temperature	98.9°F (37.2°C)
Pulse	125 beats/minute
Blood pressure	153/83 mmHg
Respirations	24 breaths/minute
Oxygen saturation	98% on room air

HEENT: Pupils round, dilated to 5 mm, equal and reactive to light. EOMI without nystagmus. Oropharynx dry.

NECK: Supple, no meningeal signs.

CARDIOVASCULAR: Tachycardic rate, regular rhythm without rubs, murmurs or gallops.

LUNGS: Clear to auscultation bilaterally.

ABDOMEN: Soft, nontender, nondistended, hypoactive bowel sounds.

EXTREMITIES: No clubbing, cyanosis or edema.

SKIN: Warm, dry and flushed; no rashes.

NEUROLOGIC: Alert and oriented to person, place, and time; moving all extremities, following commands.

PSYCHIATRIC: Patient exhibited signs of acute paranoia and reported visual hallucinations; easily distractible and appeared to be responding to his own internal stimuli. He denied suicidal or homicidal ideations.

A bedside fingerstick blood glucose returned normal (100 mg/dL). The patient was placed on the cardiac monitor, a peripheral intravenous line was placed, and blood was drawn and sent for laboratory testing. Laboratory tests, including a complete blood count, chemistry panel, creatinine, serum glucose and urinalysis, were all within normal limits. A urine toxicology screen was sent, and an ECG demonstrated sinus tachycardia with normal intervals.

What is your diagnosis?

ANSWER

The diagnosis is Jimson weed poisoning (*Datura stramonium*) that caused an anticholinergic toxidrome. The patient admitted consuming several Devil's Trumpet flowers (Jimson weed) approximately eight hours prior to presentation in an attempt to "get high." Poison control was called, with recommendations for supportive care and admission to the Pediatric Intensive Care Unit (PICU) for close observation. Administration of activated charcoal was not recommended based upon the eight-hour time interval between his ingestion and presentation. The patient received 1 liter normal saline IV, a total of 3 mg lorazepam IV for agitation, and was admitted to the PICU for close observation. The following day, his symptoms had completely resolved, his vital signs had stabilized, and he was counseled and discharged home with his parents.

Jimson weed poisoning

Jimson weed is a wild herb that grows throughout the United States. It usually matures between May and September, is accessible to almost anyone, and is particularly popular among adolescents curious about the plant's hallucinogenic effects.[1] Jimson weed contains the tropane alkaloids atropine, scopolamine and hyoscyamine.[2] The plant grows to approximately 1.5 meters (5 feet) tall and has a solitary white, trumpet-shaped flower (Figure 94.1). Each autumn, a spiny capsular fruit is produced that contains up to 50 small black seeds. Although all parts of the plant are toxic, the seeds contain the highest concentration of atropine.[3] One hundred seeds contain up to 6 mg of atropine.[1,3] A dose of atropine exceeding 10 mg is regarded as potentially lethal.[1]

Any part of the plant can be eaten; usually the seeds or flowers are consumed. A common practice is to prepare tea for consumption by boiling the seeds. The toxicity of tropane compounds from Jimson weed results from competitive block-

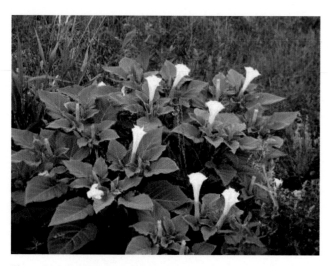

Figure 94.1 Jimson weed plant (*Datura stramonium*), from Wildflowers of Ontario Website (available at www.wildflowersofontario.ca/list1.html, last accessed January 12, 2009).

ade of acetylcholine at peripheral and central muscarinic sites. The onset of symptoms is usually within 30–60 minutes of ingestion, and may last for 24–48 hours.[4] Both central and peripheral nervous system syndromes may be seen.

Initial symptoms include hallucinations, dry mucous membranes, thirst, dilated pupils, blurred vision, and difficulty speaking and swallowing.[1] Subsequent effects may include tachycardia, urinary retention and ileus. Rarely, late symptoms may include hyperthermia, episodes of seizures and respiratory arrest.[11] The mnemonic for anticholinergic symptoms – "blind as a bat, dry as a bone, red as a beet, mad as a hatter, hot as a hare and loony as a tune" – applies to Jimson weed poisoning.

Treatment of Jimson weed poisoning is mainly supportive, including intravenous hydration, sedation with benzodiazepines and cooling measures.[5] Pediatric patients presenting with anticholinergic poisoning from Jimson weed should be admitted to the PICU for close observation and monitoring. Efforts at GI contamination may be warranted because the ingestion often results in delayed gastric emptying and the plant material often demonstrates delayed absorption.[5] Activated charcoal binds to the toxins in Jimson weed and decreases their overall absorption.[1] Administer activated charcoal (1–2 g/kg) orally or per nasogastric or orogastric tube if the patient can protect their airway and the risk of seizures or aspiration is low.[2] If medical attention is sought within several hours after ingestion or if the patient is intubated, removal of the ingested plant by gastric lavage can be considered. However, one study in pediatric patients admitted to the PICU with Jimson weed poisoning failed to demonstrate a decrease in ICU admissions or decreased length of stay for patients who underwent successful nasogastric lavage of Jimson weed seeds.[6]

Physostigmine, a cholinesterase inhibitor, may be used to reverse central nervous system manifestations of Jimson weed poisoning.[7] The use of physostigmine is warranted in severe cases, in which patients have symptoms of anticholinergic crisis (e.g., dysrhythmias, poorly controlled hyperpyrexia, clinically significant hypertension, seizures or coma).[1] The initial dose of physostigmine is 0.5–2.0 mg in adults or 0.02 mg/kg in children; the drug is given slowly by the intravenous route.[1] Physostigmine can induce life-threatening cholinergic crisis (e.g., seizures, respiratory depression, asystole), and preferably should be used in consultation with a poison control center and only in patients exhibiting signs of anticholinergic crisis described previously.[2] Physostigmine is contraindicated in patients receiving tricyclic antidepressants, disopyramide, quinidine, procainamide, cocaine or other agents that may produce cardiac conduction abnormalities.[2] Relative contraindications to physostigmine use include reactive airway disease, intestinal obstruction and administration of depolarizing agents. In one study, pediatric patients admitted to the PICU with Jimson weed poisoning who received physostigmine did not demonstrate a decrease in ICU admissions or decreased length of stay compared to patients not receiving this medication.[6]

KEY TEACHING POINTS

1. Jimson weed contains the tropane alkaloids atropine, scopolamine and hyoscyamine; poisoning from this plant presents as an anticholinergic toxidrome.

2. Initial symptoms of Jimson weed poisoning include hallucinations, dry mucous membranes, thirst, dilated pupils, blurred vision, and difficulty speaking and swallowing. Subsequent effects may include tachycardia, urinary retention and ileus. Rarely, late symptoms may include hyperthermia, seizures and respiratory arrest.

3. Treatment of patients presenting with Jimson weed poisoning is primarily supportive (intravenous hydration, sedation with benzodiazepines and cooling measures).

4. The use of physostigmine is warranted only in severe cases, in which patients have symptoms of anticholinergic crisis (e.g., dysrhythmias, poorly controlled hyperpyrexia, clinically significant hypertension, seizures or coma).

5. All pediatric patients presenting with Jimson weed poisoning (anticholinergic toxidrome) should be admitted to the PICU for close observation and monitoring.

REFERENCES

[1] Chan K. Jimson weed poisoning – a case report. *Permanente J* 2002;6:28–30.

[2] Wagner RA, Keim SM. Plant poisoning, alkaloids – tropane. eMedicine Website. Available at http://www.emedicine.com/emerg/topic438.htm. Accessed June 26, 2008.

[3] Richardson WH, Slone CM, Michels JE. Herbal drugs of abuse: an emerging problem. *Emerg Med Clin N Am* 2007; 25:435–57.

[4] Froberg B, Ibrahim D, Furbee RB. Plant poisoning. *Emerg Med Clin N Am* 2007;25:375–433.

[5] Haynes JF. Medical management of adolescent drug overdoses. *Adolesc Med* 2006;17:353–79.

[6] Salen P, Shih R, Sierzenski P, et al. Effect of physostigmine and gastric lavage in a Datura stramonium-induced anticholinergic poisoning epidemic. *Am J Emerg Med* 2003;21: 316–7.

[7] Shervette RE, Schyldower M, Lampe RM, et al. Jimson "loco" weed abuse in adolescents. *Pediatrics* 1979;63:520–3.

95

Lethargy and bradycardia in a 14-year-old male

HISTORY OF PRESENT ILLNESS

A 14-year-old developmentally delayed male with a medical history significant for cerebral palsy, seizure disorder and autonomic instability was brought to the ED by his mother after one week of worsening lethargy and fatigue. The patient was nonverbal and nonambulatory at baseline. According to his mother, he had not experienced cough, shortness of breath, fevers, abdominal pain or vomiting, and his oral intake had been good. At triage, his heart rate was 45 beats/minute. The patient was placed on the cardiac monitor, which revealed sinus bradycardia.

PHYSICAL EXAMINATION

GENERAL APPEARANCE: The patient was awake, alert, shivering and nonverbal (baseline).

VITAL SIGNS

Temperature	92°F (33°C) rectal
Pulse	45 beats/minute
Blood pressure	110/70 mmHg
Respirations	22 breaths/minute
Oxygen saturation	97% on room air

HEENT: Unremarkable.

NECK: Supple, no meningeal signs.

CARDIOVASCULAR: Bradycardic rate, regular rhythm without rubs, murmurs or gallops.

LUNGS: Clear to auscultation bilaterally.

ABDOMEN: Soft, nontender, nondistended.

EXTREMITIES: No edema, cool to touch with delayed capillary refill, peripheral pulses palpable, slow and weak.

NEUROLOGIC: Patient was awake, tracking with his eyes, unable to follow commands (according to his mother, this was his neurologic baseline).

A peripheral intravenous line was placed, and a bedside blood glucose was within normal limits (75 mg/dL; normal range 60–159 mg/dL). A 12-lead ECG was obtained (Figure 95.1).

What is your diagnosis?

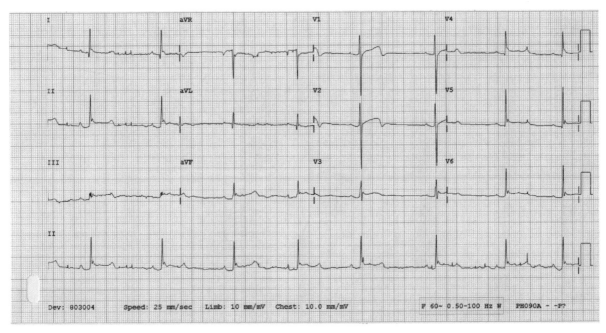

Figure 95.1 12-lead ECG from a developmentally delayed 14-year-old male with increased lethargy for one week.

ANSWER

The diagnosis is hypothermia, in this case most likely brought on by autonomic instability, the exact etiology of which remained unclear. This was his third visit to the ED for the same condition, and a work-up for an infectious etiology did not reveal evidence of infection. The patient was warmed by external measures (bear-hugger) to a core temperature of 97°F/36.1°C (patient's baseline temperature) and admitted to the pediatric service for monitoring and further evaluation. The findings on the ECG consistent with the diagnosis of hypothermia are the presence of tremor artifact (from shivering), Osborn or J-waves, PR and QT segment prolongation, and sinus bradycardia.

ECG manifestations of hypothermia

The most widely accepted grading system divides hypothermia into three grades: mild (core temperature 90–95°F or 32–35°C), moderate (core temperature 82–90°F or 28–32°C) and severe (core temperature less than 82°F or 28°C).[1] Hypothermia decreases spontaneous depolarization of cardiac pacemaker cells, prolongs action potential duration (of both depolarization and repolarization), slows myocardial impulse conduction and results in abnormal repolarization.[1] Classic ECG manifestations of hypothermia include tremor artifact, slowing of the sinus rate resulting in bradycardia, the presence of J (Osborn) waves, prolonged PR, QRS and QT intervals, and atrial dysrhythmias.[1–4]

Although nonspecific, tremor artifact is one of the earliest ECG findings in patients with hypothermia.[2] The body's ability to shiver diminishes as the core temperature decreases, and is uncommon when the body temperature falls to less than 90°F (32°C). Tremor or shivering artifact on an electrocardiogram has been associated with increased survival in severe hypothermia.[3] Sinus rhythm predominates in cases of mild hypothermia.[2]

The Osborn or J wave, also known as the camel-hump sign, is an extra positive deflection noted on the ECG at the terminal junction of the QRS complex and the beginning of the ST segment takeoff.[2] The Osborn wave is usually present when the core body temperature falls to less than 90°F (32°C), and has been consistently identified when the body temperature falls to less than 77°F (25°C).[2] The exact cause of this wave is uncertain. Investigators have suggested that the J wave is related to acidosis, a hypothalamic or neurogenic factor, an injury current, delayed ventricular depolarization or early repolarization that occurs in a portion of the ventricle before delayed depolarization is completed in another portion.[4] However, none of these theories has been proven. J waves are most commonly found in the anterior and lateral precordial leads and in lead II, although they may be present in only a single lead.[4] The presence of prominent J waves is not pathognomonic of hypothermia; they have been reported in the literature in normothermic individuals with hypercalcemia, subarachnoid hemorrhage, cerebral injuries, myocardial ischemia and following resuscitation from cardiac arrest, especially in association with ventricular fibrillation.[1]

Increasing levels of hypothermia result in progressive slowing of myocardial conduction, producing prolongation of the cardiac cycle. Delayed atrioventricular (AV) conduction results in prolongation of the PR interval and various degrees of AV block.[4] Prolongation of both the depolarization and repolarization phases of the action potential produces increases in the QRS and QT intervals, respectively, as hypothermia worsens.[4]

Hypothermia is associated with various atrial and ventricular dysrhythmias. At mild levels of hypothermia (greater than 90°F/32°C), sinus rhythm predominates.[4] Decreased AV conduction velocity often causes sinus bradycardia. With progressive hypothermia (79–90°F or 26–32°C), junctional rhythms and atrial reentrant dysrhythmias may occur. More than 50% of patients with moderate hypothermia develop atrial fibrillation with a slow ventricular response.[2,4] Atrial fibrillation usually converts to sinus rhythm spontaneously during rewarming, or soon after restoration of normothermia.[4] Ventricular fibrillation may occur below 84.2°F (29°C), and becomes common as the core drops to 77°F (25°C).[3] Asystole commonly occurs at 64.4°F (18°C) but has been seen at higher temperatures; initial core temperature does not necessarily correlate with outcome.[3]

KEY TEACHING POINTS

1. Hypothermia is categorized as mild (core temperature 90–95°F or 32–35°C), moderate (core temperature 82–90°F or 28–32°C) and severe (core temperature less than 82°F or 28°C).

2. ECG manifestations of hypothermia include tremor artifact, slowing of the sinus rate leading to bradycardia, the presence of Osborn (J) waves, prolonged PR, QRS and QT intervals, and atrial and ventricular dysrhythmias.

3. The Osborn (J) wave, an extra positive deflection noted on the ECG at the terminal junction of the QRS complex and the beginning of the ST segment, is usually present when the core body temperature falls to less than 90°F (32°C).

4. More than 50% of patients with moderate hypothermia develop atrial fibrillation with a slow ventricular response.

5. Ventricular fibrillation may occur below 84.2°F (29°C); asystole commonly occurs at 64.4°F (18°C) but has been seen at higher temperatures.

REFERENCES

[1] Aslam AF, Aslam AK, Vasavada BC, et al. Hypothermia: evaluation, electrocardiographic manifestations, and management. *Am J Med* 2006;119:297–301.

[2] Wald DA. ECG manifestations of selected metabolic and endocrine disorders. *Emerg Med Clin N Am* 2006;24:145–57.

[3] Erickson T, Prendergast H. Procedures pertaining to hypothermia. In: Roberts JR, Hedges JR, Chanmugam AS, et al. (eds.). *Roberts: Clinical Procedures in Emergency Medicine*, 4th ed. Philadelphia: Saunders, 2004:1344–5.

[4] Mattu A, Brady WJ, Perron AD. Electrocardiographic manifestations of hypothermia. *Am J Emerg Med* 2002;20:314–26.

96

Acetaminophen overdose in a 17-year-old female

HISTORY OF PRESENT ILLNESS

A 17-year-old female was brought to the ED by her mother after admitting that she took an overdose of acetaminophen (Tylenol®) 24 hours prior to arrival in a suicide attempt. She stated that she had taken 48 extra-strength Tylenol® tablets (500 mg each). The patient reported mild right upper quadrant abdominal pain and two episodes of vomiting earlier on the day of presentation. She denied co-ingestions, illicit drugs or alcohol use, and the possibility of pregnancy.

PHYSICAL EXAMINATION

GENERAL APPEARANCE: The patient was a well-developed, well-nourished teenager who appeared subdued and remorseful, but in no acute distress.

VITAL SIGNS

Temperature	98.5°F (36.9°C)
Pulse	93 beats/minute
Blood pressure	120/76 mmHg
Respirations	16 breaths/minute
Oxygen saturation	99% on room air

HEENT: PERRL, EOMI, sclera anicteric, oropharynx moist.

NECK: Supple.

CARDIOVASCULAR: Regular rate and rhythm without rubs, murmurs or gallops.

LUNGS: Clear to auscultation bilaterally.

ABDOMEN: Soft, nondistended, active bowel sounds present. Mild right upper quadrant tenderness noted, no Murphy's sign present.

EXTREMITIES: No clubbing, cyanosis or edema.

NEUROLOGIC: Nonfocal.

PSYCHIATRIC: The patient endorsed suicidal ideations but denied homicidal ideation, visual or auditory hallucinations. She was acutely depressed over recent family and social situations, as well as poor school performance and perceived pressure from her parents to succeed.

An intravenous line was placed and blood was drawn and sent for laboratory testing. Laboratory tests were significant for a total bilirubin of 1.4 mg/dL (normal 0.2–1.3 mg/dL), AST of 234 U/L (normal 14–36 U/L), ALT of 261 U/L (normal 11–66 U/L), an International Normalized Ratio (INR) of 1.2 (normal 0.8–1.2), acetaminophen level of 15 µg/mL and salicylate level of less than 1.0 mg/dL. Her serum pregnancy test was negative.

What is your diagnosis?

ANSWER

The diagnosis is acute hepatotoxicity from acetaminophen (APAP) overdose. The patient was placed on an involuntary psychiatric hold, and the Poison Control Center was consulted by phone. The patient's APAP level of 15 µg/mL fell well above the toxicity line at 24 hours on the Rumack-Matthew nomogram for acute single acetaminophen poisoning. She was started on IV N-acetylcysteine (NAC) (Acetadote®) in the ED, with an initial loading dose of 150 mg/kg over 15 minutes. During the loading dose, the patient began to experience chest and throat tightness, shortness of breath, palpitations and a flushing sensation. Her vital signs remained stable. Diphenhydramine 25 mg IV was administered and the infusion of NAC was continued with gradual resolution of her symptoms. The patient was continued on the 20-hour IV NAC regimen and admitted to the pediatric service with a psychiatric consultation. Her liver function tests peaked on hospital day #2, with an AST of 3313 U/L and ALT of 3828 U/L, as well as an elevated INR to 1.5. The patient was transitioned from IV NAC to the oral preparation once her liver function tests began to recover, based upon recommendations from Poison Control. She received a total of three doses of Vitamin K at 5 mg orally for her elevated INR. NAC therapy was discontinued once her ALT fell below 1000 U/L, and the patient was transferred to a psychiatric facility on hospital day #6, at which time her AST had fallen to 80 U/L, ALT to 935 U/L, and INR had normalized to 1.0.

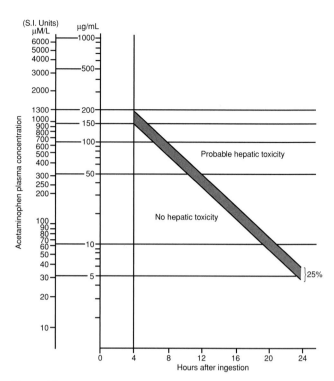

Figure 96.1 Rumack-Matthew nomogram for single acute acetaminophen poisoning (from Merck Manuals, Online Medical Library, Acetaminophen Poisoning, available at http://www.merck.com/mmpe/sec21/ch326c.html, accessed June 22, 2008).

Acetaminophen overdose and toxicity

The first priority in evaluating any overdose patient is a rapid assessment of the airway, breathing and circulation. Once the patient is stabilized, the next priority should involve consideration of gut decontamination with activated charcoal, depending on the ingested material and time from ingestion. In the case of acetaminophen overdose, activated charcoal has been shown to significantly reduce acetaminophen absorption when given after one hour of ingestion in healthy volunteers, but not when administered longer than four hours following ingestion.[1] All patients presenting with an intentional overdose should be placed on a psychiatric hold by an emergency physician.

Typically, the potentially toxic dose of acetaminophen (acetyl-para-aminophenol, or APAP) in an acute poisoning is 150 mg/kg (children) or 7.5–10 gm (adults).[2–4] With therapeutic dosing, 90% of APAP is conjugated with glucuronide or sulfate to form nontoxic metabolites. Approximately 5% of APAP is metabolized by the hepatic cytochrome p450 mixed-function oxidase enzyme to a toxic metabolite, N-acetyl-p-benzoquinone imine (NAPQI). In normal dosing, NAPQI is rapidly detoxified by glutathione (GSH) to nontoxic metabolites. Acetaminophen overdoses overwhelm conjugation pathways, resulting in increased use of the cytochrome p450 pathway and increased formation of NAPQI, increased depletion of GSH and ultimately hepatic injury.[2,3] As GSH stores are

reduced in acetaminophen overdoses, the highly reactive NAPQI can bind to cellular macromolecules that contain cysteine. This covalent binding of NAPQI causes hepatocellular damage at many sites in the liver, although centrilobular necrosis predominates.[4] Finally, because APAP is metabolized to NAPQI (its toxic metabolite) by the cytochrome p450 system, any agent that induces this system theoretically increases the risk for APAP hepatotoxicity. Ethanol is the best-studied inducer. Chronic alcohol ingestion induces the cytochrome p450 enzyme system and in turn makes the liver capable of metabolizing more APAP to the toxic metabolite NAPQI.[3]

The Rumack-Matthew treatment nomogram is the primary tool used to guide treatment after acute single dose ingestion of APAP (Figure 96.1). The nomogram was first studied retrospectively in 64 cases of acute ingestion of APAP in an attempt to correlate APAP serum levels with hepatotoxicity.[3,5] Hepatotoxicity was defined arbitrarily as an aspartate aminotransferase (AST) level of 1000 IU/L. Serum APAP levels at or above a line connecting 200 µg/mL at four hours postingestion and 6.25 µg/mL at 24 hours postingestion consistently predicted hepatoxicity.[5] This line is referred to as the "probable toxicity line." When the nomogram was introduced in the United States, the Food and Drug Administration (FDA) insisted on a 25% reduction of this treatment threshold. A line connecting 150 µg/mL at four hours and 4.7 µg/mL at 24 hours, considered the "possible toxicity line," is therefore used for treatment.[6] This nomogram was later validated in a large trial using the 72-hour NAC treatment protocol.[7]

Laboratory indicators of hepatic injury should be measured initially and daily during therapy in any patient with a serum acetaminophen concentration above the possible toxicity line. With progressive hepatic failure, testing should be done every 12 hours.[3] Subclinical elevation of serum liver transaminases (ALT, AST) occur about 12 hours after ingestion, whereas most patients who develop liver toxicity have an elevated AST level within 24 hours of ingestion.[2,4] The demonstration of a normal AST 36 hours after an acute acetaminophen ingestion is considered sufficient to eliminate the possibility of liver toxicity.[4] However, transaminase levels do not predict the clinical course. They may decline during hepatic recovery or with progressive fulminant hepatic failure.[4] During recovery, it is common for declining serum transaminases to precede the decline of serum bilirubin. Thus, the patient's liver function tests should be followed and may rise over time. Development of a coagulopathy (indicated by elevations of PT and INR) is an indicator of APAP hepatotoxicity. These levels should be monitored in a patient with a toxic overdose of APAP.

Patients with acetaminophen-induced hepatotoxicity present in four clinical phases. In Phase 1 (0–24 hours), patients may present with anorexia, nausea, vomiting, malaise and diaphoresis. Because these clinical signs are nonspecific, patients might inadvertently be given additional doses of an acetaminophen-containing product for treatment.[2] Although some patients remain asymptomatic during this phase, they may still develop clinically significant toxicity. Phase 2 begins 24 hours after ingestion, lasting for an additional 48 hours. Symptoms during this phase become less apparent and may resolve. Patients generally present with pain and tenderness in the right upper quadrant, hepatomegaly can be present, and some patients report decreased urine output during this phase. Phase 3 develops three to five days after ingestion. Symptoms seen during Phase 1 may reappear (e.g., anorexia, nausea, vomiting, malaise). Patients may have symptoms of hepatic failure with jaundice, hypoglycemia, bleeding or encephalopathy; renal failure and cardiomyopathy may occur.[2] Hepatic centrilobular necrosis is evident on liver biopsy; nearly 4% of patients who develop this degree of hepatotoxicity progress to fulminant hepatic failure. Death may occur from cerebral edema, sepsis, or multi-organ failure. Finally, Phase 4 occurs 5–14 days after ingestion, and can last as long as 21 days; patients have either complete recovery of liver function or die.[2]

The accepted antidote to treat toxic ingestions of acetaminophen is NAC. NAC works in the liver by a number of proposed mechanisms.[8] First, NAC increases the synthesis and availability of GSH by itself being converted to cysteine and then GSH. Second, NAC (via its reduced sulfur group) can substitute for GSH and directly bind NAPQI, thus detoxifying it. Finally, NAC can supply a substrate for sulfation, increasing the percentage of nontoxic metabolites produced.[8] NAC is an extremely effective antidote when administered within eight hours of ingestion of a potentially toxic dose of APAP.[3] Because it takes significant time to deplete body stores of GSH, NAC is equally effective whether started immediately following or within eight hours of ingestion. Evidence exists that NAC is effective no matter how late it is initiated or how profoundly the patient's clinical toxic effects.[3] Proposed mechanisms to explain improved outcomes of late presenters treated with NAC include improved oxygen delivery by means of increased hepato-splanchnic circulation and increased oxygen extraction, improved cerebral blood flow, a protective antioxidant effect of NAC, and NAC's limitation of lipid peroxidation minimizing the hepatotoxic effect of APAP.[3]

Prior to 2004 in the United States, the standard treatment for APAP toxicity was a 72-hour protocol using oral NAC. Using the FDA guidelines, the oral dosing protocol of NAC (Mucomyst®) is a 140 mg/kg loading dose followed by a maintenance dose of 70 mg/kg every four hours for 17 doses.[2–4,6–8] Given that nausea and vomiting are reported in 33% of APAP overdoses before NAC and in an estimated 51% during oral NAC therapy, vomiting within one hour of dosing requires a repeat dose.[3] In 2004, the FDA approved a 20-hour protocol for using intravenous NAC (Acetadote®) that had been in use in Europe, Australia and Canada for more than 20 years.[3] In this 20-hour protocol, NAC is administered as a loading dose of 150 mg/kg over 15 minutes, followed by 50 mg/kg infused over four hours. Over the remaining 16 hours, an additional 100 mg/kg is administered as a constant infusion.[2,3] Intravenous NAC is recommended for use in selected patients, including those with an altered mental status, GI bleeding, obstruction, a history of caustic ingestion, potential fetal toxicity from maternal toxicity, or an inability to tolerate oral NAC because of refractory emesis despite proper antiemetic use.[2]

Although there is general agreement that IV administration is preferable in the setting of intractable vomiting, to date no study shows clear evidence that IV therapy is more or less effective than oral NAC therapy.[3] Some evidence suggests that longer courses of NAC are more effective in late presenters, especially in the face of fulminant hepatic failure. In cases with documented elevations in AST and ALT, NAC therapy should be continued indefinitely until significant improvement, liver transplantation or death.[3]

Anaphylactoid reactions to IV NAC have been reported in 3–6% of acetaminophen-poisoned patients, although the rate may be as high as 48%.[9] These are likely the result of histamine release. Symptoms include pruritus, rash, angioedema, bronchospasm, tachycardia, hypotension, nausea and vomiting. Anaphylactoid reactions generally occur within 30 minutes after infusion of the loading dose. In most reported cases, antihistamine therapy was effective, and these transient reactions did not preclude the completion of the NAC course.[7] Kao et al. have suggested that increasing the infusion time for the loading dose of NAC to one hour can attenuate the anaphylactoid response, based on a retrospective study of patients receiving IV NAC.[10] Finally, after any adverse reaction, a critical reassessment of the need for NAC therapy is warranted.

If treatment remains indicated, evidence demonstrates that restarting the infusion at a slower rate is safe.[11]

Although increased AST and ALT levels are frequently the first laboratory signs of liver injury in APAP toxicity, their rate of rise and peak level give no indication of prognosis.[3] A collection of clinical parameters and laboratory findings known as the King's College Criteria have been established and validated to predict poor outcome from APAP toxicity. Patients who have acute isolated APAP overdoses and develop significant metabolic acidosis (pH less than 7.3 after adequate fluid resuscitation), a serum creatinine greater than 3.3 mg/dL, a prothrombin time greater than 1.8 times control (more than 100 sec), an INR greater than 6.5, or grade III or higher encephalopathy have the poorest prognosis.[12] Any patient meeting any one of these criteria should be transferred to a tertiary care center in anticipation of fulminant hepatic failure and possible transplantation. Institution of NAC therapy alone is not an indication for ICU admission.

KEY TEACHING POINTS

1. Initial management of patients presenting with an intentional acetaminophen (APAP) overdose includes attention to the airway, breathing and circulation (ABCs), placement of the patient on a psychiatric hold, and phone consultation with the Poison Control Center.
2. The potentially toxic dose of APAP in an acute poisoning is 150 mg/kg (children) or 7.5–10 gm (adults).
3. The Rumack-Matthew treatment nomogram is the primary tool used to guide treatment after acute ingestion of APAP. A line connecting 150 μg/mL at four hours and 4.7 μg/mL at 24 hours, known as the "possible toxicity line," is used as the treatment threshold.
4. The accepted antidote for ingestion of toxic levels of acetaminophen is N-acetylcysteine (NAC); the intravenous and oral preparations are equally effective but are most effective if administered within eight hours of the ingestion.
5. According to the King's College Criteria, patients with acute APAP overdoses who develop significant metabolic

acidosis (pH less than 7.3 after adequate fluid resuscitation), a serum creatinine greater than 3.3 mg/dL, a prothrombin time greater than 1.8 times control (more than 100 sec), an INR greater than 6.5, or grade III or higher encephalopathy have a poor prognosis.

REFERENCES

[1] Yeates PJA, Thomas SHL. Effectiveness of delayed activated charcoal administration in simulated paracetamol (acetaminophen) overdose. *Br J Clin Pharmacol* 2000;49: 11–4.
[2] Defendi GL. Toxicity, acetaminophen. eMedicine Website. Available at http://www.emedicine.com/ped/topic7.htm. Accessed June 22, 2008.
[3] Rowden AK, Norvell J, Eldridge DL, et al. Updates on acetaminophen toxicity. *Med Clin N Am* 2005;89:1145–59.
[4] Anker A. Acetaminophen. In: Ford MD (ed.). *Clinical Toxicology*, 1st ed. Philadelphia: Saunders, 2001.
[5] Rumack BH, Matthew H. Acetaminophen poisoning and toxicity. *Pediatrics* 1975;55:871–6.
[6] Rumack BH. Acetaminophen hepatotoxicity: the first 35 years. *Clin Toxicol* 2002;40:3–20.
[7] Smilkstein MJ, Knapp GL, Kulig KW, et al. Efficacy of oral N-acetylcysteine in the treatment of acetaminophen overdose. Analysis of the national multicenter study (1976 to 1985). *N Engl J Med* 1988;319:1557–62.
[8] Marzullo L. An update of N-acetylcysteine treatment for acute acetaminophen toxicity in children. *Curr Opin Pediatr* 2005;17:239–45.
[9] Kanter MZ. Comparison of oral and i.v. acetylcysteine in the treatment of acetaminophen poisoning. *Am J Health-Syst Pharm* 2006;63:1821–7.
[10] Kao LW, Kirk MA, Furbee RB, et al. What is the rate of adverse events after oral N-acetylcysteine administered by the intravenous route to patients with suspected acetaminophen poisoning? *Ann Emerg Med* 2003;42:741–50.
[11] Bailey B, McGuigan MA. Management of anaphylactoid reactions to intravenous N-acetylcysteine. *Ann Emerg Med* 1998;31:710–5.
[12] O'Grady JG, Alexander GJ, Hayllar KM, et al. Early indicators of prognosis in fulminant hepatic failure. *Gastroenterology* 1989;97:439–45.

97

Headache and rash in a 21-year-old male

HISTORY OF PRESENT ILLNESS

A 21-year-old male presented to the ED with the chief complaint of a throbbing bilateral headache. He also complained of facial flushing, palpitations, transient severe shortness of breath, a rash over his arms and trunk, and red eyes. He had just eaten dinner at a local seafood restaurant. He denied any previous similar symptoms or ingestion of new or different foods or medications.

PHYSICAL EXAMINATION

GENERAL APPEARANCE: The patient was awake and alert in no acute discomfort.

VITAL SIGNS

Temperature	97°F (36.1°C)
Pulse	121 beats/minute
Blood pressure	112/66 mmHg
Respirations	22 breaths/minute
Oxygen saturation	99% on room air

HEENT: PERRL, EOMI, sclera injected bilaterally, facial flushing noted.

NECK: Supple, no jugular venous distension.

CARDIOVASCULAR: Tachycardic rate, regular rhythm without rubs, murmurs or gallops.

LUNGS: Clear to auscultation bilaterally.

ABDOMEN: Soft, nontender, nondistended.

EXTREMITIES: No clubbing, cyanosis or edema.

SKIN: An erythematous, macular rash on the extremities and trunk, slightly warm to touch (Figure 97.1)

NEUROLOGIC: Nonfocal.

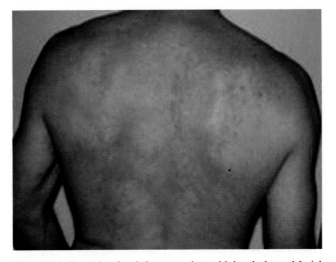

Figure 97.1 Example of rash from a patient with headache and facial flushing (from eMedicine Website, available at http://www.emedicine.com/emerg/topic523.htm, accessed June 23, 2008).

What is your diagnosis?

The diagnosis is scombroid fish poisoning. The patient reported that approximately 30 minutes before the onset of symptoms, he had eaten mahi mahi fish from a local restaurant, which tasted normal. He had eaten the same food in the past without subsequent symptoms. The patient was given diphenhydramine 25 mg IV and cimetidine 300 mg IV, which resulted in resolution of his symptoms over two hours. The patient was discharged home, and the County Public Health Department was notified by phone regarding the scombroid fish poisoning.

Scombroid fish poisoning

Scombroid fish poisoning (scombrotoxism, scombroid ichthyotoxicosis) is a food-related illness typically associated with the consumption of fish.[1] Originally, the illness was associated with Scombroidea fish (e.g., marine tuna, albacore, mackerel); however, the Centers for Disease Control and Prevention (CDC) have identified the largest vector to be nonscombroid fish, such as mahi mahi and amberjack. Epidemiologic data from the CDC suggest that scombroid poisoning is the principal chemical agent type of food-borne disease found in the United States; the second most common is ciguatera poisoning.[1]

Symptoms of scombroid fish poisoning are related to the ingestion of biogenic amines, especially histamine.[1,2] The histamine is produced via bacterial decarboxylation of histidine, normally present at levels less than 0.1 mg per 100 gm of fish. In contrast, samples of fish that produce poisoning contain histamine levels of at least 20–50 mg per 100 gm fish. Serum histamine levels and urinary histamine excretion are elevated in humans with acute illness.[2] Antihistamines (H1- and H2-blockers) have been used safely, with good efficacy abating the symptoms.

Scombroid poisoning is relatively uncommon (although it is likely highly underreported), comprising up to 5% of food-borne disease outbreaks reported to the CDC.[1,4] The illness is usually self-limited but may cause significant discomfort. The onset of symptoms is typically 10–30 minutes following ingestion, but may occur up to three hours after ingestion of the implicated fish, which is said to sometimes have a characteristic peppery and bitter taste.[3–5] The symptoms are nonspecific and include flushing, palpitations, headache, nausea, diarrhea, sense of anxiety, prostration or loss of vision (rare).[1,3,4] Findings on physical exam may include a diffuse, macular, blanching erythematous rash (most common), tachycardia, wheezing (generally only in histamine-sensitive asthmatics), hypotension or hypertension, and conjunctivitis. The magnitude of symptoms are related to individual differences in sensitivity to histamine, size of the portion consumed, whether the portion was from the same fish, and how cold the fish was before cooking. Scombroid fish poisoning can be avoided if the offending fish species are promptly refrigerated below 59°F (15°C)

or iced after catch and maintained until the fish is cooked or processed for storage.[4] Cooking does not inactivate the toxin.

If the patient has only minimal symptoms, reassurance and observation may be the only treatment necessary. Acute illness should be treated with antihistamines as needed, such as H1-blockers (e.g., diphenhydramine 25–50 mg PO/IV/IM q4–6h) and H2-blockers (e.g., ranitidine 150 mg PO q12h or 50 mg IV q8–12h, or cimetidine 300mg PO/IV q6–8h). If the patient is symptomatic enough to require treatment, antihistamines are used to counteract the excessive histamine-induced effects. Epinephrine or other adrenergic agents are rarely necessary because the entire cascade of mediators released by a true allergic reaction is not found in scombroid poisoning.[1] Blockade of histamine, the sole pharmacologic mediator of scombrotoxism, is generally the only treatment necessary.[1] Although bronchospasm is rare, bronchodilators or other adrenergic agents are recommended if it occurs. Patients receiving antihistamine therapy (particularly diphenhydramine) in the ED should not be allowed to drive at discharge. Scombroid fish poisoning is an "immediately" reportable disease to the local public health department, requiring a completed Confidential Morbidity Report form to be faxed to the health department, as well as timely notification of the public health department by phone.

KEY TEACHING POINTS

1. Symptoms of scombroid fish poisoning are related to the ingestion of biogenic amines, especially histamine. The onset of symptoms of scombroid fish poisoning usually occurs 10–30 minutes after ingestion of the implicated fish, which sometimes has a characteristic peppery and bitter taste.

2. The symptoms of scombroid fish poisoning are nonspecific, and may include flushing, palpitations, headache, nausea, diarrhea, sense of anxiety, prostration or loss of vision (rare).

3. Findings on physical examination can include a diffuse, macular, blanching erythematous rash (most common), tachycardia, wheezing (generally only in histamine-sensitive asthmatics), hypotension or hypertension, and conjunctivitis.

4. Treat acute illness with antihistamines as needed; H1-blockers (e.g., diphenhydramine 25–50 mg PO/IV/IM q4–6h) and H2-blockers (e.g., ranitidine 150 mg PO q12h or 50 mg IV q8–12h, or cimetidine 300 mg PO/IV q6–8h).

5. Scombroid fish poisoning must be immediately reported to the local public health department.

REFERENCES

[1] Patrick JD. Toxicity, Scombroid. eMedicine Website. Available at http://www.emedicine.com/emerg/topic523.htm. Accessed June 23, 2008.

[2] Morrow JD, Margolis GR, Rowland J, Roberts LJ. Evidence that histamine is the causative toxin of scombroid-fish poisoning. *N Engl J Med* 1991;324:716–20.

[3] Perkins RA, Morgan SS. Poisoning envenomation, and trauma from marine creatures. *Am Fam Phys* 2004;69:885–90.

[4] Matteuci MJ, Ly BT, Clark RF. Seafood toxidromes. In: Auerbach PS (ed.). *Wilderness Medicine*, 5th ed. Philadelphia: Mosby, 2007:1534–36.

[5] Diseasedex™, Scombroid Fish Poisoning, Anaphylaxis – Acute. In: Klasco RK (ed.). Diseasedex™, General Medicine, Thomson Micromedex®, Vol. 131. Greenwood Village, CO: Thomson, 1974–2007.

98

Bilateral foot pain and swelling in a 47-year-old male

HISTORY OF PRESENT ILLNESS

A 47-year-old male with no significant medical history presented to the ED complaining of six days of gradually worsening pain and swelling of his feet and ankles bilaterally. The patient reported great difficulty ambulating secondary to pain, as well as pain in his leg muscles bilaterally. He also reported that he had begun jogging six days prior to presentation. In the ED, he admitted to using methamphetamine five days prior to presentation, both by nasal insufflation and smoking. He also drank alcohol on a regular basis. He was seen by his primary care physician (PCP) one day earlier with the same complaints, was diagnosed with bilateral plantar fasciitis and given ketorolac 30 mg IM for pain. The patient was prescribed nabumetone and Vicodin® for pain, and furosemide for swelling prior to discharge. In the ED, he denied chest pain, shortness of breath, abdominal pain, nausea, vomiting or dysuria. He did note that his urine had become darker recently.

PHYSICAL EXAMINATION

GENERAL APPEARANCE: The patient was an obese male who appeared well nourished, well hydrated and in no acute discomfort.

VITAL SIGNS

Temperature	98.4°F (36.9°C)
Pulse	76 beats/minute
Blood pressure	159/93 mmHg
Respirations	18 breaths/minute
Oxygen saturation	100% on room air

HEENT: Unremarkable.

NECK: Supple, no jugular venous distension.

CARDIOVASCULAR: Regular rate and rhythm without rubs, murmurs or gallops.

CHEST: Clear to auscultation bilaterally.

ABDOMEN: Soft, nontender, nondistended.

EXTREMITIES: 3+ pitting edema to the mid-tibial region bilaterally over his lower extremities.

NEUROLOGIC: Nonfocal.

A peripheral intravenous line was placed, blood was drawn and sent for laboratory testing, and a 12-lead ECG (Figure 98.1) and clean catch urine were obtained. The urine was noted to appear tea-colored, and the dipstick reagent test turned positive for blood.

What is your diagnosis?

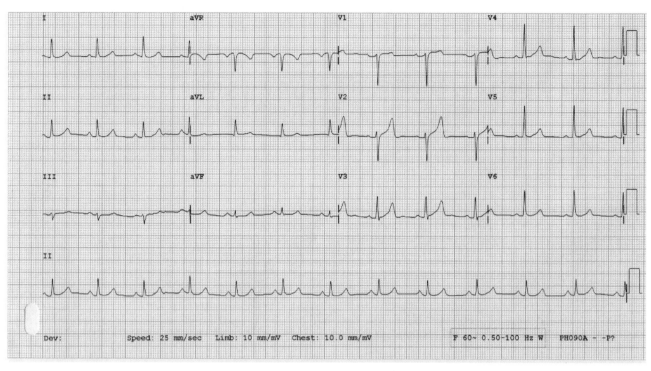

Figure 98.1 12-lead ECG from a 47-year-old male with bilateral foot pain and swelling.

ANSWER

The diagnosis is acute renal failure secondary to rhabdomyolysis, most likely resulting from recent methamphetamine use. The laboratory results were significant for a serum creatinine of 14.5 mg/dL (normal 0.8–1.5 mg/dL), BUN of 145 mg/dL (normal 9–20 mg/dL), potassium of 6.6 mEq/L (normal 3.5–5.3 mEq/L) and sodium of 124 mEq/L (normal 137–145 mEq/L). The serum creatine kinase was markedly elevated at 114,720 U/L (normal less than 170 U/L). The ECG demonstrates early peaked T waves, particularly in leads V_2 and V_3. The patient received 1 ampule D50 IV, 10 units regular insulin IV and kayexelate 30 gm orally for his hyperkalemia. A Foley catheter was placed, and a sodium bicarbonate drip (3 ampules sodium bicarbonate in 1 liter D5/water) was administered intravenously to treat the rhabdomyolysis, as well as continued intravenous hydration with normal saline. The nephrologist was consulted, a dialysis catheter was placed by interventional radiology and the patient underwent emergent dialysis and admission to the hospital. The patient was discharged on hospital day #13, with continued dialysis for one more week until his kidney function normalized.

Rhabdomyolysis and acute renal failure

Rhabdomyolysis is a clinical syndrome caused by injury to skeletal muscle. It results in the release of cellular contents into the extracellular fluid and circulation.[1] The diagnosis rests on measuring these released substances in either plasma or urine. The injury can be irreversible, leading to disability, renal failure or death. The most common causes of rhabdomyolysis are crush injury, overexertion, alcohol abuse, certain medicines, drugs and toxic substances.[2] Rhabdomyolysis accounts for an estimated 8–15% of acute renal failure.[3] The overall mortality rate for patients with rhabdomyolysis is approximately 5%; however, the mortality rate of any single patient is dependent upon the underlying etiology and any existing comorbidities.[3]

The etiologies of rhabdomyolysis may vary but the outcome is the same; as cellular membrane integrity is lost, intracellular sodium and calcium levels rise, resulting in cell breakdown and death.[4] In turn, various intramuscular components, including creatine phosphokinase (CPK), are released into plasma. Clinically, an elevated CPK is the primary marker used to identify rhabdomyolysis. It is postulated that the breakdown products of myoglobin may have a directly toxic effect on the renal system. This may be responsible for the potential renal complications of rhabdomyolysis.[4] Screening for rhabdomyolysis may be performed with a urine dipstick in combination with urine microscopy. A positive urine myoglobin test provides evidence of the diagnosis.[2]

Patients with rhabdomyolysis classically present with complaints of muscle weakness, swelling and pain.[1] The myalgias may be focal or diffuse, depending on the underlying etiology. The patient may also note dark- or tea-colored urine.[1,2] However, a high clinical suspicion for rhabdomyolysis must be maintained in patients at risk because up to 50% of those with serologically proven rhabdomyolysis do not report myalgias or muscle weakness.[1]

Along with measuring the serum CPK and urine myoglobin in patients with suspected rhabdomyolysis, potassium, BUN and creatinine levels should be measured and closely monitored. Hyperkalemia, an immediate threat to life (particularly in the hours immediately after injury), occurs in 10–40% of cases.[3] Hypocalcemia is another early complication that can be potentiated by the release of large amounts of phosphate from the lysed muscle cells.[2] Hepatic dysfunction occurs in approximately 25% of patients with rhabdomyolysis. Finally, acute renal failure and disseminated intravascular coagulation (DIC) are late complications of rhabdomyolysis (i.e., beyond 12–24 hours).[2]

Methamphetamine use causes elevated levels of serum norepinephrine and dopamine, which result in increasing adenosine triphosphate (ATP) demand.[5] Methamphetamine abusers frequently neglect eating and drinking during "binges." This combination of decreased intake of calories, dehydration and the sympathomimetic effect of methamphetamine may play a large role in the high incidence of rhabdomyolysis seen in this population.[5]

Patients with CPK elevation in excess of two to three times the reference range, an appropriate clinical history and risk factors should be suspected of having rhabdomyolysis.[3] Administer isotonic crystalloid 500 mL/h and titrate to maintain a urine output of 200–300 mL/h. Creatine kinase (CK) assay should be repeated every 6–12 hours to determine the peak CK level.[3] Urinary alkalinization is recommended for a patient with rhabdomyolysis and CK levels in excess of 6000 IU/L.[3] Alkalinization should be considered earlier in patients with acidemia, dehydration or underlying renal disease. A suggested regimen is half-normal saline solution (0.45% NaCl) with one ampule of sodium bicarbonate administered at 100 mL/h, titrated to a urine pH greater than 7.[3]

Mannitol may have beneficial effects in the treatment of rhabdomyolysis. It acts as an osmotic diuretic, an intravascular volume expander, a renal vasodilator and possibly a free radical scavenger.[1] However, the use of mannitol remains controversial, as it is mostly supported by experimental animal and retrospective clinical studies.[2] Loop diuretics (e.g., furosemide) should not be used because they may acidify the urine and do not improve (and may actually worsen) ultimate renal outcome.[1,2] Despite treatment, patients with rhabdomyolysis often develop oliguric acute tubular necrosis (ATN). In this situation, a nephrologist should be consulted for aggressive hemodialysis, often on a daily basis.[2] Over time, many patients partially or completely recover renal function.

KEY TEACHING POINTS

1. Rhabdomyolysis is a potentially life-threatening syndrome resulting from the breakdown of skeletal muscle, with leakage of muscle contents into the circulation.
2. The most common causes of rhabdomyolysis are crush injuries, overexertion, alcohol abuse, certain medications, drugs and toxins.

3. Patients with rhabdomyolysis classically present with complaints of muscle weakness, swelling and pain.
4. Elevated CPK levels and a positive urine myoglobin test support the diagnosis of rhabdomyolysis.
5. Treatment of rhabdomyolysis includes aggressive intravenous hydration, alkalinization of the urine with sodium bicarbonate and emergent hemodialysis in cases of acute renal failure. Mannitol may be of some benefit, but its use remains controversial.

REFERENCES

[1] Bontempo LJ. Rhabdomyolysis. In: Marx JA, Hockberger RS, Walls RM, et al. (eds.). *Rosen's Emergency Medicine: Concepts and Clinical Practice*, 6th ed. Philadelphia: Mosby, 2006;1975–83.

[2] Sauret JM, Marinides G, Wang GK. Rhabdomyolysis. *Am Fam Physician* 2002;65:907–12.

[3] Craig S. Rhabdomyolysis. eMedicine Website. Available at http://www.emedicine.com/emerg/topic508.htm. Accessed June 26, 2008.

[4] Fernandez WG, Hung O, Bruno GR, et al. Factors predictive of acute renal failure and need for hemodialysis among ED patients with rhabdomyolysis. *Am J Emerg Med* 2005;23:1–7.

[5] Richards JR, Johnson EB, Stark RW, et al. Methamphetamine abuse and rhabdomyolysis in the ED: a 5-year study. *Am J Emerg Med* 1999;17:681–5.

99

Snakebite in a 55-year-old female

HISTORY OF PRESENT ILLNESS

A 55-year-old female with a medical history significant for asthma and hypertension presented to the ED by ambulance after being bitten by a snake. The patient was walking on a trail in a wooded area wearing sandals when she accidentally stepped on the snake, which bit her right mid-foot. The patient felt sudden, sharp pain to her foot, and was able to shake the snake off. She reported hearing a rattling sound after the bite, and saw the snake slither away. She quickly developed severe pain, redness and swelling of her foot, followed by sensations of numbness and tingling in her hands and tongue. A companion called emergency services, and she was transported to the ED. In the ED, she complained of worsening pain and swelling to her right foot, as well as nausea. She denied chest pain, shortness of breath, abdominal pain or throat swelling. The patient's tetanus immunization status was unknown.

PHYSICAL EXAMINATION

GENERAL APPEARANCE: The patient was a well-developed, middle-aged female in moderate discomfort.

VITAL SIGNS

Temperature	98.6°F (37°C)
Pulse	95 beats/minute
Blood pressure	175/74 mmHg
Respirations	18 breaths/minute
Oxygen saturation	100% on room air

HEENT: PERRL, EOMI, oropharynx moist, no uvular swelling.

NECK: Supple.

CARDIOVASCULAR: Regular rate and rhythm without rubs, murmurs or gallops.

LUNGS: Clear to auscultation bilaterally, no rales, rhonchi or wheezes.

ABDOMEN: Soft, nontender, nondistended, active bowel sounds present.

RIGHT FOOT: Edema with erythema of the entire foot, extending to the mid-calf (panel A, Figure 99.1). Two small puncture wounds present on the medial aspect of the foot (panel B, Figure 99.1). Diffuse tenderness to palpation and warmth; palpable dorsalis pedis pulse, normal sensation and motor function of the toes and foot. No increased pain on passive extension of the toes.

NEUROLOGIC: Nonfocal.

A peripheral intravenous line was placed, and blood was drawn and sent for laboratory testing. Morphine sulfate and Zofran® were administered IV for pain and nausea, respectively. The wound was cleaned with normal saline, the foot was elevated and ice packs were applied. Laboratory results, including a complete blood count (CBC), electrolytes, BUN, creatinine, glucose, prothrombin time (PT), activated partial thromboplastin time (aPTT), International Normalized Ratio (INR), fibrin split products, fibrinogen and creatine kinase (CK), were all within normal limits.

What is your diagnosis?

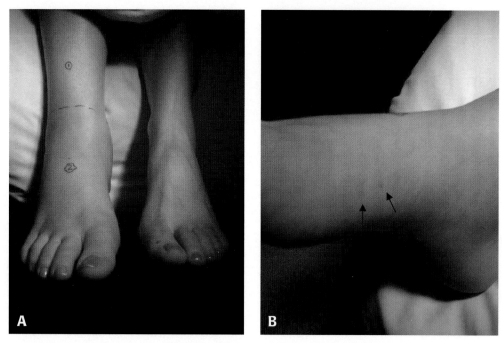

Figure 99.1 Feet from a 55-year-old female following a snakebite to the right foot (panel A); medial view of the right foot demonstrating two small puncture wounds (panel B, arrows).

ANSWER

The diagnosis is snake envenomation from a Northern Pacific rattlesnake (subfamily of *Crotalinae*, pit vipers) (Figure 99.2). The patient's tetanus status was updated, and she was given an initial four vials of Crotalidae polyvalent immune Fab antivenom (CroFab™) IV after consultation with the Poison Control Center. Six hours after the initial infusion of antivenom, the swelling and erythema appeared to increase, and an additional four vials of antivenom was administered. The patient was admitted to the ICU by the podiatry service. Laboratory tests including CBC, PT, aPTT, INR and CK remained within normal limits. By hospital day #3, the swelling, erythema and pain had reduced considerably, and the patient was discharged home weight-bearing on the right foot, with close follow up arranged.

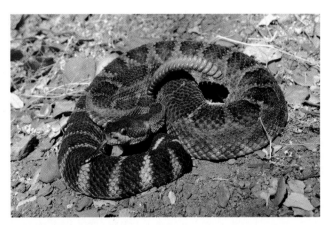

Figure 99.2 Northern Pacific rattlesnake (photograph courtesy of Robert Norris, MD, Division of Emergency Medicine, Department of Surgery, Stanford University).

Venomous snakebites in the United States

Approximately 15% of the 3000 species of snakes found worldwide are considered dangerous to humans.[1,2] Data from the American Association of Poison Control Centers for 2003 included 2911 bites by indigenous venomous snakes in the United States.[3] However, the total is clearly greater because a significant number of such bites are never reported to poison control centers. The medically important New World (North and South America) venomous snakes may be divided into the families *Viperidae* (subfamily *Crotalinae*, the crotalines or pit vipers) and *Elapidae* (elapids, the coral and sea snakes).[3] Pit vipers are found throughout most of the New World south of southern Canada. For example, in the United States all 48 contiguous states except Maine have at least one pit viper species.[3] Rattlesnakes are the most widespread of pit vipers, found throughout most of the Western hemisphere. The eastern and western diamondback rattlesnakes account for most fatalities.[4] Deaths typically occur in children, the elderly and in victims to whom antivenom is not given because envenomation is not recognized, is given after a delay or is administered in insufficient quantities.[4]

The majority of snakebites victims are men between the ages of 17–27 years.[2] Alcohol intoxication is a contributing factor in many envenomations.[3,5] More than 95% of bites are on extremities (lower more than upper) and most occur between April and October, with peak months July and August.[2,3] These months coincide with the times when native snakes are active. Humans are more prone to be bitten during outdoor activities, especially during these months. Twenty-five percent of all pit viper bites are "dry" (i.e., do not result in envenomation).[1,3] The cardinal characteristic of the rattlesnake is the tail rattle, which is formed by a group of interlocking keratin rings that vibrate against each other, producing the characteristic buzzing sound when the snake is aroused.[2] Although rattlesnakes are generally quick to sound out a warning when threatened, it is a misconception that they always do so before striking.[3] Most bites result from the

eastern diamondback rattlesnake (*C. atrox*), the prairie and Pacific rattlesnakes (*C. viridis*), the timber rattlesnake (*C. horridus*) and the pygmy rattlesnake (*S. miliarius*).[2]

Snake venoms are complex chemical cocktails of approximately 100 distinct molecular moieties.[3] The best characterized of these include the phospholipase A_2 neurotoxins, metalloproteinases and thrombin-like enzymes. Phospholipase A_2 neurotoxins competitively bind to presynaptic calcium channels, inhibiting acetylcholine release, thereby blocking neurotransmission at the neuromuscular junction and inactivating the muscle.[3] Phospholipase A_2 also damages muscle cell membranes, causing calcium influx and release of creatine and CK, which can result in diffuse myonecrosis and rhabdomyolysis. Metalloproteinases activate tumor necrosis factor alpha (TNF-α) and stimulate endogenous human metalloproteinases, intensifying inflammation.[3] Thrombin-like enzymes cause a consumptive coagulopathy but do not directly activate coagulation factors or complex with antithrombin III.[3]

Definitive diagnosis of snake-venom poisoning requires positive identification of the snake and clinical manifestations of envenomation.[1] Patients may bring the snake into the ED, alive or dead, in parts or whole, for identification. Snake parts should never be handled directly because the bite reflex in recently killed or decapitated snakes remains intact, rendering them capable of inflicting a bite.[1,2] The most common reaction to any snakebite is impending doom. Fear might cause symptoms such as nausea, vomiting, diarrhea, fainting, tachycardia or cold, clammy skin.[2] The primary local clinical findings after most pit viper bites emerge within 30–60 minutes. Common characteristics of crotaline envenomation include the presence of one or more fang marks or puncture wounds, pain, edema, erythema, or ecchymosis of the bite site and adjacent tissue.[2] Localized burning pain and early progressive edema around the bite site are common. Over a period of hours to days, the patient may develop hemorrhagic or serous vesicles and bullae at the bite site that may extend proximally.[3]

Early manifestations of snakebite envenomations typically include nausea, vomiting, perioral paresthesias, tingling of the fingertips and toes, lethargy and weakness.[1] Victims may complain of a numb sensation of the mouth or tongue.[3] More severe systemic effects include hypotension, tachypnea, respiratory distress, severe tachycardia and altered sensorium. Most pit viper snake venoms are hemotoxic (attacking tissue and blood), resulting in damage to capillary endothelial cells. This causes a third-spacing of plasma and extravasation of erythrocytes.[6] Bites by rattlesnakes and the resulting envenomation may result in a consumptive coagulopathy manifested by a prolonged or immeasurable INR, PT or aPTT, hypofibrinogenemia, the presence of fibrin-degradation products, or a platelet count less than 20,000 per cubic millimeter.[1] Muscle damage can result in elevated serum potassium and CK levels.[3] Envenomations can result in severe systemic reactions, including a syndrome similar to disseminated intravascular coagulation (DIC), acute renal failure, hypovolemic shock and death.[6]

The factors that most reduce snakebite-related injuries and mortality in the United States are rapid transport, intensive care and antivenom.[3] Once airway, breathing and circulation have been assessed and secured, a rapid, detailed history should be obtained. Key points include the time and circumstances of the bite, a general description of the snake, first-aid measures used, coexisting medical conditions, drug and food allergies, allergy to horse or sheep products, and history of snakebite and therapy.[1] The bite should be examined for fang or tooth marks and scratches, edema, erythema and ecchymosis. All rings, watches, and constrictive clothing should be removed.[2] Baseline circumferential measurements at several points above and below the bite should be documented, with measurements at the same sites repeated every 20–30 minutes until the swelling subsides.[1,2] Laboratory studies should include a CBC with platelet count, coagulation profile (PT, aPTT, INR, fibrinogen), electrolytes, BUN, serum creatinine and urinalysis.[1,2] Tests such as CK, blood typing and crossmatching, chest radiography, and electrocardiography might be indicated based on age, comorbid history and severity of the envenomation.[2] Tetanus prophylaxis should be administered based on the patient's immunization history.

The mainstay of therapy for pit viper envenomation is the early and judicious use of antivenom. Antivenom therapy is predicated on imparting passive immunity against circulating snake venom antigens.[3] Two antivenoms are currently available in the United States for use in pit viper bites: Crotalidae Polyvalent Immune Fab (CroFab®, Savage Laboratories, Melville, NY) and Antivenin Crotalidae Polyvalent (ACP®, Wyeth-Ayerst Laboratories, Philadelphia, PA).[3] ACP was introduced in the United States in 1954 and contributed to a remarkable decrease in the mortality rate from crotaline (pit viper) snakes, from an estimated 5%–25% in the nineteenth century to less than 0.5% currently.[1] CroFab® is a mixed, monospecific, polyvalent antivenom produced by immunizing sheep with the venoms of crotaline snakes.[1] In animal testing, CroFab® was 5.2 times as potent as ACP®. Current experience indicates that CroFab® is more effective for most North American pit viper species and safer to use than ACP®.[3,7]

Indications for the use of antivenom in cases of rattlesnake bites include progressive venom effects, such as worsening local injury (e.g., pain, swelling, ecchymosis), abnormal coagulation profile or systemic effects (e.g., hypotension, altered mental status).[2] Antivenom should be given as soon as possible after the bite (preferably within four to six hours) to be most effective.[3] CroFab® is administered according to the concepts of initial control and maintenance of therapy. The starting dose is four to six reconstituted vials further diluted in 250 mL of normal saline, administered to achieve initial control (defined as reversal or marked attenuation of local injury, systemic effects and coagulopathy).[2,3,8] If there is evidence of progression of local finding one hour after initial antivenom administration, or if coagulation studies and systemic signs and symptoms fail to improve, this dose should be repeated until stabilization occurs.[3] After initial control has been established, an additional two vials of CroFab® are infused at 6, 12 and 18 hours to prevent local recurrence.[1–3,8] Monitoring of patients for response to treatment and possible adverse events (e.g., anaphylaxis) in an ICU is recommended for all patients treated with antivenom.[1]

KEY TEACHING POINTS

1. The reported incidence of venomous snake bites in the United States is 7000–8000 per year, with five or six annual deaths.[1]
2. Victims of venomous snakebites require aggressive supportive care, baseline circumferential measurements at several points above and below the bite, and a CBC with platelet count, coagulation profile, electrolytes, BUN, serum creatinine, CK and urinalysis.
3. Indications for treatment of rattlesnake bites with antivenom include progressive venom effects, such as worsening local injury, abnormal coagulation profile or systemic effects (e.g., hypotension, altered mental status).
4. All patients treated with antivenom should be monitored in an ICU.

REFERENCES

[1] Gold BS, Dart RC, Barish RA. Bites of venomous snakes. *N Engl J Med* 2002;347:347–56.
[2] Gold BS, Barish RA. North American snake envenomation: diagnosis, treatment and management. *Emerg Med Clin N Am* 2004;22:423–43.
[3] Norris RL, Bush SP. Bites by venomous reptiles in the Americas. In: Auerbach PS (ed.). *Wilderness Medicine*, 5th ed. Philadelphia: Mosby, 2007:1052–6.
[4] Gold BS, Wingert WA. Snake venom poisoning in the United States: a review of therapeutic practice. *South Med J* 1994;87:579–89.

[5] Wingert WA, Chan L. Rattlesnake bites in Southern California and rationale for recommended treatment. *West J Med* 1988;148:37–44.

[6] Juckett G, Hancox JG. Venomous snakebites in the United States: management review and update. *Am Fam Physician* 2002;65:1367–74, 1377.

[7] Consroe P, Egen NB, Russell FE, et al. Comparison of a new ovine antigen binding fragment (Fab) antivenin for United States Crotalidae with the commercial antivenin for protection against venom-induced lethality in mice. *Am J Trop Med Hyg* 1995;53:507–10.

[8] Package insert, CROFAB® Crotalidae Polyvalent Immune FAB (ovine). Available online at http://www.fougera.com/products/crofab˙digifab/crofab˙packageinsert.pdf. Accessed June 30, 2008.

100

Facial swelling in a 62-year-old female

HISTORY OF PRESENT ILLNESS

A 62-year-old female with a history of type II diabetes and hypertension presented to the ED with several hours of facial swelling after eating Mexican food. Soon after her meal, the patient began experiencing generalized pruritus; over the next few hours, she developed progressive facial edema with mild shortness of breath and chest tightness. She denied throat tightness, difficulty swallowing or taking a breath. The patient reported two similar episodes over the past two months, both occurred shortly after eating tomatoes. She reported eating tomatoes her entire life without similar occurrences. The patient's medications included Prinizide® (lisinopril/HCTZ), glipizide and trazodone; none of these were new medications and no recent dose changes had occurred. She denied any known drug allergies.

PHYSICAL EXAMINATION

GENERAL APPEARANCE: The patient was a well-developed female with obvious facial swelling who appeared to be in no acute distress.

VITAL SIGNS

Temperature	98.1°F (36.7°C)
Pulse	80 beats/minute
Blood pressure	130/80 mmHg
Respirations	20 breaths/minute
Oxygen saturation	98% on room air

HEENT: PERRL, EOMI, obvious swelling of the lips and tongue appreciated (Figure 100.1). The oropharynx was moist without lesions; mild uvular swelling was noted. The patient had a coarse voice on phonation.

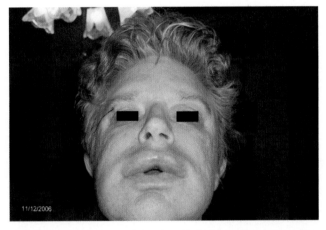

Figure 100.1 A 62-year-old female with facial swelling after eating Mexican food.

NECK: Supple, no jugular venous distension, no stridor on auscultation.

CARDIOVASCULAR: Regular rate and rhythm without rubs, murmurs or gallops.

LUNGS: Clear to auscultation bilaterally, no wheezes.

ABDOMEN: Soft, nontender, nondistended, active bowel sounds present.

EXTREMITIES: No clubbing, cyanosis or edema.

SKIN: Warm, dry, well perfused, without rashes.

NEUROLOGIC: Nonfocal.

What is your diagnosis?

ANSWER

The diagnosis is angioedema. In the ED, the patient received Solu-Medrol® 125 mg IV, Benadryl® 25 mg IV, Pepcid® 20 mg IV and nebulized racemic epinephrine with some improvement of her symptoms. After several hours, significant lip and tongue swelling persisted, and the patient was admitted to the medical service for further observation. ACE inhibitors were held, and the patient was continued on IV steroids, Benadryl® and Pepcid®. Laboratory tests were all within normal limits on admission, as well as normal tryptase and C1-esterase inhibitor levels obtained during the hospitalization. Radioallergosorbent tests (RAST) for allergy to foods returned negative to tomatoes and mildly reactive to wheat. She was discharged on hospital day #2 with nearly complete resolution of symptoms, with instructions to continue a prednisone taper, Pepcid® and Benadryl® as an outpatient. An EpiPen® was prescribed, with instructions for its use in an emergency given.

Angioedema

Angioedema (AE) is the result of interstitial edema from mediators affecting capillary and venule permeability.[1] Upward of 50% of patients with urticaria may have AE concurrently.[1] The swelling due to AE involves tissues deeper than the dermis and thus appears and feels different than urticaria. The mechanisms responsible for the swelling in both urticaria and AE are generally similar. However, a major exception to this is AE associated with C1-esterase inhibitor deficiency, which is caused by a distinct pathophysiologic mechanism and is not accompanied by urticaria.[1]

AE occurs in approximately 15% of the general population, and is more common in females than males.[2] Common locations of swelling include the periorbital region, lips, tongue, extremities and bowel wall.[2,3] Bowel wall AE may occur without skin involvement and cause abdominal pain, nausea, and possibly (although rare) bowel obstruction. The leading cause of death is airway obstruction from laryngeal edema, with a mortality of 25–40%.[2] Episodes of AE typically last between two to three days, and may be isolated or recurrent. Recurrent episodes of AE and urticaria that last less than six weeks are considered acute (90%); those that persist longer than six weeks are classified as chronic (10%).[3]

Allergic (histamine-induced) AE is a hypersensitivity reaction to various antigens, such as drugs, foods and insect venoms.[4] Kinin-induced AE is believed to be caused by bradykinin-induced activation of endothelial cells resulting in vasodilatation and capillary leakage. Two different types of kinin-induced AE are known, hereditary and drug-induced forms.[4] Hereditary AE (HAE) is an autosomal-dominant disorder that results from C1-esterase inhibitor (C1-INH) deficiency, which regulates the activity of the complement component C1, the first step in the classic component cascade.[2] C1-INH deficiency results in unregulated activity of the vasoactive mediators bradykinin, kallikrein and plasmin.[2]

ACE inhibitors precipitate attacks of AE by directly interfering with the degradation of bradykinin, thereby potentiating its biological effect.[5] The incidence of AE with ACE inhibitors is highest (25%) during the first month of taking the medication, although the first event can occur spontaneously after many years of use.[2]

The clinical evaluation of AE starts with a focused search for emergency conditions, followed by a detailed history aimed at identifying the underlying cause.[3] Life-threatening airway compromise can occur if the AE involves the upper airway. Following stabilization of the patient, a detailed history should be aimed at eliciting exposures to foods, drugs, physical stimuli, infection, occupational elements and insect stings. The differential diagnosis includes evolving anaphylaxis syndrome, erythema multiforme minor, bullous pemphigoid and dermatitis herpetiformis, urticarial vasculitis, mastocytosis, HAE (C1-esterase inhibitor deficiency), ACE inhibitor-associated AE and serum sickness.[3] Family history can assist in determining whether a hereditary component exists. Diagnosis of IgE-mediated AE is usually made historically; however, epicutaneous skin testing or RAST testing for foods may be confirmatory.[5] Hereditary AE is characterized by low levels of C1-INH, whereas serum tryptase levels are often elevated in persons with acute allergic reactions.[5]

The first priority of acute management of AE is airway protection. Providers must have a low threshold for intubation at the first signs of airway compromise.[2] For allergic AE, allergen avoidance is the standard of treatment; antihistamines (H1- and H2-blockers) and glucocorticoids improve symptoms during an acute episode.[2] Intramuscular epinephrine (0.3 cc of a 1:1000 concentration) should be the first line of treatment when laryngeal edema is suspected or airway compromise is evident. Life-threatening acute attacks of HAE do not usually respond satisfactorily to treatment with epinephrine (normal dosage), antihistamines or steroids.[3] The treatment of choice for acute episodes of HAE is plasma-derived C1-INH concentrate or fresh-frozen plasma, which contains C1-INH (and has been shown to be as effective as C1-INH concentrate).[2] Stanazol, an anabolic steroid, and danazol, a gonadotropin inhibitor, may be used for the acute phase of an attack of HAE.[5]

KEY TEACHING POINTS

1. The initial goal of therapy for angioedema (AE) is airway management. Most patients with mild acute angioedema may be treated similarly to those with an allergic reaction, although an extended observation period is recommended.
2. Severe symptoms of AE require epinephrine, H1- and H2-blockers, and glucocorticoids.
3. Drugs associated with urticaria and AE include radiocontrast agents, opiates, dextran, ACE inhibitors, aspirin and NSAIDs.
4. ACE inhibitors precipitate attacks of AE by directly interfering with the degradation of bradykinin, thereby potentiating its biological effect.

5. Patients with severe symptoms of AE that do not respond to initial treatment in the ED should be admitted to the ICU for close observation and definitive airway management (if necessary).

REFERENCES

[1] Weldon D. Differential diagnosis of angioedema. *Immunol Allergy Clin N Am* 2006;26:603–13.

[2] Temino VM, Peebles RS. The spectrum and treatment of angioedema. *Am J Med* 2008;121:282–6.

[3] Tran TP, Muelleman RL. Allergy, hypersensitivity, and anaphylaxis. In: Marx JA, Hockberger RS, Wall RM, et al. (eds.). *Rosen's Emergency Medicine: Concepts and Clinical Practice*, 6th ed. Philadelphia: Mosby, 2006:1834–5.

[4] Kulthanan K, Jiamton S, Boochangkool K, et al. Angioedema: clinical and etiological aspects. *Clin Dev Immunol* 2007;2007:26438.

[5] Dodds N, Sinert R. Angioedema. eMedicine Website. Available at http://www.emedicine.com/emerg/topic32.htm. Accessed July 6, 2008.

101

Intentional alkali ingestion in a 65-year-old female

HISTORY OF PRESENT ILLNESS

A 65-year-old female with a history of mental illness presented to the ED after consuming two glasses of liquid Drano™ approximately three hours prior to presentation in a suicide attempt. Fifteen minutes after consuming the drain cleaner, the patient developed epigastric pain and difficulty swallowing and called emergency services. On presentation, she complained of sharp epigastric pain rated at a level of 8 (on a scale of 0 to 10), nausea and difficulty swallowing. She denied shortness of breath or throat tightness, or any other co-ingestions.

PHYSICAL EXAMINATION

GENERAL APPEARANCE: The patient was awake and alert and appeared to be in no acute discomfort. She was speaking full sentences in a normal voice, tolerating her secretions.

VITAL SIGNS

Temperature	98°F (36.6°C)
Pulse	80 beats/minute
Blood pressure	145/90 mmHg
Respirations	22 breaths/minute
Oxygen saturation	99% on room air

HEENT: PERRL, EOMI; posterior oropharynx erythema without swelling, exudates or ulcerations.

NECK: Supple, no anterior tenderness to palpation or crepitance.

CARDIOVASCULAR: Regular rate and rhythm without rubs, murmurs or gallops.

LUNGS: Clear to auscultation bilaterally.

ABDOMEN: Soft, nondistended, epigastric tenderness to palpation without rebound or guarding.

RECTAL: Brown stool, hemoccult negative.

EXTREMITIES: No clubbing, cyanosis or edema.

NEUROLOGIC: Nonfocal.

PSYCHIATRIC: Suicidal ideations; denied homicidal ideations, visual or auditory hallucinations.

A peripheral intravenous line was placed, and blood was drawn and sent for laboratory testing. The patient was not allowed to have anything by mouth, and a 1-liter normal saline IV bolus was administered. Laboratory tests revealed a leukocyte count of 19 K/μL (normal 3.5–12.5 K/μL); the remainder of her laboratory tests (including hematocrit, electrolytes, BUN, creatinine, glucose, anion gap, aspirin and acetaminophen levels) were within normal limits.

What is your diagnosis?

ANSWER

The diagnosis is caustic alkali ingestion. The patient was placed on a psychiatric hold in the ED for danger to self, under close supervision for suicide precautions. Gastroenterology was urgently consulted. The patient was transferred to the endoscopy suite, where upper GI endoscopy was performed under procedural sedation. Endoscopy revealed significant edema, hyperemic mucosa and hemorrhagic exudates in the distal esophagus (Figure 101.1), with moderate edema and exudates present in the proximal to mid-esophagus without ulceration. Endoscopy of the stomach also revealed areas of moderate to severe erythema and edema with associated hemorrhagic mucosa, without evidence of ulcerations or erosions.

Following endoscopy, the patient was admitted to the medicine service with suicide precautions and continued close supervision. Intravenous antibiotics (ciprofloxacin and metronidazole) and omeprazole were begun, the patient was not allowed to eat or drink, and she received maintenance IV fluids. The patient's diet was slowly advanced over the next few days. By the time she was transferred to an inpatient psychiatric facility on hospital day #4, she was tolerating a mechanical soft diet without abdominal pain or dysphagia.

Alkali ingestions

Acids and alkalis are known to produce different types of tissue damage. Acids generally cause coagulation necrosis, with eschar formation that may limit substance penetration and injury depth.[11] In contrast, alkalis combine with tissue proteins to cause liquefactive necrosis and saponification, and tend to penetrate deeper into tissues. Additionally, alkali absorption leads to thrombosis of blood vessels, impeding blood flow to already damaged tissue.[1]

From a clinical perspective, exposure to alkali is a relatively common occurrence. In the United States, poison centers receive more than 100,000 calls annually for alkali exposures; nearly one-quarter are evaluated in a health care facility.[2] Overall, alkali injuries remain a leading cause of death from nonpharmaceuticals. Ingestion of a single identified alkali accounts for approximately 1–2% of all poisoning-related deaths reported to poison centers.[2] The most common substances encountered clinically are sodium hydroxide, sodium hypochlorite (bleach), sodium carbonate, phosphate, silica and ammonia. These are found primarily in cleaning products, disinfectants, automatic dishwasher detergents and mildew removal products.[2] Other sources of alkali include Clinitest® tablets, denture cleaning tablets, hair dyes, cement (lime) and alkaline batteries.

Tissue injury from alkali ingestion occurs rapidly; severe injury may occur within minutes of contact.[3] The most severely injured tissues are the squamous epithelial cells of the oropharynx, hypopharynx and esophagus (the most commonly involved organ). The stomach is involved in only 20% of alkali ingestions.[3] Tissue edema occurs immediately and may persist for 48 hours, eventually progressing to airway obstruction. Over time, granulation tissue replaces the necrotic tissue. Mucosal sloughing occurs four to seven days after the initial insult, and is followed by enhanced fibroblast activity.[4] The esophageal wall is weakest 7–21 days after alkali exposure. Symptomatic stricture usually occurs three weeks after the injury, but may present several years later.[4]

ED management of alkali ingestions begins with careful assessment of the airway, breathing and circulation (ABCs). After alkali ingestions, the most important task is to monitor the patient and intervene as necessary to treat complications, such as esophageal perforation. Early endotracheal intubation is warranted when airway compromise is suspected (hoarseness, throat pain, drooling or edema).[5] Intubation should occur early if significant exposure is suspected, before edema and secretions threaten the airway and make intubation difficult or impossible. Patients should have intravenous access and vigorous fluid resuscitation.

In alert patients who are not vomiting and can tolerate liquids, small volumes (1–2 cups) of water or milk are recommended within the first few minutes after ingestion.[5] Because injuries occur almost immediately, later dilution is not warranted. Emesis induction and activated charcoal administration are contraindicated in the treatment of alkali ingestions

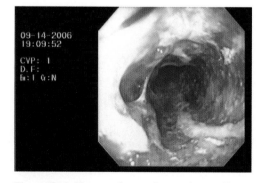
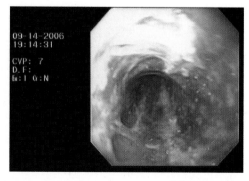

Figure 101.1 Upper endoscopy images from a 65-year-old female after ingesting liquid Drano™ demonstrate significant edema and hyperemic mucosa to the distal and mid-esophagus, along with the presence of hemorrhagic exudates.

because of the likelihood of further injury on re-exposure (emesis) or obscuring findings on endoscopy. Indications for immediate operative intervention include the presence of hemodynamic instability associated with clinical evidence of peritonitis, mediastinitis or massive hemorrhage.[2]

Flexible esophagogastroduodenoscopy (EGD) has been established as a safe and reliable tool for assessing esophageal damage up to 96 hours after caustic ingestion, as long as gentle insufflation of the upper gastrointestinal tract is used during the procedure (to avoid perforation).[1] Only clinical or radiologic suspicion for perforated viscus is a contraindication for EGD. Classifying burn degree by findings on EGD is important for prognosis and management. Generally, patients who have grade 0 (normal) and 1 (mucosal edema or hyperemia) lesions do not develop delayed sequelae, such as stricture or gastric outlet obstruction.[1] These patients with accidental ingestions can be safely discharged home after complete resolution of symptoms and confirmation of their ability to tolerate ingestions of solids and liquids (those with intentional ingestions in an attempt to cause harm still require a psychiatric evaluation). Grade 2a burns involve localized, superficial friability with blisters or ulceration, whereas grade 2b burns involve features of grade 2a burns but with circumferential ulceration. Following a grade 2b burn, stricture incidence may be as high as 71%. After grade 3 burns (necrosis ranging from small, scattered areas to extensive areas), stricture incidence can be as high as 100%.[1]

Although previously felt controversial, steroids are recommended in patients with circumferential esophageal burns and those with strongly suspected injury who cannot undergo endoscopy.[4] Antibiotics should be administered to patients with evidence of perforation or to those receiving steroids.[3,5] Psychiatric consultation should be obtained for any patient presenting with a nonaccidental ingestion in an attempt to cause personal harm. Patients deemed to be a danger to themselves or others, or those who are gravely disabled, should be placed on a psychiatric hold with urgent psychiatric evaluation.

KEY TEACHING POINTS

1. Ingestion of a single identified alkali accounts for approximately 1–2% of all poisoning-related deaths reported to poison centers.
2. Alkalis combine with tissue proteins to cause liquefactive necrosis and saponification, penetrating deep into tissues and leading to thrombosis of blood vessels, impeding blood flow to already damaged tissue.
3. Early endotracheal intubation is warranted when airway compromise is suspected (hoarseness, throat pain, drooling or edema).
4. Indications for immediate surgical intervention in alkali ingestions include the presence of hemodynamic instability associated with clinical evidence of peritonitis, mediastinitis or massive hemorrhage.
5. The gastroenterologist should be consulted early in the management of patients with alkali ingestions for consideration of urgent EGD.
6. Psychiatric consultation should be obtained for any patient presenting with an ingestion in an attempt to cause personal harm.

REFERENCES

[1] Salzman M, O'Malley RN. Updates on the evaluation and management of caustic exposures. *Emerg Med Clin N Am* 2007;25:459–76.

[2] Sivilotti MLA, Ford MD. Alkali ingestions. In: Ford MD, Delany KA, Ling LJ, et al. (eds.). *Ford: Clinical Toxicology*, 1st ed. Philadelphia: Saunders, 2001:1002–7.

[3] Kardon E. Toxicity, caustic ingestions. eMedicine Website. Available at http://www.emedicine.com/emerg/topic86.htm. Accessed June 28, 2008.

[4] Howell JM. Alkaline ingestions. *Ann Emerg Med* 1986; 15:820–5.

[5] Wax PM, Schneider SM. Caustics. In: Marx JA, Hockberger RS, Walls RM, et al. (eds.). *Rosen's Emergency Medicine: Concepts and Clinical Practice*, 6th ed. Philadelphia: Mosby, 2006:2380–5.

102

Symptomatic bradycardia in an 85-year-old female

HISTORY OF PRESENT ILLNESS

An 85-year-old female with a medical history significant for hypertension, congestive heart failure, atrial fibrillation and Alzheimer's dementia was brought to the ED from her skilled nursing facility (SNF) by paramedics following a syncopal episode, at which time she was found to be bradycardic and hypotensive. Her medications included atenolol, digoxin, captopril, aspirin and acetaminophen as needed. Per the nurse at the SNF, the patient was found unresponsive in her wheelchair; she regained consciousness upon being transferred to her bed, but remained somnolent and more confused than her baseline. When the paramedics arrived, they found her bradycardic, with an irregular heart rate ranging from 30–40 beats/minute and a blood pressure of 102/palp. An intravenous line was placed by the paramedics and 1 mg atropine was administered, after which her heart rate increased to 60–70 beats/minute.

PHYSICAL EXAMINATION

GENERAL APPEARANCE: The patient was an elderly, cachectic female who was arousable but confused and slow to respond.

VITAL SIGNS

Temperature	98.5°F (36.9°C)
Pulse	50–60 beats/minute
Blood pressure	113/34 mmHg
Respirations	22 breaths/minute
Oxygen saturation	100% on room air

HEENT: PERRL, EOMI, oropharynx dry.

NECK: Supple, no jugular venous distension.

CARDIOVASCULAR: Bradycardic rate with irregular rhythm, no rubs, murmurs or gallops.

LUNGS: Clear to auscultation bilaterally.

ABDOMEN: Soft, nontender, nondistended.

RECTAL: Normal tone, brown stool, hemoccult negative.

EXTREMITIES: No clubbing, cyanosis or edema.

NEUROLOGIC: Alert, confused, oriented to name only. Patient was able to move all extremities and follow simple commands.

A 12-lead ECG was obtained (Figure 102.1) and the patient was placed on the cardiac monitor. A peripheral intravenous line was placed and blood was drawn and sent for laboratory testing.

What is your diagnosis?

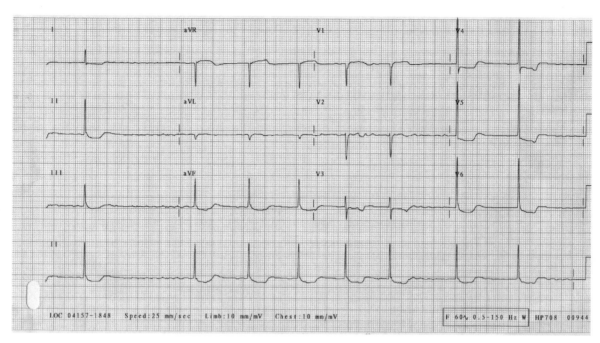

Figure 102.1 12-lead ECG from an 85-year-old female with syncope and altered mental status.

ANSWER

The diagnosis is syncope from bradycardia secondary to digoxin toxicity. The ECG shows atrial fibrillation with ventricular rate of 50 with longer pauses (lead II), narrow QRS complexes with coved, down-sloping ST segments (digitalis effect). The patient's digoxin level was 3.0 ng/mL (normal range 0.9–2.0 ng/mL), potassium was 4.8 mEq/L (normal range 3.5–5.3 mEq/L) and creatinine was 1.1 mg/dL. The patient was admitted to the medicine service, where she received gentle IV hydration and no additional digoxin or atenolol. The following day, the digoxin level was 1.4 ng/mL, and her heart rate and symptoms had improved. She did not require further doses of atropine, nor were digoxin-Fab fragments (Digibind®) administered, as her heart rate remained 50–60 beats/minute with systolic blood pressures consistently above 110 mmHg. The decision was made not to place a pacemaker during this hospitalization based on the patient's advanced dementia. The digoxin and atenolol were withheld indefinitely prior to discharge. The patient remained in atrial fibrillation with a ventricular rate in the 60s, and was discharged back to her SNF with resolution of her symptoms.

Digoxin toxicity

Digoxin is a member of the class of drugs known as cardiac glycosides, which act by inhibiting active transport of Na^+ and K^+ across cell membranes by inhibiting the Na^+/K^+ ATPase (sodium pump). This results in an increase in extracellular K^+ and intracellular Na^+. An increased intracellular Na^+ reduces the transmembrane Na^+ gradient and subsequently increases activity of the Na^+-Ca^{2+} exchanger. In turn, this activity increases the intracellular calcium concentration, which augments myofibril activity in cardiac myocytes resulting in positive inotropy. The cardiac glycosides also increase vagal tone that may lead to direct atrioventricular nodal depression.[1] Therapeutically, digitalis derivatives are used to increase myocardial contractility or slow atrioventricular conduction. However, these actions can result in significant cardiac disturbances and ECG abnormalities in the setting of toxicity.

Digitalis derivatives at therapeutic doses have been associated with several electrocardiographic changes.[1] These findings include the "digitalis effect" (abnormal inverted or flattened T waves coupled with ST-segment depression, frequently described as a sagging or scooped ST segment/T wave complex). These findings are most pronounced in leads with tall R waves. In addition, other findings on ECG with therapeutic doses of digitalis include QT-interval shortening (the result of decreased ventricular repolarization time), PR-interval lengthening (the result of increased vagal activity) and increased U wave amplitude. These electrocardiographic manifestations are also seen with therapeutic digoxin levels and do not correlate with toxicity.

ECG abnormalities with cardiac glycoside toxicity are the result of the propensity for increased automaticity (from increased intracellular calcium) accompanied by slowed conduction through the atrioventricular node. As a result, cardiac glycoside toxicity may result in a wide array of dysrhythmias. Excitant activity (atrial, junctional, ventricular premature beats, tachydysrhythmias and triggered dysrhythmias), suppressant activity (sinus bradycardia, bundle branch blocks, first-, second- and third-degree atrioventricular blocks), or any combination of excitant and suppressant activity (atrial tachycardia with atrioventricular block, second-degree atrioventricular block with junctional premature beats) have been reported.[2–4]

The most common dysrhythmia associated with toxicity induced by these agents is frequent premature ventricular beats. Paroxysmal atrial tachycardia with variable block or accelerated junctional rhythm is highly suggestive of digitalis toxicity. Marked slowing of the ventricular response in a patient with a history of atrial fibrillation on digoxin should suggest the possibility of toxicity.[1]

The ECG may demonstrate findings associated not only with cardiac glycoside toxicity but also with hyperkalemia. Acute digoxin toxicity may be associated with hyperkalemia because the Na^+/K^+ ATPase is inhibited and extracellular K^+ increases. In chronic digoxin toxicity, hyperkalemia may not be seen because the slower extracellular increase in K^+ allows for renal compensation.[1]

Drug-drug interactions are one of the most common causes of digoxin toxicity.[5] Some medications directly increase digoxin plasma levels; other medications alter renal excretion or induce electrolyte abnormalities. For example, clarithromycin, erythromycin and tetracycline have been shown to increase digoxin level by altering the gut flora that is important in digoxin metabolism.[6] Some of the most important drugs causing interaction with digoxin are antiarrhythmic agents. Quinidine, amiodarone and verapamil cause an increase in digoxin levels by reducing its renal clearance.[6]

Pre-hospital care for patients with suspected digoxin toxicity includes supplemental oxygen, cardiac monitoring, IV access, and transport to the nearest ED. Atropine is indicated for symptomatic bradyarrhythmias; lidocaine is indicated for ventricular tachycardia.[5] In the ED, activated charcoal is indicated for acute overdose or accidental ingestions. Bradyarrhythmias that are hemodynamically stable may be treated with observation and discontinuation of the drug. Proper hydration should be ensured to optimize renal clearance of excess drug. Hemodynamically stable supraventricular dysrhythmias may be treated conservatively with observation and discontinuation of digoxin. In the setting of rate-related ischemia or hemodynamic instability, Digibind® (digoxin-Fab fragments) is the treatment of choice.[5]

Hyperkalemia should be treated when K^+ levels are greater than 5.5 mEq/L. Calcium is contraindicated to treat hyperkalemia in the setting of digoxin toxicity because ventricular tachycardia or ventricular fibrillation may be precipitated.[5] Unless the patient is in extremis, other measures should be preferentially used to treat hyperkalemia (e.g., sodium bicarbonate, insulin and glucose, Kayexalate®

or Digibind®). Digoxin-Fab fragments (Digibind®) are generally indicated in digoxin toxicity for dysrhythmias associated with hemodynamic instability, altered mental status attributed to digoxin toxicity, hyperkalemia with K^+ greater than 5 mEq/L, serum digoxin level greater than 10 ng/mL in adults at steady state, or acute ingestion greater than 10 mg in adults (40×0.25 mg tablets) or greater than 0.3 mg/kg in children.[5]

In an acute overdose, the dose of Digibind® given can be calculated using the following equation:

Number of vials = (total amount ingested in mg $\times$ 0.8)/0.5

For example, a patient who overdosed on 30×0.25 mg tablets would receive ($30 \times 0.25 \times 0.8$)/0.5 vials, or 12 vials of Digibind®.[5] (Each vial contains 40 mg digoxin-specific antibody fragments).

In patients presenting with chronic digoxin toxicity, the calculation is:

Number of vials = digoxin level (ng/mL) $\times$ weight(kg)/100

For example, a 50-kg patient with a digoxin level of 5 ng/mL would be given 2.5 vials of Digibind®.[5]

If the amount ingested is unknown or the digoxin level is unavailable, rapid administration of 10 vials is generally adequate to reverse toxicity; a repeat dose with 10 vials is indicated if there is no or partial clinical response.[5] In the setting of chronic toxicity, where the drug level is not immediately available, administration of six vials is generally recommended. The calculated IV dose should be administered over 30 minutes; effects should occur within 30 minutes.[5]

KEY TEACHING POINTS

1. Cardiac glycoside toxicity may result in almost any rhythm disturbance, from premature ventricular beats to third-degree atrioventricular block.
2. Marked slowing of the ventricular response in a patient with a history of atrial fibrillation who is taking digoxin should suggest the possibility of toxicity.
3. Calcium is contraindicated to treat hyperkalemia in the setting of digoxin toxicity because it may precipitate ventricular tachycardia or ventricular fibrillation.
4. It is important to correct electrolyte abnormalities, especially hypokalemia and hypomagnesemia, in patients presenting with digoxin toxicity.
5. Important drug interactions with digoxin include clarithromycin, erythromycin and tetracycline, as well as quinidine, amiodarone and verapamil.
6. Digoxin-Fab fragments (Digibind®) are generally indicated for the following:
   a. Dysrhythmias associated with hemodynamic instability
   b. Altered mental status attributed to digoxin toxicity
   c. Hyperkalemia (K^+ greater than 5 mEq/L)
   d. Serum digoxin level greater than 10 ng/mL in adults at steady state
   e. Ingestion of greater than 10 mg in adults (40×0.25 mg tablets) or greater than 0.3 mg/kg in children.

REFERENCES

[1] Holstege CP, Eldridge DL, Rowden AK. ECG manifestations: the poisoned patient. *Emerg Med Clin N Am* 2006;24: 159–77.
[2] Chen JY, Liu PY, Chen JH, et al. Safety of transvenous temporary cardiac pacing in patients with accidental digoxin overdose and symptomatic bradycardia. *Cardiology* 2004;102:152–5.
[3] Harrigan RA, Perron AD, Brady WJ. Atrioventricular dissociation. *Am J Emerg Med* 2001;19:218–22.
[4] Behringer W, Sterz F, Domanovits H, et al. Percutaneous cardiopulmonary bypass for therapy resistant cardiac arrest from digoxin overdose. *Resuscitation* 1998;37:47–50.
[5] Schreiber D. Toxicity, digitalis. eMedicine Website. Available at http://www.emedicine.com/emerg/topic137.htm. Accessed July 7, 2008.
[6] Prybus KM. Deadly drug interactions in emergency medicine. *Emerg Med Clin N Am* 2004;22:845–63.

PART XIII

MISCELLANEOUS

103

Bilateral leg swelling in a 30-year-old male

HISTORY OF PRESENT ILLNESS

A 30-year-old male with no significant medical history presented to the ED complaining of three days of bilateral leg swelling that had progressed up his thighs, as well as facial and hand swelling. The face and hand swelling had resolved, but the leg swelling remained. He denied shortness of breath, chest pain, cough, fevers, chills, dysuria, hematuria, decreased urination, recent sore throat or abdominal pain. He denied similar episodes in the past. He took no medications. He denied alcohol or illicit drug use, and smoked three cigarettes per day. Family history was significant for hypertension. His fluid and food intake were reported as normal.

PHYSICAL EXAMINATION

GENERAL APPEARANCE: The patient appeared well developed, well hydrated and in no acute discomfort.

VITAL SIGNS

Temperature	98.2°F (36.8°C)
Heart rate	84 beats/minute
Blood pressure	160/113 mmHg
Respiratory rate	18 breaths/minute
Oxygen saturation	97% on room air

HEENT: Unremarkable.

NECK: Supple, no jugular venous distention.

CARDIOVASCULAR: Regular rate and rhythm without rubs, murmurs or gallops.

LUNGS: Clear to auscultation bilaterally without rales, rhonchi or wheezes.

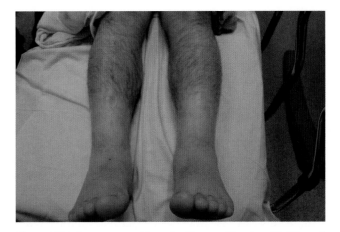

Figure 103.1 Lower extremities of a 30-year-old male with bilateral leg swelling for three days.

ABDOMEN: Soft, nontender, nondistended.

EXTREMITIES: Examination of the hands and face did not reveal edema, whereas examination of the lower extremities demonstrated pitting edema from the feet up through the pre-tibial region to the knees bilaterally (Figure 103.1). Mild edema was noted to the mid-thighs bilaterally.

A peripheral intravenous line was placed, and blood was sent for laboratory testing. While awaiting the laboratory test results, a clear, yellow urine sample was obtained, and a bedside dipstick reagent test demonstrated 4+ protein.

What is your diagnosis?

The diagnosis is nephrotic syndrome. Laboratory tests results were significant for a serum total protein of 3.9 g/dL (normal 6.3–8.2 g/dL) and serum albumin of 1.6 g/dL (normal 3.4–4.8 g/dL). The blood urea nitrogen, creatinine and electrolytes (including potassium) were within normal limits. The urinalysis demonstrated 600 mg/dL protein (range 0–9 mg/dL). The nephrologist was consulted and the recommendation was made to start the patient on furosemide 20 mg orally daily, with follow up in nephrology clinic the following day. The patient's lower extremity edema improved dramatically following initiation of furosemide, and a kidney biopsy performed two weeks after initial presentation demonstrated minimal change nephrotic syndrome (MCNS). The patient was prescribed steroid therapy (prednisone), with close follow up arranged with the nephrologist.

Nephrotic syndrome and minimal change disease

Nephrotic syndrome is characterized by the presence of proteinuria greater than 3.5 g/day/1.73 m^2, with accompanying edema, hypoalbuminemia, hypertension and hyperlipidemia.[1] It leads to a multitude of other sequelae, such as predisposition to systemic infection and hypercoagulability. In general, the diseases associated with nephrotic syndrome cause chronic kidney dysfunction, but only rarely cause acute renal failure.[1] Acute renal failure may be seen with minimal change disease, HIV-associated nephropathy and bilateral renal vein thrombosis. The causes of nephrotic syndrome can be divided into primary and secondary causes.[2] The causes of idiopathic (primary) nephrotic syndrome (in decreasing order of prevalence) are focal and segmental glomerulosclerosis, membranous nephropathy, minimal change disease and membranoproliferative glomerulonephritis.[1] Secondary causes include diabetic nephropathy, amyloidosis and systemic lupus erythematosus (SLE) with membranous nephropathy. Of these, diabetic nephropathy is the most prevalent cause of nephrotic proteinuria and end-stage renal disease in the United States.[1]

Minimal change nephropathy is responsible for 90% of nephrotic syndrome in children and about 20% in adults.[3] Clinical onset is usually abrupt, and the glomeruli are normal on light microscopy. Fusion of epithelial foot processes may be identified on electron microscopy.[3] Nephrotic syndrome may also be caused by a wide range of relatively rare diseases (e.g., amyloidosis, SLE, various infections including HIV and preeclampsia), as well as malignancy and drugs (e.g.,

probenecid, captopril, lithium, warfarin, penicillamine).[2,3] Edema, the predominant clinical feature, is ultimately the result of urinary loss of large amounts of albumin from the serum with a consequent lowering of the serum albumin concentration.[4] Definitive diagnosis of the cause of nephrotic syndrome is made by renal biopsy (which can be performed on an outpatient basis following initiation of treatment). Initial treatment of patients with nephrotic syndrome should include loop diuretics (furosemide) in consultation with a nephrologist. Adults with MCNS are treated initially with steroids (1 mg/kg/day) but respond more slowly than children; approximately 25% of adults fail to respond within three to four months.[3] Patients who frequently relapse or are dependent on steroids should be treated with cyclophosphamide, as this agent has been shown to result in long-term remission without the side affects inherent to chronic steroid therapy.[3]

KEY TEACHING POINTS

1. Nephrotic syndrome is characterized by the presence of proteinuria, with accompanying edema, hypoalbuminemia, hypertension and hyperlipidemia.
2. Evaluation of the urine by a simple urine dipstick in the ED provides qualitative information on the amount of protein in the urine. This offers preliminary evidence (along with history, physical examination and further laboratory testing) of nephrotic syndrome.
3. The causes of idiopathic nephrotic syndrome include focal and segmental glomerulosclerosis, membranous nephropathy, minimal change disease and membranoproliferative glomerulonephritis.
4. Definitive diagnosis of the cause of nephrotic syndrome is made by renal biopsy.
5. Treatment of minimal change nephrotic syndrome includes initiation of loop diuretics and steroids, in consultation with a nephrologist.

REFERENCES

[1] Bazari H. Approach to the patient with renal disease. In: Goldman L, Ausiello D (eds.). *Cecil Medicine*, 23rd ed. Philadelphia: Saunders, 2007:812.
[2] Orth SR, Ritz E. Medical progress: the nephrotic syndrome. *N Engl J Med* 1998;338:1202–11.
[3] Mason PD, Pusey CD. Glomerulonephritis: diagnosis and treatment. *Brit Med J* 1994;309:1557–63.
[4] Travis L. Nephrotic syndrome. eMedicine Website. Available at http://www.emedicine.com/ped/topic1564.htm. Accessed June 29, 2008.

104

Headache and bruising in a 33-year-old female

HISTORY OF PRESENT ILLNESS

A 33-year-old female presented to the ED complaining of several days of a constant, severe headache and bruising to her extremities. Her headache was throbbing, located over the forehead, rated at a level of 8 (on a scale of 0 to 10), and not relieved with acetaminophen. She reported associated nausea without vomiting and fatigue, but denied fevers, neck stiffness, photophobia, visual changes, focal numbness or weakness. She also noted bruising and small, red dots to her arms and legs for the past week. She denied any bleeding episodes. Her last normal menstrual period was three weeks earlier.

PHYSICAL EXAMINATION

GENERAL APPEARANCE: The patient appeared well nourished, well hydrated and in no acute discomfort.

VITAL SIGNS

Temperature	99.5°F (37.5°C)
Pulse	102 beats/minute
Blood pressure	120/82 mmHg
Respirations	18 breaths/minute
Oxygen saturation	100% on room air

HEENT: PERRL, EOMI, pale conjunctivae, oropharynx pink and moist.

NECK: Supple, no meningeal signs.

CARDIOVASCULAR: Tachycardic rate, regular rhythm without rubs, murmurs or gallops.

LUNGS: Clear to auscultation bilaterally.

ABDOMEN: Soft, nontender, nondistended.

EXTREMITIES: No clubbing, cyanosis or edema; small areas of ecchymosis on the upper and lower extremities, as well as areas of petechiae more prominent on the lower extremities (Figure 104.1).

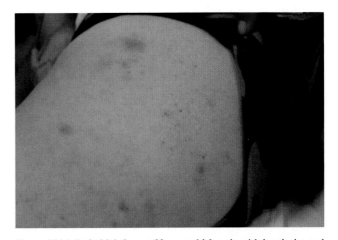

Figure 104.1 Left thigh from a 33-year-old female with headache and bruising.

NEUROLOGIC: Alert and oriented to person, place and time; cranial nerves II–XII grossly intact; upper and lower extremity strength 5/5 bilaterally, proximally and distally; no pronator drift, finger-to-nose intact, normal gait.

A peripheral intravenous line was placed, and blood was drawn and sent for laboratory testing. A noncontrast CT scan of the brain did not demonstrate an acute bleed or ischemic changes. Laboratory tests were significant for a hematocrit of 21% (normal 34–46%) with schistocytes on a peripheral smear, platelet count of 15,000/µL (normal 140,000–400,000/µL), total bilirubin of 3.4 mg/dL (normal 0.2–1.3 mg/dL) and lactate dehydrogenase (LDH) of 4151 U/L (normal 313–618 U/L). The fibrinogen, prothrombin time (PT) and activated partial thromboplastin time (aPTT) were all within normal limits, and a serum pregnancy test was negative.

What is your diagnosis?

ANSWER

The diagnosis is thrombotic thrombocytopenic purpura (TTP). The patient was admitted to the ICU. Hematology was consulted, and the patient received a transfusion of fresh frozen plasma as well as prednisone 60 mg orally. Plasmapheresis was initiated the following day, and continued on a daily basis. By hospital day #5, the patient's hematocrit and platelet count had normalized to 35% and 162,000/μL, respectively, and the LDH was 817 U/L (normal range 313–618 U/L), with dramatic improvement in her symptoms. She was discharged on hospital day #8 with close follow up arranged, and instructed to continue prednisone 60 mg daily.

Thrombotic thrombocytopenic purpura

Thrombotic thrombocytopenic purpura (TTP) is a life-threatening disease characterized by thrombocytopenia, microangiopathic hemolytic anemia, fluctuating neurologic signs, renal failure and fever. The condition is rare, with an annual incidence of 3.7 cases per million adults.[1] It is seen predominantly in females, usually between 30 and 40 years of age. Untreated, TTP has a mortality rate of 90%.[2] Neurologic and hemorrhagic presentations are the most common.

The pathogenesis of TTP is attributed to the presence of unusually large von Willebrand factor (vWF) multimers that lead to platelet clumping and subsequent microvascular thrombosis.[1] Normally, vWF circulates in plasma as large multimers that allow platelets to adhere to vascular surfaces. These are cleaved into smaller units by ADAMTS-13, a zinc-containing metalloproteinase (also known as von Willebrand factor-cleaving protease).[3] If ADAMTS-13 is lacking, the very high-molecular-weight vWF multimers accumulate, causing platelet agglutination and vascular occlusion that results in the manifestations of TTP.[3] TTP is mostly idiopathic but may be triggered by clinical situations such as bacterial or viral infections, pregnancy, drugs (e.g., clopidogrel, ticlopidine, quinine, cyclosporine) and autoimmune disorders, such as systemic lupus erythematosus, thyroiditis and antiphospholipid syndrome.[1]

The most common symptoms of TTP at presentation are nonspecific, and include abdominal pain, nausea, vomiting and weakness.[4] Neurologic abnormalities range from headache, confusion, and somnolence to focal deficits and coma.[2] Hemorrhagic presentations such as purpura, epistaxis, hemoptysis and gastrointestinal bleeding are often seen because thrombocytopenia (84%) is a frequent finding.[2] Fever is present at admission in approximately 50% of patients but may develop in additional cases during the course.[5] A temperature greater than 102°F (38.9°C) and chills suggests infection rather than TTP.[4] Patients may have renal abnormalities, including oligoanuria, acute renal failure, albuminuria and microscopic hematuria.[1]

The key diagnostic clues to this condition are from laboratory evaluation. The presence of both anemia and thrombocytopenia (platelet count less than 50,000/μL) in the absence of leukopenia suggests the diagnosis.[4] The following evidence of microangiopathic hemolytic anemia provides support (but is not specific) for the diagnosis: fragmented red cells (schistocytes) and polychromatophilic red cells (reticulocytes), increased serum levels of LDH and indirect-reacting bilirubin, and a negative direct Coombs' test.[4] Routine coagulation tests are usually normal, although slight increases in D-dimer, fibrin degradation products and thrombin-antithrombin (TAT) complexes may be seen.[6] However, in the case of severe or protracted episodes, secondary disseminated intravascular coagulation (DIC) may occur as a result of overactivation of the coagulation pathway.[6]

Plasma exchange is the treatment of choice for TTP. Approximately 80% of patients who are treated aggressively with exchange plasmapheresis survive the initial episode of TTP.[5] Platelet transfusion should be avoided because bleeding complications are uncommon in TTP, and marked deterioration in neurologic status has been reported in association with platelet transfusions.[5] The effectiveness of plasma exchange has been attributed to the removal of ADAMTS-13 autoantibodies and replacement of ADAMTS-13 activity.[4] However, plasma exchange seems to be effective for patients who do not have a severe deficiency of ADAMTS-13 activity. Daily plasma exchange should be continued until the platelet count is normal.[4] LDH levels, which reflect tissue ischemia as well as hemolysis, also serve as markers of response to treatment.[4] Although benefit has been demonstrated with high-dose plasma infusions for the treatment of TTP, problems can arise with volume overload if the patient develops renal insufficiency.[5] Plasma infusion should be reserved for two situations: if plasma exchange cannot be started promptly, and for patients with severe or refractory disease between plasma exchange sessions.[5]

The use of glucocorticoids in patients with TTP is based on clinical experience and case series alone. Clinical trials have not been carried out to guide the use of immunosuppressive agents in treating TTP. Thus, although widely used, only weak recommendations for these agents in TTP treatment exist.[4,5] Finally, relapses are rare in patients with TTP, except in those with a severe deficiency of ADAMTS-13 activity; half of such patients may have a relapse, most within a year.[4]

KEY TEACHING POINTS

1. Thrombotic thrombocytopenic purpura (TTP) is characterized by the pentad of thrombocytopenia, microangiopathic hemolytic anemia, fluctuating neurologic signs, renal failure and fever.

2. The most common symptoms of TTP at presentation are nonspecific, including abdominal pain, nausea, vomiting, weakness and neurologic abnormalities (e.g., headache, confusion, somnolence, focal deficits and coma).

3. Laboratory findings providing evidence of TTP include thrombocytopenia (platelet count less than 50,000/μL), microangiopathic hemolytic anemia, elevated LDH and indirect-reacting bilirubin, and a negative direct Coombs' test.

4. Plasma exchange is the treatment of choice for TTP; approximately 80% of patients treated aggressively with exchange plasmapheresis survive the initial episode of TTP.
5. Patients with TTP should not be treated with platelet transfusions because bleeding complications are uncommon in TTP and marked deterioration in neurologic status has been reported in association with platelet transfusions.

REFERENCES

[1] Aksay E, Kiyan S, Ersel M, et al. Thrombotic thrombocytopenic purpura mimicking acute ischemic stroke. *Emerg Med J* 2006;23:e51.

[2] Bridgman J, Witting M. Thrombotic thrombocytopenic purpura presenting as sudden headache with focal neurologic findings. *Ann Emerg Med* 1996;27:95–7.

[3] Crowther MA, George JN. Thrombotic thrombocytopenic purpura: 2008 update. *Clev Clin J Med* 2008;75:369–75.

[4] George JN. Thrombotic thrombocytopenic purpura. *N Engl J Med* 2006;354:1927–35.

[5] Tsai HM. Thrombotic thrombocytopenia purpura: a thrombotic disorder caused by ADAMTS13 deficiency. *Hematol Oncol Clin N Am* 2007;21:609–32.

[6] Franchini M. Thrombotic microangiopathies: an update. *Hematology* 2006;11:139–46.

105

Total body rash in a 33-year-old male

HISTORY OF PRESENT ILLNESS

A 33-year-old male with a medical history significant for gout and Stevens-Johnson syndrome at the age of 20 secondary to allopurinol presented to the ED complaining of a red and irritating rash on his face, torso and extremities for the past six days. The patient had been started on probenecid for gout one month earlier. The patient stopped taking the probenecid when his rash began. He was seen by his primary care provider two days prior to presentation to the ED, and started on prednisone 40 mg orally daily, hydroxyzine 10 mg orally daily and fluocinonide 0.05% cream to affected areas twice per day. One day prior to arrival, the rash worsened with increased redness, irritation and itching, and the patient also developed mild throat tightness. He denied shortness of breath, wheezing, difficulty swallowing, abdominal pain, nausea, lightheadedness or dizziness.

PHYSICAL EXAMINATION

GENERAL APPEARANCE: The patient was a well-developed, well-nourished male, alert and in no acute distress.

VITAL SIGNS

Temperature	100.1°F (37.8°C)
Pulse	130 beats/minute
Blood pressure	140/90 mmHg
Respirations	22 breaths/minute
Oxygen saturation	100% on room air

HEENT: Facial erythema and mild swelling; conjunctivae clear without erythema or discharge; no oral lesions, erythema or uvular swelling in the oropharynx.

CARDIOVASCULAR: Tachycardic, regular rate without rubs, murmurs or gallops.

LUNGS: Clear to auscultation bilaterally without wheezes.

ABDOMEN: Soft, nontender, nondistended, active bowel sounds present.

EXTREMITIES: No clubbing, cyanosis or edema.

SKIN: Red, raised papules at the distal extremities that coalesced into red macules present on the upper extremities, trunk, back, neck and face. The skin was warm to touch and mildly tender to palpation. No blisters were noted (Figure 105.1).

What is your diagnosis?

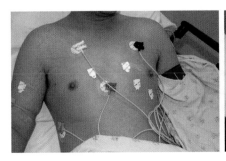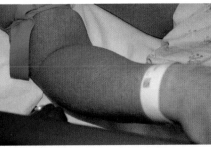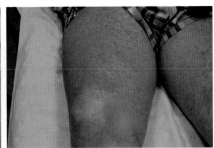

Figure 105.1 A 33-year-old male with a rash for six days.

ANSWER

The diagnosis is morbilliform drug eruption. The patient received epinephrine 0.3 mL of a 1:1000 dilution subcutaneously, Solu-Medrol® 125 mg, ranitidine 50 mg and Benadryl® 50 mg intravenously in the ED. The patient experienced mild improvement in symptoms following administration of these medications. Laboratory tests were significant for a leukocyte count of 13.6 K/µL (normal range 3.5–12.5 K/µL) with a differential of 83% neutrophils, 6% lymphocytes, 7% monocytes and 4% eosinophils. The electrolytes, creatinine and glucose were within normal limits. The patient was observed overnight in the ED with continuation of steroids and antihistamines and discharged to the dermatology clinic the following morning. A punch biopsy of the affected skin was obtained that demonstrated a superficial perivascular lymphohistiocytic infiltrate with eosinophils, consistent with a dermal hypersensitivity reaction as can be seen in a drug reaction. The patient was continued on a prednisone taper, triamcinolone ointment and hydroxyzine as an outpatient, with close follow up in dermatology arranged. The rash resolved completely over the next two weeks.

Drug eruptions

In cases of adverse drug reactions involving the skin, it is important for the clinician to distinguish between self-limited exanthematous drug eruptions and more severe presentations of drug reactions. Examples of severe drug eruptions include DRESS syndrome (drug rash with eosinophilia and systemic symptoms), Stevens-Johnson syndrome (SJS) or toxic epidermal necrolysis (TEN). These are associated with significant mortality and may necessitate treatment beyond just the withdrawal of the inciting medication.[1] Morbilliform (exanthematous) eruptions most often start 7–14 days after initiation of a new medication. These are composed primarily of erythematous macules and papules that are symmetrically distributed on the trunk and extremities, with coalescence of the lesions over the course of several days.[1] Fever, facial involvement, or pruritus may or may not be present, and resolution of the skin lesions within one to two weeks after recognition and discontinuation of the offending drug is generally seen.

Although any medication is capable of causing a morbilliform drug eruption, beta-lactam antibiotics are the most commonly implicated agents.[1,2] Skin biopsy of morbilliform drug eruptions is nonspecific, but may reveal perivascular inflammation composed of lymphocytes and eosinophils (though eosinophils are not always present). Treatment consists of symptom control with topical corticosteroids and systemic antihistamines for pruritus. Systemic steroids are frequently given on the presumption that this will expedite resolution of the rash; however, no randomized trials have been done to assess the efficacy of such therapy.[1]

DRESS syndrome describes a severe systemic drug reaction. The most common causal medications are certain anti-convulsants (phenytoin, carbamazepine and phenobarbital), sulfonamides, allopurinol, azathioprine, dapsone, minocycline, terbinafine, gold salts and antiviral agents (abacavir, efavirenz and nevirapine).[3,4] Patients typically present with a morbilliform rash that can progress to erythroderma two to six weeks after onset of the new medication, much later than the onset of other types of drug reactions. Diffuse exfoliation can occur following the erythroderma.[4] Facial edema may progress to widespread diffuse edema. Although the edema may lead to the formation of bullae, there is a negative Nikolsky's sign and epidermal necrosis typical of TEN is not seen. Mucosal involvement, elevated liver enzymes, and thyroid, renal, pulmonary and cardiac abnormalities are often noted. Lymphadenopathy occurs in 75% of cases, whereas the most characteristic finding that helps differentiate DRESS from other forms of cutaneous drug eruptions is the presence of eosinophilia in the peripheral leukocyte count (present in 70% of cases).[4] Evaluation of a patient for DRESS syndrome should include a thorough drug history, chest radiograph to evaluate for pulmonary involvement, assessment for lymphadenopathy and laboratory tests (CBC, liver enzymes, BUN, creatinine and urinalysis). Treatment of DRESS syndrome includes oral and topical corticosteroids, which improve the rash, fevers and systemic abnormalities.[4]

The spectrum of severe cutaneous adverse reactions, which may represent variants of the same disease process, includes SJS and TEN. Key components of both SJS and TEN include epidermal detachment, fever, skin tenderness, and erythema and erosions of mucous membranes (genital, ocular, oral and respiratory).[1] Classically, SJS and TEN often present with prodromal symptoms, such as malaise, rhinitis, odynophagia, myalgias and arthralgias, which may often be mistaken for a viral syndrome.[5] This prodromal state may last up to two weeks, and is followed by the abrupt development of a macular rash that may or may not be "targetoid" (as classically described). This macular exanthem generally starts centrally, then spreads to the extremities. The exanthem becomes confluent and significant dermal-epidermal dissociation ensues, resulting in a positive Nikolsky's sign (denudation with shear stress).[5]

Differentiation between cases of SJS and TEN depends on the nature of the skin lesions and extent of body surface area involvement.[6] SJS is diagnosed when the extent of involvement is less than 10%; TEN is diagnosed when the body surface area (BSA) involved is greater than 30%.[5] The incidence of SJS runs anywhere between 1.1–7.1 cases per million person-years, with a mean age of patients between 25–47 years.[5] Older age is associated with an increased degree of skin loss. Mortality has been reported at less than 5% in SJS, and as high as 50% for TEN.[5] The most frequent drugs cited as causes for SJS and TEN are anticonvulsants, sulfonamides, nonsteroidal anti-inflammatory drugs (especially piroxicam) and allopurinol.[6] Treatment of patients with SJS and TEN involves discontinuation of the offending medication and early transfer to a burn unit, where experienced personnel can care for the patient to prevent electrolyte abnormalities and infections that may occur as a result of an impaired cutaneous barrier.[1] Although various anecdotal treatments have been reported (e.g., plasmapheresis, cyclophosphamide, tumor necrosis factor-alpha, systemic corticosteroids, intravenous immunoglobulin [IVIG]), data from large randomized trials providing evidence of these treatments efficacies is lacking.

KEY TEACHING POINTS

1. Along the spectrum of cutaneous drug reactions, the morbilliform or exanthematous drug eruption is the most common and the least severe, with essentially no associated risk of death, and little morbidity.
2. The typical manifestations of DRESS (drug rash with eosinophilia and systemic symptoms) syndrome include persistent fever, elevated liver enzymes, atypical lymphocytosis or peripheral eosinophilia, facial edema and diffuse morbilliform patches that can progress to vesicles, bullae and erythroderma.
3. Key components of both Stevens-Johnson syndrome (SJS) and toxic epidermal necrolysis (TEN) include epidermal detachment, fever, skin tenderness, and erythema and erosions of mucous membranes (genital, ocular, oral and respiratory).
4. The most frequent drugs cited as causes for SJS and TEN are anticonvulsants, sulfonamides, nonsteroidal anti-inflammatory drugs and allopurinol.
5. Treatment of patients with SJS and TEN involves discontinuation of the offending medication, careful fluid and electrolyte management, and early transfer to a burn unit.

REFERENCES

[1] Cotliar J. Approach to the patient with a suspected drug eruption. *Semin Cutan Med Surg* 2007;26:147–54.
[2] Nigen S, Knowles SR, Shear NH. Drug eruptions: approaching the diagnosis of drug-induced skin diseases. *J Drug Dermatol* 2003;2:278–99.
[3] Bachot N, Roujeau JC. Differential diagnosis of severe cutaneous drug eruptions. *Am J Clin Dermato* 2003;l 4:561–72.
[4] Hughey LC. Fever and erythema in the emergency room. *Semin Cutan Med Surg* 2007;26:133–8.
[5] Browne BJ, Edwards B, Rogers RL. Dermatologic emergencies. *Prim Care Clin Office Pract* 2006;33:685–95.
[6] Knowles SR, Shear NH. Recognition and management of severe cutaneous drug reactions. *Dermatol Clin* 2007;25:245–53.

106

Bleeding gums and fatigue in a 40-year-old female

HISTORY OF PRESENT ILLNESS

A 40-year-old female with a history of hypothyroidism, status-post radioactive iodine treatment for Plummer's disease, and thymoma presented to the ED with two weeks of bleeding from her gums after dental cleaning. On further history, she reported abnormal vaginal bleeding. The patient also complained of increasing fatigue, shortness of breath and bilateral lower extremity swelling, as well as an unintentional 10-lb (4.5-kg) weight loss over the prior two months. She had also been experiencing fevers and sweats, as well as a rash on her legs. She denied recent travel, sick contacts or starting any new medications.

PHYSICAL EXAMINATION

GENERAL APPEARANCE: The patient appeared pale, diaphoretic and ill, was awake and alert but in no acute discomfort.

VITAL SIGNS

Temperature	100°F (37.8°C)
Pulse	108 beats/minute
Blood pressure	109/71 mmHg
Respirations	22 breaths/minute
Oxygen saturation	97% on room air

HEENT: Right pupil 3 mm, left pupil 4 mm, both reactive to light and accommodation, EOMI, oropharynx dry with gingival hyperplasia, no lesions, punctate areas of bleeding on gingivae.

NECK: Supple, no jugular venous distension, no meningeal signs, anterior cervical lymphadenopathy noted.

CARDIOVASCULAR: Tachycardic rate, regular rhythm, II/VI holosystolic murmur at left upper sternal border.

LUNGS: Clear to auscultation bilaterally.

ABDOMEN: Soft, nontender, nondistended.

EXTREMITIES: No clubbing or cyanosis, 2+ pitting edema to lower extremities up to knees bilaterally.

SKIN: Petechia on bilateral lower extremities.

NEUROLOGIC: Nonfocal.

The patient was placed on the cardiac monitor, a peripheral intravenous line was started, and blood was drawn and sent for laboratory tests and cultures. An arterial blood gas performed on room air demonstrated a pH of 7.47 (normal 7.35–7.45), pCO_2 of 33 mmHg (normal 35–48 mmHg), pO_2 of 31 (normal 80–95), bicarbonate of 24 (normal 23–28) and base excess of 0.6 (normal −2.4 to +2.3), with a derived oxygen saturation of 52%.

What is your diagnosis?

ANSWER

The diagnosis is acute myelogenous leukemia (AML) with blast crisis and leukostasis. The complete blood count revealed a leukocyte count of 377 K/μL (normal 3.5–12.5 K/μL) with 92% blast cells, 1% neutrophils and hematocrit of 20% (normal 34–46%) with 53,000 platelets/μL (normal 140,000–400,000 platelets/μL). Additional labs revealed a troponin I of 0.20 ng/mL (normal 0.00–0.09 ng/mL) and INR of 1.6 (normal range 0.8–1.2), with electrolytes, BUN, creatinine and glucose within normal limits. A transfusion of packed red blood cells was started in the ED. A bone marrow biopsy performed 12 hours after admission revealed marrow replacement by blastic cells with 100% cellularity, with flow cytometry of the aspirate demonstrating myeloid lineage (acute myelogenous leukemia).

Shortly after the biopsy was performed, the patient began vomiting and became acutely altered. A noncontrast CT of the brain was performed emergently, demonstrating multifocal areas of coalescent, ill-defined, high attenuation abnormalities in the right superior and posterior frontal-parietal white matter, consistent with parenchymal hemorrhage (Figure 106.1). Significant mass effect was noted on the right lateral ventricle, with midline shift from left to right about 5 mm.

The patient was intubated for airway protection, and a post-intubation chest radiograph was obtained (Figure 106.2), demonstrating diffuse, bilateral patchy infiltrates. A neurology consultation was obtained for evaluation and prognosis. Neurologic examination at this time demonstrated no localization to physical stimuli, bilateral dilated and unreactive pupils, absence of doll's eyes and right corneal reflex, and a Babinski's sign present on the right. Neurologic diagnosis was herniation syndrome resulting from cumulative mass effect of intracranial hemorrhage. In the context of coagulopathy, this has a grave prognosis. The decision was made by the family to withdraw support, and the patient expired a short time thereafter.

Acute myelogenous leukemia and leukostasis

Acute myelogenous leukemia (AML) is a malignant disease of the bone marrow in which hematopoietic precursors are

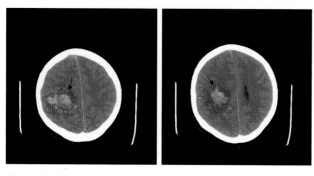

Figure 106.1 Noncontrast CT of the brain in a 40-year-old female diagnosed with acute myelogenous leukemia with blast crisis and leukostasis, demonstrating intraparenchymal hemorrhages (arrows).

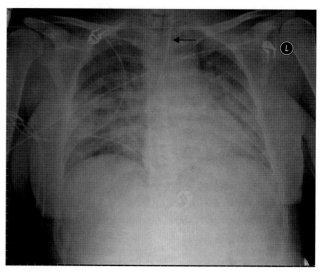

Figure 106.2 Chest radiograph from a 40-year-old female with acute myelogenous leukemia following intubation for airway protection (arrow indicates endotracheal tube).

arrested in an early stage of development.[1] Most AML subtypes are distinguished from other related blood disorders by the presence of more than 20% blasts in the bone marrow. The underlying pathophysiology consists of a maturational arrest of bone marrow cells in the earliest stages of development. The mechanism of arrest in many cases involves the activation of abnormal genes through chromosomal translocations and other genetic abnormalities.[1] There are approximately 10,500 new cases of AML each year; this incidence has remained stable over the past decade.[2] AML causes approximately 1.2% of all cancer deaths in the United States. It is primarily a disease of adulthood, with a mean age at diagnosis of 63 years; the incidence is increasing with age.[2]

The presenting signs and symptoms of AML are nonspecific, related to decreased production of normal hematopoietic cells and invasion of other organs by leukemic cells.[2] Some patients, particularly younger ones, present with acute symptoms over a few days to one to two weeks. Others have longer courses, with fatigue or other symptoms lasting from weeks to months. Symptoms of bone marrow failure are related to anemia, neutropenia and thrombocytopenia.[1] The most common symptom of anemia is fatigue.[2] Other symptoms of anemia include dyspnea on exertion, dizziness and, in patients with coronary artery disease, anginal chest pain.[1,2] Patients often have decreased neutrophil levels despite an increased total white blood cell (WBC) count. Patients may present with fever, with or without specific documentation of infection.[1,2] Patients with low absolute neutrophil counts (i.e., less than 500 cells/μL) have the highest risk of infection.

Patients may present with oozing from the gums, epistaxis, and excessive bleeding after dental procedures or minor trauma.[2] Bleeding may be caused by thrombocytopenia, coagulopathy resulting from DIC or both. Alternatively, symptoms may be the result of organ infiltration with leukemic cells. The most common sites of infiltration include the spleen, liver and gums.[1] Infiltration occurs most commonly in patients with the monocytic subtypes of AML. Gingivitis due to neutropenia can cause swollen gums, and thrombocytopenia can cause the gums to bleed.[1]

Patients with markedly elevated WBC counts (more than 100,000 cells/μL) can present with symptoms of leukostasis (i.e., respiratory distress and altered mental status).[1,2] Leukostasis is a medical emergency that requires immediate intervention. In patients with hematologic malignancies, the extremely high number of WBCs can result in hyperviscosity syndromes, as these cells are not easily deformable. They accumulate in capillaries, impairing normal function.[3–5] Anemia that accompanies many hematologic malignancies often compensates for increased viscosity due to the increased WBC count; this may account for the relative infrequency of leukostasis despite many patients with markedly elevated WBC counts.

Leukostasis is more common in acute leukemias than in chronic leukemias, with an incidence ranging from 5–13% in adult AML and 10–30% in adult acute lymphoblastic leukemia (ALL).[5] Symptoms and signs are nonspecific but usually indicate pulmonary and neurologic pathology – dyspnea, tachypnea, hypoxia, lethargy and slurred speech. WBC counts are most often greater than 100,000 (hyperleukocytosis). Even in the setting of hypoxia, a chest radiograph can be normal or show relatively unimpressive diffuse nonspecific opacities.[5] "Leukocyte larceny" can occur (pseudohypoxemia), a phenomenon of artificially low pO_2 on ABG due to markedly increased O_2 consumption by malignant leukocytes.[5] In these instances, pulse oximetry is often a better measure of oxygenation.

Pulmonary and neurologic complications are the most serious and most common causes of morbidity and mortality in leukostasis – respiratory failure, intracranial hemorrhage and coma.[3–5] Pulmonary leukostasis occurs as a result of leukocyte thrombi and plugging of pulmonary microvascular channels, leading to vascular rupture, pulmonary hemorrhage and infiltration of the lung parenchyma.[2] Intracranial hemorrhage associated with leukostasis is often multiple and intraparenchymal.[6] Hyperviscosity occurs as a result of leukostasis, and leukemic blasts plug thin-walled cerebral vessels, which results in the formation of leukemic nodules, hypoxic vasodilatation and rupture of cerebral vessels.[6,7]

Leukostasis is considered an oncologic emergency, with mortality rates as high as 40% if untreated.[5] The immediate goals of treatment after stabilization of the airway, breathing and circulation (ABCs) is to reduce the number of circulating malignant WBCs. This is done by induction chemotherapy (e.g., initiating treatment of AML), hydroxyurea (inhibits DNA synthesis of malignant cells) or leukapheresis (removal of WBCs from the circulation by a filtration machine).[5] Definitive cytoreductive therapy (chemotherapy) must be administered within a short time of leukapheresis, as malignant cells can rapidly replicate, rendering leukapheresis ineffective.

KEY TEACHING POINTS

1. Bleeding gums in a patient may be a sign of thrombocytopenia or disseminated intravascular coagulation from undiagnosed AML with blast crisis.
2. Leukostasis (WBC counts greater than 100,000) is a medical emergency requiring immediate intervention; it has a mortality rate as high as 40%.
3. The immediate goal in patients with AML blast crisis and leukostasis is aggressive stabilization of the ABCs.
4. Once the ABCs are stabilized, the immediate therapeutic goal in patients with leukostasis from AML is to reduce the number of circulating malignant WBCs by induction chemotherapy, hydroxyurea or leukapheresis.

REFERENCES

[1] Seiter K. Acute myelogenous leukemia. eMedicine Website. Available at http://www.emedicine.com/med/topic34.htm. Accessed June 23, 2008.

[2] Miller KB, Daoust PR. Clinical manifestations of acute myeloid leukemia. In: Hoffman R, Benz EJ, Shattil SJ, et al. (eds.). *Hematology: Basic Principles and Practice*, 4th edition. Philadelphia: Elsevier, 2005;1059–74.

[3] Kushinka J. Leukocytosis: an example of hyperviscosity syndrome. Conference Handout, Virginia Commonwealth University Internal Medicine Residency Program, September 19, 2005. Available online at http://www.eric.vcu.edu/home/conferences/0506handout.html. Accessed June 23, 2008.

[4] Hemingway TJ, Savitsky EA. Hyperviscosity syndrome. eMedicine Website. Available at http://www.emedicine.com/emerg/topic756.html. Accessed June 23, 2008.

[5] Majhail NS, Lichtin AE. Acute leukemia with a very high leukocyte count: confronting a medical emergency. *Cleve Clin J Med* 2004;71:633–7.

[6] Hess EP, Sztajnkrycer MD. Images in emergency medicine. *Ann Emerg Med* 2005;46:314, 322.

[7] Chou SH, Singhal AB. Multiple punctate cerebral hemorrhages in acute leukemia with blast crisis. *Neurology* 2007; 68:953.

107

Vomiting and dizziness in a 47-year-old male

HISTORY OF PRESENT ILLNESS

A 47-year-old male with no significant medical history presented to the ED complaining of nausea, vomiting, diffuse abdominal pain, and dizziness with associated general body weakness for one day. He recently experienced a mild cough, runny nose and flu-like symptoms, as well as increased urination and thirst. He was found to be ataxic earlier that day by his primary care provider (PCP), and was urgently referred to the ED for further evaluation of a possible cerebellar stroke. The patient smoked cigarettes but denied drugs or alcohol. His family history was significant for hypertension. He took no medications.

PHYSICAL EXAMINATION

GENERAL APPEARANCE: The patient appeared acutely ill, was hyperventilating and had a fruity odor on his breath.

VITAL SIGNS

Temperature	95°F (35°C)
Pulse	110 beats/minute
Blood pressure	75/35 mmHg
Respirations	35 breaths/minute
Oxygen saturation	97% on room air

HEENT: PERRL, EOMI, oropharynx with dry mucous membranes.

NECK: Supple, flattened jugular veins.

CARDIOVASCULAR: Tachycardic, regular rate without rubs, murmurs or gallops.

LUNGS: Rales at the bases bilaterally, mild expiratory wheezes throughout.

ABDOMEN: Mildly distended, diffusely tender to palpation, hypoactive bowel sounds.

RECTAL: Normal tone, brown stool, hemoccult negative.

EXTREMITIES: Cool to touch, delayed capillary refill, weak peripheral pulses.

SKIN: Cool, pale and dry, no rashes.

NEUROLOGIC: The patient was somnolent but arousable, minimally followed commands, and was moving all extremities.

A peripheral intravenous line was placed and blood was drawn and sent for laboratory testing. A 12-lead ECG (Figure 107.1) and a portable chest radiograph (Figure 107.2) were obtained.

What is your diagnosis?

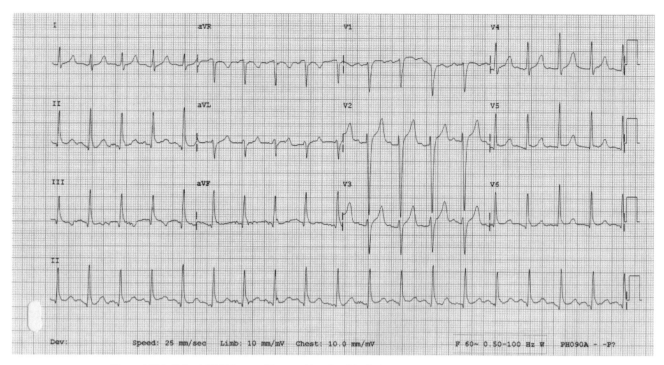

Figure 107.1 12-lead ECG from a 47-year-old male with dizziness, vomiting and abdominal pain.

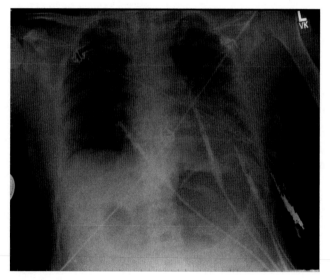

Figure 107.2 Portable chest radiograph from a 47-year-old male with
dizziness, vomiting and abdominal pain.

ANSWER

The diagnosis is diabetic ketoacidosis (DKA). A bedside glucometry test (finger-stick blood glucose) was obtained which read "critical high" (indicates more than 500 mg/dL). An arterial blood gas was also quickly obtained, which returned with results of pH of 6.95 (normal 7.35–7.45), pCO_2 of 10 mmHg (normal 35–45 mmHg), pO_2 of 132 mmHg (normal 80–95 mmHg) and base excess −28 mmol/L (normal −2.4 to +2.3 mmol/L). The 12-lead ECG demonstrated sinus tachycardia, rate 108, with peaked T waves prominent in leads V_2–V_4. The chest radiograph showed low lung volumes without infiltrate.

Two large-bore intravenous lines were placed, with normal saline boluses rapidly infusing in each line. Initial laboratory tests revealed a blood glucose level of 1419 mg/dL (normal 66–159 mg/dL), sodium of 126 mEq/L (normal 137–145 mEq/L), potassium of 7.3 mEq/L (normal 3.5–5.3 mEq/L), chloride of 83 mEq/L (normal 98–107 mEq/L), CO_2 of less than 5 (normal 22–30), anion gap greater than 45 (normal 5–16), creatinine of 4.7 mg/dL (normal 0.8–1.5 mg/dL), blood urea nitrogen of 68 mg/dL (normal 9–20 mg/dL), troponin I of 0.06 ng/mL (normal 0.00–0.09 ng/mL) and positive serum ketones. Peaked T waves in the anterior leads of the 12-lead ECG were consistent with hyperkalemia. A lactic acid level was elevated at 3.4 mmol/L (normal 0.8–2.1 mmol/L). A complete blood count showed a leukocyte count of 34.5 K/μL (normal 3.5–12.5 K/μL) and hematocrit of 47% (normal 39–51%). An insulin drip was begun at 0.1 units/kg body weight, and intravenous antibiotics were administered for possible pneumonia. A Foley catheter was placed to monitor urine output.

Shortly after beginning the intravenous fluids and insulin therapy, his heart rate and blood pressure improved to 100 beats/minute and 95/45 mmHg, respectively. However, the patient began wheezing and gradually became hypoxic. Nebulized albuterol was administered. Shortly after transfer to the ICU, the patient was urgently intubated for acute respiratory distress. A repeat chest radiograph was obtained (Figure 107.3), which demonstrated infiltrates in the left perihilar and right lower lung zones. The patient's blood pressure continued to drop; he developed septic shock despite aggressive fluid resuscitation, so a norepinephrine IV drip was begun.

Seventeen hours following presentation to the ED and aggressive fluid replacement with insulin therapy, the patient's serum glucose was 173 mg/dL, creatinine was 1.6 mg/dL, sodium was 146 mEq/L and CO_2 was 13 mEq/L, with an anion gap of 8 mEq/L. A venous blood gas obtained on 80% inspired oxygen showed a pH of 7.25, pCO_2 of 31 mmHg and PO_2 of 40 mmHg, with bicarbonate of 14 mmol/L and base excess −12 mmol/L. His blood pressure improved to 110/70 mmHg, at which time the norepinephrine drip was discontinued. Intravenous antibiotics and fluids were continued. The patient remained intubated until hospital day #7. He was discharged on hospital day #14 with instructions to continue insulin therapy for diabetes and complete an oral course of antibiotics for pneumonia.

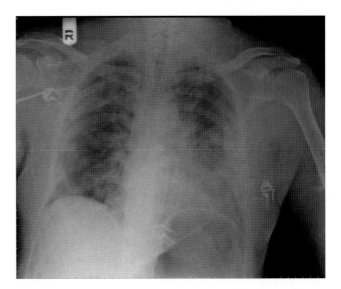

Figure 107.3 Portable chest radiograph from a 47-year-old male with DKA following endotracheal intubation.

Diabetic ketoacidosis

Diabetic ketoacidosis consists of a triad of hyperglycemia, ketonemia and acidemia, each of which may be caused by other conditions. DKA is a potentially fatal metabolic disorder that can have significant mortality if misdiagnosed or mistreated; it may be the first presentation of diabetes.[1] The incidence of DKA is between 4.6–8.0 per 1000 person-years among patients with diabetes; currently mortality is approximately 4–10%.[2] DKA occurs most commonly when an intercurrent illness or stress develops (e.g., infection, GI bleed or myocardial infarction) in a person with known diabetes, when a patient's insulin dose is inappropriately decreased or discontinued, or when an individual has new-onset type I diabetes.[3] Although DKA most commonly occurs in patients with type I diabetes, it may also occur in patients with type II diabetes.[2,3]

The main features of DKA are hyperglycemia, metabolic acidosis (pH less than 7.35 and bicarbonate less than 15 mEq/L) with a high anion gap and heavy ketonuria (3+). This contrasts with hyperosmolar nonketotic hyperglycemia (formerly known as hyperosmotic nonketotic coma, HONC), where there is no acidosis, absent or minimal ketonuria, but often very high glucose and serum sodium levels (greater than 150 mEq/L).[1] Major components of the pathogenesis of DKA are reductions in effective concentrations of circulating insulin and concomitant elevations of counter-regulatory hormones (catecholamines, glucagon, growth hormone and cortisol).[2,4] These hormonal alterations bring about three major metabolic events: hyperglycemia resulting from accelerated gluconeogenesis and decreased glucose utilization, increased proteolysis and decreased protein synthesis, and increased lipolysis with ketone production.

Hyperglycemia initially causes the movement of water out of cells, with subsequent intracellular dehydration, extracellular fluid expansion and hyponatremia. It also leads to diuresis, in which water loss exceeds sodium chloride loss. Urinary loss then leads to progressive dehydration and volume deple-tion, which causes diminished urine flow and greater reten-tion of glucose in plasma. The net result of these alterations is hyperglycemia with metabolic acidosis and an increased plasma anion gap (difference between the sum of cations and anions in plasma or serum).[4]

The diagnosis of DKA is comparatively straightforward when there is a clear history that the patient has diabetes. However, this diagnosis can be challenging when the patient is unconscious or DKA is the first presentation of diabetes. The possibility of DKA should be considered whenever assessing a patient who presents with "hyperventilation" or "anxiety." It is essential to measure the blood glucose rapidly, especially in the resuscitation of any unconscious or altered patient.[1] Polyuria, polydipsia and weakness are usually present. Nau-sea, vomiting and abdominal pain may predominate. If the patient is already being treated with insulin, there may be a history of reduced or omitted doses. Chest pain may be described if DKA complicates acute myocardial infarction, although silent infarction may occur. Therefore, a rapid 12-lead ECG is essential in the initial evaluation of patients pre-senting with DKA.

On examination, the patient may have an increased depth and rate of respiration (known as Kussmaul breathing). The mouth, tongue and lips are usually dry, and the odor of keto-nes may be noted on the patient's breath.[1] Body temperature tends to be low or normal, even in the presence of infection.[3] A fever almost always indicates infection. Patients can present with generalized neurologic abnormalities, usually in the form of depressed mental status. They may present with symptoms resembling acute stroke. The patient's level of consciousness is related to serum osmolality, not to the degree of acidosis.[4]

Successful therapy for DKA requires correcting hypo-volemia, hyperglycemia, metabolic acidosis and electrolyte imbalances.[5] This also requires vigilant hemodynamic mon-itoring. The treatment of DKA consists of providing fluid, insulin, potassium and phosphate (if needed) while managing any precipitating illnesses. Rehydration with intravenous nor-mal saline is the most important step in treating DKA – with-out adequate fluid replacement, insulin will not work effec-tively and blood glucose concentrations will remain elevated.[3] Initial fluid rates should be 500–1000 mL/h, decreasing to 200–500 mL/h once orthostatic changes in blood pressure resolve.[3] Once blood glucose concentrations fall to less than 250 mg/dL, intravenous fluids should be changed to contain 5% dextrose (D5 with 0.45% sodium chloride) to prevent blood glucose levels from falling too rapidly, which may have a role in the development of cerebral edema.

An insulin infusion rate should be started at a rate of 0.1 units/kg/hour if the serum potassium is normal or elevated.[1–3] If the patient's serum glucose level is not responding (less than 10% fall in blood glucose levels) after two or three hours (with adequate hydration), the infusion rate should be doubled. Although the typical potassium deficit in DKA is 500–700 mEq, most patients are hyperkalemic at the time of initial presentation because of the effects of insulino-

penia, hyperosmolality and acidemia.[3] During rehydration and insulin therapies for DKA, the serum potassium concen-tration typically declines rapidly as potassium re-enters the intracellular compartment. A reasonable protocol for potas-sium replacement in DKA entails using intravenous fluids and insulin until the potassium concentration is less than 5.5 mEq/L. At this time, potassium chloride is added to the intravenous fluids in the amount of 20–40 mEq/L. The goal is to maintain the serum potassium concentration in the range of 4–5 mEq/L while carefully monitoring the rate of potassium infusion (rapid infusion can cause life-threatening dysrhythmias).

Bicarbonate therapy does not improve the outcome in DKA, and is not recommended regardless of the severity of the acidemia.[4] Insulin administration inhibits ongoing lipolysis and ketone production while promoting the regeneration of bicarbonate. Phosphorus depletion is common in DKA, aver-aging 1.0–1.5 mmol/kg. However, phosphorus replacement seems to have little impact on outcome in DKA, and therefore is not routinely recommended.[4] The serum phosphate level should be measured four hours after the start of therapy. If the level is severely depressed (less than 1mg/dL), phosphate replacement is advised.

KEY TEACHING POINTS

1. The main features of DKA are hyperglycemia, metabolic acidosis with a high anion gap, and significant ketonuria.
2. The possibility of DKA should be considered whenever assessing a patient who presents with "hyperventilation" or "anxiety."
3. Successful therapy for DKA requires correcting hypo-volemia, hyperglycemia, metabolic acidosis and electrolyte imbalances, and necessitates vigilant and frequent moni-toring.
4. Potassium and glucose levels should be checked immedi-ately in patients in DKA. Ensure that serum potassium lev-els are not low prior to insulin administration, which may result in life-threatening dysrhythmias.
5. Consider and treat precipitating conditions which may be responsible for DKA (e.g., infection, GI bleeding, myocar-dial infarction).

REFERENCES

[1] Hardern RD, Quinn ND. Emergency management of dia-betic ketoacidosis in adults. *Emerg Med J* 2003;20:210–3.
[2] Fernandez-Frackelton M. Diabetic ketoacidosis. *Emerg Med Clin N Am* 2005;23:609–28.
[3] Andreoli TE, Carpenter CJ, Bennett JC, et al. Diabetes mellitus. In Andreoli TE, et al. (eds.). *Cecil Essentials of Medicine*, 4th ed. Philadelphia: Saunders, 1997:539–42.
[4] Kitabchi AE, Wall BM. Management of diabetic ketoacido-sis. *Am Fam Phys* 1999;60:1–13.
[5] Bull SV, Douglas IS, Foster M, et al. Mandatory protocol for treating adult patients with diabetic ketoacidosis decreases intensive care unit and hospital lengths of stay: results of a nonrandomized trial. *Crit Care Med* 2007;2007:41–6.

108

Right leg swelling in a 50-year-old male

HISTORY OF PRESENT ILLNESS

A 50-year-old male with a medical history significant for depression and restless leg syndrome presented to the ED complaining of three days of progressively worsening right leg swelling. He reported some redness associated with the swelling, as well as lower leg pain. He denied recent long travel or prolonged immobility, chest pain, shortness of breath, light-headedness or dizziness. He worked as a manager at a local supermarket and spent most of his time on his feet. His medications included zolpidem, trazodone, ropinirole and fluoxetine. He denied any family history of clotting disorders.

PHYSICAL EXAMINATION

GENERAL APPEARANCE: The patient appeared well nourished, well developed and in no acute discomfort.

VITAL SIGNS

Temperature	99°F (37.2°C)
Pulse	75 beats/minute
Blood pressure	131/93 mmHg
Respirations	16 breaths/minute
Oxygen saturation	97% on room air

HEENT: Unremarkable.

NECK: Supple, no jugular venous distension.

CARDIOVASCULAR: Regular rate and rhythm without rubs, murmurs or gallops.

LUNGS: Clear to auscultation bilaterally.

ABDOMEN: Soft, nontender, nondistended.

EXTREMITIES: Right lower extremity swelling from the ankle to the knee involving the calf anteriorly to the shin, with mild erythema and warmth to the calf and shin (Figure 108.1). Leg circumference 10 cm below the tibial tuberosity measured

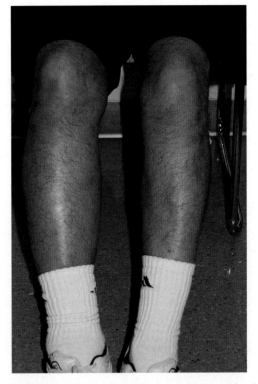

Figure 108.1 Bilateral lower extremities from a 50-year-old male with right leg swelling.

44 cm on the right and 38 cm on the left. The right calf was tender, with a positive Homan's sign. Dorsalis pedis and posterior tibialis pulses were 2+ on the right foot and ankle, respectively.

A peripheral intravenous line was placed, and blood was drawn and sent for laboratory testing.

What is your diagnosis?

ANSWER

The diagnosis is deep vein thrombosis (DVT) of the right popliteal vein. A D-dimer test returned positive, and a presumptive diagnosis of DVT was made in the ED pending ultrasound. The patient received 10 mg fondaparinux (Arixtra®) subcutaneously, and was started on warfarin 5 mg orally daily. He returned the following morning for a formal right lower extremity ultrasound, which demonstrated thrombus in the right popliteal vein (Figure 108.2). The patient continued fondaparinux 10 mg subcutaneously daily, along with warfarin 5 mg daily until his International Normalized Ratio (INR) fell into the range of 2–3, at which time the fondaparinux was discontinued.

Deep vein thrombosis

Venous thromboembolism (VTE) is estimated to affect approximately 2 million Americans per year. It is a frequently encountered problem in the ED.[1] To minimize the risk of fatal pulmonary embolism (PE), accurate diagnosis and prompt therapy are crucial.[2] Long-term complications include the post-thrombotic syndrome and recurrent VTE. The pathogenesis of venous thrombosis involves three factors, referred to as Virchow's triad. Those factors are damage to the vessel wall, venous stasis and hypercoagulability.[2]

The signs and symptoms of DVT are often nonspecific; thus clinical diagnostic accuracy is poor. Extremity swelling, pain and edema place the patient at risk for DVT.[3] Significant thrombus can be present in asymptomatic patients, however. The clinical accuracy for the diagnosis of acute DVT has been reported to be about 50% in symptomatic patients.[3] Homan's sign (pain associated with forced dorsiflexion of the ankle) remains part of the traditional physical examination of patients with suspected DVT. Numerous studies have documented the unreliability of this sign, with estimates of Homan's sign accuracy ranging from being positive in 8–56% of cases of proven DVT, yet being positive in greater than 50% of symptomatic patients without DVT.[4]

Wells and coworkers have developed the first clinical model for the diagnosis of patients presenting with suspected DVT.[5] This model includes a thorough clinical examination and the identification of risk factors that predispose patients to having increased risk of VTE (Table 108.1).[6] In accordance with this model, patients are first divided into three risk categories (low, moderate and high), then further assessed through the use of D-dimer and ultrasonography. In 15 studies that evaluated Wells DVT prediction rule, patients whose test scores put them in the highest strata of pretest probability had a prevalence of DVT, across studies, ranging from 17–85%.[7] Patients with a moderate pretest probability had a prevalence of 0–38%, and those with the lowest pretest probability had a prevalence of 0–13%.

Plasma D-dimers are specific cross-linked derivatives of fibrin, produced when fibrin is degraded by plasmin. Concentrations are raised in patients with VTE.[8] Although sensitive for VTE, high concentrations of D-dimers are insufficiently specific for making a positive diagnosis because they occur

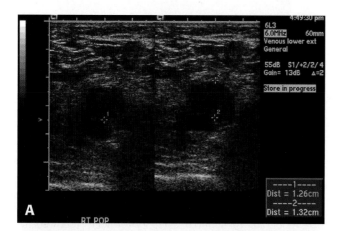

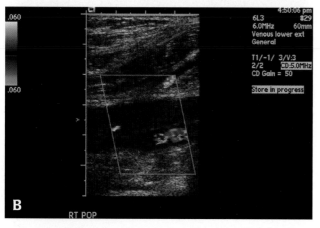

Figure 108.2 Right lower extremity Doppler ultrasound from a 50-year-old male with right leg swelling, demonstrating lack of compressibility of the popliteal vein (right image, panel A) and lack of flow in the popliteal vein (panel B).

TABLE 108.1 Wells clinical prediction rule for deep vein thrombosis (DVT)

Clinical feature	Points
Active cancer (treatment within 3 months or palliation)	1
Paralysis, paresis or immobilization of lower extremity	1
Bedridden for more than 3 days because of surgery (within 4 weeks)	1
Localized tenderness along distribution of deep veins	1
Entire leg swollen	1
Unilateral calf swelling of greater than 3 cm (below tibial tuberosity)	1
Unilateral pitting edema	1
Collateral superficial veins	1
Alternative diagnosis as likely as or more likely than DVT	−2

Risk score interpretation (probability of DVT):

- high risk: 3 points or more
- moderate risk: 1 to 2 points
- low risk: less than 1 point

in other disorders, such as malignancy, pregnancy and following surgery. Nevertheless, D-dimer tests generally have a high negative predictive value and are useful to rule-out disease in low-risk patients. Diamond et al. measure D-dimer levels followed by venous duplex examination in 148 patients seen in the ED for suspected DVT.[9] Nineteen patients (12.8%) had positive venous duplex examinations and 129 (87.2%) duplex examinations were negative. None of the 19 patients with positive venous duplex studies had D-dimer levels within the normal range. The sensitivity, specificity, positive predictive value and negative predictive value were 100%, 48.8%, 22.4% and 100%, respectively.[9]

Compression ultrasound is now recognized as the most appropriate primary initial imaging modality for evaluating patients at risk for peripheral DVT. Its accuracy in diagnosing acute or chronic DVT is well established in patients who have lower extremity symptoms (average sensitivity and specificity of 97% for proximal DVT).[3,8] However, the need for evaluation of calf veins remains controversial. The advantages of ultrasound include it is noninvasive, it lacks ionizing radiation and the need for intravenous nephrotoxic contrast media, it has a relatively low cost, and the equipment is portable.[3] The most simple ultrasound criterion for diagnosing VTE is noncompressibility of the vascular lumen under gentle probe pressure (compression ultrasound).[8] If no residual lumen is observed, the vein is considered to be fully compressible, indicating the absence of venous thrombosis.

Prior to the introduction of low-molecular-weight heparins (LMWH), unfractionated heparin (UFH) and warfarin were considered the standard treatment for DVT. The use of UFH required continuous intravenous application and frequent monitoring, thus precluding the possibility of outpatient therapy or early discharge.[10] Clinical use of LMWH has revolutionized the treatment of DVT by offering many treatment advantages over UFH, including less frequent dosing, fixed dosages, and the opportunity to initiate outpatient or short-stay inpatient programs for DVT treatment, with a subsequent reduction in costs to patients and the healthcare system.[10] LMWH has been shown to have a higher benefit-to-risk ratio than treatment with UFH, and is at least as effective as UFH in terms of major bleeding, PE and recurrent VTE risks.[10]

Fondaparinux (Arixtra®) is a novel synthetically derived agent that exerts its antithrombotic activity by selective inhibition of factor Xa.[11,12] The predictable and sustained anticoagulant effect of fondaparinux for 24 hours allows once-daily injection. Because fondaparinux does not cross-react with heparin-induced antibodies, platelet count monitoring may no longer be necessary.[12] The dose is 7.5 mg subcutaneously once daily (patients 50–100 kg) or 10 mg subcutaneously once daily (patients over 100 kg). In a randomized, double-blind study comparing fondaparinux with enoxaparin for the initial treatment of symptomatic DVT, 43 (3.9%) of 1098 patients randomly assigned to fondaparinux had recurrent thromboembolic events compared with 45 (4.1%) of 1107 patients randomly assigned to enoxaparin.[12] Major bleeding occurred in 1.1% of patients receiving fondaparinux and 1.2% of

patients receiving enoxaparin. Mortality rates were 3.8% and 3.0%, respectively. The researchers concluded that once-daily subcutaneous fondaparinux was at least as effective (not inferior) and as safe as twice-daily, body weight-adjusted enoxaparin in the initial treatment of patients with symptomatic DVT.

Not all patients are suitable for outpatient treatment of DVT. According to Douketis, four questions can be asked to identify patients for whom outpatient treatment might be inadvisable.[11] First, does the patient have massive DVT? Second, does the patient have objectively confirmed symptomatic PE? Third, is the patient at high risk of anticoagulant-related bleeding complications? Fourth, does the patient have major comorbidity or other factors that might warrant hospitalization? If the answer to any of these questions is yes, hospitalization for treatment should be considered.[11]

Whether LMWH, unfractionated heparin or factor Xa inhibitor is initially used for the treatment of DVT, oral anticoagulation therapy with warfarin is started on the first (or second day) of treatment.[11] The usual dose of warfarin is 5–10 mg on the first day and 5 mg daily thereafter. The INR should be tested at least twice during the next two to three weeks, every two weeks during the next four weeks, and every three to four weeks thereafter.[11] Treatment with LMWH or UFH should be continued for at least five days and until the INR has been greater than 2.0 for two consecutive days. Warfarin should be administered (with a target INR of 2–3) for three months to patients with DVT following exposure to transient risk factors (e.g., surgery, trauma, immobility), and for at least six months to patients with unprovoked (or idiopathic) DVT.[11]

Finally, treatment of patients with suspected DVT is problematic if diagnostic imaging is not immediately available. Pretest clinical probability and D-dimer assessment can be used to identify patients in whom empiric protective anticoagulation is indicated.[13] Siragusa et al. demonstrated that a strategy incorporating Wells criteria to place patients in a low-, moderate- or high-risk category for VTE, followed by D-dimer testing, allows for the safe deferral of diagnostic tests for up to 72 hours.[13] In this study, patients identified as having a high or moderate pre-test probability with positive D-dimer received protective full-dose treatment with LMWH; the remaining patients were discharged without anticoagulation. All patients were scheduled to undergo tests for VTE within 72 hours. In total, 533 patients with suspected VTE (409 with suspected DVT and 124 with suspected PE) were included in the study. A total of 23.8% of patients had confirmed VTE. At follow up in 72 hours, only a single thromboembolic event (0.2%) occurred, whereas at the three-month follow-up, five events (1.2%) occurred in patients in whom the diagnosis of DVT or PE had previously been ruled out. None of the patients had major bleeding events, and 90% of the patients were treated as outpatients. The researchers concluded that this approach allows the safe deferral of diagnostic procedures for DVT and PE for up to 72 hours in selected patients with suspected VTE.

KEY TEACHING POINTS

1. The pathogenesis of venous thrombosis involves damage to the vessel wall, venous stasis and hypercoagulability, known as Virchow's triad.

2. Extremity swelling, pain and edema increase the likelihood for DVT; the presence of a Homan's sign is an unreliable clinical sign of DVT.

3. The Wells DVT prediction rule is useful in categorizing patients as low-, moderate- or high-risk for DVT.

4. The plasma D-dimer test generally has a high negative predictive value and is best used to rule out DVT in low-risk patients.

5. Compression ultrasonography is the most appropriate initial imaging modality for diagnosing DVT, with an average sensitivity and specificity of 97%.

6. Most patients diagnosed with DVT can be treated as outpatients with either LMWH or synthetic factor Xa inhibitor (fondaparinux) in combination with warfarin.

REFERENCES

[1] Hooker EA, Carver L. Outpatient delayed screening for patients with suspected deep vein thrombosis (correspondence). *Am J Emerg Med* 2005;23:227–8.

[2] Bates SM, Ginsberg JS. Treatment of deep-vein thrombosis. *N Engl J Med* 2004;351:268–77.

[3] Hamper UM, DeJong MR, Scoutt LM. Ultrasound evaluation of the lower extremity veins. *Radiol Clin N Am* 2007;45:525–47.

[4] Urbano FL. Homans' sign in the diagnosis of deep venous thrombosis. *Hosp Physician* March 2001:22–4. Available online at http://www.jcomjournal.com/pdf/hp_mar01_homan.pdf. Accessed June 26, 2008.

[5] Wells PS, Hirsh J, Anderson DR, et al. Accuracy of clinical assessment of deep-vein thrombosis. *Lancet* 1995;345:1326–30.

[6] Merli GJ. Pathophysiology of venous thrombosis, thrombophilia, and the diagnosis of deep vein thrombosis-pulmonary embolism in the elderly. *Clin Geriatr Med* 2006;22:75–92.

[7] Segal JB, Eng J, Tamariz LJ, et al. Review of the evidence on diagnosis of deep venous thrombosis and pulmonary embolism. *Ann Fam Med* 2007;5:63–73.

[8] Tovey C, Wyatt S. Diagnosis, investigation, and management of deep vein thrombosis. *BMJ* 2003;326:1180–4.

[9] Diamond S, Goldbweber R, Katz S. Use of D-dimer to aid in excluding deep venous thrombosis in ambulatory patients. *Am J Surg* 2005;189:23–6.

[10] Merli G. Anticoagulants in the treatment of deep vein thrombosis. *Am J Med* 2005;118:13S–20S.

[11] Douketis JD. Treatment of deep vein thrombosis. What factors determine appropriate treatment? *Can Fam Phys* 2005;51:217–23.

[12] Buller HR, Davidson BL, Decousus H, et al. Fondaparinux or enoxaparin for the initial treatment of symptomatic deep venous thrombosis. *Ann Intern Med* 2004;140:867–73.

[13] Siragusa S, Anastasio R, Porta C, et al. Deferment of objective assessment of deep vein thrombosis and pulmonary embolism without increased risk of thrombosis. *Arch Intern Med* 2004;164:2477–82.

109

Fever and rash in a 57-year-old male

HISTORY OF PRESENT ILLNESS

A 57-year-old male with a medical history significant for hypercholesterolemia presented to the ED complaining of fevers as high as 103°F (39.4°C) for eight days and a vesiculo-pustular, raised rash located on both arms, shoulders and face spreading to the legs bilaterally. The rash was described as tender to touch but not pruritic. The patient also complained of arthralgias most prominent in both knees. He reported a dry, nonproductive cough, but denied shortness of breath, chest pain, recent travel or sick contacts. His review of systems was negative for abdominal pain, diarrhea or constipation, nausea or vomiting, dysuria, hematuria or penile discharge. He did not take medications, and was allergic to sulfa. He reported emigrating from China 14 years earlier. He denied tobacco, alcohol and drug use, including IV drugs. His last PPD test was negative 14 years ago. The patient had recently received his routine tetanus, pertussis and diphtheria vaccinations one month prior to the onset of his symptoms.

PHYSICAL EXAMINATION

GENERAL APPEARANCE: The patient was a middle-aged male, awake, alert and in no acute discomfort.

VITAL SIGNS

Temperature	102.8°F (39.3°C)
Pulse	80 beats/minute
Blood pressure	114/63 mmHg
Respirations	18 breaths/minute
Oxygen saturation	96% on room air

HEENT: PERRL, EOMI, sclera anicteric, oropharynx pink and moist without lesions.

NECK: Supple, no jugular venous distension, anterior cervical lymphadenopathy.

CARDIOVASCULAR: Regular rate and rhythm without rubs, murmurs or gallops.

LUNGS: Clear to auscultation bilaterally.

ABDOMEN: Soft, nontender, nondistended.

GENITOURINARY: No penile lesions or discharge.

EXTREMITIES: No clubbing, cyanosis or edema.

NEUROLOGIC: Nonfocal.

SKIN: Scattered clusters of 2–3 mm vesicles, each cluster 1–2 cm in diameter. The clusters of vesicles were more confluent on the shoulders compared to those found on the face and arms (Figure 109.1). Vesicles were noted on the trunk as well as both palms, but spared the soles of the feet. Ill-defined plaques were noted on both knees, without vesicles.

A peripheral intravenous line was placed, and blood was drawn and sent for laboratory testing. Laboratory tests were significant for a leukocyte count of 10.5 K/μL (normal range 3.5–12.5 K/μL) with 84% neutrophils (normal 50–70%), erythrocyte sedimentation rate (ESR) of 89 mm/hr (normal 0–20 mm/hr), C-reactive protein (CRP) of 32.8 mg/dL (normal less than 0.9 mg/dL), sodium of 128 mEq/L (normal 137–145 mEq/L) and ALT of 101 U/L (normal 11–66 U/L).

What is your diagnosis?

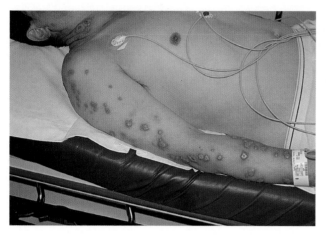 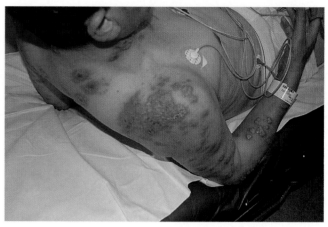

Figure 109.1 A 57-year-old male with fever and vesiculopustular rash.

ANSWER

The diagnosis is Sweet's syndrome. In the ED, the patient initially received IV ceftriaxone and acyclovir. The patient's varicella DFA samples returned negative for herpes zoster. He was seen by both a dermatologist and infectious disease specialist during hospitalization, with the presumptive diagnosis of Sweet's syndrome. The patient was prescribed prednisone 60 mg orally daily, with marked improvement of his symptoms. A skin biopsy performed one day following admission demonstrated a dense, fairly discreet infiltrate of polymorphonuclear leukocytes in the dermis to the mid-reticular dermis, confirming the diagnosis of Sweet's syndrome. The patient continued to improve clinically and was discharged on hospital day #5 to continue prednisone and to follow up as an outpatient with dermatology.

Sweet's syndrome

Sweet's syndrome (acute febrile neutrophilic dermatosis), first described by RD Sweet in 1964, is a condition characterized by the sudden onset of fever, leukocytosis and tender, erythematous, well-demarcated papules and plaques.[1–3] The lesions may appear anywhere but favor the upper body, including the face, usually sparing the trunk and back.[1,2] The individual lesions are often described as pseudovesicular or pseudopustular, but may be frankly pustular, bullous or ulcerative.[1] Oral and eye involvement (conjunctivitis or episcleritis) have been frequently reported. Arthralgias or arthritis are present in 33–62% of patients.[4] Although the condition may occur in the absence of other known diseases, Sweet's syndrome is often associated with hematologic diseases (including leukemia) and immunologic diseases (rheumatoid arthritis, inflammatory bowel disease). The condition is more common in females, with the mean age of onset in the mid- to late-fifties. Sweet's syndrome may last from one week to more than four years; recurrence is common (25–37%).[4,5]

Fever is the most frequent symptom in patients with Sweet's syndrome.[3] The cutaneous manifestations may be preceded by fever; alternatively, fever can be present throughout the duration of the dermatosis. However, in some patients with biopsy-confirmed malignancy-associated Sweet's syndrome, fever may be absent.[3] Arthralgia, general malaise, headache and myalgia are other associated symptoms that may be present. Patients with this condition can appear dramatically ill.

The erythrocyte sedimentation rate (ESR) and C-reactive protein (CRP) are generally elevated in patients with Sweet's disease.[1,2] The leukocyte count is said to be greater than 8 K/µL in 80% of affected individuals. Anemia and elevated alkaline phosphatase are present about half the time. The presence of anemia and a low platelet count have been associated with an underlying malignancy.[6]

Diagnostic criteria for classical Sweet's syndrome consist of major and minor criteria.[2,3] Major criteria include abrupt onset of painful erythematous plaques and nodules, and histopathologic evidence of a dense neutrophilic infiltrate without evidence of primary leukocytoclastic vasculitis. Minor criteria include pyrexia (greater than 38°C), association with underlying hematological or visceral malignancy, inflammatory disease or pregnancy, or preceded by upper respiratory infection, gastrointestinal infection or vaccination. Additional minor criteria include excellent response to treatment with systemic corticosteroids, potassium iodide or colchicine, and abnormal laboratory values at presentation (three of the following four): ESR greater than 20 mm/hr, positive CRP, leukocyte count greater than 8 K/µL and greater than 70% neutrophils.

Systemic corticosteroids are the treatment of choice for Sweet's disease.[1–3] Generally prednisone or prednisolone is used, with an initial dose of 0.5–1.5 mg/kg/day. The dose is reduced within two to four weeks. A good response can be anticipated, with resolution of malaise within hours; mucosal lesions and fever resolve within two days. Skin lesions of Sweet's syndrome should resolve within one to four weeks. Recurrence is common (25–37% of patients), with chronic relapsing disease seen in about 15% of patients.[1] Other medications have been used in the treatment of Sweet's disease with varying success, including topical corticosteroids, nonsteroidal anti-inflammatory drugs (e.g., indomethacin), potassium iodide, cyclosporine, doxycycline, dapsone and colchicine.[1–3]

KEY TEACHING POINTS

1. Sweet's syndrome is characterized by the sudden onset of fever, leukocytosis and tender, erythematous, well-demarcated papules and plaques.
2. Fever is the most frequent symptom in patients with Sweet's syndrome.
3. Elevated ESR, CRP and leukocyte count greater than 8 K/µL are common laboratory abnormalities in patients with Sweet's syndrome.
4. Systemic corticosteroids are the treatment of choice for Sweet's syndrome.
5. Sweet's syndrome is often associated with hematologic disease (including leukemia) and immunologic diseases (including rheumatoid arthritis or inflammatory bowel disease).
6. Diagnosis of Sweet's syndrome is confirmed histologically, with biopsies of lesions demonstrating a dense neutrophilic infiltrate without evidence of primary leukocytoclastic vasculitis.

REFERENCES

[1] Burrall B. Sweet's syndrome (acute febrile neutrophilic dermatosis). *Derm J Online* 1999;5:(1999):8. Available online at http://dermatology.cdlib.org/DOJvol5num1/therapy/sweets.html. Accessed June 19, 2008.

[2] Habif TP. Hypersensitivity syndromes and vasculitis. In: Habif TP (ed.). *Clinical Dermatology, A Color Guide to*

Diagnosis and Therapy, 4th ed. Philadelphia: Mosby, 2004: 650–2.

[3]   Cohen PR. Sweet's syndrome. Orphanet Encyclopedia Website. Available at http://www.orpha.net/data/patho/GB/uk-Sweet.pdf. Accessed June 19, 2008.

[4]   Von den Driesch P. Sweet's syndrome (acute febrile neutrophilic dermatosis). *J Am Acad Dermatol* 1994;31:535–56.

[5]   Fett DL, Gibson LE, Su WP. Sweet's syndrome: systemic signs and symptoms and associated disorders. *Mayo Clin Proc* 1995;70:234–40.

[6]   Bourke JF, Keohane S, Long CC, et al. Sweet's syndrome and malignancy in the U.K. *Br J Dermatol* 1997;137: 609–13.

110

Dehydration and general body weakness in a 75-year-old female

HISTORY OF PRESENT ILLNESS

A 75-year-old female with a medical history significant for hypertension and depression presented to the ED complaining of general body weakness and fatigue worsening over several months, as well as intermittent, bitemporal headaches. Recently, the patient reported increased difficulty getting out of bed in the morning because of her weakness. She denied chest pain, shortness of breath, abdominal pain, fevers or chills, dysuria, focal weakness, visual changes and blood-tinged or dark stools. The patient did report a decreased appetite as well as occasional nausea over the past several weeks. Her medications include paroxetine, venlafaxine, hydrochlorothiazide and verapamil. She denied tobacco or alcohol use, and lived alone.

PHYSICAL EXAMINATION

GENERAL APPEARANCE: The patient appeared fatigued, dehydrated, awake and alert, and in no acute discomfort.

VITAL SIGNS

Temperature	98.1°F (36.7°C)
Pulse	80 beats/minute
Blood pressure	80/40 mmHg
Respirations	18 breaths/minute
Oxygen saturation	98% on room air

HEENT: PERRL, EOMI, visual fields intact, oropharynx dry.

NECK: Supple, no jugular venous distension.

CARDIOVASCULAR: Regular rate and rhythm without rubs, murmurs or gallops.

LUNGS: Clear to auscultation bilaterally.

ABDOMEN: Soft, nontender, nondistended, hypoactive bowel sounds noted.

RECTAL: Normal tone, brown stool, hemoccult negative.

EXTREMITIES: Warm, well-perfused without clubbing, cyanosis or edema.

NEUROLOGIC: Alert and oriented to person, place and time; upper extremity and lower extremity strength 5/5 proximal and distal; sensation grossly intact; delayed biceps and patellar reflexes bilaterally.

The patient was placed on the cardiac monitor, a peripheral intravenous line was placed, and blood was drawn and sent for laboratory testing. A 12-lead ECG was obtained (Figure 110.1), and a 1-liter intravenous bolus of normal saline was infused. The blood pressure improved to 90/50 at completion of the NS infusion. A chest radiograph demonstrated no infiltrate, effusion or cardiomegaly. A noncontrast CT of the brain showed only age-related atrophy without evidence of hemorrhage.

What is your diagnosis?

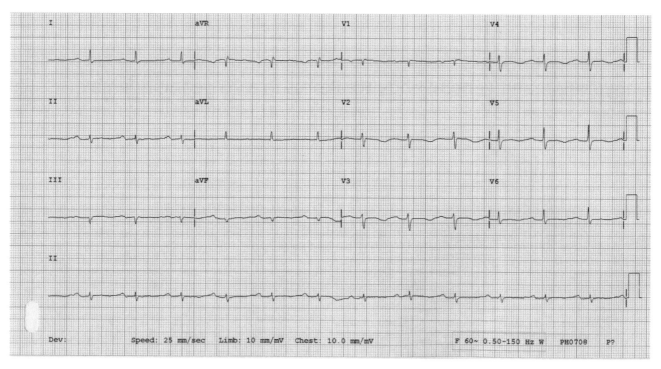

Figure 110.1 12-lead ECG from a 75-year-old female with general body weakness and fatigue.

ANSWER

The diagnosis is panhypopituitarism. The 12-lead ECG demonstrates a normal sinus rhythm, rate 80, first-degree AV block, with nonspecific ST-T wave changes and U waves. Laboratory results were remarkable for potassium of 2.5 mEq/L (normal 3.5–5.3 mEq/L) and magnesium of 1.5 mg/dL (normal 1.6–2.3 mg/dL); the remainder of the laboratory results, including a complete blood count, remaining electrolytes, BUN, creatinine, glucose, troponin I and urinalysis, were within normal limits. The potassium and magnesium were replaced intravenously in the ED, IV hydration was continued, and the patient was admitted to the medicine service. A thyroid-stimulating hormone (TSH) level sent from the ED returned low the next day (0.068 μIU/mL; normal 0.200–5.500 μIU/mL). An endocrinology consult was obtained during hospitalization, and further laboratory testing revealed a low free T4 analog level (0.6 ng/dL; normal 0.8–1.7 ng/dL), as well as an elevated prolactin level (57 ng/mL; normal 3–30 ng/mL) and elevated total T3 level (212 ng/dL; normal 87–180 ng/dL); a random cortisol level was low (less than 1.0 μg/dL; normal 6–19 μg/dL). The patient underwent an MRI of the brain, which revealed a macrocystic pituitary sellar/suprasellar mass 1.2 cm × 1.5 cm × 1.3 cm, suspicious for cystic degeneration of a pituitary adenoma (Figure 110.2).

The patient was started on Levothroid® 75 μg orally daily and a hydrocortisone oral taper prior to hospital discharge. Following discharge, the patient was seen by the neurosurgeon to consider treatment options for her pituitary mass. It was decided to repeat the MRI in three months, which demonstrated substantial regression of the cystic sellar/suprasellar space-occupying lesion.

Panhypopituitarism

Hypopituitarism is a clinical syndrome of deficient pituitary hormone production.[1] This may result from disorders involving the pituitary gland, hypothalamus or surrounding structures. The incidence and prevalence of hypopituitarism are estimated to be 4.2 per 100,000/year and 45.5 per 100,000, respectively.[2] Panhypopituitarism refers to involvement of all pituitary hormones; however, not all pituitary hormones are always involved, resulting in partial hypopituitarism. Pituitary hormones of clinical significance include adrenocorticotropic hormone (ACTH), follicle-stimulating hormone (FSH), luteinizing hormone (LH), growth hormone (GH), prolactin, thyroid-stimulating hormone (TSH) and antidiuretic hormone (ADH).

Of the various causes of hypopituitarism in adults, pituitary adenoma or its treatment by surgery or radiotherapy is by far the most common.[3] Other causes include traumatic brain injury, subarachnoid hemorrhage, stroke, nonpituitary tumors, infections, pituitary infarction, autoimmune disorders and idiopathic causes.[2,4] Clinical presentation of pituitary adenomas is dominated by visual impairment followed by endocrine symptoms (hypopituitarism).[5] Visual impairment due to chiasmatic compression occurs in 60–80% of nonfunctioning pituitary adenomas, whereas headache is reported in 5–25% of all patients.[5] Pituitary apoplexy has been reported in 6% of cases of nonfunctioning pituitary adenomas.[5]

When pituitary hormone production is impaired, target gland hormone production is reduced because of the lack of trophic stimulus.[1] Pituitary hormone deficiencies can be caused by the loss of hypothalamic stimulation (tertiary hormone deficiency) or by direct loss of pituitary function (secondary hormone deficiency).[6] Normally, subphysiologic target hormone levels stimulate the pituitary gland to increase trophic hormone production. However, in hypopituitarism the pituitary gland response is absent, suboptimal or inappropriate with biologically inert hormone production. This results in progressive secondary failure of the target glands. Patients with hypopituitarism typically present with low target hormone levels accompanied by low levels of the corresponding trophic hormone.

Presentation of panhypopituitarism varies from asymptomatic to acute hemodynamic collapse, depending on the etiology, rapidity of onset, and predominant hormones involved. Individuals with the following deficiencies typically present with the indicated conditions (Table 110.1).[1] Other presenting features of panhypopituitarism may be attributable to the underlying cause. A patient with a space-occupying lesion involving the pituitary may present with headaches or visual field deficits. A patient with large lesions involving the hypothalamus may present with polydipsia and syndrome

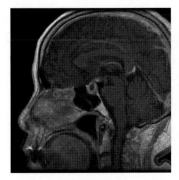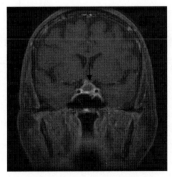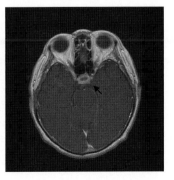

Figure 110.2 MRI of the brain from a 75-year-old female demonstrating a macrocystic pituitary sellar/suprasellar mass (arrows).

TABLE 110.1 Hormone deficiencies and associated conditions in panhypopituitarism

Hormone deficiency	Condition
Adrenocorticotropic hormone (ACTH)	Adrenal insufficiency
Thyroid-stimulating hormone (TSH)	Hypothyroidism
Gonadotropin	Hypogonadism
Growth hormone (GH)	Failure to thrive and short stature in children, fatigue and weakness in adults
Antidiuretic hormone (ADH)	Polyuria and polydipsia

of inappropriate antidiuretic hormone (SIADH).[1] Physical examination findings may be normal in subtle presentations. Patients may present with features attributable to deficiency of target hormones, including hypothyroidism, adrenal insufficiency, hypogonadism and failure to thrive.

ACTH deficiency causes adrenocortical insufficiency, with clinical features resembling those of primary adrenal failure.[7] Weakness, nausea, vomiting, anorexia, weight loss, fever and postural hypotension may occur. Patients with pituitary failure are usually slightly overweight. Their skin is fine, pale and smooth, with fine wrinkling of the face. Body and pubic hair may be deficient or absent, and atrophy of the genitalia may occur. Postural hypotension, bradycardia, decreased muscle strength and delayed deep tendon reflexes occur in more severe cases. Neuro-ophthalmologic abnormalities may occur if a large intrasellar or parasellar lesion results in compression of the optic chiasm.

Hormone studies aimed at both the target gland and their respective stimulatory pituitary hormone should be performed for proper interpretation (i.e., ACTH and Cortrosyn® stimulation test; TSH and thyroxine; FSH, LH, and either estradiol or testosterone as appropriate for gender; prolactin; GH provocative testing). MRI or CT of the brain is useful for imaging the pituitary gland.

Medical care consists of hormone replacement as necessary and treatment of the underlying cause. The goal is to replace hormones in a physiologic manner, with efforts to avoid consequences associated with overreplacement.[6] Glucocorticoids (e.g., hydrocortisone) are required if the ACTH-adrenal axis is impaired. This is particularly important in sudden vascular collapse due to pituitary apoplexy, or acute obstetric hemorrhage with pituitary insufficiency (Sheehan's syndrome). In such cases, appropriate hormone replacement therapy should not be delayed pending a definitive diagnosis. Secondary hypothyroidism should be treated with thyroid

hormone replacement. Surgical treatment depends on the underlying cause and the severity of hypopituitarism. In pituitary apoplexy, prompt surgical decompression may be lifesaving if brain imaging reveals tumor mass effect.[1]

KEY TEACHING POINTS

1. Patients with hypopituitarism typically present with symptoms due to low target hormone levels accompanied by low levels of corresponding trophic hormones.
2. Presentations vary from asymptomatic, mild and chronic symptoms, to acute vascular collapse, depending on the etiology, rapidity of onset and predominant hormones involved.
3. Pituitary adenoma is the most common cause of hypopituitarism in adults, which typically presents with headache, visual impairment and symptoms related to endocrine dysfunction.
4. Medical therapy for hypopituitarism consists of hormone replacement (as indicated) and treatment of the underlying cause. Glucocorticoids are required if the ACTH-adrenal axis is impaired.
5. Unless contraindicated, neurosurgery is the primary treatment option for symptomatic pituitary tumors.

REFERENCES

[1] Mulinda JR. Hypopituitarism (panhypopituitarism). eMedicine Website. Available at http://www.emedicine.com/MED/topic1137.htm. Accessed July 5, 2008.

[2] Schneider HJ, Aimaretti G, Kreitschmann-Andermahr I, et al. Hypopituitarism. *Lancet* 2007;369:1461–70.

[3] Prabhakar VKB, Shalet SM. Aetiology, diagnosis, and management of hypopituitarism in adult life. *Postgrad Med J* 2006;82:259–66.

[4] Urban RJ. Hypopituitarism after acute brain injury. *Growth Hormone IGF Res* 2006;16:S25–9.

[5] Minniti G, Esposito V, Piccirilli M, et al. Diagnosis and management of pituitary tumors in the elderly: a review based on personal experience and evidence of literature. *Eur J Endocrinol* 2005;153:723–35.

[6] Molitch, ME. Anterior pituitary. In: Goldman L, Ausiello D (eds.). *Cecil Medicine*, 23rd ed. Philadelphia: Saunders, 2007:1675–7.

[7] Tyrrell JB, Findling JW, Aron DC. Hypothalamus and pituitary. In: Greenspan FS, Baxter JD (eds.). *Basic and Clinical Endocrinology*, 4th ed. Norwalk, CT: Appleton & Lange, 1994:96–7.

111

Left arm swelling in a 95-year-old female

HISTORY OF PRESENT ILLNESS

A 95-year-old female was sent to the ED from the orthopedic clinic for left arm swelling. The patient had fallen on her left shoulder two weeks earlier, sustaining a left humeral neck fracture. Her left arm was placed in a sling, and she was transferred to a skilled nursing facility for care issues. Upon recheck of her left arm at the orthopedic clinic, significant swelling from the mid-humerus to the fingertips was noted. A left shoulder radiograph was obtained (Figure 111.1), and the patient was subsequently transferred to the ED. The patient had been keeping her left arm in the sling since her fall. She had noted increasing swelling to her arm and hand, but denied pain or numbness. She reported weakness in that arm since the fall, and was unable to raise her arm against gravity.

PHYSICAL EXAMINATION

GENERAL APPEARANCE: The patient appeared well nourished, well hydrated and in no acute discomfort.

VITAL SIGNS

Temperature	98.6°F (37°C)
Pulse	88 beats/minute
Blood pressure	145/90 mmHg
Respirations	18 breaths/minute
Oxygen saturation	99% on room air

HEENT: Unremarkable.

NECK: Supple, no jugular venous distension or midline tenderness.

CARDIOVASCULAR: Regular rate and rhythm without rubs, murmurs or gallops.

LUNGS: Clear to auscultation bilaterally.

ABDOMEN: Soft, nondtender, nondistended.

EXTREMITIES: Left upper extremity in sling, 4+ pitting edema of the arm noted from the mid-humerus to the fingers. Radial

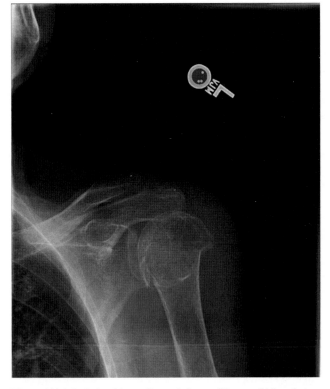

Figure 111.1 Left shoulder radiograph from a 95-year-old female two weeks after a fall on her left shoulder.

pulse was palpable, sensation and motor function of the left hand grossly intact. The patient was unable to abduct her arm against gravity secondary to weakness.

NEUROLOGIC: Significant for left arm weakness, otherwise nonfocal.

What is your diagnosis?

ANSWER

The diagnosis is deep vein thrombosis (DVT) of the left internal jugular vein, in addition to a left humeral neck fracture. The radiograph (Figure 111.1) demonstrated an impacted humeral neck fracture. The patient underwent Doppler ultrasound evaluation of the left upper extremity, which demonstrated incomplete occlusion of the left jugular vein due to intraluminal thrombus (Figure 111.2). The remaining veins of the deep venous system, including the left subclavian, axillary, basilic, cephalic and brachial were patent.

The patient was admitted to the medical service and started on anticoagulation with low-molecular-weight heparin (enoxaparin) subcutaneously and Coumadin® orally. The patient was discharged to the skilled nursing facility the following day to continue enoxaparin and Coumadin® until her International Normalized Ratio (INR) fell into the range of 2–3, at which time the enoxaparin would be discontinued.

Isolated internal jugular vein thrombosis after upper extremity trauma

Deep vein thrombosis (DVT) of the upper extremity occurs infrequently, constituting only 10% of all deep vein thromboses.[1] Upper extremity DVT is characterized by pain, edema and functional impairment; however, it may be completely asymptomatic.[2] Both isolated or combined thrombosis of internal jugular and subclavian veins may occur.[2] Central venous catheters (CVC) contribute to the risk of upper extremity venous thrombosis in 7–14% of all cases.[3] Other specific risk factors are effort-related compression of the deep veins of the upper extremity and compression caused by the thoracic outlet syndrome (Paget-Schroetter syndrome).[3] Complications associated with upper extremity venous thrombosis include pulmonary embolism (11–26%), superior vena cava syndrome (21–23%) and post-thrombotic syndrome (27–50%).[3]

Clinical symptoms of upper extremity DVT include peripheral edema, prominent superficial veins and discoloration.[4] Neurologic symptoms including pain, paresthesias and motor weakness may also be present.[4] In particular, swelling and extremity discomfort are the most common complaints, present in approximately 80% and 40%, respectively.[5] Duplex ultrasound is the initial imaging test of choice for diagnosing upper extremity DVT because it is noninvasive and has a high sensitivity for peripheral (jugular, distal subclavian, axillary) upper extremity DVT.[6] However, acoustic shadowing from the clavicle limits visualization of a short segment of the subclavian vein and may result in a false-negative study.[6] Contrast venography provides excellent characterization of venous anatomy but has several drawbacks, including possible technical difficulty in cannulating the vein, requirement of iodinated contrast agent and radiation exposure.[6] Other imaging modalities for diagnosing upper extremity DVT include CT scan (requires contrast dye) and magnetic resonance angiography.

Anticoagulation is the mainstay of treatment for upper extremity DVT, alone or in association with fibrinolytic treat-

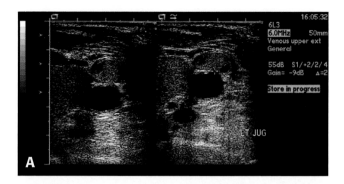

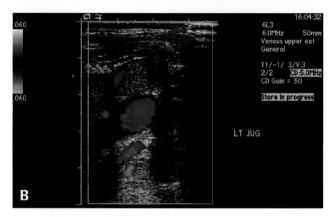

Figure 111.2 Ultrasound of the left jugular vein of a 95-year-old female demonstrating thrombus (panels A and B) and incompressibility of the jugular vein (right image, panel A).

ment or surgery.[2] Anticoagulation has been shown to significantly decrease the acute and chronic morbidity rates compared with conservative treatment alone in upper extremity DVT, and has been recommended as initial therapy for all cases.[4] Treatment with unfractionated or low-molecular-weight heparin (LMWH), followed by oral anticoagulant (e.g., Coumadin®) for at least three months is well supported and should be regarded as the option of choice.[5] Home treatment with LMWH is feasible in many patients, and can reduce hospitalization rates and their associated costs. Although internal jugular vein thrombosis following CVC placement, surgery or trauma to the neck is more frequently reported, isolated jugular venous thrombosis following upper extremity trauma is rare. Only one similar case could be found in the literature, in a patient with internal jugular vein thrombosis following surgical treatment of a humeral nonunion.[4]

KEY TEACHING POINTS

1. Risk factors for upper extremity DVT include the presence of central venous catheters, effort-related compression of the deep veins of the upper extremity or compression from thoracic outlet syndrome, trauma to the neck or humerus, neck surgery and acquired clotting disorders.

2. Clinical symptoms of upper extremity DVT classically include peripheral edema, prominent superficial veins and discoloration, with swelling and extremity discomfort being the most common complaints.

3. Upper extremity DVT is uncommon, constituting only 10% of all DVTs.

4. Duplex ultrasound is the initial imaging test of choice for diagnosing upper extremity DVT because it is noninvasive and has a high sensitivity.

5. Anticoagulation with unfractionated or LMWH and oral Coumadin® is the initial treatment of choice for upper extremity DVT.

REFERENCES

[1] Har-Noy O, Meltzer E. Upper-extremity deep-vein thrombosis in an elderly man. *CMAJ* 2007;176:1078–9.

[2] Oymak FS, Karahan OI, Gulmez I, et al. Thrombosis of internal jugular and subclavian veins: a possible complication of cough. *Turk Resp J* 2001;2:40–3.

[3] Blom JW, Doggen CJM, Osanto S, et al. Old and new risk factors for upper extremity deep venous thrombosis. *J Thromb Haemost* 2005;3:2471–8.

[4] Pearsall AW, Stokes DA, Russell GV, et al. Internal jugular deep venous thrombosis after surgical treatment of a humeral nonunion: a case report and review of the literature. *J Shoulder Elbow Surg* 2004;13:459–62.

[5] Bernardi E, Pesavento R, Prandoni P. Upper extremity deep venous thrombosis. *Semin Thromb Hemost* 2006;32:729–36.

[6] Joffe HV, Goldhaber SZ. Upper-extremity deep vein thrombosis. *Circulation* 2002;106:1874–80.

Answer index

64. Open both bone forearm fracture
65. Jones fracture (base of the 5th metatarsal)
66. Occult radial head fracture with associated fat pad signs
67. Open Monteggia fracture-dislocation of the left forearm
68. Depressed tibial plateau fracture
69. Septic arthritis of the hip
70. Closed femur fracture

IX. Hand

71. Subungual abscess of the thumb
72. High-pressure injection injury to the hand
73. Felon of the distal phalanx of the finger
74. Extensor tendon laceration of the finger
75. Infected cat bite to the finger

X. Pediatrics

76. Paroxysmal supraventricular tachycardia (PSVT)
77. Dilated cardiomyopathy
78. Subdural hematoma
79. Colocutaneous fistula from PEG tube placement
80. Respiratory syncytial virus (RSV) bronchiolitis with concomitant bacterial pneumonia
81. Hydrocephalus from a posterior fossa brain tumor
82. Esophageal coin
83. Ileocolic intussusception
84. Hemolytic uremic syndrome (HUS)
85. Moyamoya disease
86. Third-degree heart block from Lyme carditis
87. Intracranial hemorrhage from an arteriovenous malformation (AVM)

XI. Infectious Disease

88. Vertebral osteomyelitis
89. *Plasmodium vivax* malaria
90. Purpura fulminans from *S. pneumoniae* sepsis
91. Sepsis from a liver abscess
92. Psoas muscle abscess with vertebral osteomyelitis
93. Miliary tuberculosis

XII. Toxicology/Environmental

94. Jimson weed poisoning
95. Hypothermia with ECG changes
96. Intentional acetaminophen overdose
97. Scombroid fish poisoning
98. Rhabdomyolysis and acute renal failure from methamphetamine abuse
99. Pit viper (rattlesnake) envenomation
100. Angioedema
101. Intentional alkali ingestion with caustic esophageal injury
102. Digoxin toxicity

XIII. Miscellaneous

103. Nephrotic syndrome
104. Thrombotic thrombocytopenic purpura (TTP)
105. Morbilliform drug eruption
106. Acute myelogenous leukemia (AML) with blast crisis and leukostasis
107. Diabetic ketoacidosis (DKA)
108. Right leg deep vein thrombosis (DVT)
109. Sweet's syndrome
110. Panhypopituitarism from a pituitary adenoma
111. Left internal jugular vein DVT

Subject index